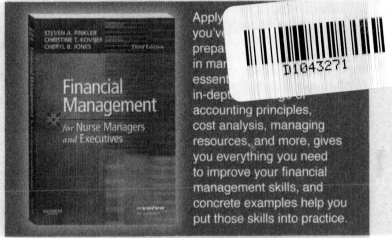

FOURTH EDITION

Budgeting Concepts for Nurse Managers

Steven A. Finkler
PhD, CPA
Professor Emeritus of Public and Health Administration,
Accounting, and Financial Management
Program in Health Policy and Management
Robert F. Wagner Graduate School of Public Service
New York University
New York, New York

Mary L. McHugh
PhD, RN, BC (Informatics)
Associate Professor, School of Nursing
University of Colorado at Denver and Health Science Center
Denver, Colorado

SAUNDERS

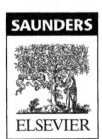

ELSEVIER

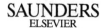

SAUNDERS
ELSEVIER

11830 Westline Industrial Drive
St. Louis, Missouri 63146

Acquisitions Editor: Yvonne Alexopoulos
Senior Developmental Editor: Lisa P. Newton
Publishing Services Manager: Jeffrey Patterson
Project Manager: Jeanne Genz
Design Direction: Louis Forgione

Transferred to Digital Printing 2011

About the Authors

STEVEN A. FINKLER, PhD, CPA

Steven A. Finkler is Professor Emeritus of Public and Health Administration, Accounting, and Financial Management in the Program in Health Policy and Management at New York University's Robert F. Wagner Graduate School of Public Service. At the Wagner School he teaches courses in budgeting and financial management. He led the Wagner specialization in health care financial management for more than 20 years. He is a past member of the National Advisory Council for Nursing Research at the National Institute of Nursing Research, NIH, and currently serves as Treasurer and Board member of a large not-for-profit nursing home in New Jersey. Dr. Finkler is one of the founding faculty members of the Johnson & Johnson—Wharton Fellows Program in Management for Nurse Executives and is the only faculty member to have taught in that program for every year since it began in 1983.

Dr. Finkler has won a number of awards for his teaching and research. They include the 2002 Pioneering Spirit Award from the American Association of Critical-Care Nurses (AACN), the 2003 Sigma Theta Tau International Research Award in the Health Policy and Systems category, and the 2006 *American Journal of Nursing* Book of the Year Award in the Nursing Management and Leadership category for *Accounting Fundamentals for Health Care Management* (with David M. Ward).

In addition to this book, Dr. Finkler has authored 17 other books, among them *Financial Management for Nurse Executives* (third edition, 2007, with Christine T. Kovner and Cheryl Bland Jones); *Essentials of Cost Accounting for Healthcare Organizations* (third edition, 2007, with David M. Ward and Judith Baker); *Accounting Fundamentals for Health Care Management* (2006, with David M. Ward); *Financial Management for Public, Health, and Not-for-Profit Organizations* (second edition, 2005); and *Finance and Accounting for Nonfinancial Managers* (third edition, 2003). He has also published more than 200 articles in *The Journal of Nursing Administration, The New England Journal of Medicine, Nursing Economic$, Journal of Neonatal Nursing, Western Journal of Nursing Research, O.R. Nurse Managers' Network, Health Services Research, Medical Care, Healthcare Financial Management, Health Care Management Review,* and other journals and contributed a chapter to *Managing Hospitals: Lessons from the Johnson & Johnson—Wharton Fellows Program in Management for Nurses.*

Dr. Finkler received a BS degree in economics with joint majors in accounting and finance (summa cum laude) and an MS degree in accounting (with highest honors) from the Wharton School at the University of Pennsylvania. His master's degree in economics and PhD in business administration were awarded by Stanford University. Dr. Finkler, who is also a Certified Public Accountant, worked for several years as an auditor with Ernst and Young and was on the faculty of the Wharton School for 6 years before joining New York University. He was Editor of *Hospital Cost Management and Accounting* from 1984 through 1997.

MARY L. McHUGH, PhD, RN, BC

Mary L. McHugh is an Associate Professor of Nursing at the University of Colorado at Denver and Health Science Center in Denver, Colorado. Dr. McHugh received a BS in nursing from Wichita State University in Wichita, Kansas. She earned an MS in nursing (psychiatric nursing with a minor in nursing administration), and was awarded a PhD in clinical nursing research from the University of Michigan in Ann Arbor, Michigan. She has experience as a staff nurse, charge nurse, unit manager, department manager, and director of nursing. In her various hospital management roles, she has had responsibility for budgets ranging from a few hundred thousand dollars to a hospital nursing budget of $50 million.

Dr. McHugh has also won grants and awards for her research and teaching and is a member of the American Nurses Association, Sigma Theta Tau International, the Council on Graduate Education for Administration in Nursing (CGEAN), the American Medical Informatics Association (AMIA), and the Healthcare Information and Management Systems Society (HIMSS) at the national level and of a variety of state-level nursing groups. She has developed and managed nursing administration programs at two universities as well as having developed the first totally on-line nursing informatics course in the United States in 1995 (with the assistance of Dr. Rob Gibson, an expert in educational media support). She has published extensively in the fields of nursing administration, informatics and statistical analysis for nurses. She has worked as a statistical consultant and as a consultant in computer systems analysis and design and has consulted with hospital administrators and directors of operating rooms in productivity enhancement and cost reduction efforts.

Dr. McHugh has published numerous book chapters in informatics texts, distance learning texts, and nursing administration textbooks. She has published in diverse journals, including *Nursing Economic$, AORN Journal, Research in Nursing and Health, Dimensions of Critical Care Nursing, Proceedings of the Symposium on Computer Applications in Medical Care, Applied Nursing Research, The American Journal of Nursing, Matrix,* and the *Journal for Specialists in Pediatric Nursing,* among others.

REVIEWER

Paula Antognoli, PhD, RN, CNAA
Assistant Professor
Division of Nursing
West Texas A & M University
Canyon, Texas

Preface

We are extremely pleased to present the fourth edition of *Budgeting Concepts for Nurse Managers*. Nurse managers face tremendous challenges in performing their administrative responsibilities. In the past decade, the roles of nurse managers have greatly expanded and their responsibilities increased—particularly in the area of financial management. Most nurse managers entered their management jobs directly from positions as bedside nurses. Few had formal education in management and leadership prior to their new roles. Typically, they were recognized as excellent clinicians, and therefore most of their education in management was acquired through on-the-job experience, management training sessions at their place of work, and conferences and seminars. However, these kinds of learning opportunities have significant limitations, especially in the more technical areas of budgeting and financial management, forecasting, quality management, and information management. Today's managers must be adept in a variety of managerial skills, and knowledge of the use of a variety of tools, strategies, and techniques must be gained from formal education. Budgeting is a prime example of a situation in which a manager can get by with the assistance of the organization's finance department staff, but the manager's performance in the budgeting domain can improve considerably with formal education.

The goal of this book is to expand and improve nurses' knowledge about and skills in budgeting. Its mission is to assist nurse managers to gain knowledge of budgeting concepts and skill in applying that knowledge to the management of clinical and administrative operations. It should be noted, however, that the basic principles of budgeting apply to all the arenas in which nurses work, including education, and research. The book is designed to serve all nurses because the authors believe that an understanding of the budgeting process is valuable for every nurse, from new graduate nurses just beginning their nursing careers to nurses at the pinnacles of their careers in roles such as vice president or chief nursing executive (CNE), chief operating officer (COO), or chief executive officer (CEO). Deans of nursing certainly need this knowledge; the budgets of schools of nursing are every bit as constrained as hospital budgets. Moreover, nurse researchers must understand budgeting because they are legally and ethically responsible for managing the budgets of their research projects.

In order to serve such a wide audience, the conceptual and tactical budgeting issues presented in this book range from the most basic, "How do I begin?" all the way to sophisticated treatment of topics of interest to midlevel and top managers. For example, the chapters on revenue budgeting, on benchmarking and productivity, on budgeting for computer systems, and on budgeting for the operating room will certainly be of interest to CNEs, who are responsible not only for nursing, but also for many other clinical support departments, and for CEOs, who are responsible for the financial success of the entire organization. The content will assist nurses in all settings, not merely hospital nurse managers. The book includes information relevant to clinics, surgery centers, private practice nursing, hospices, home health agency nurses, and other health care settings.

Budgeting Concepts is written specifically for students in graduate nursing administration programs and for nurses in roles at all levels of management. For its examples, it draws upon situations in which nurse managers find themselves. The book is written at a level that assumes no previous financial management education or experience on the part of the reader. It is not, however, designed to create a level of expertise that will allow the nurse to dispense with the advice and assistance of professional financial managers. Rather, it should improve nurses' ability to communicate and collaborate with the people in the organization's finance department. It is designed to improve the performance of nurse managers in the budget process and perhaps provide them with the knowledge that will enable them to introduce some innovative uses of budgets into their organizations.

What about *Financial Management for Nurse Managers and Executives*,[1] written by Finkler (one of this book's authors), Kovner, and Jones? That book exists, so why is this book on budgeting needed? This budgeting book is one of great depth but limited scope. It considers only issues related to budgeting. The financial management book's content extends beyond the realm of budgeting to issues such as financial statements, economics, marketing, and business plans. We view these two books as complementary, with this book focused more on budgeting per se, and *Financial Management for Nurse Managers and Executives* providing a broader review of budgeting for those who are already familiar with many aspects of budgeting. In addition, it addresses many other aspects of financial management that are of growing interest to nurses.

As in any book, some areas are discussed in greater depth than others. The level of detail for each topic reflects our belief about the depth of knowledge required by today's nurse manager. Each chapter has an extensive list of references and suggested readings if the reader wants more in-depth knowledge in a particular subject area. In an attempt to provide a coherent whole, chapters refer to pertinent material in other chapters. However, each chapter is virtually self-contained, so the reader can choose to read a single chapter on a particular topic or read chapters in an order different from that presented.

We envision that this book will be used in graduate courses in financial management for nurses. But it should be noted that this information is also important for non-nurse managers of health care institutions. There are many health care disciplines (radiology, laboratory, emergency department, etc.) in which managers need budgeting skills, but in which there has been a lack of formal education. This book can help managers in those areas as well as nurse managers. Further, a careful study of this book might help non-nurse managers avoid some of the pitfalls associated with their attempts to control nursing costs without understanding the nature of nursing services.

The content covered in this book is appropriate for all levels of nursing education and for nurse managers at all levels in the hierarchy. It is also appropriate for advanced practice nurses because the principles of budgeting apply to office practices as well as to hospitals, nursing homes, and other health care settings. The content of this book is also appropriate for programs that prepare chief nurse executives (CNEs) and for programs that prepare first- and mid-level nurse managers as well. Instructors teaching courses in programs preparing various levels of managers may want to assign

[1]Finkler, S.A., Kovner, C.T., Jones, C.B. (2007). *Financial Management for Nurse Managers and Executives,* ed 3, St. Louis: Saunders.

chapters that are most relevant to the level of the students in their program. Individual instructors also may choose to modify their coverage of chapters based on their students' specific needs.

Note On Changes in the Fourth Edition

The first edition of *Budgeting Concepts for Nurse Managers* was published in 1984. At that time, many nursing administration master's degree programs were just beginning to add courses in financial management to their curricula. This book was a forerunner of the many books on financial management for nurses that have been written since the 1980s. The second edition was published in 1992. DRGs (Diagnosis-Related Groups) were well entrenched, but managed care had not yet taken over the majority of health insurance plans as it did in later in the 1990s, and much medical care was still located in hospitals. The third edition was published in 2001, and so much has changed in the 7 years since the third edition! In 2001, even though quality management was a part of the health care scene, it was not a major basis upon which health insurance companies based their decisions about which health care facilities to include in their networks. The Institute of Medicine report *To Err is Human: Building a Safer Health System* was published in November of 1999, and its full effect had not even begun to be realized. Computer systems were beginning to become more commonplace, but they did not have the pervasive impact on clinical care that they have today.

This edition builds on the successes of the first, second, and third editions and takes advantage of the many helpful comments that we have received over the years from colleagues and students. As we thought about writing the fourth edition of this book, we reflected on what has worked well in prior editions and on the changes made necessary by rapid changes in the health care environment. Certainly, the importance of careful budgeting has grown with time, with increasing pressure on the health care system to control costs and deliver quality care, with the widespread implementation of new computer systems in clinical settings, and with the seriousness of the nursing shortage. Nevertheless, as we reread the book, we discovered that the foundational concepts of budgeting have not changed over time.

That said, we have made substantial revisions to the fourth edition of the book. Numbers and facts throughout the book were updated. In addition, we have added two exciting new chapters—the first on budgeting for information systems, and the second, under the leadership of an experienced operating room leader, Marilyn Bowman-Hayes, focuses on special issues in budgeting for perioperative departments. Several new features in this edition were based on feedback solicited from nursing students and other users of the third edition.

First, we have added a new coauthor! Dr. Mary McHugh brings knowledge of computer and information systems and a special interest in successful budgeting processes for nursing. She is certified in Informatics by ANCC and has a certificate in Quality Management from the Frank Barton School of Management. She has been responsible for budgets at the nursing unit level and at the departmental level in both hospitals and schools of nursing, and she has managed hospital nursing department budgets as large as $50 million dollars. She is an award-winning teacher and author in the fields of Informatics, Nursing Administration, and Statistics and Data Analysis. She brings knowledge of current issues in budgeting for hospitals, clinics, and ambulatory care centers as well as schools of nursing. Her teaching in administration includes content related to nursing leadership and management, nursing financial management, patient care services management, and management decision support systems. She is also responsible for teaching master's- and doctoral-level statistics courses and informatics courses in the system lifecycle, in database management, systems, and expert decision support systems.

Second, we have updated the content in every chapter and added two new chapters on the critical functions of budgeting for information systems and for the perioperative department.

- **Chapter 1** has incorporated a new emphasis on quality management as a budgeting concern. That enhanced focus on quality management has been extended throughout the book.
- **Chapter 2** directly addresses strategies for managing nursing operations in a time of budget reductions or when a shortage of nurses leads to insufficient staffing. It also addresses the need to *manage* changes in unit operations associated with reductions in budget and staffing that are not secondary to reductions in nursing workload.
- **Chapter 4** adds new content on the calculation and presentation of information related to determining the break-even point for a new business or a new program within an existing institution.
- **Chapter 5** incorporates additional concepts and strategies related to managing a nursing operation in the face of increasing nursing shortages. It presents information on budgeting for traveler nurses and per diem nurses when regular staff cannot be employed in sufficient numbers to cover the need. In addition, it presents new information on general differences among nurses and on managing an intergenerational nursing staff.
- In **Chapter 7**, content on business planning has been greatly expanded, and content on quality management has been updated and expanded. The impact of the Institute of Medicine's landmark report *To Err Is Human* is discussed, and the role of the nurse manager in using strategic planning and budgeting skills to manage quality in an era of nursing shortages is addressed.
- **Chapter 8** has added information about the use of spreadsheets in planning and budgeting, and it provides a list of Websites with free online tutorials to assist the nurse manager in learning to use this most important management tool. Additional information on full-time equivalent calculations has been added, along with a new emphasis on clinic staffing, including a sample staffing plan for an orthopedic clinic.
- **The Capital Budgeting Chapter (10)** has been expanded to further explicate the process decision makers are increasingly forced to apply when funds are too constrained to allow for the purchase of even necessary items. Additional material on how to justify a capital item has been included with more extensive discussion of item prioritization processes and vendor bidding.
- The chapters on variance analysis (**Chapters 13 and 14**) now incorporate a discussion of the use of statistical process control techniques to determine the materiality of a budget variance. They emphasize that some variation between the budgeted amount and the actual amount spent is inevitable. The new materiality section presents a method for determining when a variance represents a normal (and minor) fluctuation versus when it represents an important and unexpected deviation from budget.
- **Chapter 15** is a new chapter that covers planning and budgeting for computer systems. Content is presented concerning the process for evaluating the need

for a new computer system and then designing or purchasing and implementing the system. Topics include budgeting for project management, staff training, costs of purchasing the hardware and software, expenses involved in system integration, and contracting for system support and system upgrades.

- **Chapter 16**, also a new addition to the book, focuses on the very complex issues of budgeting for the operating room. A wide range of topics is covered, ranging from obtaining buy-in from key stakeholders and budgeting for on-call staff to implants, instruments, equipment, maintenance and repair contracts, and computer service and support contracts. The special issues related to staffing in the operating room are addressed, as are the unique capital budgeting problems faced by directors of operating rooms. They and other nurses will be interested in learning about some of the nonstatistical forecasting techniques used to plan for operating room budgets and in the new section on marketing the services of the operating room to the community.
- **Chapter 17**, on benchmarking, productivity, and cost-effectiveness analysis has been expanded by the addition of new examples and discussions of benchmarking. A more in-depth discussion of productivity measurement and management increases the utility of this chapter for nurse managers.
- Finally, **Chapter 18**, on costing nursing services, has been updated and new content relevant to emerging technology such as radio-frequency identification (RFID) chips that could be used to track nursing activity is presented.

One of the things we are most excited about with the publication of this edition is the availability of several online resources to accompany the text. There are discussion questions and budgeting problems available on line for student and instructor use, and problem solutions and test questions are available to instructors. These materials are available for homework assignments, class discussions, and examinations. The Glossary, previously included in the text, is available online with this new edition. **Also** available online are PowerPoint class notes. Despite having made every effort to get this edition as near perfect as possible, our past experience tells us that mistakes do happen. Thus, we also will post errata online as they are discovered. To access these valuable resources, please visit our website at http://evolve.elsevier.com/Finkler/budgeting/.

Acknowledgements

We express our thanks to the many people who helped with the preparation of this book. First we thank the many nurses whom we have taught and with whom we have worked over the years. They have shared their knowledge and insights about the real world of financial management encountered by nurses in all kinds of health organizations.

Next, our thanks go to Christina Graf, RN, who originally wrote Chapter 8 on operating budgets. She also prepared the appendix of budget forms and instructions. We would also like to thank Marilyn Bowman-Hayes, RN, who led the development of Chapter 16 on operating room (OR) budgeting. Her years of experience as an OR nurse, an OR Clinical Nurse Specialist and as Director of Perioperative Services have provided an extremely wide-angled view of surgery department operations and of the special issues relevant to budgeting for a perioperative department. We thank our many students who, over the years, have provided feedback and suggestions about what would make the book a more valuable learning tool. And we thank our families, who have tolerated the many hours we have taken from them to devote to the development of this new edition.

We would like to thank Paul Antognoli who reviewed the book for the publisher and provided the authors with helpful comments.

We are grateful to Yvonne Alexopoulos, Lisa Newton, and Jeanne Genz for their efforts in transforming our work from a raw manuscript into a published text.

Finally, we thank our readers. We thank you not only for reading this book but also for helping to improve it. We encourage you to contact us with comments, suggestions, examples, or corrections.[2] All material we receive that is used in a subsequent edition will be acknowledged in that future edition.

Steven A. Finkler and Mary L. McHugh

---

[2]Send errata and other communications to Dr. Mary McHugh at mary.mchugh@uchsc.edu. Dr. Finkler may be contacted at steven.finkler@nyu.edu.

Contents

Introduction
The Different Types of Budgets

1

■ WHY BUDGET?

Traditionally, most nurse managers relied on the organization's financial managers to produce and manage the nursing department budget. Since about the early 1990s, that has no longer been the case. Nurses in management positions have increasingly taken control of planning, implementing, and controlling their own departmental budgets. This is appropriate because the manager closest to the operation is the manager most likely to have intimate knowledge of the budgetary requirements of the area, and of the best ways to use and control financial resources. Because of the transfer of budgetary responsibility and control to the nurse manager, it has become essential for nurses to develop sophisticated skills in the administration of their department's budget. In a survey of 43 nurse leaders at the Institute for Nursing Healthcare Leadership national invitational conference in June 2001, budgeting and financial management were at or close to the top priorities in virtually every area surveyed (Scobel & Russell, 2003).

Health care services are costly to provide. Only health care organizations that are financially sound can provide high-quality services. Organizations that do not pay adequate attention to their finances may find themselves in difficult positions. They suffer financial losses and do not have sufficient resources to continue normal operations. They have to choose between cutting quality and cutting services—which they realize may lead to such a poor competitive stance that they will ultimately fail anyway. In the past, administrators have typically chosen to cut quality of care by replacing RNs with unlicensed assistive personnel or by simply cutting staff and expecting the remaining staff to assume heavier workloads, which actually forced the remaining staff to reduce the amount of care provided. Ultimately, the institution acquired a reputation for poor care and patients abandoned it for better facilities. Then the institution commonly failed and closed. Therefore, the results of poor financial management are serious for both patients and staff: poor quality of care for the patients and ultimately, perhaps, loss of jobs, benefits, and seniority for the staff.

Good budgeting processes can help an institution avoid failure. Budgeting provides the organization with the ability to plan its activities and control its costs. It allows choices to be made that will allow it to provide the best care possible while staying within the financial means of the organization. Budgeting provides managers with the tools needed to ensure that the resources benefit patients and the institution rather than being wasted.

That explains why health care organizations must budget. But why have nurses become so much more involved in budgeting at every level of health care, from the hospital unit to strategic planning at the enterprise level in multi-health-care systems? The answer, quite simply, is that no one knows what resources are needed to provide quality nursing care better than nurses. With the publication of the landmark report on preventable medical errors (IOM, 1999), there has been a marked shift from a focus only on cost savings in health care to a primary focus on quality and safety of care first and then on cost savings second. In fact, third-party payers may not reimburse a health care facility at all if it cannot prove that it meets certain quality standards (Leapfrog Group, 2005; Oermann, 2004; Sloane, 2002).

At one time financial managers tried to provide nursing departments and units with their budgets. Nurse managers were simply told how many staff members they could hire and how much they could spend. However, such an approach to budgeting was doomed to failure. Financial managers do not have the ability to monitor the dynamic forces that affect the need for nursing care. Nurses are often the first to recognize shifts in patient demographics, patient acuity, types of illness, environmental effects on health, and changes in health care technology. Nurses know whether physicians and nurse practitioners are expanding their practices or retiring and whether health care practitioners are opening practices in underserved areas. Nurses know which patients have shorter lengths of stay and where admissions are rising or falling. Only nurses working in each nursing unit or in the administration of the health care organization can reasonably assess the nursing resource requirements.

Nurses must get involved in the budget process to make certain that they have the resources needed to provide high-quality clinical care. Budgeting is not separate from clinical caregiving. If anything, budgeting has a direct bearing on the amount of clinical care provided and the way it is provided. Just as a blood pressure cuff and a thermometer are tools nurses use in providing clinical care, so is a budget. Just as nurses prepare a patient care plan for the clinical care of a single patient, developing a budget acts as a plan to determine the overall clinical care that all patients will receive. It determines whether care will be provided by a nurse or an aide—or not at all. It determines which clinical supplies will be available. The elements of the budget are intertwined with the care patients receive.

In essence, for health care organizations to be efficient, they must involve nurses in the budgeting process. Only then can they ensure that resources are not wasted, perhaps causing an organization-wide financial crisis, while at the same time being aware of the specific needs that nursing has in order to provide patients with quality health care services. This book provides the essential budgeting techniques that nurses require in order to determine their needs and to most effectively communicate their needs to those individuals who make the final decisions about how to allocate an organization's limited resources.

■ DEFINITION OF BUDGETING

A *budget*[1] is a plan. To many individuals, budgeting is so onerous an activity that merely the word "budget" has taken on many negative connotations. A budget, however, is simply a plan. The plan is formalized (written down) and quantified (e.g., stated in dollar terms). It represents management's intentions or expectations. In financial terms, an organization-wide budget generally compares expected *revenues* to expected *expenses* in order to determine the organization's expected financial results. Revenues are the amounts of money the organization has earned by providing its services. Expenses are the costs of the services provided. Individual departments' budgets look at only a portion of the organization's overall revenue and expense information.

Budgeting forces managers to plan ahead. The focus on the future instead of the present allows managers to anticipate problems or opportunities far enough ahead of time to respond appropriately. Budgeting can greatly enhance communication and coordination among units and departments. This can allow units or departments to work together efficiently instead of duplicating efforts or failing to share critical information. Waste can be avoided through the knowledge developed and shared by involvement in the budget process. Budgets can be used to provide both managers and staff with the motivation to work positively for the organization. They can also show how well both management and units or departments are performing. These benefits of budgeting are discussed in greater detail in Chapter 2.

Budgeting does not happen automatically. It requires great effort and commitment from all levels of management. Often a facility budget committee (which should include the *Chief Nurse Executive*) is formed to ensure maximum cooperation and coordination throughout the budget process. Many organizations produce a budget calendar that indicates the various specific activities to be carried out in the budget process, identifies the responsible individuals (e.g., finance office, unit or department managers, Board of Trustees), and provides deadlines for the completion of each budget activity. Larger organizations have budget manuals. These manuals include uniform instructions and forms to be used throughout the organization, a copy of the budget calendar, and a statement of organizational mission. They also generally include a variety of other pieces of information relevant to the process of budget preparation. For instance, inflation rates, specific measurable goals, and an environmental statement are often included.

Budget manuals or packages are institution-specific, differing substantially from one organization to another. This book focuses primarily on concepts that are applicable to the budgeting process in a wide range of health care organizations, rather than providing a specific set of forms for the reader to fill in. The book's Appendix provides a sample set of forms, with instructions, for a unit's operating and capital budget. However, understanding the budgeting process is more important than learning how to complete one specific set of forms. The reader should understand that each organization will have its own set of forms that will differ from the examples presented in the Appendix. Managers must be able to think conceptually about budgets and budgeting in order to develop sensible, workable, efficient budgets. The focus of budgeting is not on filling in a standard set of forms.

Further, this book is about budgeting rather than just budgets. Budgets are plans. They represent an educated guess about what might be accomplished.

---

[1] Definitions of all words that appear in italics are provided in the Glossary on the book's website at http://evolve.elsevier.com/Finkler/budgeting/

Budgeting is a process whereby plans are made and then an effort is made to meet or exceed the goals of the plans. This latter effort is referred to as the *control* process. Control of costs requires a concerted effort by both managers and staff. This book will thus have its primary focus on the preparation of budgets and a second, well-emphasized focus on the topics that surround control, such as *variance analysis*, which determines how and why the actual results are varying from the budget. Such analysis uncovers problems that may have a negative financial impact on the organization and allows actions to be taken to correct those problems at an early stage.

A budget without a formal control system to ensure that actual results conform as closely as possible to the plan loses much of its managerial value. The budgeting process as a whole is of great importance because it can improve the organization's control over its use of scarce resources. This improved control can ensure that inefficiency is minimized and that the amount of dollars available for the provision of high-quality patient care is maximized.

Budgets are critical tools for any health care system, whether it be an acute care hospital, an ambulatory care facility, a visiting nurse association (VNA), a Public Health Department, or a privately owned nursing business. Nurse entrepreneurs starting new ventures need budgets and budgeting skills every bit as much as managed care organizations, clinics, hospitals, or nursing homes. The concepts discussed in this book are relevant to nurse managers in all health care organizations.

■ TYPES OF BUDGETS

Many managers tend to think of the budget as simply a cap on expenses that tells them how much they may spend. This is a very limited view of just the *operating budget*. The operating budget, in turn, is only a part of the overall budget of the organization. A well-managed organization has a *master budget*. The master budget is a set of all the major budgets in the organization. It generally includes the operating budget; a *long-range budget*, a *program budget*, a *capital budget*, and a *cash budget* (see Figure 1-1). Some organizations also use another type of budget referred to as a *performance budget* or *outcomes budget*, as well as a number of *product-line budgets*. From time to time the organization will also need to budget for some additional special project that is not part of its normal activities. In these cases it will prepare a *special-purpose budget*. This chapter provides an introduction to each of these types of budgets.

The Operating Budget

Those readers who already have some budgeting experience are probably most familiar with the operating budget. It is the plan for day-in and day-out operating revenues and expenses for a period of 1 year. If the budget shows an excess of revenues over expenses, it means that the organization expects to make a *profit* from its activities for the year. If the organization is a *for-profit* company, some of the profits can be paid to the owners of the company in the form of a *dividend*. Even *not-for-profit* organizations need to earn profits. These profits can be used to replace worn-out equipment and old buildings or to expand the services available to the community. If any health care organization, for-profit or not-for-profit, consistently fails to earn profits, it will not survive unless it is supported by outside funding such as public tax monies that may be used to support a state or county hospital. Without profits, no organization

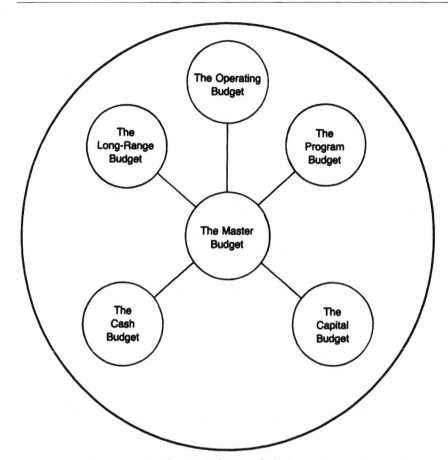

Figure 1-1 The master budget.

can keep current by adding necessary new technologies, nor can it continue to provide high-quality care.

If there is a budgeted excess of expenses over revenues, it means that the organization expects to have a loss for the budgeted year. Over time, losses mean that equipment and buildings cannot be replaced and that there are restrictions on the organization's ability to expand—or perhaps even maintain—its quantity and quality of services. If losses occur for too many years in a row, eventually the organization will have to cease operations.

The operating budget includes the revenues that are expected to be received from *Medicare, Medicaid, managed care organizations*, other *private insurers, self-pay patients*, and contributions. In some cases, contributions are sufficient to offset losses from routine operations and to keep a health care organization in business despite losses. The operating budget also plans for the routine costs of operating each department and unit in the organization, including the purely administrative departments that do not directly provide services. The operating budget is discussed in detail in Chapter 8.

Long-Range Budgets

Budgets help managers plan for the future. An operating budget provides a detailed plan for the coming year. However, many of the changes that occur in an organization require long lead times and take a number of years to be implemented fully. To avoid suffering from short-sightedness, many organizations employ a long-range plan or budget. Such 3-, 5-, or 10-year plans allow management to ignore the trees temporarily and focus on the whole forest. Where is the organization relative to its peer group? What improvements can be made over the next 3, 5, or 10 years? What must be done each year to move toward those goals?

In many organizations, the primary focus of the budgeting process is on the development of the operating budget. Managers tend to look at what happened during the past year and what is happening during the current year. They then add an increase for inflation and produce a budget for the next year. The problem with this approach is that it contains no vision. There is no way to make a major leap forward, because what has been done in the past is simply being projected into the future. If one would like to be able to look back 5 years from now and say, "Look how far we have come," it is necessary to have a way to make major strides forward. Otherwise, 5 years from now the organization will have made little if any advancement.

That is where long-range plans are helpful. Their focus is not on how to get through next year but rather on what major changes ought to be made over the coming years. Long-range plans frequently are not extremely detailed. When a plan is laid out for the next 5 years, it does not go into how many employees will be needed or what exact piece of equipment will be bought. It may be as general as to say that over the next 5 years three new tertiary care services will be added to the organization's services for the community. It may not even specify which ones.

Long-range plans help to give the organization a sense of commitment to the future. They provide long-term goals so that the organization is not always working only on things that can be accomplished within the arbitrary fixed time period of 1 year. Such long-range budgets serve a vital function in allowing the organization to prepare each year's detailed operating budget on the basis of an overall sense of purpose and direction. The operating budget becomes more than just the next year's survival plan; it becomes a link between where the organization has been and where it is going. To develop long-range plans, we employ a strategic planning process. Strategic planning links the overall mission of the organization to its activities. Strategic planning and long-range budgets are discussed in Chapter 7.

Program Budgets

Program budgets are special budgeting efforts analyzing specific programs. Generally, the orientation is toward evaluating a planned new program or closely examining an existing program, rather than merely planning the revenues and expenses for the program for the coming year. Often the program involved is in some way optional. The purpose of the program budget is to make a decision. Should the new program be undertaken or not? This question has somewhat less relevance for the types of programs and services that are considered to be essential to the organization and that are in no way optional.

Even for essential programs, however, there is the question of how the program's goals can best be accomplished. For example, a hospital must have laboratory services.

This may not be seen as being optional. However, the hospital may maintain a large, fully equipped laboratory or it may have minimal equipment for tests that must be done immediately, while sending the rest of the tests to an outside laboratory service. The extent of the in-house laboratory might be the subject of a special program budgeting effort or evaluation. Once the program evaluation has been performed and the program accepted, the revenues and expenses of the program will become part of the regular operating budget.

Often, program budgets are developed for specific programs as a result of the long-range budgeting process. The long-range budget for a same-day surgery organization may determine that three additional same-day surgery locations should be added over the next 5 years. Because new locations often require a year to plan and sometimes more than a year to implement once the planning phase is complete, one result of the long-range plan may be to select one location to be added immediately. Frequently, new services involve labor and equipment from numerous departments. By setting up a program budget process for the new location, all the information related to the addition of that location can be considered and evaluated.

Because program budgets often cut across departments, they generally must be developed with committee input from at least the major departments that will be affected by the change. Program budgets also cut across years. The financial impact of a change must be assessed not just in the coming year but over a reasonably long period of time. The operating budget is a 1-year budget, so this is another reason for special budget treatment for new programs or services.

In recent years, the *business plan* has become a vital tool for the evaluation of new programs or projects. The elements of such plans, along with long-range budgets and other aspects of program budgeting, are discussed in Chapter 7.

Capital Budgets

Many expenditures made by health care organizations are for the acquisition of items that will last for more than 1 year. Such acquisitions are defined as capital expenditures. Frequently, these purchases do not concern the introduction of an entire program and therefore do not warrant a full-scale program budget effort. Often, capital budget items will concern only one department or unit and may be part of an already existing program. Yet capital expenditures frequently concern large outlays of money that deserve special attention. The multiyear life of capital assets also creates the need for a focus on such items, separate from the operating budget.

Capital expenditures are made to purchase items that will provide benefits for a number of years into the future. If capital items are evaluated based only on their benefits for the coming year, their value to the organization will be understated. The operating budget has the capability to look at only the coming year's revenues and expenses. Therefore, capital items must be put into a separate budget that can evaluate their benefits over their entire useful lifetime.

For example, suppose that a nursing home were to entirely renovate one wing of its building. Patients will use the wing and the organization will receive revenues from patients in that wing for a number of years. If the entire renovation cost were charged as an expense in this year's operating budget, the project would appear financially infeasible. Patients could never be charged enough in 1 year to recover the full construction costs. The new wing will be available for many years, however, and patients can be charged for the renovation well into the future.

If this were treated as an operating budget expense, it might show a $1,000,000 expense for the renovation this year but only $100,000 of revenues from the patients who benefited from the renovation. The operating budget cannot match future revenues to current outlays to see if the project is feasible. It looks only at revenues and expenses for the coming year. The capital budget seeks to bridge this gap for projects or purchases with a multiyear life.

The capital budget looks at a capital investment—whether it is a renovation, a new wing for the nursing home, or a new refrigerator for a nursing station—to determine whether the expenditure is feasible economically over the lifetime of the asset. Thus, even though an item may cost only $600 or $800, by recognizing its 3-, 5-, or 10-year expected lifetime, it is more likely that a fair assessment will be made concerning whether it is reasonable to spend the money for this specific purpose.

This does not mean that all acquisitions that are not warranted on a financial basis would be rejected. The capital budget can go beyond simply dollars and cents and look at costs and benefits in a broader sense. The general benefit provided to the community can be considered. Often, capital items will be purchased even if they lose money. However, for the organization to survive there must be an understanding of which things generate a profit and which things lose money. Enough profit-making activities must be selected to cover those expenditures that result in losses. The key thrust of capital budgeting is that the evaluation of the expenditure should be based on its impact over its full lifetime, rather than simply looking at the costs and benefits in the first year. Capital budgets are discussed in Chapter 10.

Product-Line Budgets

A product line is a set of products or services that have some commonality that allows them to be bundled together, such as a common diagnosis or a specific set of surgical procedures. For example, Cardiac Surgery might be one product line, and Women's Health might be another. Budgeting in health care organizations is focused largely on departments and units. In all hospitals, for example, radiology has a budget; dietary has a budget; nursing has a budget. However, it is becoming more and more common for there to be budgets for specific types of patients, such as heart surgery patients or childbearing women. These budgets include the costs of surgery, recovery, delivery room, radiology services, meals, nursing care, and other costs.

A product-line budget cuts across multiple departments that provide services to the patients served by a particular product line. In today's tight financial environment, it is often of great managerial interest to be able to budget for the planned revenues and expenses of specific patient groups, such as heart surgery patients. This makes a great deal of sense because Medicare and many insurance companies pay according to a particular *Diagnosis Related Group (DRG)* code and not for separate, individual services delivered to the patient. Product-line budgeting has the potential to reveal the profitability involved in treating various types of patients.

The move toward product-line budgeting has also gained impetus because of active pressure by *Health Maintenance Organizations (HMOs)* negotiating with health care providers for discounted rates for specific groups of patients. It is difficult to negotiate sensible revenue rates unless the related costs of the patients are known.

Health care organizations have therefore been moving in the direction of product-line budgeting, while not abandoning department budgets. However, the process is a difficult one. Measuring the cost of nursing care for patients in any one category is complicated. Yet, to determine a budget, such information is essential. Product-line costing is therefore discussed in Chapter 16, along with the issue of costing-out nursing services.

Cash Budgets

Cash is the lifeblood of any organization. Survival depends on the ability to maintain an adequate supply of cash to meet the monetary obligations of the organization as they become due for payment. Operating budgets focus on the revenues and expenses of the organization. If the organization is expected to lose money, that will be reflected in the operating budget. It is possible, however, for the organization to have a cash crisis even if it is not losing money. Many of the expenses that an organization incurs are paid currently. Wages are typically paid at least monthly and frequently biweekly or weekly. However, revenues may take several months to collect because of the internal lags in processing patient bills and the external lags before organizations such as HMOs or Medicare make payment. Thus an organization can literally run out of cash even though it is making a profit!

Oddly enough, this problem tends to be most severe for an organization with an increasing number of patients. Although an increasing patient volume is normally thought of as a healthy development, it results in growing expenses as well as growing revenues. The revenues may well increase by a greater amount than the expenses. The expenses, however, typically have to be paid much sooner than the revenues are received. Without careful management, such growing profitability can easily bankrupt an organization.

These problems tend to be particularly severe for start-up ventures. A nurse entrepreneur must carefully consider the timing of cash flows, even if a profit is made on every unit of service. Rent, phone bills, and employees have to be paid currently even though insurance companies are known to delay payments to health care providers. A cash budget is a critical tool in the day-to-day survival of an organization.

Another cash problem relates to major capital expenses. Only a 1-year portion of capital outlays will show up in the operating budget as a current-year expense. If the organization budgets to add a wing for $10,000,000, and it is expected to have a 20-year life, then there will typically be a charge of one twentieth of the cost, or $500,000 per year, as an expense called *depreciation* in the operating budget. However, the entire $10,000,000 will have to be paid in cash in the coming year when the wing is built. Thus there will be a cash outlay of $9,500,000 more than is shown in the operating budget as an expense.

For these reasons, a cash budget is prepared. Cash budgets plan for the monthly receipt of cash and disbursement of cash by the organization. If a shortage is predicted for any given month, appropriate plans can be made for short-term bank financing or long-term bond financing. Cash budgets are discussed in Chapter 12.

Performance Budgets

This book introduces an approach to budgeting that is not yet widely used in health care organizations. The budget is called a performance budget, and it attempts to make plans for units, departments, and organizations that will better provide the ability to evaluate whether the unit, department, or organization is accomplishing what it wants to do. An operating budget does a pretty good job of detailing the resources that will be needed. However, the measures in that budget, as you will see as you read this book, are fairly simplistic.

Nursing organizations or units have many objectives besides generating patient days, visits, or encounters. They want to ensure quality of care and cost-effectiveness. But such goals are rarely explicit in the budget process. How much spending is budgeted to improve patient care? How much for reduction in the number of medication errors?

A performance budget attempts to determine how much money is being budgeted to provide direct care, to provide indirect care, to ensure quality of care, to control costs, to provide patient satisfaction, to provide staff satisfaction, and so on. One still cannot easily measure direct outcomes, such as how much health has been produced. But the nursing profession has made great strides in looking at process, such as preparing patient care and discharge plans. It is possible to create a performance budget that examines whether the prescribed process is in fact being carried out and that relates that process to its share of the costs budgeted for the unit. A look at this new approach, called performance or outcomes budgeting, is provided in Chapter 11.

Special-Purpose Budgets

A budget is a plan. There is not a great deal of rigidity in the definition of a budget. Therefore, there is also not a great limitation placed on the types of budgets that are possible. Any health care organization can prepare a budget for any activity for which it desires a plan.

In recent years, a number of health care organizations have offered screening for high cholesterol, colon cancer, diabetes, and HIV. In some cases, these screenings have been free, and in others there has been a charge. What will it cost to provide the service free (i.e., to help the community and at the same time get some favorable press)? How much would you have to charge just to cover the costs of such a program?

Often these programs are not part of the yearly operating budget. They are special programs, put together on the spur of the moment in response to a current need. A special-purpose budget can be prepared any time a plan is needed for some activity that is not already budgeted as part of one of the ongoing budget processes. The budget does not need any formal system or set of forms. It is desirable, however, to know in which department the special budget is to be managed and the nature of the impact on staffing and on the morale of the staff that will be assigned to carry out the work of the special activity. One would also want to know whether a profit, a loss, or neither is anticipated. The key to developing a special-purpose budget is to try to consider rationally all human and financial consequences of the proposed activity.

■ BUDGETING METHODOLOGY

The previous discussion centered on the types of budgets. This topic should be contrasted with the wide variety of budgeting methodologies. Methodologies are different approaches for developing and using the types of budgets that have been discussed in this chapter. For example, these methodologies include *Zero-Base Budgeting* and business plans (two techniques widely used to develop program budgets). They include variable or *flexible budgeting*. These and other methodologies are discussed throughout this book.

■ RELEVANT TIME PERIODS FOR BUDGET PREPARATION

Budgeting is often viewed as a necessary evil rather than as a labor of love. Therefore, the questions that arise are when and how often budgets must be prepared. The answer depends on the type of budget being considered. Some budgeting is done once and once only. Other budgets can be relegated to just several times per decade. Some budgeting must be done annually. Finally, there are proponents of performing some budgeting activities on a continual (monthly) basis.

One-Shot Budgets

Special-purpose budgets such as those discussed earlier need to be prepared only once. There is no particular time of the year when they are prepared. Similarly, program budgets are commonly prepared on a one-shot basis. Program budgets are concerned primarily with the evaluation of major new services that the organization is considering offering. Preparing a program budget is generally needed only once for any given program. However, that initial budget covers a number of years. If the project, program, or service is rejected, there is no need to review it on a regular basis. If the program is approved, it is often reviewed periodically, comparing actual outcomes to the budgeted projections.

Program budgets do not have to be prepared at any specific time during the year. Generally, because the program does not currently exist, there is no experience to draw upon in making up the budget. A number of assumptions must be made. Further, numerous options and alternatives must be considered. As a result, a program budget commonly requires a number of months and many meetings to prepare.

Infrequently Prepared Budgets

Long-range budgets are generally prepared on an infrequent basis. Such budgets generally cover a span of 3, 5, or 10 years. Although some organizations may make annual adjustments to or modifications of a long-range plan, the main body of the budget typically remains unchanged over its lifetime. This provides a sense of stability and direction for the organization. Nevertheless, long-range budgets should be reviewed annually to determine whether any major unexpected changes in the organization's environment require modification to the plan.

Long-range plans are much less detailed than program budgets. Therefore, they do not necessarily require the long preparation time that a program budget requires. However, rather than simply being related to one department, one program, or one part of the organization's existence, the long-range plan gets to the core of why the organization exists and where it wants to go. If the organization is having difficulty in assessing where it wants to head in the future, it may take many months before there can be agreement on a challenging yet realistic plan that meets the needs of the community, the organization, and the organization's employees.

Annual and Monthly Budgets

Most individuals are familiar with budgeting as an annual phenomenon. Operating, capital, cash, and performance budgets fall into this category. Each of these budgets must be prepared every year. However, it is necessary to divide the annual budgets into smaller time periods in order to have an adequate basis for controlling costs during the year. It is undesirable to have to wait until the end of the year to find out whether the unit, department, or organization as a whole has been keeping to the budgeted expectations. By the end of the year it is too late to do anything about problems that arose and could have been corrected midstream. Certainly, any problems can be corrected as part of the process of budgeting for the next year—but even then, one would not know whether they were successful until the end of the subsequent year. Accurate monthly plans are vital to the control of operations on a timely basis.

Furthermore, the nature of the health care field is such that it is an inadequate approach for hospitals and most other health care facilities to simply take an annual budget and divide by 12 to get expectations for each month of the year. The number of days, number of weekends, type of weather, and other factors can create substantial differences in patient care demand and staff workload patterns from month to month. Normal seasonality will create some months with peak demands on the organization and other months when workload levels are lower than average. Therefore, each month typically must be planned for individually.

In many cases, a nursing unit or department will be required to submit only a total budget for the year. In these cases, the organization will probably provide monthly reports comparing the budget and the actual results, based on dividing the annual budget into 12 equal months (or in some cases 13 months, each with 28 days).[2] Even if this is the case, the nurse manager should take the annual budget and prepare a set of monthly budgets that take into account factors such as seasonality. In order to manage staff and supplies efficiently, the nurse manager needs to understand how unit resource consumption is likely to vary from month to month.

Continuous Budgeting

In a system that focuses on annual preparation of operating and cash budgets, there are a number of weaknesses that could be cured if budgets were prepared more frequently. Continuous budgeting is a system in which a budget is prepared each month for a month 1 year in the future. For example, once the actual results for January are known, ideally by mid or late February, the budget for the next January can be prepared. There are four major problems with the traditional annual budgeting approach that are addressed by continuous budgeting: attitude toward budgeting, time-management concerns, accuracy of budgets, and increasing myopia regarding the future.

Attitude

Many managers find budgeting to be very disruptive to their work. Budgeting comes once a year and requires a major diversion from routine activities. Several weeks or longer of full-time effort are devoted to preparing the budget for the entire next year. It is a mammoth process that often is faced quite reluctantly. On the other hand, if a much smaller effort is required on a regular monthly basis, the process may not seem so onerous. It may become a part of normal routine rather than an interruption of it. The result is greater familiarity and comfort with the process, which leads to a much better attitude toward the entire budgeting process. This in turn leads to a better

[2] Some health care providers use 13-month years. The major benefit of this approach is that each month has exactly 4 weeks.

effort by managers in preparing the budget. More important, it leads to more successful budgets.

Time Management
The problem of attitude goes hand in hand with the problem of time management. There are so many things to be done. Nothing else seems to get done during the most intensive period of budget preparation. With continuous budgeting, the bulk of the process is spread evenly throughout the year. One or two days of effort each and every month, instead of several weeks of full-time effort in one or two months, reduces the disruptive nature of the process.

Several days can be given up each month without important functions going undone that month. Giving up several weeks in one month is inherently so disruptive that many things get pushed off, and it takes several months of overtime effort to catch up. It is important to manage the time spent on budgets, rather than letting the budget process disrupt day-in and day-out management functions.

Accuracy
By the time the budget is prepared using the annual approach, most of the current year has passed; with it, the crises of the year have seemed to dim. The months start to run together and appear to be very much alike in the manager's memory. By preparing a budget for the next July right after this July has passed, the chances are that the budget for the subsequent July will be a much more realistic and accurate reflection of what typically happens during July. It will capture peculiarities of the month with a much higher degree of precision than would be possible if the next July's budget were not prepared until February or March.

In practice, the monthly budgets developed under a continuous budgeting approach do not constitute finalized, approved budgets. The negotiation and approval process would not be done more than once a year. The budget prepared each month for the same month one year in the future allows for the compilation of a more accurate budget when the entire next year's budget is developed once a year. At the same time, as discussed previously, the time it takes to compile the budget will be substantially reduced because it simply puts together all of the monthly budgets that have been prepared during the year.

Further, accuracy is improved because if changes occur during this year that affect some basic assumptions that were made in planning the next July's budget, it is not too late to modify, adjust, or correct the budget for the next July. Managers are not left with only their thoughts at one point in time. There is time before the budget is finalized to reflect on the budgets that have been prepared for the months of the next year and to revise them as ways to improve operations arise.

Myopia
One of the beneficial elements of a budget is the opportunity it gives management to peer into the future. If an annual budget for the year beginning next July (assuming we use a June 30 year-end for *fiscal* purposes) is completed by April of this year, one can see 14 months into the future. Expectations regarding this May and June (i.e., the last 2 months of this year) are known, as are those for all 12 months of next year.

This foresight allows managers to take expectations of the future into account when making current decisions. Projections of workload, inflation, future capital equipment acquisitions, and so on help managers to manage effectively in the present.

By the time the next year begins, however, the horizon has decreased from 14 months to 12 months. Halfway into the year, the horizon is only 6 months. The resulting effect is creeping myopia. Each month, one sees less far into the future. Uncertainty increases, and the efficiency of decision making decreases. Decisions that would easily be made in August must be postponed if they arise in March because the manager does not know enough about the future. Continuous budgeting ensures that at any point there is a horizon of approximately 1 year.

■ BUDGETING BEYOND THE HOSPITAL

By the end of the twentieth century, it was clear that the hospital was no longer the be-all and end-all provider of health care services. The last few decades of the twentieth century saw hospitals lose their dominant position. Hospitals, without question, still serve a vital role as a part of the overall health care system. However, organizations providing ambulatory care, such as clinics, ambulatory surgery centers (ASCs), VNAs, hospice, managed care organizations, and long-term care providers, have also become important players in the health care marketplace.

All health care organizations have an important need for high-quality budgeting. The remainder of this book will at times use examples of hospitals. At other times the budgeting examples will focus on nonhospital health care organizations. In all cases the role of the book is to provide the reader with sound concepts of budgeting. The techniques taught in this book can then be applied in a wide variety of situations and organizations.

An alternative approach was considered. The book could have provided a chapter on budgeting for long-term-care organizations, another chapter on budgeting for home care organizations, and so on. However, the fundamentals of budgeting apply across all health care organizations. A book providing a chapter on budgeting for each type of organization would basically provide a limited amount of information repeated over and over using a different specific example. Instead, it was decided to integrate a variety of examples throughout a book that provides both breadth and depth in budgeting, without excessive repetition. Based on the authors' experience in the field, this approach will best serve the wide readership of the book, providing the foundations that nurse managers need to prepare and control budgets in many different health care settings.

Summary and Implications for Nurse Managers

A budget is basically a plan that provides a formal, quantitative expression of what the organization's management plans to accomplish. The development of the budget helps the organization to establish goals and a plan for the future.

The various types of budgets within an organization together constitute the master budget. The most familiar part of this master budget is the operating budget, which details the day-to-day operating revenues and expenses of the organization. Additionally, other budgets that are part of the master budget include a long-range plan, program budgets, capital budgets, performance budgets, and a cash budget.

Although one thinks of budgeting as an annual event, this is really a broad generalization. A budget that evaluates whether to add, expand, contract, or delete an entire program may be prepared only once. Long-range budgets providing overall organizational direction are generally prepared only every 3, 5, or 10 years. Capital, operating, performance, and cash budgets are prepared annually.

Summary and Implications for Nurse Managers—cont'd

Operating and cash budgets must have detailed information regarding each month within the year because not all months will be the same. The detailed monthly information is vital if one wishes not only to have a plan but also to use that plan for controlling operations.

Continuous budgeting, a technique with several advantages over more traditional budget approaches, calls for preparing the budget for each month nearly 1 year before that month arrives.

What implications do these basic concepts about the different types of budgets have for nurse managers? First, as one prepares any budget, whether it is a program budget or a unit operating budget, it is important to have an understanding of how that budget fits into the overall scheme of things. This chapter should have provided the reader with a sense of the different types of budgets, why they exist, and how the capital and operating budgets fit into this picture. This book allows the reader to think about each of the types of budget in terms of the information it requires from and provides to the nurse manager and the organization and how that information relates to the other types of budgets the organization prepares.

This chapter should also serve to introduce nurse managers to the fact that budgeting is a tool for planning and controlling what happens within a nursing unit, department, or organization. Budgeting is not inherently complex. A budget is a plan. After the plan is made, it must be implemented and used to try to control results.

In order to maximize the benefit of budgeting, many organizations have developed lengthy budget processes with dozens of complex forms. The budgeting process in many organizations has become complicated. But the underlying concept is not. Budgeting requires the development of a plan. It must then be determined whether the plan results in a feasible financial outcome for the organization. If it does not, the plan must be revised until there is a feasible result.

Sometimes the result will not be as good as one would like. However, it is necessary to balance the long-term financial needs of the organization so that it can remain in business, with the short-term quality-of-care needs for patients and the other needs of the organization's employees. It is this balancing act that requires substantial information. Much of the rest of this book focuses on how to generate the information needed to make effective decisions about the use of scarce resources available to the organization.

References and Suggested Readings

Campbell, C., Schmitz, H., and Waller, L.C. (1998). *Financial Management in a Managed Care Environment (Delmar's Health Information Management Series)*. Albany, NY: Delmar.

Cleverley, W.O. (2002). *Essentials of Health Care Finance*, ed 5. Boston: Jones and Bartlett.

Cripps, M., Studdard, A., and Woodhall, G. (2004). *Financial Management: Budgeting in Hospitals and Financial Trusts*, ed 2. (Essentials of Nursing Management Series). New York: Palgrave McMillan.

Gapenski, L.C. (2004). *Healthcare Finance: An Introduction to Accounting and Financial Management*. Washington, D.C.: Alpha Press.

Henderson, E. (2003). Budgeting: Part I. *Nursing Management* 10(1), 33-37.

Henderson, E. (2003). Budgeting: Part II. *Nursing Management* 10(20), 32-36.

Kleinman, C.S. (2003). Leadership Roles, Competencies, and Education: How Prepared Are Our Nurse Managers? *Journal of Nursing Administration* 33(9), 451-455.

Kohn, L.T., Corrigan, J.M., Donaldson, M., Eds. (1999). Institute of Medicine (IOM), Committee on Quality of Health Care in America. *To Err Is Human: Building A Safer Health System*. Washington, DC: National Academy Press; (Reissued, 2000). Also available online at: http://www.nap.edu/books/0309068371/html/

Leapfrog Group. (2005). How and why Leapfrog started. *The Leapfrog Group: Getting Healthcare Right*. Downloaded September 15, 2005 from: http://www.leapfroggroup.org/about_us/how_and_why

McLean, R.A. (2002). *Financial Management in Health Care Organizations*, ed. 2. Delmar Series in Health Services Administration. Albany, NY: Delmar.

Oermann, M. (2004). Interview With Suzanne Delbanco, PhD, Executive Director of The

Leapfrog Group. *Journal of Nursing Care Quality* 19(2), 85-87.

Pelfrey S. (1997, March). Managing financial data. *Seminars for Nurse Managers* 5(1), 25-30.

Scoble, K.B., and Russell, G. (2003). Vision 2020, Part I: Profile of the Future Nurse Leader. *Journal of Nursing Administration* 33(6), 324-330.

Sloane, T. (2002). Follow the guidelines to the money. *Modern Healthcare* 32(50), 22.

Zelman, W.N., McCue, M.J., Milikan, A.R., and Glick, N. (2003). *Financial Management of Health Care Organizations: An Introduction to Fundamental Tools, Concepts, and Applications,* ed 2. Maiden, MA: Blackwell Publisher.

The Budgeting Process

LEARNING OBJECTIVES
The goals of this chapter are to:

- Describe the budgeting process
- Discuss the elements of planning
- Explain the role of communication and coordination in budgeting
- Introduce the concept of a budget timetable
- Describe the use of PERT and CPM scheduling tools
- Emphasize the importance of controlling results
- Introduce the concept of budget flexibility
- Introduce the concept of organizational philosophies of fiscal affairs
- Explain the role of information gathering
- Discuss the specific steps in the budgeting process, including programming; developing unit, department, and cash budgets; negotiation and revision; and feedback

■ INTRODUCTION

Each organization has its own specific budget forms, timetables, and specific budget processes. Conceptually, however, there are certain elements and specific steps that should be undertaken as part of the budget process (Box 2-1). Four key elements exist throughout the budgeting process. These are planning, controlling, establishing an underlying organizational philosophy of fiscal affairs, and gathering information. In addition to those four elements, this chapter also discusses specific steps in the budgeting process: programming; developing unit and departmental budgets; developing the cash budget; negotiating and revising budget proposals; budget approval and implementation; and feedback.

■ PLANNING

Preparing a budget should provide impetus for the organization's managers to plan ahead. Past management experience has shown that, in general, organizations that are actively managed will do better than those that just let things happen. Properly planned, the budgeting process forces managers to establish goals. Without goals, organizations tend to wander aimlessly, rarely improving the results of their operations or the services they offer (see Box 2-1).

Organizations that are not serious about the budget process often move from crisis to crisis. This is basically a managerial version of fire fighting taking precedence over fire prevention. If managers push off careful attention to budget preparation because of current emergencies at hand, they are setting themselves up for the next

BOX 2-1 The Budgeting Process

Underlying Elements of Budgeting
1. Planning
2. Controlling results
3. Philosophy of fiscal affairs
4. Information gathering

Specific Steps in Budgeting
1. Programming
   A. Budget foundations
      • Environment scan
      • General goals, objectives, and policies
      • Organization-wide assumptions
      • Specifying program priorities
      • Specific measurable operating objectives
   B. Long-range and program budgets
2. Developing unit and department budgets
   A. Operating budget
   B. Capital budget
3. Developing cash budgets
4. Negotiating and revising the budget
5. Budget approval and implementation
6. Feedback

round of emergencies. Careful planning provides an opportunity for examining options and alternatives in a calm, rational setting. The result is generally a more satisfactory outcome and fewer crisis situations arise.

By requiring managers to prepare a budget at least annually, organizations compel their management to forecast the future. Changes in factors that affect the organization's business can be anticipated and their impact predicted. Typically, these factors include patient demographics, stability or change in medical practices, availability of specialists, provider referral patterns, technology and development, or closure of competitor facilities in the organization's service area. Careful study of these aspects of the organization's business environment enables managers to anticipate changes that will affect the organization and to plan actions accordingly. When one responds to changes after the fact, alternatives may be limited. By considering the impact of changes during the planning phase, the broadest possible range of alternative actions can be considered. Often the result of careful planning is that more cost-effective approaches can be found and put into place than are possible when managers are responding to crises.

If management's initial plans indicate that revenues are not expected to be great enough to cover expenses, there is time during the budget planning process to consider actions that might increase revenues or reduce costs. Alternatively, investigation of the business environment may reveal that much higher demands will be placed on the organization than has been the case in the past. Both downturns and upturns in demand for health care services require health care managers to respond to what may become a profoundly changed business environment. Business downturns are generally viewed as undesirable problems. But a sudden surge in demand also causes managers serious problems in delivering needed services. One may think of these as "bad problems" and "good problems," but they constitute management problems just the same. Solutions to problems caused by changes in the business environment may be difficult to generate in the best of circumstances. Without the type of information most typically obtained during the budget planning process, managers may not be aware that a change is imminent. By the time the organization recognizes that a loss has occurred or that demand is outstripping the organization's ability to serve the needs of its patients, it may be too late to do anything about it.

Is it an important problem if the organization loses money? Many organizations that nurses work for are not-for-profit.[1] Does it matter if a not-for-profit organization loses money in some years? It clearly does matter. If revenues are less than expenses, then ultimately cash receipts from revenues will be less than the cash needed to pay expenses. If losses persist, a point will come when there is not enough cash to meet routine obligations such as payroll. Lenders may not loan the organization money to pay those expenses out of fear that the organization will not be able to repay the loan. For every organization there is the question of survival. If losses occur a number of years in a row, bankruptcy could result.

Nor is long-term survival the only consideration. Hospitals, nursing homes, home care agencies, and other health care organizations are providing service to their communities. If money is wasted through lax management, the quality and breadth of services offered will have to be lower than they might otherwise have been. The degree of care exercised in budgeting can make a difference in the quality of care that patients receive. It can be the difference between money spent on unneeded or wasted supplies versus money spent on hiring one additional nurse on each shift.

Communication and Coordination

An effective planning process requires a high level of communication among the managers of the organization. The managers of the organization should act as a group to develop the overall goals and directions of the organization as well as its specific measurable goals for the coming year. Once decided upon, these goals should be communicated clearly to all managers and staff. The planning process should be based on this common set of objectives, and the managers of the various units and departments of the organization should coordinate their plans with each other.

These two managerial functions of communication and coordination go hand in hand. Many managers feel that they know their objectives, so they have no need to formalize those goals as part of the budget process. Yet the fact that a given manager has certain goals and objectives does not mean that everyone in the organization knows what those goals are. The budget, if communicated to other managers and staff, provides a document that systematically informs all managers and staff of exactly what they and their units or departments are expected to accomplish. It also provides a basis for discussion if some of those expectations appear to be unreasonable.

---

[1] Not-for-profit or non-profit health care organizations are formed primarily to provide service to the community. For-profit health care organizations have the primary goal of earning a profit for their owners through the services they provide. Both types of organizations generally do make profits. For-profit organizations must distribute a reasonable profit to their owners or the owners may close the organization so they can move their money to better investment opportunities. Not-for-profits may reinvest all profits back into the organization (for expansion of services and replacement of plant and equipment) or may have to provide funds for supporting uninsured members of the community. In some cases, a not-for-profit must render funds to a larger sponsoring organization such as a religious order.

Communication among various levels of management should be more than simply a statement of overall goals. Organizational policies, constraints, and assumptions must be communicated to all managers working on the budget. Staffing cannot be planned efficiently without an assumption about patient-load expectations. Nursing salary costs cannot be planned without assumptions about anticipated pay raises. Over time, Travelers,[2] and part-time employee needs cannot be calculated without assumptions about staff availability and costs. All this information has little value in budget preparation unless it is communicated to the managers who are preparing the detailed elements of the budget. The budget preparation process should bring together information in a formalized manner and disseminate it to the individuals who need that information to operate their units or departments.

Communication is also a requirement for employee motivation and evaluation. Using budgets for motivation and evaluation is discussed in Chapter 3. Budgets can be an effective motivational tool if they have been communicated to the individuals that they are aimed at motivating. One can hope to get individuals to work toward accomplishing the organization's objectives only if they have been informed as to what those objectives are. A sense of equity requires that individuals be told what is expected of them if they are going to be subsequently evaluated on how well they have met those expectations. The budget lays out in black and white the organization's goals and expectations. The budget can communicate the organization's expectations directly to its managers.

Budget Timetable

It is important to have a plan for the planning process. Managers should have a road map that tells them what steps must be taken in the planning process and when they should be undertaken. Table 2-1 presents a sample budget timetable. Each organization will have its own timetable. In small organizations, the entire process described by the timetable may take only a few months. In large health care systems, the budgeting process often takes more than 6 months.

Just as the length of time to complete the budget process varies from organization to organization, so do the specific elements of the budget timetable. Table 2-1 assumes a budget process for an organization with a July 1 through June 30 fiscal year. As one reviews this sample timetable, it becomes clear why budgeting is a complex task and one that is constantly subject to deadlines.

The first step is appointing the supervisory Budget Committee and a Chair for the committee. This committee is usually selected by the Chief Executive Officer (CEO) but may be appointed by the Board. The Chair may be either the CEO or the Chief Financial Officer (CFO). Members typically include the CEO, the CFO, the Chief Operations Officer (COO), and the Vice Presidents or Division Managers of each operational division of the organization. For example, in a large organization, the Chief Nursing Officer or Nursing VP (CNO) may have responsibility for all of Nursing, Pastoral Care, the Dietary Department, and perhaps other areas. The CFO will have responsibility for payroll, billing, financing, and perhaps other areas such as the Legal Department. In a very small organization, the committee may consist of the CEO, the CFO, and the managers of each department. What is most important is that the Budget

---

[2] "Travelers" in this context means staff obtained through a temporary staffing company. They typically receive an hourly wage much higher than that of regular staff, but have no job security or seniority.

TABLE 2-1 Sample Budget Timetable

Activity	Responsibility	Deadline for Completion
Appointment of the Budget Committee	Chief Executive Officer	December
First meeting of Budget Committee	Budget Committee; Chair	January 5
Completion of budget foundations activities and communication to department heads	Budget Committee	February 28
Completion of long-range and program budgets	Budget Committee and subcommittees	March 31
Submission of unit capital and operating budgets	Unit managers	April 15
Negotiation between nursing units and nursing administration	Chief Nurse Executive and unit managers or department supervisors	April 22
Compilation of all nursing unit budgets	Chief Nurse Executive	April 30
Development of cash budget	Chief Financial Officer	May 15
Negotiation and revision process	All managers	June 15
Approval of the budget	Chief Executive Officer	June 16
Final approval of the budget	Board of trustees	June 20
Implementation of the budget	All managers	July 1

Committee—which makes decisions about how the organization will spend money during the following fiscal year—include those people who will have to manage the major divisions of the organization according to the requirements of that budget.

The selection of the Budget Committee and its Chair should take place as early as possible. Then the committee should meet promptly. In this example, it is assumed that the committee first meets no later than the first week in January, a full 6 months before the next fiscal year. Generally, serving on the Budget Committee is a responsibility of the CEO, CFO, and several other positions, so the persons who will be appointed should plan for this duty and manage their calendars accordingly. In fact, it is not uncommon for the Budget Committee meeting schedule to be available from the CEO's office well before the time that the committee is expected to meet. The committee must go through all the steps of *budget foundations* (discussed later in this chapter) to ensure that department heads will have the information needed to prepare their budgets. In this example, 2 months are allowed for that process.

The long-range plan and program budgets cannot be completed without having, at the very least, information about the organization's environment, as well as its goals, objectives, and policies. This information is prepared by the Budget Committee as part of the foundation's activities. During the month of March, the long-range plan must be formulated (or reviewed) and specific programs considered. The decisions regarding these programs must be known early in the budget process so that all department heads can take the impact of new programs or program changes into account in preparing their operating and capital budgets. In actuality, the long-range plan and new programs are generally considered at some length even before the budget process begins, and the month of March in this example is used to finalize decisions based on months of consideration and data collection and analysis.

Each organization creates its unique set of budget forms to meet its particular needs and situations. Before departmental or unit managers can begin to prepare their operating and capital budgets, these documents must be reviewed, modified, and distributed to all managers involved in budget preparation. Unit managers will have started preparing their budgets in early March. However, the long-range and program budgets may cause some changes to be made. This leaves just a 2-week period for a unit manager to finish preparing a first draft of the unit's budget. However, this may be sufficient because she or he has previously been provided with information about the unit's activities and performance during the prior year. Unless it is known that changes in patient census, acuity or some other factor can be expected during the next year, the new budget is most commonly prepared using the prior year's data.

Once the Nursing Unit Managers submit their proposed budgets to the CNO, there is often a brief but intense period of negotiation between the nursing administration and its units. Managers may have been asked to cut their operating budgets by a few percentage points. If so, managers of units that expect an increase in activity will certainly need to negotiate a budget consistent with the expected new activity. In the area of operating budgets, the negotiation may address new staff needed for an expected increase in workload. This negotiation should be relatively straightforward if the facility uses a variable budget that bases expenditures on activity. Clearly, it costs more to provide care for an expected census of 48 patients per day than for 39 patients per day.

Another area of negotiation is the capital budget. There is usually a specific capital budget dollar amount; it is the limit of the capital dollars the nursing department may spend in the next fiscal year. All of the various Unit Managers will try to get their own capital items approved, and it will be up to the CNO to decide which capital items to submit in the final nursing department budget. Typically, the items that are accompanied by the best justification data and narrative get approved. Therefore, Unit Managers need to be skilled in preparing their capital budget requests. It is naïve to assume that a CNO will divide the capital budget dollars evenly among the various nursing units. In fact, it would be irresponsible for the CNO to fund capital requests on a dollar-per-unit basis. The CNO needs to evaluate each request in light of the value to the organization of each item, regardless of the unit requesting the item. So Unit Managers **must** expect to negotiate vigorously for their requests.

In Table 2-1, only 1 week is available for this negotiation process. If this time could be expanded, there would be less likelihood of an atmosphere of crisis and more time for reasoned discussions. Because the time is typically short, wise Unit Managers will have taken the time to document thoroughly the need for any increases in personnel to be requested in the new budget. Additionally, they should research any capital items to be included in the budget. This means that the request will be accompanied by an explanation of the need for the item, the consequences if the item is not purchased, and two or three bids for the item. Knowing that the budgeting process is a *negotiation* process, the wise Unit Manager will not wait until just before the budget is due to begin gathering the information needed to justify additional personnel and capital equipment items. It is not unreasonable to begin the process of justification and bid acquisition at any time throughout the year when needs are identified. Then when it is time to submit the budgets, the groundwork will have been done and all the data needed for the negotiation process will be well in hand.

The nursing department has 1 week in this timetable to compile all the unit budgets into a final nursing department budget. Finance has 2 weeks to take the information from all the budgets of the organization and develop a unified cash budget.

One month is then allowed for organization-wide negotiation and budget revision. If all goes well, the budget can be approved by the Board at its June meeting so that it can be put into effect on July 1. Even with this 7-month process, it would not be unusual for there to be delays (especially in negotiation and revision) that prevent an acceptable budget from being developed by July 1. To avoid such a situation, the process could be started earlier. However, to start the process any earlier would mean that the information collected at the very start of the budget process would be outdated by the start of the year.

Because many aspects of the budgeting process cannot be undertaken without information generated by one of the previous activities, the budget timetable becomes a crucial guide in the budget process. Failure to meet one deadline may impact all remaining deadlines.

◼ PERT AND CPM

The budget timetable provides an indication of the complexity of the budgeting process. However, the timetable gives information about just the major events in the process. As one works on preparing the budget, there are many other elements of the planning process that must be worked into that time frame. Unit managers must receive information, such as admissions or patient-day projections, as well as planned changes in services offered. Communication must take place concerning recruiting efforts planned by the personnel department (or nurse recruiting office). Many other pieces of the process must come together at just the right time in order for each phase of the budget to be completed by its deadline. *CPM* and *PERT* are two techniques that can be used to aid in this process.

CPM, or *Critical Path Method*, and PERT, or *Program Evaluation and Review Technique*, are two industrial engineering approaches to scheduling that are widely used in industry. The two approaches are similar in many respects. Both were developed in the 1950s. Both techniques use an arrow diagram to indicate the various events or activities that must take place in a complex project. They both identify a critical path that represents the shortest time to complete the project. And both use time estimates for each activity. Based on those activity-time estimates, a project schedule is developed. Such techniques could be used to determine the most efficient budget timetable. They could also be helpful to managers who are working on specific projects such as getting a new program or system from the planning stage to the active patient care stage.

In developing these systems, there is a planning phase in which the activities are identified. Then there is a scheduling phase in which the length of time for each activity is estimated and a determination is made regarding which activities must be completed before others can be started. A control phase is sometimes used to monitor progress along the path and make schedule revisions as needed.

In most projects, certain activities can take place concurrently with each other. These form different parallel branches in the diagram (Figure 2-1 is a simplified example). Some activities must precede other activities. For example, suppose that activity A provides basic information that all departments need to begin forming their budgets. Once activity A has been completed, activities B, C, and D can all start at the same time and continue on parallel courses.

Suppose further that there is a department that needs information from activity B before it can complete its budget. For instance, the dietary department might have to wait for the nursing department's operational budget in order to know the total

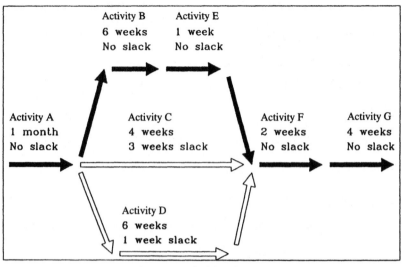

Figure 2-1 Scheduling diagram.

number of patient days in the budget, so that its workload can be predicted. Activity E (e.g., dietary budget) will follow activity B (nursing operational budget) on the same path.

All department budgets will have to be completed before a cash budget (Activity F) can be completed. Therefore, all parallel paths will have to come together. Then activities F and G can be completed. Activities B and E together require 7 weeks. This is more than activity C or activity D. Activity C has 3 weeks of slack. A delay of up to 3 weeks would have no impact on the overall process. Activity B has no slack because the Nursing Department's operational budget and budget assumptions must be available to ancillary departments for their budget to be prepared on time. However, Activity D, final preparation of the Capital Budget, and negotiations among the Unit Managers and Nursing Administration has 3 weeks of slack. It can be delayed 3 weeks—and may not even be begun until 4 weeks into that time period, when the operational budget is submitted, with no negative impact. Activities A, B, and E are critical. A delay of even 1 day in that path will create a delay in the entire process. Therefore, the path from A to B to E to F to G (in boldface in Figure 2-1) is said to be the critical path. One of the major benefits of CPM and PERT is the identification of where delays are critical and where they are not.

In recent years, a number of software programs have been developed to enable a manager to do project planning more efficiently on a personal computer. Programs such as Microsoft Project incorporate the essentials of PERT and CPM, while making the computational aspects substantially easier for the manager.

In order to get everything done most efficiently, it is useful to have a system to track how much time is available for each activity and to determine which activities will create roadblocks in the process if they are not completed on time. Both of these methods provide such systems, and both are useful not only for scheduling the budgeting process but also for a wide variety of other time-dependent projects. A more detailed discussion of CPM and PERT is contained in most industrial engineering and operations research texts.

■ CONTROLLING RESULTS

Just as planning is a critical element of the budgeting process, so is the control of the organization's financial results (see Box 2-1). Control is an attempt to keep the organization functioning in accordance with its plan. It is desirable for all employees to act in an efficient manner within the constraints of the budget. If the agreed-upon budget calls for a 10% reduction in staffing, then that reduction should take place.

The budget itself should be arrived at on the basis of the best overall interests of the organization and the community it serves. The development of the budget should be a give-and-take process that results in the elimination of only nonessential costs. In extremely hard financial times, the final budget may even cut essential items. In this case, top management would choose to eliminate the least essential of the essential items. Prioritization is crucial. Once a budget has been agreed upon, managers are obligated to do their best to follow it, even if it calls for undesirable cuts. How can management ensure that the reduction will take place? This is the role of the control process. Through the use of motivational tools, management can give the employees of the organization incentives to try to carry out the budget (see Chapter 3). Through the use of *variance reports,* managers can examine how well they are succeeding and can assess where and why the organization is not meeting its budgeted expectations (see Chapter 13).

A time of budget reduction requires especially skillful management on the part of the unit-level managers. It is a time when, if clinical operations are not meticulously supervised, the quality of care will be seriously compromised. Unit managers cannot simply assume that nurses know how to prioritize patient care activities and leave them to it when staffing is reduced—as it almost always is when there is a serious budget reduction. What the Unit Manager must do is meet with the unit's staff and together, come to some decisions about exactly which nursing activities may be cut and which must be maintained at all costs. This is a good time for consultation with the management engineers if available. Examples of this kind of decision making include:

- Deciding to dispense with the night shift's review of all the chart orders every night because the computer-based clinical order-entry system already has error traps.
- Eliminating routine bed baths because patients have much shorter lengths of stay, and pain is well controlled, so they are far less likely to perspire heavily enough to need daily baths.
- Consulting with the medical staff to review the unit's routines for assessments. For example, can vital signs be taken routinely in noncritical patients every 8 hours instead of every 4 hours?
- Working with medical staff to develop standing order sets for commonly encountered clinical problems (such as fever, new-onset shortness of breath, pain management, etc.) so that time-consuming calls to physicians can be reduced without compromising patient care.

Budget Flexibility

The control process can do more than provide incentives to follow the budget and assess whether the budget is being met. If actual results start to vary substantially from the budget, the control process will alert the manager that there may be a need to make midstream corrections. For example, if the state government were suddenly to cut Medicaid payment levels, what should the organization do? Even though the patient workload may remain the same, the cut in revenue may be significant enough to require layoffs or some other belt-tightening actions.

As painful as such actions are, it would be foolhardy to simply ignore the implications of the revenue change until the next budget year. This would allow the organization to be out of control. By year-end, the accumulated losses could be devastating to the organization. By alerting managers to the problem, the control process has given the organization a choice: make no cost changes now or make an immediate budget response. In some cases, taking no immediate action may be an appropriate choice. However, it is desirable to avoid the chance of being in a situation in which an immediate budget response is required but in which managers are unaware of that fact because of the lack of a working control system. The role of the control process is to make managers aware so that they can decide whether or not some action is in fact needed immediately.

Many budgeting experts believe that once in place, budgets should not be revised. They are the original plan, and all results should be compared to that plan. Certainly, if budget revisions were allowed on an unlimited basis, an enormous amount of time might be spent developing new budgets and getting them approved throughout the year. Even if the budget is not revised, however, that does not mean that actions must remain as planned. If census drops sharply, it may be necessary to reduce staffing to be financially prudent. The fact that a certain staffing level has been budgeted does not mean that a unit is entitled to that staffing level no matter what else happens.

On the other hand, a great rise in patient census may require more staffing to ensure provision of quality care. The budget should not be viewed as an arbitrary dictator. A budget should be a flexible guide to actions. When some uncontrollable events occur that were not considered in the budgeted expectations, actual actions should contain appropriate responses to actual events. Such responses sometimes justify additional spending above budget. In other cases, spending the amount called for in the budget may be excessive, based on what the actual events dictate.

The key is not whether or not the budget is revised. The budget is simply the plan. The essential issue is what actions are taken throughout the year. If the budget is ignored, the value of the plan is largely lost. But by revising actions from those called for in the budget in response to actual occurrences, the original budget is not being ignored. Rather, it becomes a base that is built upon. The revised actions should produce a better result than even strict adherence to the budget would obtain. For a summary of the elements of planning and control, see Figure 2-2.

■ PHILOSOPHY OF FISCAL AFFAIRS

The budgeting process in any organization depends as much on the specific individuals working in that organization as it does on the formalized mechanical steps involved in budget preparation and use. The role of individual human beings in the budget process cannot be overemphasized. Not only do organizations have their own forms and procedures, they also tend to have specific philosophies of fiscal affairs. The philosophical underpinnings of the budget process constitute the third key element in the budget process (see Box 2-1). The amount of participation that any individual manager has in the budget process depends on the approach or philosophy of the organization's top management. Some organizations are top-down—allowing unit managers limited control over their budgets. Other organizations delegate substantially all

BUDGETING

PLANNING

Think Ahead
Anticipate Change
Establish Goals
Forecast Future
Examine Alternatives
Communicate Goals
Coordinate Plans

CONTROLLING

Keep to Plan
Motivate Employees
Evaluate Performance
Alert Management to
  Variations
Take Corrective Action

Figure 2-2 Summary of the elements of planning and control.

budget preparation and control duties. Many managers have to suffer with unrealistic budgets imposed upon them from above, whereas other managers are given full responsibility but little guidance.

Teachers of budgeting often stress the importance of participation in the budget process by individuals at all levels in the organization. The further basic budget preparation is removed from the top management, the more likely the budget is to reflect a full understanding of why the cost structure is as it is. If the budget is expected to be a useful tool for managing, it must be realistic. It is hard for managers high in the organization to make correct determinations of what is realistic minimal spending that will allow for maintaining efficiency and high-quality care. It is impossible for top-level managers to be aware of all the specific circumstances and conditions that exist in the day-to-day operations throughout the organization. Unit managers work for years to gain the insight and understanding they have attained. They have the experience, judgment, and specific information about their units that lets them put together a sensible budget. They are in the best position to be able to plan for that unit for the coming year.

■ GATHERING INFORMATION

The fourth critical element in preparing budgets (see Box 2-1) is gathering key information. One type of information needed is cost information. Whether one is preparing a program budget, capital budget, or operating budget, an understanding of how costs relate to the item being budgeted is needed. One must be able to collect and use information about costs in order to prepare the budget. A second major area of data collection concerns personnel issues. Given a history of alternating periods of nursing surpluses and shortages, managers must plan their budgets with an understanding of issues related to recruiting and retaining nurses. Finally, budget preparation requires managers to peer into the future. To do so, they need to be armed with adequate forecasting techniques.

Cost Information

Cost behavior is a particularly complicated area. If patient workload rises by 10%, can costs be expected to rise by 10% as well? This relationship would imply that costs are directly proportional to patient volume. However, this assumption is generally a poor one. Some costs do not change at all as volume changes. For example, the salary of the top nurse administrator in a community health center will not vary if the average number of patient visits rises or falls by 5% or 10%. Other costs do, of course, vary as there are more or fewer patients. Understanding how and why costs vary and being able to predict costs are critical parts of the budgeting process.

Additionally, when budgets are prepared, it would be helpful to be able to predict the patient volume necessary for the service not to lose money. The so-called break-even point at which one neither makes nor loses money requires a costing technique commonly referred to as *break-even analysis.*

Cost behavior, *cost estimation,* and break-even analysis are discussed in Chapter 4.

Personnel Issues

In the area of nursing, the single greatest cost relates to personnel. During nursing shortages, issues of nursing recruitment and retention become critical to most health care organizations. Operating budgets in many health care organizations lose much of their effectiveness if they do not fully take into account the costs and difficulty of attracting and keeping nurses.

During nursing shortages it is not at all uncommon for positions to remain unfilled. In place of the new staff members, agency nurses and overtime are often used. Frequently, these stopgap measures are more costly than filling the position would be if it were possible to attract a nurse to take the job. Chapter 5 looks at issues of personnel and staff recruitment and retention. A thorough understanding of this topic is necessary to be able to prepare an operating budget that allows (1) sufficient resources for recruitment and retention costs to keep all positions filled or (2) a realistic personnel budget that considers the costs related to temporary staffing of vacant positions. This personnel information is important not only to operating budgets but also as a consideration when preparing long-range and program budgets.

Forecasting

To determine the amount of staff needed (which is calculated as part of the operating budget process in Chapter 8), it is first necessary to have some idea of how many patients there will be and how sick they will be. Therefore, a critical step in gathering information for the budgeting process is *forecasting.* This can provide many pieces of the information needed to design a budget that will allow for the programs and services to be provided.

Will there be the same number of patients next year as this year? How do you forecast the number of patient days? These are critical questions for the preparation of the budget. If more patients are expected, it will be necessary to budget for more staff. How do you forecast the number of discharges by *case-mix*? When using DRGs, this becomes vital to the organization. How do you forecast the level of patient acuity? How do you know how many chest tubes to order for inventory? Forecasting allows prediction of any items that will help in the planning process. Chapter 6 looks at several forecasting techniques.

Integration of Information

Although costs, personnel, and forecasting have been discussed as distinct topics, they are in fact interrelated. A nurse manager is unlikely to predict a unit's or a department's costs for the coming year without introducing some knowledge of recruiting and retention plans and without using forecasting techniques. Chapters 4 through 6 work together to provide a conceptual foundation and specific workable techniques that allow the reader to generate the information that is needed for preparing the different types of budgets.

It should also be noted that the budget process does not require a manager to gather all the information needed for all types of budgets before preparing any of the budgets. Some cost information and forecasts may be developed as a guide to the managers who are preparing the organization's long-range plan. That plan may well be completely finished before any cost information, personnel calculations, or forecasts are prepared for the operating budget.

In fact, in many cases managers begin to prepare a particular type of budget and then realize that they need certain background information that has not been gathered. A nurse manager creating an operating budget for a unit might start to put together the operating budget described in Chapter 8. However, before staffing could be determined, the unit would need a forecast of patient workload. At this point, the manager would have to forecast the next year's workload, if this has not already been done.

The budgeting process does not have a rigid path that first requires that costs be conceptualized, then recruitment issues considered, then forecasts made, and then a given type of budget prepared. To the contrary, the process is highly integrated. However, in this book the chapters related to gathering information (Chapters 4 through 6) precede the chapters about the preparation of each type of budget. This is because, at a minimum, managers should be aware of these concepts and the availability of the techniques as budgets are prepared.

■ PROGRAMMING

So far, this chapter has focused on essential elements that are integral to all aspects of budgeting. These elements are planning, controlling, organizational philosophy, and information gathering. The remainder of this chapter is concerned with specific steps in the process of budgeting. These steps are listed in Box 2-1.

A common approach to budgeting is to start initially on the compilation of the operating budget. However, a bit of preliminary thought and background work will improve the budget outcome substantially. The first part of the budget process is *programming*. It should be started well before the actual operating budget is begun.

Programming includes a total organizational review, with a focus on where the organization is headed. Programming also includes determining which specific programs should be undertaken. The programming process can be viewed as consisting of two major phases. The first phase provides the foundations for all budget preparation. Essentially, these foundations are established by determining the organization's goals and its relative strengths and weaknesses within its environment. The second phase is concerned with strategic planning.

Budget Foundations

The foundations of the budgeting process consist of a scan of environmental position; a statement of general goals, objectives, and policies; a list of organization-wide assumptions; specification of program priorities; and, finally, a set of specific, measurable operating objectives (Figure 2-3).

Environmental Scan

No organization exists in a vacuum. The community, its economy, shifting demographics, inflation, the role of a key employer, the socioeconomic setting, and other external factors play vital roles in the organization's success or failure. Each organization must understand its position within the community and its relative strengths and weaknesses. Once they have been determined, the organization can move forward to fulfill a particular role or mission.

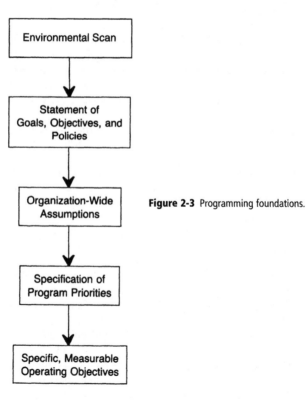

Figure 2-3 Programming foundations.

The environmental scan must analyze the needs of the community. It must also assess the competition that exists. Based on knowledge of the needs of the community, the characteristics of the population, the existing competition, and other similar factors, the organization can determine its relative strengths and weaknesses and set its overall goals and objectives.

The potential dangers of not examining the environment cannot be stressed too much. If a community hospital opens an open-heart surgery facility in spite of the existence of several high-quality, high-volume open-heart surgery facilities at nearby tertiary care centers, there is the potential for a medical disaster (if high mortality rates are associated with low volume) as well as an economic disaster (due to the inability to recover all the high equipment costs associated with the open-heart surgery program) at the new facility. The fact that several thoracic surgeons want the hospital to offer open-heart surgery does not mean that it is in the best interests of the organization.

It is only by carefully reviewing the needs of the community and examining its own relative strengths and weaknesses that a health care organization can establish a set of goals, objectives, and policies that will serve to enhance the comparative strengths of the organization and to minimize its weaknesses. Reviewing the environment may result in eliminating weaknesses. For example, a relatively weak maternity service can be improved and expanded if the community needs that type of care, or it can be totally eliminated.

If there is adequate maternity care in the community, then providing maternity services at the hospital may simply deprive other services at the hospital from having adequate resources. Sometimes the choice is between doing two things very well or doing three things only adequately. If the community urgently needs all three things, it may well be better to do all three than to eliminate any one of them. If one of the three is readily available elsewhere, however, then the long-run interests of both the community and the organization may be served best by eliminating one of the three services and devoting greater attention and resources to the remaining two.

What data can a nurse manager collect to contribute to the organization's environmental review? Although much of the demographic data will be collected by the marketing and other nonclinical staff, nurse managers can contribute some critical information. For example, they can get a sense about changing physician attitudes toward the use of the organization's facilities as opposed to those of a competitor. Based on their industry contacts, they may be aware of changes taking place at other organizations that will affect the competitiveness of their own facilities. This information forms part of the overall picture that the organization requires so as to assess its position in the community correctly.

Many health care organizations would benefit by getting all levels of nursing management more actively involved in the environmental review process. The starting point for this activity would be for the Chief Nurse Executive (CNE) to solicit this type of information from the various nurse managers well before the operating budget is prepared. The CNE could then use this information when participating in the major planning sessions that precede the specific preparation of the operating and capital budgets.

The environmental review serves as the guiding force for determining the organization's long-run direction. The total environmental statement need not be prepared annually. It is to be hoped that the major direction of the organization will not change each year. However, the environmental statement should be reviewed annually for two major reasons.

First, an annual review of the environmental statement is necessary so that it can be modified as significant changes in the environment occur. Some changes may occur only rarely, such as the addition of a major new competitor, but other elements of the environment are much more subject to change. For example, the overall state of the economy is one environmental element subject to frequent change. Some health care organizations tend to be relatively immune to the impact of economic change, but others must seriously consider economic fluctuations in preparing their various budgets.

The second reason for an annual review of the environmental statement is that it serves as a good review of where the organization is and where it wants to be going. Having done that review, it is more likely that the prepared budget will take into account the organization's desired long-term direction during the coming year.

General Goals, Objectives, and Policies

Once the organization's position in the environment is understood, the overall goals of the organization can be established. These goals are broad, long-term objectives, established in light of the organization's strengths and weaknesses.

For example, based on the environmental review, a home health agency may decide that the adjacent communities are underserved and may decide to institute a 5-year period of geographic expansion. A nursing home may set a goal of substantially increasing its occupancy. A hospital may decide to phase out its maternity service.

The key to long-run objective setting is that it is basically more of a qualitative direction-setting process than a quantitative exercise with specific numerical goals. The detailed numbers can be worked out later. First, the overall direction must be set.

Objectives need not always point to growth. Maintaining the current high level of care is a possible objective. Contraction is also a possible direction; an organization may have a goal of retreating from areas of care in which losses are occurring in order to ensure financial survival. As was the case with the environmental statement, the overall goals, objectives, and policies of the organization may not change each year. They should be reviewed annually, however, if only to place in the minds of budget preparers the picture of the forest before they start to plan for the individual trees.

Organization-Wide Assumptions

Throughout the budget process it will be necessary for all managers to work on the basis of some explicit assumptions. How large will salary increases be during the next year? What will be the impact of inflation on the purchase price of supplies? Will the government change its policies with respect to reimbursing Medicare and Medicaid patients? Probably the most crucial of assumptions concerns workload. What will be the occupancy or patient volume in the coming year? How about for the next 5 or 10 years?

These critical questions are sometimes ignored at the organizational level, but when they are, each manager has to make independent assumptions when preparing the portion of the budget for the department or unit. It is highly likely that the various individual managers will come up with different assumptions in many areas. For purposes of coordination, it makes more sense if the managers in the organization agree upon an entire set of assumptions for all managers to use when the budgets are prepared. In this way, the assumptions can be questioned, corrected, adjusted, improved, or at the very least, made uniform before they are employed in actual budget preparation.

Specifying Program Priorities

The next fundamental step is to establish a set of priorities for the entire organization. It is not unusual for the long-range plan, program budget, and capital budget to contain proposed spending for more things than the organization will be able to afford. There is a tendency to want to achieve all elements of a long-range plan immediately. When it becomes clear that the organization cannot do everything, how can a choice be made between what is to be done and what is to be postponed?

If the setting of priorities takes place after long-range plans, program budgets, and capital budgets have already been prepared, a ferocious battle may ensue. In preparing detailed budgets, special-interest groups are formed, and they take on vested interests in the projects they have helped to plan. Trying to make rational choices at this stage becomes quite difficult. Politics may make more of a difference than common sense.

Therefore, it is advisable to try to set a generalized hierarchy of priorities at an early stage—before detailed program budgets are developed. When it is necessary to make choices, top management can use the formalized guidelines that have been developed from the perspective of long-term growth and development, as opposed to letting power politics rule the budgeting process.

Specific, Measurable Operating Objectives

One of the most frustrating elements of budgeting occurs for unit and department managers when they are expected to develop budgets totally unaided by any communicated goals or guidelines and then find their budgets rejected because they do not provide adequately for achieving such goals as improved efficiency or reduced cost per patient day.

Organizations should provide a set of specific, measurable goals that the budget should accomplish. This set of goals should be communicated before the units and departments prepare their budgets. Managers can then attempt to prepare budgets that achieve these goals. If the goals are unattainable, managers can be prepared to explain why they feel that is the case.

The established goals should be consistent with the overall general policies and goals of the organization, but they should be much more specific. For example, staffing reductions of 5% or ceilings on spending increases of 3% provide firm, specific goals. After individual budgets are prepared, a negotiation process will occur. Some units and departments may successfully argue for increases in excess of the specific guidelines. If the financial position of the organization is tight, this may mean that other units and departments will have to accept less than the specific guidelines. However, at least everyone will have a common starting point and a reasonable knowledge of what is expected from each budget.

Strategic Planning

Programming represents a total organizational review. This includes reviewing the programs the organization uses to carry out its mission. It requires establishing certain foundations for the budget process, as described earlier. Once these foundations have been laid, the organization can employ a strategic planning process to establish a long-range plan or budget, deciding on the direction that the organization should be taking over the next 3, 5, or 10 years. This long-range plan will focus on the types of major programmatic changes the organization must undertake to continue to meet its mission.

One outcome of the long-range plan is the decision to prepare specific program budgets. Program budgets are used primarily to evaluate new programs being considered to help the organization attain its long-range plan. Strategic planning and long-range and program budgets are discussed in Chapter 7.

■ UNIT AND DEPARTMENT BUDGETS

Once the programming process is completed, the next step is preparing unit or departmental budgets (see Box 2-1). There are two different types of budgets that are generally prepared at this level of the organization. These are the operating budget and the capital budget, which were introduced in Chapter 1 and are discussed more fully in Chapters 8 and 10, respectively.

The operating and capital budgets are generally prepared at the same time. Decisions concerning one budget are also likely to affect the other. For example, if the capital budget includes computer equipment for the nursing stations, there may be some impact on staffing. Perhaps less overtime from the clerical staff is expected to be needed because of efficiencies created by having a computer. Therefore, it is not appropriate to create either the operating budget or the capital budget without reference to the other.

Once a decision has been made to purchase a capital asset, a calculation must be made to allocate its cost into the various years during which it will provide useful benefits. The amount allocated to each year is called the *depreciation*. The operating budget of an organization must reflect all costs of providing services for the coming year. The entire purchase price of a capital asset is not a cost of the coming year because only a portion of the capital asset will be used up during the year. However, one year's share, the annual depreciation, is treated as a cost for the budgeted year. This depreciation becomes one element in the operating budget.

■ THE CASH BUDGET

Having completed an operating and capital budget, the next step in the budget process is preparing a cash budget (see Box 2-1). Most nurse managers are not directly involved in the annual cash budgeting for their organization. However, there will be times when nurse managers will be preparing a business plan for a new venture or service and will need to prepare a cash budget in conjunction with that plan. Whether nurse managers are directly involved in the preparing of cash budgets or not, it is vital to understand the cash budgeting process because it does impact nursing services.

Chapter 12 gives the reader some understanding of how the financial manager handles the organization's cash resources.

■ BUDGET NEGOTIATION AND REVISION

The fourth specific step in the budgeting process is negotiation and revision (see Box 2-1). Conceptually, most yearly budgets are prepared on the basis of one of three fundamental approaches: (1) annual increments; (2) negotiation; or (3) detailed evaluation. All these approaches result in at least some negotiation and revision of proposed budgets.

The first approach assumes that initially each department or unit is assigned a percentage increase that will be allowable for the coming year. For example, a nursing home might indicate that all departments can plan to spend 4% more in the coming year than was allocated in the current year. The second approach is based on political power rules and the fact that each unit or department can request whatever it wants and then negotiate the best deal it can manage. The third approach follows the rule of reason. A unit or department should request what it actually needs to provide its services in a high-quality, cost-effective manner. The budget will be evaluated to check that all expenses proposed are in fact essential.

In actuality, the third, and on the surface most sensible, approach often tends to be too time-consuming and costly to use. Top-level managers cannot review in detail each budget each year to evaluate whether each element is indeed justified. The negotiation approach does not seem to be an equitable approach. Therefore, the use of a flat percent increase is the most common approach to budgeting. However, preparing budgets based on a flat percentage increase represents just a starting point in the budget negotiation, revision, and approval process.

As a result of limitations on the resources available to health care organizations, budgets often cannot be accepted as submitted. Even if everyone is told to assume a certain percentage increase, some needs will be so critical that they will have to receive more than the flat percentage. Often, approval of a larger increase in one department results in adjustment downward in other departments. This leads to a series of negotiations, with managers having to defend their proposed budgets and state why they should not be cut. This creates substantial complexity because most of the budgets that comprise the organization's master budget are interrelated. Changes in one type of budget can have direct ramifications on the other budgets of the organization.

For example, the capital budget for the various units and departments of the organization cannot be finalized until all program budgets have been prepared because a new program may require departments to purchase additional capital items. This is why program budgets are prepared earlier in the budget process than are unit and department budgets.

The operating budget, in turn, must contain revenues and expenses related to capital items to be purchased during the coming year. The cash budget cannot be prepared until after the operating budget has been established. Because the cash budget must be prepared in time for the financial officers to arrange any necessary short-term borrowing to start the year, the operating budget preparation and the subsequent cash budgeting cannot be left until the last minute. Therefore, first make the long-range plan. Then make decisions regarding program budgets, and follow up with the necessary capital and the operating budgets. Finally, prepare the cash budget. This represents the first round of budget preparations.

However, the *master budget* is prepared in a series of repeating rounds, as seen in Figure 2-4. Because most managers are not involved in preparing all the different types of budgets, they do not observe this cycling process. Instead, they observe only a back-and-forth process in which their budgets are submitted and come back for either cuts or additional justifications. The managers revise and resubmit the budgets with explanations of why the requested expenses should be allowed. This process of negotiation over the operating and capital budgets may occur several times.

From the organizational point of view, the back-and-forth negotiations are part of a larger effort to gain consistency and feasibility across all parts of the master budget. Often, the outcome of the first attempt at preparing the master budget is not feasible. For example, the cash budget may show that there will not be enough cash for all the proposed capital expenditures and new programs. The operating budget may have an excess of expenses over revenues that is deemed unacceptable. The next

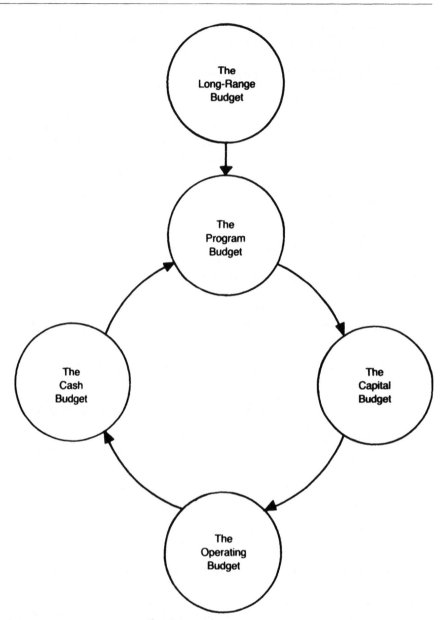

Figure 2-4 Budget preparation cycle.

step might be to ask various departments to tighten up on their operating costs so that the organization will at least break even. A revised operating budget will be prepared. That operating budget can be used to project a new cash budget.

Even with cuts in the operating budget, the cash budget may still show an unacceptable cash shortfall. This will necessitate reevaluating which programs and capital budget items provide the most benefit and which can be postponed or disapproved. Some capital expenditures may be put off until the future or scrapped. This may result in an acceptable set of budgets that make up the master budget.

On the other hand, there may be so many vital capital expenditures that it is preferable to go back and increase revenues or cut the operating budget expenses again, rather than cut enough capital items to make the cash budget balance. Or perhaps more borrowing will be planned. The repetitive process must continue until the program and capital expenditures contained in the master budget can be paid for within the structure of the operating and cash budgets. Note in Figure 2-4 how this results in a clockwise cycling until all of the budgets are compatible.

■ BUDGET APPROVAL AND IMPLEMENTATION

Once all budget negotiations and revisions have been completed, the budget must be approved. In most organizations, management must take the budget to a board of trustees or directors, who formally vote on whether to adopt it. Even after extensive revisions by management, the board may change the budget before finally approving it. The final approved budget must then be implemented. Management must actively take steps to carry out the budget as approved and achieve all its revenue and expense targets.

■ FEEDBACK

The last step in the budget process is *feedback* (see Box 2-1). Information about actual results that is used to improve future plans is called feedback. A critical element of the budget process is to provide such information or feedback. During the year, many things will not happen according to budgeted plans. Some variations from the budget will be due to random uncontrollable events that establish no pattern. A particularly cold winter may cause the census to rise unexpectedly.

At the very least, the unusual nature of the winter must be recognized. When planning for the next year's budget commences, should it be based on the most recent year or on prior years? It is known that the past winter was unusual. Therefore, the patient volume during that winter should be discounted as next year's budget is prepared. This is called a feedback process. The information generated by the control system allows for more effective planning for the coming year.

In some cases, such as the example just given, the feedback information will lead managers to ignore the current year's actual results when preparing the next year's budget. In other cases, feedback information may stress the current year's results for preparing the next year's budget. In all cases, this feedback approach can be used when the following year's budget is prepared so as to improve its accuracy.

Summary and Implications for Nurse Managers

Budgeting consists of planning and controlling. The planning phase of the budget process requires that managers think ahead, anticipate changes, establish goals, forecast the future, examine alternatives, communicate goals, and coordinate plans. The controlling phase of budgeting requires that managers work to keep actual results close to the plan, motivate employees, evaluate performance of staff and units, alert the organization to major variances, take corrective actions, and provide feedback for future planning.

Continued

Summary and Implications for Nurse Managers—cont'd

Each organization has its own approach to budgeting and its own philosophies regarding the budget process. Some health care organizations treat budgeting as a highly centralized process. This approach tends to generate frustration by the managers asked to carry out the budget. Other organizations call for more participation by managers throughout the organization. Such budgets tend to gain more support by the staff and are more likely to result in targets that can be achieved.

The actual budgeting process requires that the organization consider its environment, define goals and policies, make assumptions for use throughout the organization, specify priorities, and define specific, measurable objectives. Managers within the organization must collect information on costs and personnel and must prepare forecasts for items in the future. All of the various types of budgets in the master budget must be prepared, and they are generally not approved without a process of review, justification, and revision. Finally, once budgets have been approved and are in place, a system must be created to control the results of operations.

Some of the concepts discussed in this book are not used in all organizations. That is a simple reality. Some of the budgeting concepts and techniques that are not already being widely used are new, advanced techniques. You have the opportunity to be one of the first nurse managers to employ them. This will require that you act as an innovator. Trying to innovate is often the most frustrating—and rewarding—part of being a manager.

Many nurse managers are frustrated because they find that real-life health care organizations have a variety of budgeting weaknesses. Often, these weaknesses are not even in areas that require particularly high levels of sophistication. Instead of becoming frustrated by the lack of a perfect system, managers should act to improve the system. If this book is successful, readers will not only learn from it but will also begin to use the knowledge to improve the budget process in their respective organizations. Such use will lead to a personal sense of accomplishment (for both the nurse manager and the authors of this book). In addition, health care organizations will be placed in a better position to meet the financial challenges of the future.

In reading this book, consider the following questions: Why must a nurse manager understand the budget process? How will such an understanding affect a nurse manager's performance and the performance of the manager's subordinates? Finally, how will such knowledge affect the performance and evaluation of the nursing unit or nursing department?

This chapter has provided no more than an overview of the budgeting process. Each of the chapters in the remainder of this book provides more detail about the process of budgeting. Even when the reader has completed the book, many specific details of the budget process will have gone without discussion. These details tend to be elements of the process that are specific to each institution. As a manager works within an organization, many specific details will have to be learned about the budget system in place in order to supplement the information contained in this book. We recognize that there is an inherent limitation on what one can learn from a book. We hope, however, that having read this book, the nurse manager will find that the details that must be learned on the job will make more sense and be substantially easier to grasp.

References and Suggested Readings

Dunham-Taylor, J. (2005). *Healthcare Financial Management for Nurse Managers.* Sudbury, MA: Jones and Bartlett.

Gapenski, L.C. (1997). *Financial Analysis and Decision Making for Healthcare Organizations: A Guide for the Healthcare Professional.* Chicago: Irwin.

Gross, M., Larkin, R., and McCarthy, J. (2000). *Financial and Accounting Guide for Not-For-Profit Organizations,* ed. 6. Hoboken, NJ: Wiley.

McLean, R.A. (2002). *Financial Management in Health Care Organizations,* ed. 2. Albany, NY: Delmar.

Nowicki, M. (2004). *The Financial Management of Hospitals and Healthcare Organizations,* ed. 3. Chicago: Health Administration Press.

Zelman, W., McCue, M., Milliken, A., and Glick, N. (2003). *Financial Management of Health Care Organizations: An Introduction to Fundamental Tools, Concepts, and Applications,* ed. 2. Ames, IA: Blackwell Publishing.

Motivation and Incentives

3

- Explain the role of budgets in employee motivation
- Identify the issues of goal divergence and goal congruency
- Explore alternative incentive systems, including their strengths and weaknesses

- Consider the negative implications of unrealistic expectations
- Reiterate the role of communication in the control process
- Clarify the importance of using budgets for interim evaluation

■ INTRODUCTION

The planning process and the resulting budget lay the groundwork for motivating managers and other staff members and for providing a yardstick that will allow for their evaluation. Managers can tell from the budget exactly what financial performance is expected of them. Actual results are compared to the budget. If managerial performance is evaluated on the basis of that comparison, the budget can be an effective motivational tool. This assumes that continued employment as a manager, as well as pay raises and promotions, depend at least in part on the evaluation of the manager's performance in the budgeting arena.

However, the effectiveness of budgeting in motivating managers and staff depends largely on the organization's approach to budgeting. If a budget is so tight as to be impossible to meet without causing harm to patients or the organization itself, it can discourage managers and cause a negative result. On the other hand, a challenging but attainable budget can draw out the best effort from individuals. By setting goals, managers tend to be more efficient because they are striving to reach a specific end. This is true only if at least part of the budget is under the manager's control. It is especially true if there is some structure designed to reward the meeting or surpassing of budget requirements. In addition to raises and promotions, budget performance can be tied to bonuses.

■ THE BUDGET AS A TOOL FOR MOTIVATION

The budgeting process concerns primarily individuals, not numbers. If the employees of an organization do not work to make the organization succeed, the numbers constituting a budget have little relevance. Motivating staff and managers cannot be overemphasized. If people are not motivated to carry out the budget, it is likely to fail.

This is why budgets that are arbitrarily imposed from above, without fair consideration of input from those expected to carry out the budget, tend to do so poorly. It is why such a sense of frustration exists when managers are denied the authority needed to go along with their responsibility. It is why there is a need to have budget flexibility in the face of changing realities. Moreover, it is why clinical budgets need to reflect the variability that exists when patient visits and patient days may be variable. Motivation is the critical underlying key to budget success.

One of the attractive motivational features of budgets is that they present a specific, measurable goal. When there is a clearly stated goal, or set of expectations, managers and staff can work toward meeting that goal. Individuals are much more likely to work efficiently if they have a clear and realistic target to shoot for. Most people are motivated to do a good job. They need to feel a sense of accomplishment in a job well done. Setting demanding but realistic budget goals combined with public praise and even rewards when the goals are met or exceeded is one way to enhance motivation and performance

Compare the likely progress of a dieter with specific weight-loss goals to one who simply wants to lose a lot of weight, or compare an athlete with measurable objectives to one who just wants to be strong or run fast. Setting specific goals and working toward them is a tremendous self-motivator. This holds true in the workplace as well.

Motivation is also related to the problems of nurse retention. Turnover is a costly problem in the nursing profession. It costs money to recruit and train new nurses. Why do nurses leave? Research shows that few nurses leave solely because of salary levels (Bowles & Candela, 2005; Gardulf et al., 2005; Hart, 2005). The research shows issues such as patient care quality, staffing levels, leadership style, and opportunities for professional advancement, in addition to salary and other issues are all related to turnover and retention (Bowles & Candela, 2005; Gardulf et al., 2005; VanOyen, 2005). Individuals who seek out professions for reasons other than solely the monetary return are particularly likely to be looking for personal satisfaction in their jobs.

A feeling of accomplishment in helping patients improve clinically is of predominant importance in generating job satisfaction among nurses. However, helping the organization stay within its financial constraints can also add to a nurse's job satisfaction. Most employees want to have a sense of pride in their organization and want their organization to do well. Nevertheless, a goal of "staying within financial constraints" is no better than the dieter's hope to "lose weight." A more specific goal, such as "Let's use fewer than six ABD pads per abdominal surgery patient this month, because that's all we're budgeted for and the average patient needs only three," is likely to be a better motivator. Then if the nurses spend the month being careful not to waste ABD pads, they can see at the end of the month that they have reached the goal and helped the organization. To control results, there must be clearly defined goals.

Control is complicated by the fact that even when the primary goal of the nursing staff is to help patients, it is the basic nature of individuals that their own personal goals will often be different from the goals of the organization they work for (Figure 3-1). This does not mean that human nature is bad—just that there is such a thing as human nature and it is foolish to refuse to recognize it.

For example, other things being equal, most employees of a hospital would prefer a salary that is substantially larger than the salary they are currently receiving. Most would be quite content if the hospital were to double their salary overnight. There is nothing particularly wrong in their wanting more money. In fact, ambition is probably a desirable trait among staff. On the other hand, hospitals will not provide

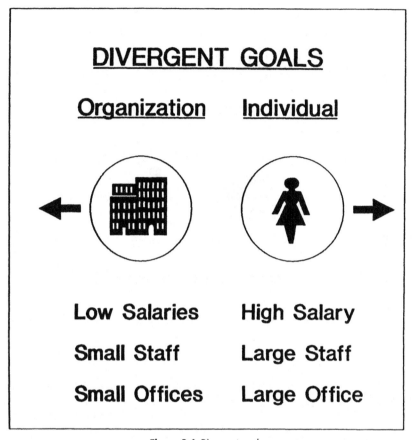

Figure 3-1 Divergent goals.

employees with 100% raises because they lack the revenues to pay for those raises. Although the nursing staff is not wrong to desire the raises, the hospital is not wrong to deny such raises. Inherently, a tension or conflict exists as a result.

Most nurse managers would like more resources. They would like larger offices with new furniture and remodeled facilities. They would certainly like more staff to carry out the existing functions. Introductory economics books clearly indicate that society has limited resources. All organizations must make choices concerning how to spend their limited financial resources. Thus, the fact must be faced that even when morale is generally excellent and is not considered to be a problem, an underlying tension naturally exists. Even though the employees may want to achieve the mission of the organization in providing care, their personal desires will be for things the organization cannot or will choose not to provide. This is referred to as *goal divergence* (see Figure 3-1).

The organization must bring together the interests of the individual with its own interests so that they can work together. In the budgeting process, the manager is attempting to control the amount the organization spends. But it is not the organization that controls costs; it is the human beings involved in the process. There must be some motivation for the human beings to want to control costs. Bringing the

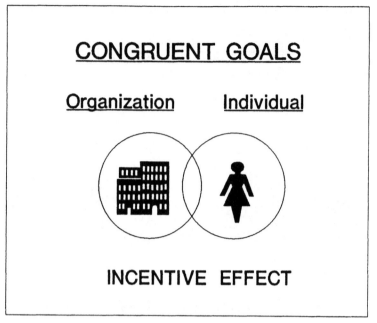

Figure 3-2 Congruent goals.

individuals' desires and the organization's needs together is referred to as *goal congruence* (Figure 3-2).

In order to be certain that the human beings will in fact want to control organizational costs, the manager needs to make sure that it is somehow in their direct best interests for costs to be controlled. The key is to establish some way that the normally divergent desires of the health care organizations and their employees become convergent or congruent. For example, nurses must go to some personal trouble to avoid the spread of infections in the hospital through meticulous handwashing, gloving, and other universal precautions. However, one study found less than 40% compliance with hand hygiene in a neonatal intensive care unit, with the result of an unacceptably high rate of hospital-acquired infections (Won et al., 2004). Further research on the rate of nosocomial infections and handwashing hygiene in hospitals demonstrates that infection-control procedures are, overall, not meticulously followed (Helios, 2005; Panhotra, 2004; Won et al., 2004). Given that the result of failure to wash hands between patients is not immediately obvious, and that nurses are so busy that they have to prioritize their actions, it is not surprising that these studies have shown many violations of infection-control procedures—in one study compliance was as low as 23.8% among some health care workers (Panhotra, 2004). The rewards on the violation side of the equation exceed the rewards for meticulously following procedures at all times. For this to change, the manager must change the system so that it is more rewarding to follow infection-control procedures than to ignore them. The goal is for both the organization and the employee to want the same thing.

Management by Objectives (MBO) is one approach that can help to accomplish this end. The superior and subordinate (supervisor and manager or manager and staff) sit down and develop a set of objectives that form the basis for performance evaluation. By allowing participation in the process of determining the objectives to be achieved, people are likely to work harder to achieve them. (MBO is discussed further in Chapter 11.)

Because congruent goals are not always the norm, and because divergent goals frequently exist, it is necessary to address formally how convergence is to be obtained. Organizations generally achieve such convergence or congruence by setting up a system of incentives that makes it serve the best interests of the employees to serve the best interests of the organization.

■ MOTIVATION AND INCENTIVES

Although nurses are motivated by factors other than money, it would be foolish to ignore the potential of monetary rewards to influence behavior. Health care organizations are searching for the proper mix of incentives that will motivate managers and staff to control costs. Financial incentives are frequently employed. The most basic financial incentives are the ability to retain one's job and to get a good raise.

In industry, another common motivating tool is a bonus system. Managers have many desires that relate to spending money (e.g., larger offices, fancier furniture, larger staffs), so formalized approaches must be developed that will provide incentives to spend less money. For example, one could tell a nurse manager that last year her department spent $2,000,000, but next year her budget is $2,080,000 (a 4% increase). However, if her department spends less than $2,080,000, she and her staff can keep 10% of the savings. If the department spends only $1,950,000, the nurse manager and the staff will get a bonus of $13,000 (i.e., $2,080,000 less $1,950,000, multiplied by 10%) to share. The total cost to the organization is $1,963,000, including the bonus, as opposed to the $2,080,000 budgeted. The nurses benefit and the organization benefits. In this case, goal congruence is likely to be achieved.

Many health care organizations have in fact added bonus systems. The use of bonus systems has both positive and negative aspects. The positives relate primarily to the strong motivation employees have to reduce costs. The negatives relate to the potential detriment to quality of patient care and to the potentially negative effect on employee morale.

Incentive approaches such as bonuses have complex implications. When an incentive is given to accomplish a particular end, sometimes the responses to that incentive are unexpected. In the case of Medicare, it has been found that DRGs, intended to reduce hospital spending, increase spending on nursing homes and home care agencies. In the case of a 10% bonus for spending reductions, a nurse manager may have an incentive to provide less staff nurse time per patient day. The organization must be concerned about the impact the incentives will have on the quality of patient care. If incentives cause nurse managers to reduce staff to save money, they may unexpectedly reduce the quality of care as well.

These are not insurmountable problems. However, managers must try to anticipate unintended consequences when developing incentive systems. The quality issue requires that a strong internal quality assurance program be in place. Part of the bonus process would have to place restrictions on bonuses when quality of care has declined. The other major problem with a set bonus for a fixed budget is that patient census and acuity are variable. A fixed budget incentive may merely drive the unit management to act to reduce census by telling Admissions that beds are not ready when they are or by otherwise trying to have patients sent to other units.

An incentive to treat fewer patients can be solved by making the incentive dependent on patient volume, adjusting automatically for changes in volume. This adjustment is important even if volume is totally outside the control of the manager and the unit. If patient volume and revenues are falling, costs should decline commensurate with the decline in workload. The bonus system should not reward a manager simply because there are fewer patients. On the other hand, increasing costs resulting from rises in patient volume should not cause bonuses to be lost. When volume is variable, a better incentive might relate to the unit's average cost per patient day.

For example, suppose that a department has a budget of $2,080,000. Suppose further that half of that represents costs that remain constant regardless of volume (*fixed costs*) and that half represent costs that vary in direct proportion with volume (*variable costs*). If the volume of patients drops by 10%, one would expect the variable costs to fall by $104,000 (i.e., 10% of the half of the $2,080,000 that varies with volume). Therefore, costs should have been $2,080,000 less $104,000, or a total of $1,976,000. If actual costs were $1,950,000, the bonus would be based on the $26,000 difference between the adjusted budget of $1,976,000 and the actual cost, rather than being based on the full difference between the original budget and the actual result. In this case, the bonus would be only $2,600, rather than the $13,000 calculated earlier.

Volume adjustment budgets such as this should be particularly appealing to managers if workload is rising. It is hard to convince managers that a bonus based on reduced costs will help them if each year the patient volume increases and costs rise with patient load. No matter how hard the manager and staff work to reduce costs, a large increase in workload will undoubtedly keep them from spending less than was budgeted. A bonus based on a fixed budget will never yield a payoff for hard work. On the other hand, if the budget basis for the bonus adjusts with patient volume, then as workload increases, the allowed spending increases. It would become possible to earn a bonus even if more money was spent than had been budgeted originally. And in a typical facility, this benefits both the facility and the staff because the higher volume means more revenue.

This does not mean that bonuses are the solution to all motivational problems. Bonus systems have a variety of other problems. Some bonus systems reward all employees if spending is reduced. But if everyone gets a bonus, no one feels that her or his individual actions have much impact. As long as everyone else holds costs in check, individuals may feel that they do not have to work particularly hard to reap the benefits of the bonus. In that case, probably very few will work hard to control costs. On the other hand, bonuses given only to some employees may create jealousy and discontent. It is also possible that bonuses may create a competitive environment in a situation in which teamwork is needed to provide quality care.

There are incentive alternatives to bonuses. For example, one underused managerial tool is a letter from supervisor to subordinate. All individuals responsible for controlling costs should be evaluated explicitly with respect to how well they control costs. That evaluation should be communicated in writing. This approach, which is both the carrot and the stick, costs little to implement but can have a dramatic impact. Most people respond well to praise and other forms of positive feedback about their personal performance and their department's performance. Framed certificates of achievement along with a moderate monetary reward for an outstanding achievement can be a strong motivator. Some successful managers keep a small trove of inexpensive toys, pens, coffee mugs, and other similar items that they can present to a staff member who has gone beyond expectations to help save money or in some other way improve the department's performance. Although the monetary value of the items may be small, the sense of pride and joy in being appreciated that these gifts can bring to staff are very large indeed.

Telling individuals that they've done a good job and that their boss knows they've done a good job can be an effective way to get people to continue trying to do a good job in the future. Managers are the people who hear all the complaints, but in some institutions, people forget that the managers need to be commended for a job well done too. Although end-of-year evaluation is a good time to praise a highly performing manager, supervisors of managers should remember that every manager—like every other employee—needs to hear something positive about his or her performance more than once a year. In the real world, praise is both cheap and, in many cases, effective. On the other hand, fair criticism, especially in writing, can have a stinging effect that managers and staff will work hard to avoid in the future. Ultimately, however, people tend to respond better to praise than to criticism.

■ MOTIVATION AND UNREALISTIC EXPECTATIONS

Although motivational devices can work wonders at getting an organization's staff to work hard for the organization and its goals, they can also backfire and have negative results. This occurs primarily when expectations are placed at unreasonably high levels.

There is no question that many people do attempt to *satisfice*—to do just enough to get by. One thing incentives are used to accomplish is to motivate those individuals to work harder. A target that requires hard work and stretching, but that is achievable, can be a useful motivating tool. If the target is reached, there might be a bonus, or there should be at least some formal recognition of the achievement, such as a letter. At a minimum, the worker will have the self-satisfaction of having worked hard and reached the target. However, some kind of tangible reward is important and should be provided.

It is important to recognize that positive outcomes of reward systems can occur only if the target is reachable. Some health care organizations have adopted the philosophy that if a high target makes people work hard, a higher target will make them work harder. This may not be the case. If targets are placed out of reach, they will probably **not** result in people reaching to their utmost limits to come as close to the target as possible. In fact, that approach may lead to cynicism and hostility toward a management that promises to make bonuses available and then places them out of reach.

It may seem that the organization is short-changing itself whenever someone achieves a target. The executive may think, "We set the target too low. Perhaps if the target were higher, this manager would have achieved the higher target. The target we set was achieved, so we do not know just how far this person can go. We haven't yet realized all of his or her potential." The problem with that logic is that there are risks associated with it.

If a nurse manager fails to meet a target because of incompetence or because of insufficient hard work, the signal of failure that is sent is warranted. In fact, repeated failure may be grounds for replacing that individual in that job. But if a manager is both competent and hard working, failure is not a message that should be sent. Even though it is desirable to encourage the individual to achieve even more, the signal of failure will be discouraging.

When people work extremely hard and fail, they often question why they bothered to work so hard. If hard work results in failure to achieve the target, then why not ease off? If they are going to fail anyway, why try very hard? And when people get discouraged, they may become angry. This situation can lead to turnover in the management group and even sabotage by angry persons who feel their supervisors are against them and that they are being set up to fail. Thus managers at every level of the organization must be extremely careful to ensure that all goals assigned are reasonable, or results may be less favorable than they otherwise would be.

■ THE BUDGET AS A TOOL FOR COMMUNICATION

Of course, for motivation to really exist, the budget goals must be communicated. This concept was introduced in Chapter 2. It is important enough to warrant a few additional comments. The earlier examples should make it clear that this discussion does not relate to motivating only the managers of the organization. Costs are incurred because of the actions of all individuals in an organization. A nurse manager will have little success in controlling costs without the cooperation of all the nurses and other staff on the floor.

A good practice is to sit down once a year and review all aspects of the budget on which the staff nurses have some impact. However, communication should also be an ongoing process. When a manager has a once-a-year meeting with the staff concerning the budget, it is quickly forgotten. In order to reinforce that meeting, a short weekly or monthly meeting should be held to discuss the budget relating to one or several items, such as bandage tape, diapers, chest tubes, disposable gloves, or sponges. It does not even have to be a separate meeting; it can be a 2-minute note made at any regularly scheduled meeting. The key is to make the staff aware of specific, definite, attainable goals that they can work toward. Further, by having the budget mentioned every week, an awareness is created, and it becomes second nature to conserve the organization's resources.

Note that in no way does this imply reducing quality of care. The focus is on reducing inefficient and wasteful use of resources. To the staff nurse, this means, for example, taking care not to rip off 2 feet of tape when 6 inches would do the trick. For the nurse manager, it means setting a staffing schedule that minimizes overtime and agency nurse costs. The point that careful use of resources benefits patients should be made to the nursing staff. Approximately 40 million Americans are without health care coverage because they cannot afford to buy health insurance. If nurses understand that by conserving resources they are helping to keep health care costs affordable, they are more likely to collaborate with the manager and each other in conserving supplies and other resources.

Conservation of resources is the key, and it should become second nature. The benefits of once-a-year meetings wear off in a few weeks. If the manager does not mention the budget again until a month of excessive use has occurred, a strong admonition at that time will tend to create budget antagonism rather than cost control. It is critically important that the manager emphasize that conservation of resources does not mean that patients should not receive needed materials and services. Rather, the nurses are asked to assist in controlling wastage and excessive use of resources. When a nurse manager conveys specific, measurable goals in a routine manner, cost control can become a routine part of the way a nurse functions. The best control of resource use requires that the staff view control of resource use to be a key part of their job—and part of quality patient care.

■ USING BUDGETS FOR INTERIM EVALUATION

Evaluation is a necessary element of controlling costs. The organization must evaluate how well managers are keeping to their budgets. In this respect, interim evaluations are of particular importance.

If the manager simply prepares a budget, tells everyone what it is, and then puts it in a drawer until it is needed to help prepare the next year's budget, an important element of motivation and control is lost. Even if the manager takes the budget out of the drawer each month and tells the unit's staff, "This is how much we have budgeted for bandage tape for this month, that's your goal," the last major step toward controlling costs has not been taken. The budget has not been used to evaluate how well the unit, staff, and manager are doing.

Many organizations would argue that at the end of each year they compare the budgeted amounts to the actual results to see how well they did. The problem is that by then it is too late to do anything about it. The budget should be a living document; it should be used as a motivational and control tool throughout the year.

Each month there should be comparisons between what was expected and what has been accomplished. First, this will allow managers to give feedback to the staff nurses, their supervisors, and themselves as to whether the budget's goals are being attained. The person attempting to lose 10 pounds quickly gives up if there is no available scale on which progress can be observed. Telling the nurses the goals without giving timely reports on whether they are being attained will weaken their motivation.

Second, these monthly evaluations help to bring any unanticipated results to the manager's attention. Then the manager may be able to make adjustments in staffing or take other action so that the budget will be met in future months. And it should be recognized that a budget can be too low. If there is any concern that nurses are denying patients needed care in order to achieve budget goals, the mission and purpose of the health care organization are being violated. The important point is that the budget should be appropriate to the patient care workload and should reflect both conservation of resources and quality patient care. To ensure that resources are used wisely and well, a monthly review of census, patient acuity, and the budget is in order. That kind of frequent review will assist the manager and the staff to make midstream corrections so that budget and patient care goals are jointly met.

This, of course, assumes that the situation is under the manager's control. Perhaps the manager will watch month after month as the unit fails to meet the budget because something outside the unit's or the manager's control is affecting the results. For example, if the organization uses a fixed monthly budget that does not take account of patient volume, the manager with a consistently growing patient volume will typically be over budget. The situation is out of the manager's control. The unit and the manager will probably be blamed if the budget goals are not met, so monthly information allows a manager to serve early notice that a problem outside of her or his control exists.

In evaluating any individual in an organization, there is one primary rule that must be followed: responsibility should equal control. If managers are held responsible for things they have no control over, the organization will reward and punish the wrong individuals. The results are invariably an unhappy group of individuals and, in nursing, higher turnover, which is extremely costly to the institution. Of course, a key result will be that the manager and the department never meet goals, and that typically means the organization is not exerting control—or is exerting control in a way that will not help the organization to succeed.

Summary and Implications for Nurse Managers

Budgets can help to control costs if they are used to motivate all staff members, not just managers. This requires communication of specific, measurable financial and care-quality goals on a regular and frequent basis. Such a process will improve results as individuals make self-motivated efforts to achieve specified, attainable goals.

However, it is necessary to understand the incentives needed to inspire individuals to work toward the overall well-being of the organization. When a health care organization asks a nurse to accomplish something, it is important to be concerned with why that person would want to do it. Perhaps the nurse's reason is to benefit patient care. Effective managers have some understanding of human motivation in general and of the kinds of things that motivate the staff they supervise. Effective managers also make sure that achievement of one goal does not mean another goal is sabotaged. Too strong an emphasis on cost control can have the undesirable result of lowering the quality of patient care. But quality patient care and cost control can go hand in hand among nursing staff. Excellence in patient care is a motivator for most nurses, but often they don't understand the role of cost conservation in the larger picture of health care. Without managerial influence, there can be little motive among nurses to work for cost control. Perhaps the nurse will control costs out of loyalty to the organization or out of fear of losing a job. Or perhaps it will be done in the hope of earning a promotion. But for most nurses, understanding that patient care is served by controlling costs is the best motivator.

Reaching an understanding of what people tend to want to do and what they tend not to want to do is important. Once a manager knows what they do not want to do, a careful attempt should be made to develop some clear motivational device that will give them an incentive to do what they otherwise might not want to do. After all, how many people would work if they did not get paid at all? Some psychologists view paychecks as a bribe to get people to come to work. Once they are at work, additional incentives should be provided to make sure that the organization benefits from their efforts to the greatest extent possible. For nurses, the pride of knowing they provide quality patient care can serve as a very strong motivator.

References and Suggested Readings

Bowles, C., and Candela, L. (2005). First job experiences of recent RN graduates: Improving the work environment. *Journal of Nursing Administration* 35(3), 130-137.

Brady, D.J., Cornett, E., and DeLetter, M. (1998, September-October). Cost reduction: What a staff nurse can do. *Nursing Economic$* 16(5), 273-274, 276.

Caroselli, C. (1996, September-October). Economic awareness of nurses: Relationship to budgetary control. *Nursing Economic$* 14(5), 292-298.

Crowell, D.M. (1998, May). Organizations *are* relationships: A new view of management. *Nursing Management* 29(5), 28-29.

Gardulf, A., Soderstrom, I., Orton, M., Eriksson, L., Arnetz, B., and Nordstrom, G. (2005). Why do nurses at a university hospital want to quit their jobs? *Journal of Nursing Management* 13(4), 329-337.

Goode, C., Krugman, M., Smith, K., Diaz, J., Edmonds, S., and Mulder, J. (2005). The pull of magnetism: a look at the standards and the experience of a western academic medical center hospital in achieving and sustaining magnet status. *Nursing Administration Quarterly* 29(3), 202-213.

Hart, S. (2005). Hospital ethical climates and registered nurses' turnover intentions. *Journal of Nursing Scholarship* 37(2), 173-177.

Helios, K. E. (2005). Management of serious nosocomial bacterial infections: do current therapeutic options meet the need? *Clinical Microbiology & Infection* 11(10), 778-787.

Girvins, J. (1998). Satisfaction and motivation. *Nursing Management* 5(4), 11-15.

JCAHO. (2005). Improving quality via pay-for-performance programs: will it work? *Joint Commission Benchmark* 7(1), 6-7, 11.

Jones, D. (2005). Savings sharing: Rewarding staff for responsible decision-making. *Journal of Nursing Administration* 35(4), 199-204.

Judge, T., Thoresen, C., Bono, J., Patton, G. (2001). The job satisfaction–job performance relationship: A qualitative and quantitative review. *Psychological Bulletin* 127(3), 376-407.

Murphy, L. (2005). Transformational leadership: a cascading chain reaction. *Journal of Nursing Management* 13(2), 128-136.

Panhotra, B., Saxena, A., and Al-Arabi Al-Ghamdi, A. (2004). The effect of a continuous educational program on handwashing compliance among healthcare workers in an intensive care unit. *British Journal of Infection Control* 5(3), 15-18.

Porter-O'Grady, T. (2004). Overview and summary: shared governance: is it a model for nurses to gain control over their practice? *Online Journal of Issues in Nursing* 9(1), 1-3.

Sims, C. (2003). Increasing clinical, satisfaction, and financial performance through nurse-driven process improvement. *Journal of Nursing Administration* 33(2), 68-75.

VanOyen, F. (2005). The relationship between effective nurse managers and nursing retention. *Journal of Nursing Administration* 35(7/8), 336-341.

Won, S., Chou, H., Hsieh, W., Chen, C., Huang, Shio-Min H., Tsou, K., Tsao, and Po, N. (2004). Handwashing program for the prevention of nosocomial infections in a neonatal intensive care unit. *Infection Control and Hospital Epidemiology* 25(9), 742-746.

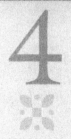

CHAPTER

4

Cost Concepts

LEARNING OBJECTIVES
The goals of this chapter are to:

- Define service units
- Define basic cost terms
- Explain the underlying behavior of costs and the importance of that behavior
- Provide tools for cost estimation

- Explain how costs can be adjusted for the impact of inflation
- Provide tools for break-even analysis
- Explain the activity-based costing technique

■ BASIC COST CONCEPTS

To prepare a budget that can provide a good plan of expenses for the coming year, it is necessary to have an understanding of the nature of costs. Revenues are also important. (Revenues are discussed in Chapter 9.)

Service Units

Costs are generally collected for *service units* or units of service. A service unit is a basic measure of the item being produced by the organization, such as clinic visits, discharged patients, patient days, home care visits, and hours of operations. Most measurements of cost relate to the volume of service units. Within one health care organization, a number of different types of service units may exist.

Fixed Versus Variable Costs

A critical basic cost issue is the distinction between fixed and variable costs. The total costs of running a unit or department can be divided into those costs that are fixed and those costs that are variable.

Fixed costs are those costs that do not change in total as the volume of a service unit changes. For instance, the salary of the Chief Nurse Executive does not change day by day as the census changes. *Variable costs,* on the other hand, vary directly with the volume of service units. For example, linen-use costs are higher on a day when the unit is full than they are on a day when the unit is only at 50% of capacity. The definition of the service unit measure is crucial in defining fixed and variable costs. Most clinical supplies used in a hospital vary with the number of patient days.

However, surgical supplies are more likely to vary with the number and type of surgical procedures, and clinic supplies are likely to vary with the number of clinic visits.

The concepts of fixed and variable costs are often conceptualized by the use of graphs. Figure 4-1 gives an example of fixed costs. Specifically, the graph shows the annual salary of a unit nurse manager for the coming year. The salary is $60,000.[1] That salary is a fixed cost for the organization. The salary paid to a nurse manager is not dependent on any patient-volume statistic. In Figure 4-1, the vertical axis shows the cost to the institution. The higher the place on the vertical axis, the higher the costs. The horizontal axis shows the number of patients. The further to the right a point is on the horizontal axis, the more patients the institution has.

Note that the fixed costs appear as a horizontal line. This is because, regardless of the volume, the salary for the nurse manager remains the same. Thus the cost is the same for 8,000 patients, or for 10,000, or for 12,000.

Variable costs, on the other hand, vary with the volume of service units. Suppose that each hospital patient's temperature is taken twice a day. If the hospital's thermometers use disposable thermometer covers, one would expect use of disposable covers to vary directly with patient volume. Assuming that each thermometer cover costs $.50 and that two a day are used for each patient, the cost of these items would be $1 for each patient each day. The more patient days, the more the cost for that disposable item in the total nursing unit budget.

Consider Figure 4-2. This graph plots the cost of disposable thermometer covers as it varies with patient volume. As in Figure 4-1, the vertical axis represents the cost, and the horizontal axis represents the patient volume. Because the thermometer cover example relates to inpatients, the label on the horizontal axis has been changed from "Annual number of patients" in Figure 4-1 to "Annual number of patient days" in Figure 4-2. Unlike Figure 4-1, which shows some positive amount of cost even at a volume of zero, Figure 4-2 shows zero cost at a volume of zero because zero patient days implies that none of this particular supply will be used. The total variable cost increases by $1 for each extra patient day.

[1] This is a hypothetical number, Nurse manager salaries vary over time, and vary by geographic region, institution size, and institution type.

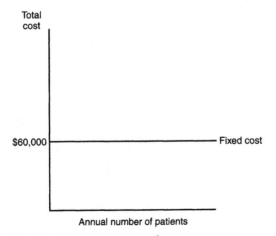

Figure 4-1 Fixed costs: cost for a nurse manager.

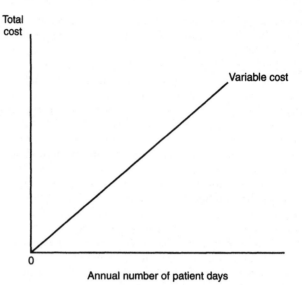

Figure 4-2 Variable costs: the costs of a disposable supply.

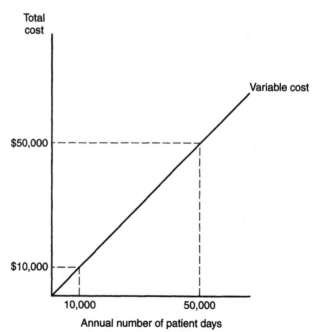

Figure 4-3 Variable costs: the costs of a disposable supply at volumes of 10,000 and 50,000 patient days.

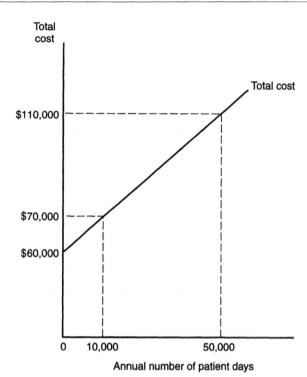

Figure 4-4 Total costs for the unit.

For instance, in Figure 4-3, dotted lines have been inserted to show the cost when there are 10,000 patient days and the cost when there are 50,000 patient days. As you can see, $10,000 would be spent on the disposable item if there were 10,000 patient days and $50,000 if there were 50,000 patient days.

The total of the fixed and variable costs is shown in Figure 4-4. This figure combines the fixed costs from Figure 4-1 with the variable costs from Figure 4-2. Note that the total costs start at $60,000, even if volume is zero, because of the fixed costs of the nurse manager.

The Relevant Range

One potential problem exists with this type of graphic analysis of fixed and variable costs. It concerns an issue accountants refer to as the *relevant range*. The relevant range represents the likely range of activity covered by a budget. For example, a unit might expect 80% occupancy. However, a range from 75% to 85% occupancy is possible. In that case, the relevant range extends from the number of patient days associated with a 75% occupancy level to the number of patient days associated with an 85% occupancy level.

Variable costs increase proportionately over the relevant range. It is unlikely that a health care organization would pay $.50 for each disposable thermometer cover at **any** volume level. If purchases increase substantially, there probably will be a price reduction per unit. On the other hand, if purchases were to decrease substantially, the hospital possibly would have to pay more per unit. However, the variable costs may reasonably be considered to increase proportionately over the relevant range.

Fixed costs are not fixed over any range of activity. If a nursing unit had zero patient days, the hospital would close the unit and would not have any fixed cost for a nurse manager. If patient volume rose substantially and exceeded the capacity of the unit, the hospital might need to open a second unit and have the additional cost of a second nurse manager. The costs are, however, fixed over the relevant range.

Essentially, variable costs do not increase by exactly the same amount per unit over any range of volume, and fixed costs do not remain fixed over any range of volume. However, for most budgets, volume expectations for the coming year do not assume drastic changes in volume.

When fixed and variable costs are graphed, the relevant range issue is often ignored (e.g., costs appear fixed over all ranges of activity in the graph). However, the user of the graph should bear in mind that the graph's information is accurate only within the relevant range.

Other Complications

In health care, there are several additional problems related to applying the concepts of fixed and variable costs. These problems generally concern issues of *step-fixed costs*, *mixed costs*, and *relevant costs*.

Many costs are step-fixed (sometimes called *step-variable*). Such costs do vary within the relevant range, but not smoothly. They are fixed over intervals that are shorter than the relevant range (Figure 4-5).

For example, staffing patterns may be such that a nursing unit will use five nurses over a range of workload. If that range is exceeded, the unit would have to use six nurses. Clearly, more patient days or greater average acuity requires more nursing care hours. However, if the staffing pattern is about 4.2 hours of nursing time per patient day, the unit would not expect to hire a nurse for an additional 4.2 hours every time the patient-day census increases by one.

As long as there is a staffing chart that indicates how many *full-time equivalent (FTE)* nurses are needed for any volume of patient days, the presence of step-variable costs does not present a major budgeting problem. Generally, because of the use of

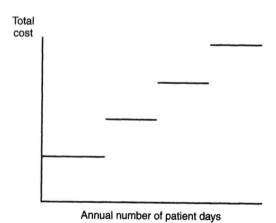

Annual number of patient days

Figure 4-5 Example of step-fixed costs.

overtime and agency nurses, a step-fixed pattern of cost is estimated by treating the staffing costs as if they were variable. Although this will not produce a perfectly precise result, it is usually a reasonable approximation.

A more difficult problem is posed by mixed costs. A mixed cost is one that contains some fixed cost and some variable cost. For instance, electricity is a mixed cost. A hospital or nursing home spends some basic amount to light the hallways and public areas of a building regardless of volume, but patient rooms will have lights on only if there is a patient in the room. Therefore, the more patient days, the higher the electricity cost—even though part of the overall cost is fixed. Most units and departments have some mixed costs.

For example, suppose that a home care agency pays some staff every day, regardless of the amount of work, and pays some staff by number of visits. This creates a mixed-cost situation. Or suppose that the intensive care unit of a hospital has highly variable patient volume. The nurse manager of the unit knows that this year the unit will have a total of 10,000 patient days, and for next year 12,000 patient days are predicted. Because the unit is busy at some times and slow at others, it is difficult to use a staffing chart based on step-fixed costs. The patient days are not incurred evenly throughout the year. Can a nurse manager simply assume that a 20% increase in patient days from 10,000 to 12,000 will cause a need for 20% higher staffing costs than the unit had in the year with 10,000 patient days?

Probably not. There is likely to be some minimum staffing level as long as the unit is open. The cost for that minimum staffing level represents a fixed cost because it does not change with volume. Then as volume increases, there will be additional staff requirements. If the nurse manager wishes to determine how much staff to budget for during the coming year, it is necessary to be able to separate the mixed cost into fixed-cost and variable-cost components. As volume increases, the fixed cost will not change and the variable costs will increase in direct proportion to the volume change. However, those cost increases may not be incurred at the average RN per-hour rate. The variable part of the staffing budget may have to be budgeted at a much higher, temporary staff hourly rate if no other options are available for staffing when workload is higher than normal.

There are several ways to separate mixed costs into their fixed-cost and variable-cost components so that future costs can be predicted. Later in this chapter there is an examination of the high-low approach and regression analysis techniques of *cost estimation* to solve that problem.

The Impact of Volume on Cost per Patient

If a nurse manager were to ask what it costs to treat patients in the unit, accountants would probably answer that it depends. Costs are not unique numbers that are always the same. The cost to treat a patient depends on several critical factors. One of the key drivers of cost is the volume of patients for whom care is being provided.

Suppose that an outpatient cardiology clinic has fixed costs of $200,000 and variable costs of $200 per patient. Using this hypothetical data, what is the total cost per patient? If there are 3,000 patients for the year, the total costs will be the fixed cost of $200,000 plus $200 per patient for each of the 3,000 patients. The variable costs would be $600,000 (i.e., $200 per patient times 3,000 patients). The total cost would be $800,000 (i.e., $200,000 fixed cost plus $600,000 variable cost). The cost per patient would be $267 (i.e., $800,000 total cost divided by 3,000 patients) per patient.

However, what if there were only 2,500 patients? Then the variable costs, at $200 per patient, would be $500,000, and the total cost would be $700,000. In that case, the cost per patient would be $280. The cost is higher because there are fewer patients sharing the fixed costs. Each patient causes the facility to spend another $200. The $200,000 fixed cost is spread among fewer patients because it remains the same, regardless of the number of patients. If there are more patients, each one shares a smaller portion of the $200,000 fixed cost. If there are fewer patients, the fixed cost assigned to each would rise. For example, suppose there were only 500 patients. The variable costs of $200 per patient would total $100,000, and the total cost would be $300,000. The cost per patient would be $600—more than double the previous results based on 2,500 and 3,000 patients.

In trying to understand costs, it is critical to grasp the concept that because fixed costs do not change in total, the cost per patient or per patient day does change as volume changes. With a greater volume, there are a larger number of patients to spread out the fixed costs. Consider a pie. If you divide a pie among 10 people, each person will receive a smaller portion than if you divide the pie among 5 people. The pie is like fixed costs. The greater the volume, the smaller the amount of fixed-cost "pie" each patient must carry. There is no single answer to the question "What does it cost the unit per patient?" That question can be answered only by stating the cost per patient given a specific number of patients. The number of patients is critical because fixed costs per patient rise as the number of patients drop; while fixed costs per patient drop as the number of patients rise.

One implication of this result is that health care organizations almost always find higher volume preferable to lower volume. As volume increases, the average cost per patient declines. If prices can be maintained at the original level, the declining cost will result in lower losses or higher profits. Of course, this assumes that the patients are insured or that they are willing and able to pay the cost of care. Increasing the volume improves the facility's financial status only if that increase involves paying patients. This is an important concern today, when there are more than 46 million uninsured Americans (NCHC, 2004; Zwillich, 2005; DeNavas-Walt, Proctor, & Lee, 2006). Many of those uninsured people are what are called the "working poor"; that is, they make too much money to be eligible for publicly financed health care services but do not make enough money to buy their own health insurance. (Typically, their employers do not offer health care as a benefit, and purchasing health insurance privately is prohibitively expensive for most people in the category of the working poor). However, assuming the facility can increase the volume of paying customers, higher volume typically means the cost per patient will be lower.

Relevant Costs

Another costing concern is the issue accountants refer to as relevant costs. Relevant costs are those costs that change as a result of a decision. Costs that remain the same regardless of a decision are not "relevant" costs for making the decision.

If someone asks a nurse manager the cost of treating a particular type of patient, the answer should be, "It depends." In the previous section it was pointed out that cost depends on the number of patients. It also depends on what the answer will be used for. If the question is just one of historical curiosity, the average cost is an adequate response. The average cost is the total cost divided by the volume. In the previous example, the total cost at a volume of 2,500 patients was $700,000, and the average cost (i.e., the total $700,000 divided by the volume of 2,500 patients) was $280 per patient. However, if the information is to be used for decision making, that response may well be incorrect.

Suppose that the health care facility were trying to decide whether to negotiate with an HMO to accept additional patients of the same average acuity and mix as the 2,500 patients it currently has. The HMO has offered $250 per patient for 500 patients. Based on the earlier calculations, the cost per patient for 500 patients is $600! However, the facility would not be providing only 500 patients with care. It already has 2,500 patients. Based on the earlier calculations, the average cost is $280 per patient at 2,500 patients. At 3,000 patients, the average cost would be $267. Given that information, would it pay to accept the additional patients at a price of only $250?

It definitely would. Why should the facility accept $250 if the additional patients will cost at least $267? Actually, the additional patients will not cost at least $267. All the patients, on average, will cost that amount. The $267 includes a share of both fixed and variable costs. If the facility is going to treat at least 2,500 patients regardless of the outcome of the HMO negotiation, the fixed costs of $200,000 will be incurred. The fixed costs will not change if the facility has the extra 500 patients.

Decisions such as this one rely on *marginal analysis*. The margin refers to a change from current conditions by even a minor amount. A patient on the margin refers to adding one more patient or reducing volume by one patient. Marginal costs are the costs of treating one more patient.

On the *margin*, if the facility were to take the additional HMO patients, it would have more variable costs but would not have any additional fixed costs (assuming that the number, 3,000 patients, is within the relevant range). Each extra patient causes the facility to spend only the variable costs of $200 per patient. That is less than the $250 the HMO has offered to pay. The facility will be better off by $50 for each additional patient.

The additional costs incurred for additional patients are often referred to as the *marginal*, or *out-of-pocket*, or *incremental costs*. If fixed costs were to rise because the relevant range was exceeded, those costs would appropriately be included in the incremental costs along with the variable costs. The key element in relevant costing is that the only costs relevant to a decision are those that change as a result of the decision.

The decision may be to add a new service or to close down an existing one. It may be to expand volume (as shown in the example of the HMO), or it may be to contract volume. In any case, when a decision is being made that contemplates changing patient load, the essential pieces of information to be considered are the revenues and costs that change. Effective managerial decisions require that the manager know the amount by which total costs will increase and the amount by which total revenues will increase or, alternatively, the amount by which both will decrease. Costs that do not change in total for the organization are not relevant to the decision. Fixed costs generally do not increase when additional patients are added (within the relevant range), and therefore they are not relevant.

In the cardiology clinic-HMO example, suppose that prior to the HMO negotiation, the clinic was receiving $275 for each of its 2,500 patients. Total revenue ($275 times 2,500) was $687,500. Total costs were $700,000 (calculated earlier). The clinic was losing $12,500 (the amount that the cost of $700,000 exceeds the revenues of $687,500). If the HMO business is accepted, the additional revenue would be $250 times 500 patient days, or $125,000. The total cost for 3,000 patients (calculated earlier) is $800,000. The cost increase of going from 2,500 patients to 3,000 patients is only $100,000 (i.e., $800,000 total cost for 3,000 patients versus $700,000 total cost for 2,500 patients).

The total costs with the HMO patients are $800,000, and the total revenues are $812,500 (i.e., the original $687,500 plus $125,000 revenue from the HMO). The unit has gone from a loss of $12,500 to a profit of $12,500. The costs have increased by $100,000 while the revenues have increased by $125,000. The amount by which the extra revenues exceed the extra costs for the 500 HMO patients accounts for the turnaround from a loss to a profit. This should not be surprising. The extra revenue per patient is $250. The additional cost per patient day is $200. The difference between the incremental revenue of $250 per patient and the incremental cost of $200 per patient is a profit of $50 per patient. This extra profit of $50 for each of the 500 HMO patients accounts exactly for the $25,000 profit from the HMO patients.

Had the facility used average cost for its decision because the $250 revenue per extra patient was less than the $267 average cost, it would have turned away the extra business and lost the chance to gain a $25,000 profit. The average cost is not relevant because it incorrectly assumes that each extra patient will cause the clinic to have additional variable and fixed costs. The incremental cost is relevant because it considers only the additional revenues and additional costs that the clinic will have as a result of the proposed change.

■ COST ESTIMATION

One of the most difficult parts of the budget process is predicting the individual elements of the budget. Trying to predict how much will be spent on each type of expenditure in the coming year presents great problems for both inexperienced and experienced managers.

One approach is simply to look to what happened this year and predict that it will occur again next year, with an increment for inflation. At the other extreme is an approach that says it is desirable to do better next year than this year, so it is appropriate to budget a certain percentage less than was spent this year. In each case, the approach is far too simplistic. A priori, there is no reason to believe that next year will be just like this year, and simply wishing to spend less than this year will not make it so.

Some sort of clear methodology is needed that will allow prediction of what will happen next year based on the past. A way of considering formally why that prediction may not come true is also needed. Finally, if costs are to be reduced below the predicted outcome, there must be a specific plan of action that the nurse manager believes can accomplish the cost cutback.

This section considers several methods of cost estimation. Not all elements of the budget are simply costs. Items such as the number of patient days must be predicted as well. A discussion of general forecasting is presented in Chapter 6. Here the focus will be solely on prediction of costs. Often, historical information about costs incurred in the past can be a great aid in predicting what costs will be in the future. This is especially true in the case of mixed costs, which have elements of both fixed and variable costs. Cost estimation techniques exist that look at historical information and compare the change in cost over time with the change in volume over time in order to isolate fixed and variable costs.

If costs rise as volume rises, what could account for the increase in costs? Fixed costs, by definition, do not change as volume changes. Therefore, any change in cost as volume changes must be attributable to the variable costs. By seeing how much costs change for each unit change in volume, it is possible to calculate the variable cost per unit. In turn, the fixed cost can be determined. The fixed and variable costs can then be used to estimate costs for the coming year based on a forecast of the volume in the coming year.

There is one critical problem in the flow of logic that allows cost estimation to take place. Changes in cost over time are assumed to be the result of changes in volume. To some extent, changes in cost over time are the result of inflation. If inflation were a constant percent that remained the same each year, one could argue that past inflation can be ignored and inflation will automatically be built into predictions for the future. However, inflation rates tend to fluctuate from year to year. Over a period of years the fluctuations can be substantial. Therefore, in order to be able to predict fixed and variable costs, the data being used should be free from the impact of inflation.

Adjusting Costs for Inflation

Suppose that a nurse manager is interested in determining how much the total RN staff cost of a unit will be for the coming fiscal year, 2009.[2] The unit is staffed with a minimum of 10 FTE RNs for any volume up to 9,000 patient days at a certain acuity level. The cost of those 10 FTEs is a fixed cost because the unit will always have at least that cost. As volume increases above 9,000 patient days, additional nursing time will be needed. In 2007, patient days numbered 9,800 and the cost, including fringe benefits, was $500,000. In 2008, the patient days totalled 11,000 and the cost was $580,000. The cost increase of $80,000 was attributable to both the increased volume and inflation.

Most readers are probably familiar with the consumer price index (CPI). This is the most widely used measure of inflation. The CPI and many other indexes of inflation, such as the hospital market basket index, were developed by or for the federal government. The CPI measures the relative cost of a typical basket of consumer goods. Whatever the basket of goods cost in the base year is considered to be 100% of the cost in that year, or simply 100. The index is revised and a new base year is established from time to time. If it costs twice as much to buy the same goods in a year subsequent to the base year, then the index would be 200% of the base year costs, or simply 200.

The U.S. Department of Commerce, Bureau of the Census, annually publishes the *Statistical Abstract of the United States*. Included in this book are Indexes of Medical Care Prices. There are several useful indexes under that heading, including the index of Medical Care Services and the Hospital Daily Room Rate index. The book may be ordered from the Website http://www.census.gov/statab/www/ and pdf files of the book may be found online at http://www.census.gov/prod/www/statistical-abstract.html.

Recall that in this example the nurse manager wants to find the variable cost per patient day of nursing labor for 2009, using current dollars as of the end of 2008. If information from 2004 through 2008 is used, the nurse manager would have to find the value of an appropriate index in each of those years. The financial managers in most health care institutions can provide nurse managers with appropriate indices adjusted for labor costs in the specific geographic area. Failing that, most library reference sections

[2] A fiscal year may have a starting point at any convenient date, not necessarily January 1. For example, a fiscal year could begin on July 1 and end on June 30. In that case, fiscal year 2009 would refer to the year from July 1, 2008, to June 30, 2009.

can be of assistance with current index information. Assume that an appropriate index for those years has values as follows:

$$
\begin{array}{ll}
2004: & 258 \\
2005: & 287 \\
2006: & 318 \\
2007: & 357 \\
2008: & 395
\end{array}
$$

Suppose also that the following cost and volume information is available:

Year	Patient Days	Cost
2004	8,000	$383,714
2005	8,700	$425,923
2006	8,850	$468,515
2007	9,800	$613,286
2008	11,000	$762,704

It appears that costs have risen from 2004 to 2008, even though volume is below 9,000 patient days in each of those years. Because the staffing is fixed at 10 FTEs for any volume below 9,000 patient days, the cost is expected to be about the same in each of those 3 years and to increase only as volume increases above 9,000 patient days, thus requiring more nursing staff. The cost information, however, is not comparable because of the impact of inflation. In order to make the numbers reasonable for comparison purposes, they must be restated in *constant dollars* (i.e., amounts that have been adjusted for the impact of inflation).

This adjustment can be made by multiplying the cost in any given year by a fraction that represents the current value of the index divided by the value of the index in the year the cost was incurred. This is not a complicated procedure. For example, in 2004 the cost was $383,714. The hypothetical index value is currently 395. In 2004 it was 258. Multiply $383,714 by the fraction 395/258. The result is $587,469, which is the 2004 cost adjusted to 2008 dollars. Now the $762,704 spent when there were 11,000 patient days in 2008 can be compared to $587,469, the constant-dollar cost of 8,000 patient days in 2004.

In a similar fashion all of the data can be restated into 2008 dollars as follows:

Year	Patient Days	Original Cost		Index Fraction		Adjusted Cost
2004	8,000	$383,714	×	395/258	=	$587,469
2005	8,700	$425,923	×	395/287	=	$586,201
2006	8,850	$468,515	×	395/318	=	$581,960
2007	9,800	$613,286	×	395/357	=	$678,565
2008	11,000	$762,704	×	395/395	=	$762,704

Note that, adjusted for inflation, there was little change in costs from 2004 to 2006, the period during which the staffing numbers were fixed because patient days were below 9,000.

High-Low Cost Estimation

The high-low approach is a relatively simple, quick-and-dirty approach to cost estimation. It is unsophisticated and therefore not terribly accurate, but in many cases it may be good enough. It certainly is better than simply taking a guess.

The key to the high-low method is the fact that fixed costs do not change at all in response to changes in volume. The way the method works is to look at the organization's cost for a specific area over the past 5 years. When you do this, remember to use costs after adjusting the original amounts spent for inflation, as described earlier.

The use of 5 years is arbitrary. It might be more appropriate to use a longer period of time, but you would not want to use data from fewer than 5 years; such a short amount of time should be used only if there have been substantial changes in the unit that would make earlier data no longer relevant. For the period of time chosen, find the highest volume and the lowest volume and compare the costs at these two volumes. These costs are readily obtained from *variance reports* of prior years.

The amount by which the costs changed should be compared to the amount by which the volume changed. In this example, the highest volume in the past 5 years was 11,000 patient days, and the cost for nursing labor that year for the department was $762,704. The lowest volume in the past 5 years was 8,000 patient days, and the constant dollar-inflation-adjusted cost in that year was $587,469. In this case, inflation-adjusted cost increased by $175,235. If $175,235 is divided by 3,000 patient days, the result is $58.41 per patient day. Although it is certainly likely that nursing labor is a step-fixed cost and therefore will not go up by $58.41 for **each** additional patient day, this volume provides a reasonable measure of the amount of additional nursing services needed per patient day when there are significant changes in volume.

If the variable cost per patient day is $58.41, what is the fixed cost? The yearly total variable cost is first found by multiplying the variable cost per patient day by the number of patient days ($58.41 × 8,000 = $467,293). The total nursing labor cost for 8,000 patient days was $587,469 in 2004; if $467,293 is the variable cost, then the remainder, $120,176, represents the fixed cost. Similarly, for 11,000 patient days at $58.41 per patient day, the variable cost is $642,528; and given a total cost of $762,704 in 2008, the fixed cost would be $120,176. The fixed cost is expected to be the same at either volume level because, by definition, it is fixed.

This fixed and variable cost information can be used in preparing the next year's budget. If 12,000 patient days are expected, costs would be expected to rise by $58.41 times 1,000 patient days, or $58,401. The fixed-cost portion will not change. Because this information has been calculated using 2008 constant dollars, both the fixed and variable costs would have to be adjusted upward for the expected 2009 salary increases or, more generally, for the expected impact of inflation during the next year.

The high-low method is not terribly accurate because it considers only the experience of 2 years. One or both of the 2 years chosen may have had some unusual circumstance that would skew the costs in that year. A superior prediction is possible if some method is used that takes more experience into account. *Regression analysis* is a method that can provide such a prediction.

Regression Analysis

The volume of patient days and the total costs for those days for a number of years can be plotted on a graph. The horizontal axis represents the volume, and the vertical axis represents the cost. The result is a scatter diagram. The series of points on the graph represent a volume and the cost at that volume. If a line is drawn through the points, it can be used for future predictions. By selecting any expected volume on the horizontal axis, it is possible to go vertically up to the line and then from the line, move horizontally across to a point on a vertical cost axis. That point represents the

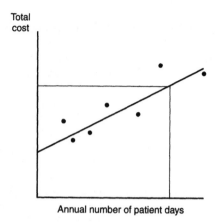

Total
cost

Annual number of patient days

Figure 4-6 Predicting costs from a scatter diagram.

prediction of cost. For example, Figure 4-6 shows a scatter diagram with a line drawn through the points.

The difficulty in drawing the diagonal line connecting those points is placing it properly so that it will provide accurate predictions. Regression analysis is a technique that applies mathematical precision to a scatter diagram. Regression technique can select the one line that is effectively closest to all the individual points on the scatter diagram and that will therefore provide the best predictions of cost for the future. This can break costs down fairly accurately into their fixed-cost and variable-cost components.

Simple linear regression analysis can take all available past information into account in estimating the portion of any cost that is fixed and the portion that is variable. The phrase "simple linear regression" refers to several issues. First, it is simple in the sense that there is only one *dependent variable* and one *independent variable*. Cost is the dependent variable that is being estimated. Cost depends on the value of the independent variable.

An independent variable is a causal factor. For example, the most significant causal factor for nursing costs in a hospital might be patient days. The more patient days, the greater the costs for nursing. For the admissions department of the hospital, it would not be patient days but rather the number of patients that is important because admission time is the same for each patient, regardless of the ultimate length of stay. For a home health agency, the most significant causal factor might be the number of home visits.

The second part of the phrase "simple linear regression" refers to the presumption that cost behavior can be shown in a linear fashion (i.e., using a straight line). What if a slightly lower price per disposable supply unit were paid for every increase in volume (e.g., \$.75 for one unit, \$.7499 per unit for two units, \$.7498 per unit for three units, and so on)? In that case, Figure 4-2 would not be an accurate reflection of how variable costs change. It would be necessary to draw a curved line in the graph—but the mathematics involved with curved lines instead of straight lines are far more complicated. Variable costs are generally treated as if they were linear, even if that is only an approximation of their true behavior.

Finally, the term "regression" refers to trying to regress, or bring all the points from the scatter diagram as close as possible to the estimated line.

For example, suppose that the CNE wanted to make a rough starting prediction for the total cost of all nursing units in a hospital for the coming year. If last year there were 50,000 patient days and this coming year patient days are expected to be 52,000, then there is a 4% expected increase in the number of patient days. However, it cannot be assumed that all nursing costs will go up by 4% because some costs, like the salary of the CNE, are fixed and will not rise in proportion to the number of patient days.

The high-low method discussed earlier would be one way to make the prediction, but the high-low method relies on only two data points. Far greater accuracy in breaking out fixed and variable costs is possible if the past years' costs are examined on a detailed basis, cost item by cost item, to determine which were fixed and which were variable. This would be a time-consuming procedure. Gathering information costs money, and even if that information were gathered, there are always some costs that cannot be separated into fixed and variable components without some estimating methodology because they are mixed costs. For example, nonmedical supplies such as paper, pens, and forms will be needed to some extent regardless of patient volume. On the other hand, the more patients, the more nonmedical supplies used. How can you separate that cost into the fixed portion and the variable portion? Even looking at past cost records cost item by cost item will not allow you to determine how much of the cost was fixed and how much was variable. In this case, how can costs be divided into their fixed and variable components and less money spent on gathering information than by examining each line item from past years? Regression analysis can help to separate these mixed costs.

Mixed Costs and Regression Analysis

Suppose it is known that last year the combined cost of the salary of the nurse manager plus the disposable supplies was $110,000 and that the number of patient days was 50,000. This uses the information represented in the graphs presented in Figures 4-1 through 4-3. The volume of patient days is expected to go up to 52,000 next year. Should the $110,000 cost be increased by 4% because volume is increasing by 4%? No, it should not. Some costs are fixed. Only variable costs would increase as volume increases.

One would expect costs to increase by $2,000, or $1 for each extra patient day, because it is known in this example that variable costs for the disposable thermometer covers were described in this simple example as being $1 per patient day. However, dealing with a more realistic example with many different fixed, variable, and mixed costs, the variable costs per patient day would not necessarily be known. Suppose that the following historical information were available (already adjusted for inflation using the indexing techniques):

Year	Patient Days	Cost
1999	40,000	101,000
2000	42,000	102,000
2001	43,000	103,000
2002	44,000	104,000
2003	45,000	105,000
2004	46,000	106,000
2005	47,000	107,000
2006	48,000	108,000
2007	49,000	109,000
2008	50,000	110,000

If the high-low technique were used to evaluate the fixed and variable costs, there would be a strange result. The highest cost is $110,000, and the lowest cost is $101,000; costs have risen by $9,000. At the same time, volume has increased from 40,000 patient days to 50,000 patient days, or an increase of 10,000. When $9,000 is divided by 10,000 patient days, a variable cost of $.90 per patient day results. Is this an accurate estimate? No, because it is known that the variable cost is $1 per patient day. What might be the cause of the discrepancy?

It is possible that 1999 was the first year that disposable thermometer covers were used. Perhaps many of them were defective and were thrown away, or perhaps some were wasted because of lack of familiarity with using them. In any case, if more than $1 per patient day was spent on disposables in the low-volume year, then the costs were unduly high in that year. Therefore, the change in cost from 1999 to 2008 looks unrealistically low, and the variable cost measure is unrealistically low.

At the other extreme, had there been unusual waste (perhaps the fault of the nurses, but possibly due to quality problems with a large batch of the disposable item) in the most recent, high-cost year, the change in cost would look especially high and the variable cost per unit would have come out to more than $1. As has been stated before, if you rely on just two data points, as the high-low method does, your results are subject to the whims of unusual events in either one of those years.

In reality, one would not expect to use exactly $1 per patient day on disposable supplies in any year. For one reason or another, some patients will have their temperature taken only once on a given day. This might be caused by admission to the hospital late in the day, for instance. On the other hand, patients running fevers will undoubtedly have their temperature taken more often. A pattern of costs that is more likely to be observed is as follows:

Year	Patient Days	Cost
1999	40,000	$101,000
2000	42,000	$101,800
2001	43,000	$103,600
2002	44,000	$103,800
2003	45,000	$105,300
2004	46,000	$106,700
2005	47,000	$106,900
2006	48,000	$108,800
2007	49,000	$108,900
2008	50,000	$110,000

Simply looking at this list does not provide a lot of insight about fixed and variable costs. Figure 4-7 shows a scatter diagram for these points. By looking at this diagram, one can roughly see how the costs are increasing as volume increases. A straight line cannot go through all the points on this scatter diagram. However, the regression technique uses all the available information to select a line that will provide the best estimate in the absence of any other information.

Regression analysis uses information about the dependent and independent variables in the past to develop an equation for a straight line. As part of that process, it calculates a constant value and a coefficient for the independent variable. If the dependent variable is the cost, the constant represents the fixed cost, and the coefficient of the independent variable represents the variable cost.

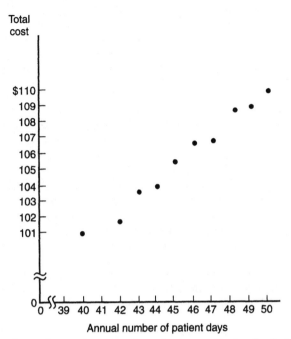

Figure 4-7 Scatter diagram of total costs for nursing (costs and patient days in thousands).

Regression analysis is a statistical technique. A detailed discussion of statistics is beyond the scope of this book. However, there are many mechanical approaches to regression that have made it a workable tool for use in health care institutions. Regression can be performed on many handheld calculators. There are also a wide variety of statistical programs and spreadsheet programs for personal computers that have regression capability.

Turn back now to the scatter diagram in Figure 4-7; it is possible to use regression analysis to predict what the costs will be for the nursing unit next year if there are 52,000 patient days. Regression analysis will determine a specific line to plot through this scatter diagram that will give the best possible estimate of fixed and variable costs and therefore allow prediction of the costs next year.

Basically, the process requires several simple steps. First, determine the cost associated with each volume of patient days. For instance, when there were 40,000 patient days, the cost was $101,000. The independent variable, patient days, is often referred to as the X variable because it is plotted on the horizontal axis. The dependent variable, cost, is often referred to as the Y variable, because cost is plotted on the vertical axis.

Any computer program used will require that you provide the X values and the Y values for each year. Having provided that information, it is generally necessary only to give a command to compute the regression in order to complete the process. It is important not to let the extremely quantitative nature of regression theory learned in a statistics course discourage you from attempting to use this tool. In practice, little mathematics is required of the user. Regression is a tool to help you manage more effectively. The major difficulty in using regression is simply a fear of the process (and this relates not only to nurses but also to most managers throughout most industries).

In the example, regression analysis predicts that the fixed cost is $62,255, and the variable cost is $.96 per unit. Figure 4-8 shows the resulting line. If extended to the left, the line would have its intercept at $62,255, increasing with a slope of .96. These figures are not exactly the expected variable cost of $1 per patient day and the fixed cost of $60,000 for the salary of the nurse manager. They are, however, better estimates than the ones the high-low method would provide. The high-low approach predicts a fixed cost of $50,000 and a variable cost of $.90 per patient day. Regression analysis is an inexpensive, potentially very useful, and relatively simple way of estimating fixed and variable costs and helping to predict the future.

For any number of patient days predicted, it is now possible to multiply by .96 and then add $62,225 to get a forecast of future costs. In many of the computer regression packages, the process is made even simpler just by requiring that the forecast volume be entered into the computer along with the historical data. The computer will then generate the estimated cost for the coming year automatically, based on the forecast volume. Remember, however, that it is necessary to adjust upward the resulting cost for expected increases due to inflation for the coming year.

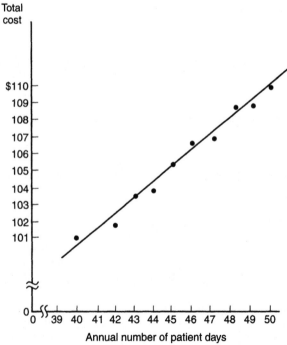

Figure 4-8 Simple linear regression of total costs for nursing (costs and patient days in thousands).

You will soon find this approach to be quite simple, but it is useful only as a tool to **aid** you in managing. It should not be allowed to take over the role of your judgment. The mathematical model is accurate in predicting the future if nothing has changed. It is your role as a manager to know if there are reasons that costs would be likely to change from their past patterns.

For instance, if you knew that during the first year that disposable thermometer covers were used there was a great deal of waste, you might want to eliminate that year from the analysis. If you did, your regression results would have shown fixed costs of $59,970 and variable costs of $1.005. Recall that the fixed costs were actually $60,000, and the variable costs were $1. As you can see, the input of judgment into the process can substantially improve the resulting estimates.

When a regression analysis is performed, one statistic that is generally provided by the calculator or the computer is the R-squared (R^2). This value can range from a low of 0 to a high of 1. If the value is close to 0, it means that the independent variable does not do a good job of explaining the changes in the dependent variable. An R-squared of .2, for example, might indicate that patient days are not a good predictor of nursing cost. On the other hand, an R-squared of .8 would indicate that it is a very good predictor. However, it is possible to become even more exact in estimating costs, by using multiple regression analysis.

Multiple Regression Analysis

There is a type of regression analysis that is more sophisticated than simple linear regression. It is called "multiple regression" because it allows for the use of multiple independent, or causal, variables. The use of simple linear regression can be a substantial aid in estimating future costs because it is so efficient at predicting the fixed cost and the variable cost per unit when there is one major independent variable. Sometimes, however, there will be several key variables. For instance, suppose that the nursing costs vary with the number of patient days but also with the number of patients. That is most probably the case.

Certainly the costs vary with the number of patient days. The more patient days, the more temperatures to be taken, pulses to be checked, medications to be administered, and so on. Yet for each patient there is a medical history to be recorded, a chart to be set up, a patient care plan to be established, valuables to be stored, orientation to be given, discharge planning to be done, discharge education to be provided, and so on. These costs are not fixed—the more patients, the more time spent on these activities—but they do not vary directly with the number of patient days. Several patients with long lengths of stay will cost less than many patients with short lengths of stay, even if the total patient days are the same. So it is likely that the cost of a nursing unit varies with both the number of patient days and the number of patients.

Most handheld business calculators do not perform multiple regressions, although some do. However, most spreadsheet and statistical programs for personal computers can handle this function easily. Instead of simply entering the X and Y values for each year into the calculator or computer, you now enter an X value for the historical information for each of the independent variables, as well as the Y value. Then when you want to predict a future cost, you provide the computer with, for example, the expected number of patient days and the expected number of patients, in order to predict the expected costs.

Sometimes, the multiple regression level of sophistication adds extra work and complexity without substantially changing the results. Recall that when all is said and done, the result is just an estimate. All types of events can happen in the future that will throw off the estimate, no matter how finely tuned it is. It is not necessary to add complexity for its own sake. At times, however, multiple regressions can produce information that would not otherwise be available.

For example, more and more attention has been placed on measures of patient acuity or the level of intensity of required nursing services. It certainly is clear that the number of nursing services vary not just with the number of patient days but also with the severity of the patients' illnesses. If data about the number of patient days and the average acuity level are used as independent variables, the accuracy of estimated costs might improve substantially.

For a home care agency, costs might vary with the number of visits. However, the nurse manager might be able to predict costs better if the number of visits by nurses were used as one variable and the number of aide visits as another variable. One might even divide nurse visits into two variables—one for short visits and one for longer visits.

Another use for multiple regressions is in investigatory work with respect to costs. Suppose that there is a strong feeling by the nursing staff that the way a particular physician practices medicine is extremely costly. This is common in the operating room (OR), where particular surgeons often exhibit out-of-the-ordinary behavior. The number of operations by that specific physician each year can be used as an independent variable. If costs do increase as a result of more cases by that physician, it would show up as a positive coefficient for that independent variable. The nurse manager would then have evidence to support the more general feelings of the staff that the physician is an unusually high resource consumer.

The readers of this book are encouraged to pursue the topic of regression analysis further. This should be done on both a conceptual basis, reviewing the underlying principles and theories of regression analysis, and on a practical basis, using a computer software package to perform some regression analyses.

■ BREAK-EVEN ANALYSIS

To this point, the general behavior of costs (fixed vs. variable) has been discussed as have the techniques of cost estimation (high-low and regression). Attention will now be focused on using cost information for understanding whether a particular unit or service will lose money, make money, or just break even. This technique is useful for the evaluation of both new and continuing projects and services. It is often used in developing a business plan. (Business plans are discussed in Chapter 7.)

In many instances nurse managers find it necessary to be able to determine whether a program or service will be profitable. One key to profitability is volume. Prices are often fixed. Average cost, however, is not fixed. As the number of patients rises, the cost per patient falls because of the sharing of fixed costs. One cannot make a simple comparison of price and average cost and determine that a program or unit will make a profit or a loss. To determine whether something will be profitable, it is critical to know the volume of patients. Break-even analysis is a technique that is used to find the specific volume at which a program or service neither makes nor loses money. Forecast information about the likely volume of the service can be compared to the break-even volume to predict whether there will be profits or losses.

Break-even analysis is based on the following formula:

$$\text{The Break-Even Quantity (Q)} = \frac{\text{Fixed Costs (FC)}}{\text{Price (P)} - \text{Variable Cost per Patient (VC)}}$$

or

$$Q = \frac{FC}{P - VC}$$

where Q is the number of patients needed to just break even, FC is the total fixed cost, P is the price for each patient, and VC is the variable cost per patient. At a quantity lower than Q there would be a loss; at a quantity higher than Q there would be a profit. The P is assumed to be the average amount collected per patient. Health care organizations commonly give discounts or have bad debts or charity care. This analysis is not based on a P equal to the charge for the service but instead considers P to be the average amount of revenue the organization ultimately receives per patient.

The basis for the formula is the underlying relationship between revenues and expenses. If total revenues are greater than expenses, there is a profit. If total revenues are less than expenses, there is a loss. If revenues are just equal to expenses, there is neither profit nor loss, and the service is said to just break even. Expenses are the sum of the total fixed costs and total variable costs.

An Example of Break-Even Analysis

For example, suppose that an integrated health care delivery system opens a new home health agency that charges, on average, $50 per visit. The agency has fixed costs of $10,000 and variable costs of $30 per patient visit. If there are no patients at all, there is no revenue, but there are fixed costs of $10,000, and there is a $10,000 loss. If there were 100 patients, there would be $5,000 of revenue ($50 times 100 patients), $10,000 of fixed cost, and $3,000 of variable cost ($30 times 100 patients). Total costs would be $13,000 ($10,000 of fixed cost plus $3,000 of variable cost), while revenues are $5,000, and the loss is $8,000. These data are hypothetical.

Each additional patient brings in $50 of revenue but causes the agency to spend only $30 more. The difference between the $50 price and the $30 variable cost, $20, is called the *contribution margin*. If the contribution margin is positive, it means that each extra unit of activity makes the organization better off by that amount. The contribution margin from each patient can be used to cover fixed costs, or if all fixed costs have been covered, it represents a profit.

In this example, when there are 100 patients, there is $20 of contribution margin for each of the 100 patients, or a total contribution margin of $2,000. Note that the loss with zero patients was $10,000, while it was only $8,000 when there were 100 patients. The loss decreased by $2,000—exactly the amount of the total contribution margin for those 100 patients.

How many visits would the agency need to have to break even? The answer is 500. If each additional patient generates $20 of contribution margin, then 500 patients would generate $10,000 of contribution margin (500 patients × $20 = $10,000), exactly enough to cover the fixed costs of $10,000. If the agency has 500 patients, it will just break even.

This could have been calculated using the following formula:

$$Q = \frac{FC}{P - VC}$$

or

$$Q = \frac{\$10,000}{\$50 - \$30} = \frac{\$10,000}{\$20} = 500 \text{ visits}$$

Break-even analysis can also be viewed from a graphical perspective (Figure 4-9). The total cost line starts at a level of $10,000 because of the fixed costs. The total revenue line starts at zero, because there is no revenue if there are zero patients. Where the revenue line and the total cost line intersect, they are equal, and the agency just breaks even. Note that at quantities of patients less than the break-even point, the cost line is higher than the revenue line. This means that for that volume, the total costs are more than the total revenues. The organization will lose money. At quantities of patients above the break-even point, the revenue line is higher than the costs, and a profit is made.

Break-even analyses can focus on the number of patient days needed to break even or on the total number of patients, surgeries, clinic visits, or other appropriate volume measures.

When there are various types of patients, break-even analysis becomes more complicated. The formula presented at the beginning of this section assumes that there are only one price and one variable cost, and therefore one contribution margin. If there are different types of patients with different prices and different variable costs,

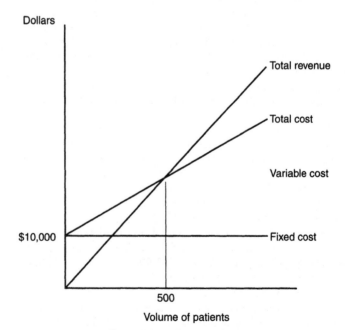

Figure 4-9 Break-even analysis.

it is necessary to find a weighted average contribution margin. This weighted average can be divided into the fixed costs to find the break-even volume for all patients.

For example, suppose that there are three classes of home care visits, which will be referred to here as complex, moderate, and simple. The prices for the visits are $80, $50, and $30, and the variable costs for the visits are $55, $30, and $20, respectively. The contribution margin for each type of patient can be calculated by subtracting the variable cost from the price, as follows:

	Price		Variable Cost		Contribution Margin
Complex	$80	–	$55	=	$25
Moderate	$50	–	$30	=	$20
Simple	$30	–	$20	=	$10

The crucial piece of information for calculating the break-even point is the relative proportion of each type of visit. The management of the home health agency expects that 20% of all visits are complex, 30% are moderate, and 50% are simple. This information can be used to determine a weighted average contribution margin. This requires multiplying each type of visit's individual contribution margin by the percentage of patients receiving that type of visit. The results are added together to get an overall weighted contribution margin, as follows:

Visit Type	Percentage of Visits		Contribution Margin		Weighted Average Contribution Margin
Complex	20%	×	$25	=	$ 5
Moderate	30%	×	$20	=	$ 6
Simple	50%	×	$10	=	$ 5
TOTAL WEIGHTED AVERAGE CONTRIBUTION MARGIN					$ 16

This $16 weighted contribution margin (CM) represents the average contribution margin for all types of visits. It can be used to calculate the break-even quantity. Assume that fixed costs are $10,000. The break-even quantity of visits is:

$$Q = \frac{FC}{P - VC} = \frac{FC}{CM}$$

or

$$Q = \frac{\$10,000}{\$16} = 625 \text{ visits}$$

Of the total of 625 visits needed to break even, 20%, or 125, would be expected to be complex; 30%, or 188, would be moderate; and 50%, or 312, would be simple.

This method works for three different types of patients. What if there were more than three types? The same weighted average approach that can be used to find the break-even volume when there are three different types of patients could be used even if there were hundreds of different types of patients, as is the case with the Medicare DRG system. Similarly, for outpatient care, patients can fall into a number of different categories.

What if there is more than one price for each type of patient? Medicaid pays one price, Medicare another, HMOs another, and self-pay yet another. This still can work within the same framework that has been presented. It would be necessary to calculate a weighted average contribution margin treating each payer for each type of patient as a separate group. For example, if Medicaid pays $40 per visit regardless of the type of visit, and the other payment rates are the same as indicated earlier, the contribution margin by type of patient by payer would be as follows:

	Price	Variable Cost	Contribution Margin
Complex Medicaid	$40	$55	($15)
Complex other	$80	$55	$25
Moderate Medicaid	$40	$30	$10
Moderate other	$50	$30	$20
Simple Medicaid	$40	$20	$20
Simple other	$30	$20	$10

If it is possible to anticipate the percentage of patients whose bills will be paid by Medicaid, a weighted average contribution margin can be estimated. Assume that 10% of all patients are in the category of complex Medicaid, and 10% are in the category of complex other. Assume that 20% of all patients are in the category of moderate Medicaid, and 10% of all patients are in the category of moderate other. Assume that 30% of all patients are in the category of simple Medicaid, and 20% of all patients are in the category of simple other. The weighted contribution margin would be:

Visit Type	Percentage of Visits		Contribution Margin		Weighted Average Contribution Margin
Complex Medicaid	10%	×	($15)	=	($ 1.50)
Complex other	10%	×	$25	=	$ 2.50
Moderate Medicaid	20%	×	$10	=	$ 2.00
Moderate other	10%	×	$20	=	$ 2.00
Simple Medicaid	30%	×	$20	=	$ 6.00
Simple other	20%	×	$10	=	$ 2.00
TOTAL WEIGHTED AVERAGE CONTRIBUTION MARGIN					$13.00

The break-even volume could then be calculated as follows:

$$Q = \frac{FC}{P - VC} = \frac{FC}{CM}$$

or

$$Q = \frac{\$10,000}{\$13} = 769 \text{ visits}$$

The number of visits of any type could be determined by multiplying the 769 break-even volume times the percent of patients in any given class. For example, because 30% of the patients are in the Medicaid simple category, 30% of 769, or 231 patients, would be expected at the break-even level.

Using Break-Even Analysis for Decision Making

If a particular service is expected to have a volume of activity well in excess of the break-even point, managers must make a clear-cut decision about starting or continuing the service. If the volume is too low to break even, several options exist.

One approach is to lower the volume needed to break even. There are three ways to reduce the required break-even level. One approach is to lower the fixed costs.

In some cases, it might be possible to do that. Another alternative would be to increase prices. Price increases would increase the contribution margin per patient. They would also have the effect of lowering the break-even point. However, price increases might reduce the expected volume. In that case, the price increases would be defeating their purpose. Also, prices are sometimes regulated and beyond the control of the organization. Finally, one could try to reduce the variable cost per unit. This might be accomplished by increased efforts to improve efficiency.

If it is not feasible to change the fixed costs, prices, or variable costs, an organization can try to attract more patients so that the volume will rise above the break-even point. In the example presented, what type of patients would be desirable? The most desirable type of visit is a complex, non-Medicaid visit. Such a patient yields a contribution margin of $25 per patient. The least desirable is a complex Medicaid visit. The contribution margin is negative. For each additional complex Medicaid visit, the agency loses money. In this particular example, the most attractive patient produces the highest revenue. However, the focus should not be on revenue. If the patient who produces the highest revenue also produces extremely high variable costs, that patient might not be as attractive as a patient who produces lower revenue but also much lower variable costs. The attractiveness of additional patients is determined by how much contribution margin they provide to the organization.

Break-Even and Capitation

As managed care has become more and more prevalent, some negotiated contracts call for capitated payments. In such an arrangement, the managed care organization pays the health care provider a set amount for each member for each month. This is called the per member per month (PMPM) payment. Under *capitation*, an increase in the number of services provided to patients will not cause revenues to increase. On the other hand, an increase in the number of members will increase revenues.

Suppose that an HMO were to offer a home health agency $1 per member per month to provide all home care services for all its members. Over the course of a year, revenue would be $12 per member ($1 PMPM times 12 months = $12). Assume that the agency's variable costs are $30 per visit. Furthermore, the agency will have increased fixed costs of $20,000 if it takes the HMO members. How many members would the HMO need to have for the home health agency to break even on the contract?

We can use break-even analysis to calculate the break-even number of members. The fixed costs are $20,000. The variable costs are $30 per visit. The price is $12 per member per year. However, we do not have enough information to calculate the break-even point. This is because we know only the variable cost per visit. We need to know the variable cost per member per year. In order to find the break-even volume of members, it is necessary to predict the utilization levels—that is, the number of home visits each member will have.

Most individuals will not need any visits in a typical year. Suppose that the average person consumes 0.3 visits in a given year.[3] The variable cost for 0.3 visits per year is $9 (the $30 variable cost per visit multiplied by 0.3 visits per year). That $9 represents the

---

[3] To avoid using fractions, HMOs often perform their analyses per thousand members. They would say they expect 300 visits per year per thousand members. That approach would not have an effect on the number of members needed to break even.

variable cost per member per year. We can now calculate the break-even point as follows:

$$Q = \frac{FC}{P - VC}$$

$$Q = \frac{\$10,000}{\$12 - \$9} = 3,333 \text{ members}$$

Both the price and the variable costs in the calculation are per member per year. The quantity calculated represents the number of members needed to break even. If the HMO guarantees 5,000 members, the agency will likely make a profit. If there are only 2,000 members, it will lose money.

What if the agency has other fixed costs as well? Are they needed for the calculation? No. The determination of whether the HMO contract is profitable depends only on the marginal costs of the contract. Fixed costs that exist whether or not the agency contracts with the HMO are not relevant to the decision or calculation. What if the HMO contract did not cause fixed costs to rise? Then the contract would be profitable for the agency as long as the revenue per member per year exceeded the variable cost per member per year.

Break-Even Table for a Start-Up Business or Program

Sometimes it is helpful to prepare a table showing all costs and expected revenue so that lenders and partners/owners can see when the enterprise will break even and start to make a profit—if ever. It should be noted that relatively few start-up programs or businesses make money during the first year or two. Sometimes health care facilities are willing to add a new program that they know will lose money for the foreseeable future, but there are other social, ethical, or financial reasons to go into that business. For example, an obstetric unit may not make money itself (especially if there are a significant number of uninsured, indigent women in the community). However, it may be worth losing some money in that unit because women often bring their whole families in for care wherever they go to give birth. Another reason to take a loss may be that there is no other nearby facility that provides obstetric services, and women and babies might be injured or even die if they have to be transported to a distant facility when they arrive in the emergency department in trouble. Another reason for going into a money-losing program may be that donors will be more generous toward a facility that has such a program, and the donations will more than make up for the direct revenue shortage. A break-even table can often assist the planners to visualize what the fixed-cost/variable cost formulas should tell them mathematically.

Additionally, a break-even table shows the planners exactly at what point the new enterprise is expected to start showing a profit, given the cost and revenue projections, so that they can use the table on a month-to-month basis to track any changes from the projections. This will give them early warning of problems and allow them to make adjustments or abandon the enterprise should the break-even point become unreachable. Table 4-1 shows how the expenses and projected revenue will affect the new enterprise on a monthly basis. It includes information about the cash flow that will be necessary to sustain the enterprise until the break-even point is reached. (And that can assist planners to determine how much money they will need to borrow to operate the business until it begins to turn a profit.)

TABLE 4-1 Break-Even Analysis Table for a New Enterprise or Program (All Numbers in Dollars)

	January	February	March	April	May[5]	June	July	August	September
PROFIT ANALYSIS									
Revenues									
Sales		5,000.00	7,000.00	10,000.00	15,000.00	20,000.00	25,000.00	30,000.00	30,000.00
Interest on Savings[1]	0.00	218.40	8.19	6.60	4.58	4.24	3.89	15.35	15.35
Total Revenues	0.00	5,218.40	7,008.19	10,006.60	15,004.58	20,004.24	25,003.89	30,015.35	30,015.35
Expenses									
Salaries	9,000.00	9,000.00	9,000.00	9,000.00	9,000.00	9,000.00	12,000.00	12,000.00	12,000.00
Office Supplies	2,000.00	800.00	500.00	100.00	100.00	100.00	100.00	100.00	100.00
Depreciation	83.33	83.33	83.33	83.33	83.33	83.33	83.33	83.33	83.33
Utilities	500.00	500.00	500.00	500.00	500.00	500.00	500.00	500.00	500.00
Office Rent	1,000.00	1,000.00	1,000.00	1,000.00	1,000.00	1,000.00	1,000.00	1,000.00	1,000.00
Interest on Loan[2]	583.33	583.33	500.00	416.67	333.33	250.00	166.67	83.33	
Total Expenses	11,583.33	11,966.67	11,583.33	11,100.00	11,016.67	10,933.33	13,683.33	13,683.33	13,683.33
Profit/(Loss)	(11,583.33)	(6,748.26)	(4,575.14)	(1,093.40)	3,987.92	9,070.90	11,320.56	16,332.01	16,332.01
CASH FLOW ANALYSIS									
Beginning Cash Balance	0.00	52,416.67	1,966.67	1,583.33	1,100.00	1,016.67	933.33	3,683.33	3,683.33
Loan Receipt	70,000.00								
Total Rev. from above	0.00	5,218.40	7,008.19	10,006.60	15,004.58	20,004.24	25,003.89	30,015.35	30,015.35
Total Exp. From above	(11,583.33)	(11,966.67)	(11,583.33)	(11,100.00)	(11,016.67)	(10,933.33)	(13,683.33)	(13,683.33)	(13,683.33)
Purchase of Furniture	(5,000.00)								
Office Deposit	(1,000.00)								
Loan Repayment[3]		(10,000.00)	(10,000.00)	(10,000.00)	(10,000.00)	(10,000.00)	(10,000.00)	(10,000.00)	
Ending Cash Balance[4]	52,416.67	1,966.67	1,583.33	1,100.00	1,016.67	933.33	3,683.33	3,683.33	20,015.35

Notes:
1. Interest revenue - it is assumed that 5% interest is earned for a period on any cash balance at the end of the previous period.
2. Interest expense - it is also assumed that 10% interest is paid on the loan for any loan balance owed at the beginning of a period.
3. Loan repayments are assumed to be paid on the last day of the month in which they are made.
4. The cash balance at the end of one month becomes the beginning cash balance for the next month.
5. May is the break-even month in this table.

A break-even analysis may be the most important part of your plan for starting a new program within an existing facility or for starting an entirely new enterprise. It identifies the period of time during which the business must be operated at a loss—and most new businesses operate at a loss for some period of time. It shows the month-to-month expenditures and revenue flows and how the income pays for the monthly expenses as well as how much of the income is used to pay off debts and start-up costs. Finally, it shows when the income has paid off the start-up costs, debts, and operating expenses and when a surplus of funds begins to accrue. The point at which the income totals finally equal all the costs is the break-even point. After that, there should be excess revenue over expenses, and of cash inflows over cash outflows. It should be noted that not all cash inflows are revenue (for example, when you borrow money, that is not considered to be revenue) and not all cash outflows are considered to be expenses (for example, when you buy furniture it is not considered to be an expense when you buy it, but rather becomes an expense, called depreciation, gradually over time as you use it).

It is important to realize that the break-even point may come early or it may come late. In an unprofitable business, it never comes at all. The break-even point is usually highly dependent upon volume of business. If every transaction produces some excess of revenue over expenses, that excess is the profit from the transaction. However, there may have been significant start-up loans that have to be paid off. The loan may be from the owners to themselves. A break-even point must be calculated for new programs in an existing business too. There is no hard-and-fast rule about how quickly a business must achieve its break-even point and start to turn a profit. However, many small programs are expected to turn a profit within a few months or a year at the outside. As a general rule of thumb, few investors will be interested in an endeavor that doesn't turn a profit within the first 2 to 3 years. There are several ways to present break-even analysis information. Table 4-1 is one good way, but there are others. It is most important that the visual presentation allow planners to understand quickly how the expenses and revenues interact to produce a financial outcome, and to understand the time periods of loss, break-even, and profitability for the new enterprise.

Preparing a break-even analysis table and cash flow analysis such as the presentation in Table 4-1 can also assist planners in determining how much money they need to borrow to ensure that they do not run out of cash to pay expenses before the enterprise begins to turn a profit. Essentially, the planners must figure out how much money they will need to cover expenses during the months when the business is increasing. Of course, the loan repayments will prolong the time needed to break even. On the other hand, the new enterprise will never have a chance to break even if it is unable to pay wages and salaries, to purchase equipment and supplies, and to pay its bills. Its creditors will quickly stop providing credit, and employees will leave if they do not receive their paychecks. Therefore, break-even analysis must be combined with cash-flow analysis (see Chapter 12) in order to develop a workable budget plan for the new enterprise.

Break-Even Analysis Cautions

A few words of caution are advisable when working with break-even analysis. First of all, once a break-even point has been calculated, one must decide whether it is likely that actual volume will be sufficient to exceed that point. This will require volume forecasts such as those shown in Chapter 6. To the extent that the forecast of volume is incorrect, the decision to go ahead with a new service may turn out to be a bad one, even if the break-even analysis is perfect.

Another potential problem is that break-even analysis assumes that prices and costs are constant. If it can be reasonably expected that prices will fall over time, a higher volume would be needed to keep a service viable unless variable or fixed costs would be falling as well. On the other hand, if prices are expected to rise faster than costs, a marginal service today may become profitable over time, even without an increase in volume.

Another consideration is that there is an assumption that the mix of patients will stay constant. Suppose that in the previous example, over time there are more and more patients in the category of Medicaid complex. The contribution margin for such patients is negative. If the demographics of the population are such that a shift in mix in that direction is likely, the results of the break-even analysis require very close scrutiny. Will there be enough of those patients to shift a profitable service over to a loss?

As with all budgeting tools, judgment is essential. The nurse manager must, through experience, insight, and thought, examine the assumptions of any modeling technique and also consider the reasonableness of the results. If a result does not seem to make sense, it is often because it does **not** make sense. However, break-even analysis is a tool that can help to provide a manager a firm starting point in understanding whether a project or service is likely to be financially viable.

■ ACTIVITY-BASED COSTING

Activity-based costing (ABC) is a relatively new approach to determining costs. In the last half of the 1990s, ABC started to become used widely by health care organizations. The approach is based on the observation that costs are incurred because of specific activities. In most costing methods, costs are assigned to cost centers and patients on the basis of some measure of volume, such as patient days, visits, or hours. For example, OR costs are assigned to patients based on minutes in the OR. From an ABC perspective, it is not necessarily the amount of time but rather the specific activities that generate costs. Based on this notion, managers need to focus on the actions that drive costs higher. The activities of an organization that cause it to incur costs are referred to as *cost drivers*.

The use of cost drivers to assign costs has the impact of improving accuracy by focusing cost measurement more on a cause-and-effect basis. For example, suppose that a health care organization has a purchasing department that orders many items on a routine basis and some items on a special-order basis. The activity is the placing of orders. However, it is quite possible that a special order will be more costly than a routine order.

The costs of the purchasing departments must be allocated to patients if the organization is to recover its full costs. One common approach to such allocation is based on the number of purchase orders. Departments that generate a lot of purchase orders are assigned a greater share of the costs of the purchasing department. In turn, those costs are allocated to the patients who use the department. This seems to be quite reasonable.

However, if a rush order is an activity that causes purchasing to spend extra money (for the time of the personnel in the department, for express freight costs, etc.), then from an ABC perspective, one would argue that the departments that generate a large number of rush orders should be charged more than the departments that don't, all other things being equal. In other words, costs should not be assigned simply on the basis of the number of purchase orders generated by each department. Within purchasing, the activity of placing a rush order is more costly than the activity of placing a regular order. Rush orders drive costs higher.

The ABC approach requires the manager to analyze the activities of each cost center or department in an organization. The various activities that are cost drivers must be identified. Then costs are assigned to departments and ultimately to patients, based on the amount of cost-driving activities they require.

For example, suppose that an OR has traditionally assigned its costs based on minutes of surgery. A patient who undergoes a 2-hour surgery is charged twice as much as a patient who undergoes a 1-hour surgery. However, one of the costs of surgery is cleaning and preparing the room after every surgery. Suppose that those costs are the same for each surgery, regardless of the length of the surgery. The activity of cleaning and preparing the room should then be charged equally to each surgical patient, rather than being based on the length of the surgical procedure.

This probably means that more allocation bases will be needed. The depreciation cost of the surgical suite may be charged to patients based on the length of the procedure. The cost of cleaning the room may be charged equally per patient. The cost of supplies consumed during the surgery should include the extra cost of any rush orders that were required for the procedure. This will complicate the costing process but will produce substantially more accurate information. ABC proponents argue that most industries really do not have a good sense of which of their products or services are profitable and which lose money. Further, employees may be more cost conscious if they use ABC information.

Consider the purchasing department/operating room examples discussed in this section. The surgery patients who require special-order items are being subsidized under the old costing system. The costs of the rush orders are being spread over all departments that order supplies. This could cause a particular type of surgery to appear more profitable than it is because the true costs of the rush orders are not assigned to the departments and patients that caused the special orders.

However, once the ABC system is in place, that will change. The OR will be charged directly for each special order. It can then assign the order to specific patients who required the rush-order items. This in turn will provide more accurate information about the cost of care for each type of patient. Further, seeing the higher costs resulting from rush orders, the manager of the OR may plan more carefully, thus avoiding the need for many of the rush orders. This will reduce the total costs for the patient, department, and organization.

In terms of routine medical or surgical nursing, using ABC requires an examination of what nurses do and why they do it. ABC works well with the concept of value-added costs. By examining everything we do to determine the cost drivers, we can also assess whether each activity adds value to the patient. If it doesn't, perhaps it can be eliminated. If it does add value, then the cost of the activity should be assigned to the patient who directly benefits from it.

One problem with ABC is deciding how minutely to define activities. Is taking a pulse or blood pressure an activity? Certainly. However, should we determine the cost of that activity and then track how many times each is done for each patient? This is not an easy question. From a clinical perspective, we already track such activities in the patient chart. However, until costing and clinical systems are fully linked, it would require additional data input to track the activity for costing purposes. And what about activities that are necessary but never enter the clinical chart? With ABC, as with any approach to costing, we must always balance the value of more accurate information against the extra cost of collecting that information.

Summary and Implications for Nurse Managers

Assessing costs is a complex topic. In general, costs do not increase in proportion to volume. The implications of this observation are that although money might be lost on a particular program, higher volume may be desired. More patients do not necessarily mean greater losses. It is possible that volume increases can turn a loss into a profit. Understanding how that can happen requires an understanding of cost behavior. Some costs are fixed, whereas other costs are variable. The result of that basic nature of costs is that the cost per patient declines as there is increasing volume. The greater the number of patients who share the fixed costs, the lower the average cost per patient. Costing is further complicated by the fact that because all costs do not vary with volume, there are times when decisions must be based solely on the costs that do vary. This is referred to as relevant costing.

An important part of the budgeting process is the prediction of costs. Estimated costs for the future can be based on historical cost information. Some estimation relies on using the historical information to isolate variable costs from fixed costs. To make such calculations, it is first necessary to convert historical cost information into common or constant dollars. This requires *indexation* of costs for the impact of inflation. Indexation is a process that adjusts a dollar value for the impact of inflation over a period of time by using a *price index*, such as the CPI. A price index is a tool that indicates year-to-year changes in prices. Using indexed historical costs, the results of the cost-estimation process will be in constant dollars. In preparing the next year's budget, the cost estimate has to be adjusted upward by the anticipated inflation rate over the next year.

Once constant-dollar information is available, cost can be estimated by using the high-low method, simple linear regression, or multiple regression analysis. Being able to estimate fixed and variable costs is potentially a valuable tool. In order to apply the results, however, projections of the estimated number of patients, patient days, acuity level, and so forth are needed. Chapter 6 focuses on the process of forecasting such data.

Break-even analysis is a tool that allows one to focus specifically on the quantity of patients needed for a program, project, or service to be financially viable. Its foundations are in fixed and variable costs. At low volumes of patients, the average cost may surpass the revenue per patient. As the number of patients increases, the cost per patient falls as fixed costs are shared. Eventually, the cost per patient falls below the revenue. Break-even analysis allows the manager to determine what the break-even quantity is so that a reasonable decision can be made about the financial viability of a program, project, or service.

From the nurse manager's standpoint, the topics of this chapter have critical implications. At the most basic levels, falling volume will mean rising cost per patient. In such cases it is likely that a revenue crisis will exist, and actions to restrain costs should be immediately contemplated. On the other hand, rising volumes represent an opportunity. They not only bring in more revenue but also decrease the average cost per patient. Therefore, there is the opportunity for profit from more patients and for more profit from each patient. Profits ultimately allow the organization to replace buildings and equipment, add services, add staff, improve quality, and raise salaries.

Additionally, in preparing budgets, nurse managers should take into account the behavior of costs. The fact that certain costs vary in proportion and others are fixed may reorient their thinking from the notion that a 10% increase in volume requires 10% more resources. This in turn can allow managers to prepare budgets in a more sophisticated and exact manner.

Similarly, the use of ABC can assist managers in obtaining a more accurate measure of costs. Accuracy in turn leads to better decisions and ultimately to improved financial results.

References and Suggested Readings

Baker, J.J. (1998). *Activity-based Costing and Activity-based Management for Health Care.* Gaithersburg, MD: Aspen.

Cokins, G. (2001). *Activity-Based Cost Management: An Executive's Guide.* Hoboken, NJ: John Wiley & Sons.

DeNavas-Walt, C., Proctor, B., and Lee, C. (2006). *Income, Poverty, and Health Insurance Coverage in the United States: 2005.* Washington, D.C.: U.S. Department of Commerce, U.S. Census Bureau. Downloaded from http://www.census.gov/ prod/ 2006pubs/p60-231.pdf on March 6, 2007.

Dodson, G.M., Sinclair, V.G., Miller, M., et al. (1998, September-October). Determining cost drivers for pediatric home health services. *Nursing Economic$* 16(5):263-271.

Eldenberg, L., and Wolcott, S. (2004). *Cost Management: Measuring, Monitoring, and Motivating Performance.* Hoboken, NJ: John Wiley & Sons.

Finkler, S.A., and Ward, D.R. (1999). *Cost Accounting for Health Care Organizations: Concepts and Applications*, ed. 2. Gaithersburg, MD: Aspen.

Horngren, C., Datar, S., and Foster, G. (2005). *Cost Accounting*, ed. 12. New York: Prentice Hall.

Leeman, J., and Mark, B. (2006). The chronic care model versus disease management programs: A transaction cost analysis approach. *Health Care Management Review* 31(1):18-25.

McBryde-Foster, M. (2005). Break-even analysis in a nurse-managed center. *Nursing Economic$* 23(1):31-34.

NCHC (National Coalition on Health Care). (2004). *Facts on Health Insurance Coverage.* Washington, D.C.: NCHC. Downloaded from http://www.nchc.org/facts/coverage.shtml on March 6, 2007.

Neumann, B.R., Clement, J.P., and Cooper, J.C. (1999). *Financial Management: Concepts and Applications for Health Care Organizations*, ed. 4. Dubuque, IA: Kendall Hunt.

Ohura, T., Sanada, H., and Mino Y. (2004). Clinical activity-based cost effectiveness of traditional versus modern wound management in patients with pressure ulcers. *Wounds: A Compendium of Clinical Research and Practice* 16(5):157-163, 189-191.

Ory, C., Vanderplas, A., Dezii, C., and Chang, E. (2005). Congestive heart failure: Attributable costs within the managed care setting. *Journal of Pharmaceutical Finance, Economics & Policy* 14(2):87-97.

Pertelle, V. (2005). Activity-based management and costing: Essential tools in competitive bidding. *FOCUS: Journal for Respiratory Care & Sleep Medicine.* pp. 38-40. Downloaded on March 7, 2007 from: http://www.allbusiness. com/government/government-procurement/ 846739-1.html

Ross, T. (2004). Analyzing health care operations using Activity-Based-Costing (ABC). *Journal of Health Care Finance* 30(3):1-20.

Sorensen, D., and Sullivan, D. (2005). Business: Managing trade-offs makes budgeting processes pay off. *Healthcare Financial Management* 59(11):54-58, 60.

Toyabe S., Cao P., Kurashima S., Nakayama Y., Ishii Y., Hosoyama N., and Akazawa K. (2005). Actual and estimated costs of disposable materials used during surgical procedures. *Health Policy* 73(1):52-57.

West, D.A., West, T.D., Balas, E.A., and Micks, L.L. (1996, May-June). Profitable capitation requires accurate costing. *Nursing Economic$* 14(3): 162-170, 150.

Wodchis, W.P. (1998). Applying activity-based costing in long-term care. *Healthcare Management Forum* 11(4):25-32.

Zwillich, T. (2005). 45.8 Million in U.S. Now Lack Health Insurance. *WebMD Health News.* Downloaded March 6, 2007 from http:// www.webmd.com/news/20050830/millions- in-us-now-lack-health-insurance.

Personnel Issues

5

LEARNING OBJECTIVES
The goals of this chapter are to:

- Explain the relationship between nursing shortages and budgeting
- Explain how to lessen the impact of nursing shortages
- Provide some insights into how an organization can work to limit its own nursing shortages through retention and recruitment

- Describe causes of nursing shortages
- Outline the various costs associated with nurse recruitment
- Identify some alternative solutions when staff nurses are in short supply

■ INTRODUCTION

This chapter focuses primarily on some key issues of personnel adequacy, including nursing shortages, nurse recruitment, and nurse retention. Personnel costs are the single largest line item in any nursing budget, and the nursing shortage is having a significant effect on personnel costs in many facilities. Readers familiar with the literature in this area may choose to skip this chapter. It is included in this book because it is critical that all nurse managers with budget responsibility have at least some exposure to these issues.

■ BUDGETING AND NURSING SHORTAGES

The largest part of most operating budgets for nursing units, departments, and organizations consists of *personnel* costs. Getting an operating budget approved is sometimes difficult. Justifying the need for a given level of staff requires careful calculations and lucid arguments. However, in preparing an operating budget, it is often assumed that hiring the amount of labor approved in the final budget is not a problem. This is not necessarily the case in nursing. Nursing shortages occurred on and off throughout the last half of the 20th century. The existence of budgeted but vacant positions is a common occurrence. It also creates a great deal of budgeting difficulty.

At the time the reader is using this book, there may or may not be a nursing shortage. However, issues related to recruitment, retention, and the impact of nursing shortages on the budget-preparation process are critical parts of budgeting. History has shown that nursing shortages occur from time to time, and at the time this book is being written, there is a growing nursing shortage in the United States—a shortage that is predicted to extend at least until near the end of the baby boom generation, approximately until the year 2020 (Buerhaus, 2000; Nevidjon & Erickson, 2001). Buerhaus made it clear that not only will there be a nursing shortage, but by 2010, the average age of RNs will be over 45 years, with more than 40% of the nurses over age 50. It is a physical reality that the average person over age 50 simply does not have the energy or physical stamina that people have in their 20s and 30s. Thus, it may be necessary to lower workloads somewhat so that the existing workforce can manage the job. This will mean higher staffing costs. Nurse managers today would do well to discuss the issue of an aging work force with the facility's top administration so that plans can be made to deal not only with the shortage, but also with a rapidly aging workforce. Finally, there is a trend among employees today to value personal leisure time over extra money (Nevidjon & Erickson, 2001). The desire for more leisure or personal time may be exacerbated by an aging workforce that is too tired to work extra shifts and double shifts to make up for shortages in the units. This factor may further exacerbate the shortage of nurses.

Nurse managers should be prepared to work through the budget process to lessen the impact of such shortages on their organizations when they occur. Therefore, this chapter considers a topic that is essential reading for the foreseeable future for nurse managers who must staff their facilities. Not only will there be an absolute shortage of nurses, the nurses one does have may not be nearly as productive as nurses were when the manager was a young staff nurse. Also conflict may arise between the older nurses who are too tired to accept a lot of overtime and for whom on-call work is a major problem. The younger nurses will not accept the total burden of covering the shortage and on-call duty. But a younger nurse isn't likely to suffer physically from the demands of extra work. Many people over 50 are simply not capable of functioning competently after working a full day and then being awakened at night to come in to staff an emergency or unexpected admission. Because of these factors, clinical facilities will almost certainly have to increase their staffing levels at least somewhat. Unfortunately, this need comes at a most difficult time when positions are going to be hard to fill, so there may be extra vacancies.

If vacant positions are left unstaffed throughout the year, two potentially serious side effects occur. The first is that the nurses working on a unit begin to suffer burnout as the result of being overburdened. Shortages of staff lead to overwork, poor morale, increased sick leave, and other stress-related problems. These stress-related problems will increase dramatically as the staff ages and many of the nurses reach ages ranging from 50 to 65. That, in turn, may well lead to even more resignations and early retirements because the older nurses will not be able to carry the excess workload caused by the vacancies. Those losses will then further exacerbate the staffing shortages on the units.

The second side effect involves one of two possibilities. One possibility is that the facility will replace the vacancies with agency nurses. In most cases, the unit must pay between 3 and 4 times the regular staff hourly rate for an agency nurse. (See Chapter 8 for a discussion of budgeting for a unit that uses agency nurses.) Obviously, heavy use of agency staff will not only greatly raise the staffing costs for the facility, but it may also engender dissatisfaction among the permanent staff, who will inevitably find out that agency nurses earn many more dollars per hour than the regular staff. The work of unit organization and quality maintenance will fall more heavily on permanent staff because agency staff are so temporary that it is not uncommon that they do not have to share the unit's committee work.

The second possibility is that the health care organization starts to assume that less money will be spent than has been put into the budget. Positions are approved with the expectation that they will never be filled. Eventually, if staff is finally available to be hired, the organization may resist filling the positions because it has made its overall plans based on the expectation that the money allocated for those positions would never be spent. The approved but vacant positions provide top management with a cushion to ease the impact of other unexpected financial problems throughout the year. Essentially, the budgeted but unfilled positions may be permanently lost. Worse, some financial managers have, in the past, gotten so used to high vacancy rates that they create, in essence, a shadow budget. Whereas the unit manager's budget shows a certain amount for staffing costs, the financial manager bases the organization-wide budget on the assumption that a certain percentage will not be spent because of vacancies. Then when the positions are filled, the financial manager tries to hold the unit manager to the staffing costs in the shadow budget rather than those in the correct budget. Sometimes the financial manager even refuses to allow the positions to be filled. This effectively lowers the nursing care hours per patient day, procedure, or visit on a permanent basis. Unfortunately, because most nurse staffing costs are based on patient care requirements, that leads to guaranteed insufficient levels of care in the unit. Nurses know when their patients are not receiving proper nursing care and may become demoralized by the poor care that is all they are permitted to provide. That situation tends to lead to even more resignations as the result of the exhaustion and demoralization of the staff.

In any case, failure to use the vacancy money to replace staff with agency or per diem nurses or to pay for voluntary overtime for nurses who want that extra work may look good to some non-nursing managers. But it is actually likely to seriously exacerbate the facility's staffing problems. Replacing permanent staff with agency staff creates additional budgeting difficulties because of the cost of overtime and agency nurses. On a per-hour basis, both overtime and agency nurses are significantly more expensive than the cost of a full-time staff member being paid on a straight-time basis. This excess hourly cost is partially offset if the position does not need to be staffed every day. However, when the hospital hires an agency nurse, the contract is typically for a period of approximately 12 to 13 weeks at a minimum. And that nurse must be paid, regardless of workload. Thus, to maintain an adequate level of quality of care, vacancies often result in higher staffing costs—but only if agency nurses can be obtained. It may be difficult to determine whether the net effect will be greater or less spending than would occur if the vacant positions were filled.

An attempt must be made to budget on the basis of the expected **actual** staffing pattern, which should be based on the expected workload. If the equivalent of 12 full-time employees is authorized in a budget, the dollars in the budget should be based on the best expectation of how those 12 full-time equivalent (FTE) employee positions will be staffed. If the most likely event is that the unit will be able to have 11 regular full-time staff members, but that the 12th position will be covered by 1,200 hours of agency nurse time, the budget should replace the cost of the 12th staff member with the cost of 1,200 agency nurse hours. In order for such a calculation to be made, it is critical to have some idea as to whether the 12th position will be staffed by hiring a staff member or using agency nurses. Alternatively, the 12th position could be covered by regular staff overtime.

Regular staff overtime can be attractive to a financial manager. It is far cheaper to pay 1.5 times the regular salary (time and one-half) than 4 times the salary of a regular staff member. Because the benefits for that full time nurse are already paid, the facility saves the benefit costs of hiring a new permanent staff member. That can be a danger to the unit managers. We have seen hospitals where the financial officer decided to approve overtime liberally instead of refilling permanent staff vacancies because doing so can be significantly cheaper for the facility. It saves the extra cost of a second person's benefits and, of course, the overtime is never used unless there is a staff shortage. When a permanent replacement person is hired, not only does the facility have to pay for another benefits package but also, that nurse will report to work as scheduled, even if workload is down. It should be noted that floating and giving excess nurses the day off will not eliminate all excess staffing on low-workload days.

Another approach is to revise the manner in which nursing care is offered. Nursing units can be reorganized to make greater use of alternative types of personnel. Or else computers could be acquired in an effort to reduce the number of nursing hours needed for documentation. It is likely that attempts to introduce shared governance, clinical ladders, case management, alternative staffing power, or computers will have an impact on the actual spending of a nursing unit. These expected changes and their costs should be built into the budget. (See Chapter 8 for a discussion of budgeting for these special staffing cases.)

Some health care organizations attempt to stretch their available staff over the existing number of patients when an adequate number of nurses cannot be recruited. Such stretching can only mean fewer nursing hours per patient day and a lower quality of care. It is the obligation of the organization and its employees to be explicit in addressing both the problem and its ultimate impact on care. Such explicit recognition is not only ethically correct but is also likely to push the organization to work harder to resolve the problem of its nursing shortages.

Therefore, before the development of operating budgets can be discussed fully in Chapter 8, it is important to address issues that are related to nursing recruitment and retention as well as to alternative models of providing patient care. This is the topic of the remainder of this chapter.

■ THE NURSING SHORTAGE AND ITS CAUSES

Has there really been a nursing shortage? The answer to this question is clearly yes. There have been unfilled positions. Many health care organizations have not been able to hire as many RNs as they have wanted to. Has this shortage been caused by drastic reductions in the number of nurses? Perhaps surprisingly, the answer to that question is no. There are more nurses working as nurses today than ever before. But there is also an increased need for nurses.

Most of this increase may be accounted for by increasing levels of patient acuity (Buerhaus, 2000). As the Medicare Diagnosis Related Groups prospective payment system began to take effect in the 1980s, lengths of stay in hospitals dropped. Because earlier discharge eliminated the least acute inpatient days, the average acuity level of the remaining inpatient days rose. On average, patients were sicker each day they were in the hospital because patients no longer stayed in the hospital as inpatients during the days when they did not need extensive nursing care. This trend increased because of pressure from managed care organizations in the 1990s, because of the pressures of the aging population in the United States, and because of advancing medical science, which has allowed many procedures to be moved to outpatient settings and has produced costly inpatient treatments for many diseases that were formerly untreatable. Therefore, the average inpatient day requires more nursing care. At the same time, demand for nurses for home care, primary care, and other types of ambulatory care has also grown at a rapid rate.

The long-term trends concerning the availability of adequate numbers of RNs do not appear to be favorable. The aging of the American population constantly increases the demand for nurses. At the other end of the spectrum, there have been a declining number of people in the college-age group. Thus, as the need for nurses will probably continue to increase, the pool of people available to become nurses will not keep pace. The shortage of nurses is projected to be at least 800,000 by 2020 (Buerhaus, 2000). Finally, the ages of nurses in the United States force us to recognize that a high retirement rate during the next 10 years will make it very difficult to increase the numbers of nurses and to replace those retiring (AACN, 2006). The average age of U.S. RNs in 2004 was 46.8 years; that is a year older than the average age in 2000 (AACN, 2007). Not only has the average age of nurses increased, but the age of students in all basic nursing programs has increased. Therefore, the nursing profession is now and will continue to be affected strongly by retirements for the foreseeable future. Worse, the median age of the full-time nursing faculty during the 2003-2004 academic year was approximately 51.4 years (AACN, 2006) and was reported to have increased to approximately 53 years in 2006. And because of low pay, nursing schools have had a difficult time recruiting nurses into the teaching field. Many nurses now choose to remain in clinical care rather than obtain a terminal degree because the cost of acquiring a doctoral degree is no longer likely to be adequately compensated by faculty pay. So the faculty positions vacated by retiring teachers are not consistently able to be filled by nurses willing to sacrifice the pay available in practice for a life in academia—even assuming that there are nurses with the requisite academic degrees available. Given these facts, the wise nurse administrator will put resources and effort into both recruitment of nurses needed to fill expected vacancies and into efforts to retain the nurses already employed.

The shortage of nurses is also at least partly the result of the feminist movement, which has inspired proportionately more women to move away from traditionally female jobs than it has encouraged men to move into such jobs. Prior to the 1970s, strange as it may seem to women of today, many schools that served a traditionally male student group refused to admit women or strongly discouraged them from applying. Scholarships were often allocated only to male students, even if women could obtain admission. Should a woman surmount the barriers in academe, male managers would often refuse to hire women, regardless of their educational levels, as lawyers, mathematicians, engineers, accountants, business managers, or other traditionally male professions. Thus, many women found themselves effectively limited to careers as school teachers, nurses, or executive secretaries if they wanted a more professional job than that of waitress or another blue-collar job. Fortunately, society has changed radically in terms of the opportunities open to women. But an unfortunate side effect has been that fewer women willing to seek post high school education are entering nursing—at least not as a first choice. As growing numbers of college-eligible women seek out employment as physicians, engineers, accountants, and lawyers, fewer women are becoming nurses. When women do choose nursing, it is often after they have tried another field. Thus, they are older when they become nurses—and this further shortens the career years for many nurses.

Another problem that occurs in recruiting and retaining nurses is that the nursing profession has not managed to overcome many serious image problems perpetuated by a wide variety of stereotypes that do not accurately reflect the profession. The actual degree of responsibility and autonomy of nurses is often depicted unfairly. This may have made it especially difficult to recruit ethnic minorities and men into nursing.

At times when a national shortage of nurses occurs, solutions have to be national in scope. They may involve major media campaigns by nursing associations to change nursing's image. They may involve federal infusions of cash to schools of nursing in the forms of scholarship money or education loan forgiveness to nurses willing to serve in faculty roles. In fact, the only times in post World War II history that the nursing shortage has been eliminated (or significantly reduced) have been during times when the federal government has underwritten the costs of nursing education for large numbers of students. Many other national approaches have been suggested. Increases in the rate of pay for nurses may have a strong enough impact to eliminate shortages, but it takes time before wage increases can have much overall impact because of the years of education required once a person decides to go into nursing. To the extent that pay raises eliminate shortages, they fail to resolve many long-range problems, and shortages may occur again in the future as raises for nurses begin to lag when there is no existing shortage.

The remainder of this chapter is confined to the actions that individual nurse managers can take or should be aware of in their management of nursing within their organizations. A given organization may be relatively helpless when it comes to overcoming the entire industry-wide nursing shortage. However, organizations have a great degree of control over the availability of nurses to fulfill their own staffing needs.

■ RETENTION OF STAFF

The most effective personnel strategy a health care organization can use is to work at retaining the staff it already has. The national shortage of nurses means that every experienced nurse recruited must be hired away from another institution, so it is clear that recruiting nurses requires a costly amount of competition. Therefore, major efforts should be made to reduce undesirable turnover. One program that has been associated with extremely high staff retention is the Magnet Award program through the American Nurses Credentialing Center (ANCC).

Magnet Hospitals

The Magnet recognition program was developed in 1993 by the ANCC. It was founded on a landmark study by a team of nurse researchers (McClure et al., 1983) who wished to study factors associated with hospitals' ability to recruit and retain nurses. They studied a group of hospitals noted for successful recruitment and retention rates of their nurses. They called these hospitals Magnet hospitals because they were magnets for nurses. McClure and her research team identified 14 factors common to the Magnet hospitals and called them forces of magnetism. These factors are the foundation of the ANCC's Magnet Hospital program (ANCC, 2005) today and are as follows:

- Quality of nursing leadership
- Management style

- Organizational structure
- Personnel policies and programs
- Image of nursing in the facility
- Autonomy of the nurses
- Nurses as teachers
- Professional development opportunities for nurses
- Professional models of nursing care
- Quality of care
- Quality improvements
- Consultation and resources available to nursing
- Community and the hospital
- Interdisciplinary relationships.

Achievement of the Magnet Award requires considerable time and effort to document how the facility has fulfilled the Magnet criteria. To be successful, a facility must allocate at least one nursing management FTE to the effort for a minimum of 1 year and more realistically, 2 to 3 years. Additionally, the entire top management team must support the effort because that Magnet manager will need their cooperation to make changes in nursing policies, practices, and procedures that may prove initially to be expensive. For example, the hospital will have to commit resources to nurses' professional development. Sending nurses to educational programs outside the hospital will be necessary in some cases, and that can be an expensive endeavor. It is not unusual for travel, lodging, meals, and registration fees to exceed $1,000 for a single conference for one attendee.

The Magnet manager will require the authority to examine all aspects of nursing practice throughout the facility. The Magnet research found that being able to provide high-quality, excellent care to patients was important to nurses. When quality problems are found, the Magnet manager must have the authority to address them. It may be a precept of quality gurus that "quality doesn't cost, quality failures cost." Unfortunately, that truism is more obvious in manufacturing where quality problems are called "wastage" than in service industries like nursing, in which quality problems may seem to have no consequences. As a result, people are sometimes very reluctant to correct quality problems—especially when the correction incurs costs that appear unnecessary to the unit manager.

The entire nursing department must commit to building strong and positive relationships among the nurses, physicians, therapists, and dietitians—in short, throughout the entire care team. Positive and collaborative interdisciplinary relationships are a key component of a Magnet facility. The traditional hospital hierarchy in which physicians give orders to nurses but may not consult with them in patient care, or in which nurses send down dietary orders but do not consult with the dietitian to provide the best possible patient care does not meet Magnet criteria.

It is not merely the Magnet study that has found that interdisciplinary collaboration is a good thing. The Magnet study found that positive interdisciplinary relationships are important for nurse retention, and another study found that such relationships have an impact on patient care outcomes. In 1986, the acute physiology and chronic health evaluation (APACHE) research team published the results of part of their research, which found a significantly lower mortality rate among patients in intensive care units that exhibited positive interactions and coordination among the staff (physicians and nurses) than in units where poor relationships existed among the physicians and nurses (Knaus et al., 1986). It has long been an unfortunate reality that relationships between physicians and nurses have been difficult in many hospitals.

An extremely unfortunate "secret" in hospitals has been the fact that some physicians feel free to verbally and even physically abuse nurses (Sofield & Salmond, 2003). All too often, when physicians abused nurses, management looked the other way or worse, threatened the nurses with termination if they attempted to obtain legal redress against physicians who abused them. In this way, hospital administrators gave tacit permission to physicians to behave badly, even criminally in some cases. Shamefully, nurse managers have participated in this cover-up of abuse of their own nurses. Abuse is highly correlated with a nurse's intent to leave the facility (Sofield & Salmond, 2003). Those who think abuse toward nurses is a rare event should review the Canadian study in which 41% of the nurses reported at least one incident of abuse during their past five shifts. Although most of the abuse was verbal, 18% involved physical abuse (Duncan et al., 2001). Patients were the most frequent offenders in the Canadian study, but physicians were also frequent abusers. In a similar study in Minnesota, 13.2% of the 4,977 nurses who returned the questionnaires claimed they had been physically assaulted at work in the previous 12 months. Worse, 51% of the victims reported that management had done absolutely nothing to address the problem or make sure that it did not happen again (Nachreiner et al., 2005).

These studies suggest that at least some hospitals that wish to seek Magnet status will have significant work to do in the area of improving physician-nurse relationships and in developing and implementing zero-tolerance policies toward physical, verbal, and sexual abuse of all members of the staff. Because abuse of nurses was found to be an important factor in turnover, the administration will have to develop zero-tolerance policies and strictly enforce those policies—regardless of the status of the offender and his or her reason for the abuse. Any administration that is not willing to tackle this issue head-on need not bother to seek Magnet status—and should expect continued high turnover rates. The cost of improved recruitment and retention will be partially monetary. But it will also involve effort, thinking, realigning some priorities and values, and the expenditure of significant human effort. The rewards, however, may astonish the hospital's administration.

Several Chief Executive Officers (CEOs) or Chief Financial Officers (CFOs) of major hospitals that had achieved Magnet certification were interviewed on video about the results of obtaining Magnet status (ANCC, 2006). Kevin Hammeran, CFO of Miami Children's hospital, claimed the program had saved their hospital millions of dollars a year in reduced turnover. Additionally, they had improved their operating margin at least 10 points since achieving Magnet status. Britt Berrett, CEO of Medical City Dallas Hospital in Dallas, Texas, noted that their hospital's patient satisfaction ratings were the best in the history of the hospital and their financial performance had never been better since they had achieved Magnet status. Dennis Brimhall, CEO of the University of Colorado, reported that their bond rating had improved as a result of achieving Magnet status.

Nursing Satisfaction

A key benefit of changing hospital operations so that Magnet certification can be achieved is that the kinds of standards involved in being a Magnet hospital are important satisfiers for the nurses. One primary element of nursing satisfaction is the development of professionalism in the delivery of health care services through a combination of increased autonomy and the availability of a variety of resources for professional growth and development. Nurses must feel like professionals and be treated as professionals in order to be happy in their employment. The improved management strategies, patient care quality, interdisciplinary collaboration, and professionalism that nurses experience in the Magnet model have consistently been cited as key factors in improved nurse satisfaction. That higher level of satisfaction, in turn, leads to better recruitment and retention.

A positive attitude toward nursing and professional treatment by physicians can be critical factors in having a satisfied staff. Indeed, these factors also have been shown to have an effect on patient survival in intensive care units (Knaus et al., 1986). The administration too must respect the nursing staff. Negative attitudes by these groups are quickly discerned by nurses and may cause significant unhappiness on the part of the staff. The view of nurses by physicians and administrators ties in with the overall issue of the image of nurses. The institution has little control over the national image of nursing. However, it can take strides toward creating a positive image internally. The way nurses are treated and the way nursing is presented to patients can make a substantial difference in the attitudes of nurses as well as the attitudes of the rest of the organization's staff—and, of course, in patient satisfaction. Image building begins with actions taken by nursing to create a positive image. Programs involving physicians and administration can be suggested by nursing administration if they are not forthcoming otherwise.

A positive attitude is demonstrated primarily by the firm expectation that all communications with nurses will be respectful and professional. Screaming at nurses, name calling, and other forms of verbal violence, as well as physical violence, toward members of the nursing staff must be recognized as being inappropriate and unacceptable and must not be tolerated. In fact, these behaviors could subject the facility to stiff fines and damage awards resulting from the creation of a hostile working environment for nurses. The law is clear: no person has to accept physical or verbal abuse as a condition of employment. Administrators who overlook or make excuses for the behavior of out-of-control physicians are giving permission for abuse of their nurses. Failure on the part of administration to discipline, immediately and firmly, physicians and anyone else who behaves abusively to nurses is a clear sign of disrespect of nurses, which can (and should) increase turnover.

The issue of financial payment is, of course, relevant. High salaries and good benefits help to keep staff from wanting to look elsewhere. It is also necessary that there be ample opportunity for advancement, either into management or on a clinical track. Many hospitals have instituted clinical ladders that allow nurses to advance in their careers while still providing patient care.

Flexible hours have also become a key element in retaining staff. A wide variety of alternative working hours have been developed by organizations attempting to recruit new nurses. These flexible arrangements must be made available to existing staff as well, or they may become dissatisfied and move to an organization that offers such hours.

From a budgeting perspective, this can become complex. The use of four 10-hour shifts to create a 4-day workweek is not necessarily a major budgeting problem. Although it may create a complicated staffing pattern for coverage, it still results in the same 40 hours of pay for 40 hours of work as 5 days of 8 hours. It will, however, require access to part-time nurses willing to work 4 to 5 hour shifts to cover the

4 or 5 hours in the day not covered by two 10-hour shifts. On the other hand, innovations such as three 12-hour shifts or two 12-hour weekend shifts, for 40 hours of pay and full benefits, can create a variety of budgeting complications. Clear decisions must be made concerning whether an FTE employee represents 40 hours of work or 40 hours of pay. (See Chapter 8 for further discussion.)

Fringe Benefits

Clearly, one of the elements of nursing satisfaction is related to the organization's employee benefits, commonly referred to as *fringe benefits*. How many weeks of vacation do staff get each year? How many paid holidays are there? Is free life insurance provided to employees? Those are several of the most obvious employee benefits. Some benefits are required by law. For example, the employer must pay the FICA tax for social security that is intended eventually to provide the employee with a social security pension. The employer must also pay unemployment insurance and workmen's compensation insurance. Most benefits, however, are voluntary or are the result of labor negotiations.

Other critical benefits concern the quality of the health insurance package offered to employees. Do nurses have to contribute to the cost of their health insurance? If so, how much? Are their family members covered? If so, what is the additional cost to the nurse? Are staff members subject to *co-payments* and *deductibles* on their health insurance? A co-payment means that the insurer bears a portion of the cost (often 70% or 80%) and the employee bears the remainder (usually 20% or 30%). A deductible means that 100% of some amount must first be paid by the employee before there are any health benefits (usually anywhere from $200 to $2,000 per year).

Most employers also offer a variety of other benefits that are somewhat less obvious and are more responsible for the term "fringe benefits" as opposed to employee benefits. For example, if the CEO belongs to a golf club and the membership is paid for by the organization, that is a fringe benefit. If the CEO drives a company-owned car, that is another example of a fringe benefit.

In terms of the budget, the fringe benefits referred to really represent several different types of cost. The vacation and holiday time for each employee is already built into the annual salary cost for that individual. There is no need to budget for that fringe benefit, except for making sure that there is adequate staff coverage for all days off. This is accounted for by budgeting additional personnel (see Chapter 8). On the other hand, the cost of life insurance, pension payments, social security taxes, tuition reimbursement, health insurance, and other fringe benefits that require cash outlays must be budgeted for explicitly.

In most organizations, the specific costs of the fringe benefits are calculated by the finance office and are assigned to departments on the basis of salaries, usually as a percentage. For example, a nursing unit might be charged 28% for fringe benefits for every dollar of salary paid to its staff. Certainly, not all employees have the same cost to the organization per dollar of salary. This is simply an average. Is it fair? It might well be that certain fringe benefits are worth more to employees of some departments than to employees of other departments. However, over the years it has been decided that it is not worth the effort to seek a more refined measure of costs. Therefore, budgeting for fringe benefits generally requires only the addition of a set percentage (provided by the finance office) to the budgeted salary amounts.

The Burnout Problem

One key reason for the failure to retain nurses is burnout. This issue is not based primarily on competition. A higher salary or more flexible hours at another institution may serve to cause staff to move from one organization to another. Burnout is more likely to cause nurses to leave nursing completely. Nurses suffering from burnout tend to be less productive, to be more error-prone, to have low morale, and to accrue a high number of sick days.

Burnout can be caused by a variety of factors. Unrealistic expectations, poor management practices, the excessive use of agency nurses who depend heavily on the regular staff, lack of a good working relationship with physicians, and inconsistent organizational policies are among the various causes. However, the most obvious cause of burnout is short-staffing. When there are simply not enough nurses to get the job done on a given day, the existing staff can push themselves. When 9 nurses are doing the work of 10, each of the 9 is very tired at the end of the shift. It is hoped that they will be able to relax a bit before their shift the next day. When some of those 9 are asked to follow the shift with an immediate second shift, the problem increases. However, over their days off, it is hoped they can relax and recuperate from the stress of trying to do more than one person's work on their regular shifts, as well as working a few second shifts. On a short-term basis, such a situation may be unpleasant but bearable.

The problems in nursing can and sometimes do become much worse, however. The general financial difficulties faced by many health care organizations already cause staffing levels to be cut to the bone. A fully staffed unit may be staffed with so few nurses as to push each nurse to the limit on a regular basis. When a vacancy occurs on top of that tight staffing situation, the extra stress caused by trying to do more than one can do on a continual basis can become unbearable. Research has repeatedly demonstrated that people have a natural work pace. The pace does differ a bit from person to person, thus there are those who are consistently high performers and others whose performance is not quite as efficient. People can work up to 30% faster and harder for short periods of time. For nurses, this means that if they are short-staffed for a day, they can usually handle the extra load. Two or three days or even a week can be managed. When the workload returns to normal, there is a period of "recuperation" during which people work more slowly. However, if the workload stays high for more than a week, or worse, if the excessive workload becomes the norm, people start to suffer exhaustion.[1] They become dissatisfied with the quality of the work they can do, and dissatisfied with the job—or even with the profession of nursing. So they leave, and staffing becomes even worse while the organization tries to recruit replacements. Effectively, lack of adequate staff causes nurses to leave the organization, resulting in even greater stress on those who remain.

What can be done to help reduce burnout? Nurses are more content if they believe that they have a caring manager who is interested in their development. Managers should be supportive and fair. Managers should be seen as using staff time wisely.

---

[1] Managers who are unfamiliar with the research on work pace may mistakenly think that staff who worked faster during a crisis should maintain that level of productivity all the time. They then think it a good idea to reduce staffing to the crisis levels without understanding that it is impossible for the staff to maintain that level of work over prolonged periods of time. When managers severely reduce staff, quality-of-care incidents occur and turnover becomes epidemic.

The overall attitude and management approach of unit managers and higher level nursing administrators can, at least to some extent, offset the problems of burnout.

Flexible hours are another measure aimed at reducing burnout. Allowing nurses to take four 10-hour shifts and have 3 days off is one approach to reduce the draining effect of the constant day-in and day-out stress related to a nurse's job. Having 3 days off may not only reduce burnout but may also be seen by nursing staff as quite desirable, thus increasing nurse satisfaction. Care must be exercised, however. A nurse may take three 12-hour shifts at one hospital and four 10-hour shifts at another. The financial rewards to the individual nurse are great, but the physical and emotional stress may be overwhelming. The impact on patient care may be negative.

The most direct approach to reducing burnout is to increase the overall staffing level. However, this may be nearly impossible, given both the financial constraints of the organization and the overall shortage of available staff. Using alternative personnel (so-called nurse extenders) for providing care presents a potential option to reduce the amount of work per staff nurse. The use of alternative providers of care is discussed later in this chapter.

■ RETENTION PROGRAMS

The problem of turnover is significant enough to warrant specific attention and direct programs aimed at staff retention. This should go beyond the basic notions of having competent managers, physicians who work on a collegial professional basis with nurses, autonomy in work, and the other elements of nurse satisfaction. Such programs should work toward making the institution one that shows caring for its staff and creates a loyalty bond that is hard to break. Some such programs involve significant financial investment, whereas others take relatively little.

First of all, employees should have a way of being recognized. There should be a formal mechanism that allows a pattern of exemplary work, or even one good deed, to gain recognition. There are a variety of ways employee behavior can be recognized. The first is in the form of performance evaluations with interviews. Such evaluations are a two-edged sword. They need to be firm enough to make clear that poor performance will not be ignored or rewarded. However, there should be a strong focus on positive aspects. This may be in terms of recognizing good performance or even in terms of offering training in areas where performance could be improved. Rather than dwelling on poor past performance, a greater amount of time should be spent on discussing ways to accomplish more and to improve future performance.

Performance evaluation meetings are often uncomfortable for evaluators and for those being evaluated. However, such meetings should not be given short shrift. Employees should leave the meeting with a feeling that they understand what is expected of them, with a sense that their individual efforts make a difference in the overall performance of the unit, and with a clear sense that their positive contributions have been noted and specifically recognized by the organization.

Another key element of performance conferences should be to elicit input. What is going on that the employees like, and what kinds of things cause the employees to complain? Open communication—with honest follow-up on suggestions and complaints—is likely to win support and loyalty. A refusal to budge from the way things are is more likely to result in resentment and, in some cases, resignations.

In addition to meetings with staff members, their specific actions may warrant letters of commendation. Such letters could be the result of favorable patient comments on a form supplied to patients for that purpose. Or they could be based on recommendations by other staff. Commendations should be presented in appropriate ceremonies and noted in organization newsletters so that as many people as possible are made aware of them. This provides further psychological benefit to the recipient and perhaps serves notice to other workers of the possibility of gaining such recognition. Achievement of such recognition should be within the reach of most staff members.

In providing motivation, the carrot can be used or the stick can be used. There are some schools of thought that argue that the stick is more appropriate than the carrot. Poor performance is unacceptable and that fact should be conveyed to workers. Other schools of thought argue that in the long run the carrot will have more positive results. By accentuating the positive and minimizing the negative, a happier and psychologically healthier work environment results. In many cases, a combination of the carrot and the stick is probably optimal. However, permitting a few nurses to violate policy, fail to complete work, report late for work, and call in sick frequently can damage the morale of the most highly performing nursing unit. Worse, if there is no "stick" to punish the slackers for their bad behavior, the good nurses may come to the following conclusion: "Why should I consistently work hard, be on time, and follow the rules when those guys don't and nothing happens to them?" In this way, one bad apple can indeed spoil the whole barrel. On the other hand, managers who are consistently punitive toward poor behavior but fail to recognize and reward excellence tend to create dissatisfaction among the staff. Almost everybody wants and needs praise for good performance from their managers. Managers who fail to provide that positive feedback are failing their staff members and are quite likely to suffer high turnover as a result.

Another program for retention involves financial remuneration. Money is not a solution to all problems. One study has shown that nurses listed the quality of nursing care they were able to provide; their relationships with other nurses and with their patients; adequate staffing levels so they had time to provide excellent nursing care; autonomy; education support; and their nursing leadership as the factors most influential in their satisfaction. Monetary compensation was not listed in the top ten satisfiers (Dunn et al., 2005).

When Dunn and colleagues listed the dissatisfiers, benefits and salary still were not among the top ten items listed in terms of importance to nurses. Nursing departments should attempt to deal with all these factors. However, although money is not the solution to all problems, financial incentives have become a major competitive factor in this era of nursing shortages. To attract and retain nurses, a health care facility must pay competitive salaries. It does not, however, have to pay substantially higher salaries than other facilities in its service region.

Higher salaries are one type of financial incentive. They can be costly to health care organizations. Other types of financial incentives can be achieved without substantially higher cost to the institution. One example is the use of salaries instead of hourly wages. This approach may make some nurses feel better about themselves and their institutions. However, a substantial number of nurses may be needed to work extra hours or extra shifts in these times of nursing shortages. Facilities will not retain their staff members if they attempt to convert to salaries and then save money by having mandatory overtime that is not paid at all (because the nurses are on salary) or by paying only straight time for those extra hours. Additional hours must be paid at the standard time-and-one-half or double-time (for holidays). Any other approach will probably lead to higher turnover.

Another financial approach is the use of bonuses. Generally, bonuses are paid only out of cost savings. Thus, the institution can afford to pay for them because the payment is only part of a larger amount that would otherwise have been spent anyway. Bonuses are becoming more and more widespread. Bonuses are discussed in Chapter 3.

Innovative employee benefits are another area that can be used to help retain nurses. For example, the use of child care centers located at the health care organization (perhaps with discounted or subsidized rates) can help retention significantly. Additionally, such centers have the capacity to reduce sick leave substantially. Much sick leave is the result of a nurse staying home to take care of a sick child. Sick leave can therefore be reduced if the child care center has facilities for mildly ill children.

These approaches to retention have already been noted in the nursing literature. However, to be truly competitive, an organization must be innovative. For example, suppose that a nurses' softball team group were formed to provide exercise, companionship, and sports activities outside work hours. Indeed, if the facility's campus is sufficiently large, perhaps a ball field could be constructed on site. Another idea may be to institute a drama club and stage a dramatic or musical play, with performances for the staff and patients every few months. A club of this type provides an excellent release from the routine work pressures. In this way it reduces the burnout syndrome. Over the years, such clubs and sports teams help nurses to develop intense loyalty to the facility. Nurses might not leave the organization because they don't want to be left out of the game or leave their dramatics group. Bridge clubs and other organization-sponsored activities (annual picnics and sponsored trips to a zoo or museum) result in the development of a sense of family and community, rather than strictly to a workplace. When times get tough, families and communities hang together.

Career Ladders

A common complaint of staff nurses is that there is little room for advancement within the clinical ranks. Nurses can go into management. However, if they choose to pursue a bedside, hands-on, clinical career, there is little difference in reward for a nurse with 30 years of experience as compared to one with 5 years of experience. The concept of career ladders or clinical ladders is one suggestion for overcoming this deterrent to nurse retention.

There are a wide variety of career ladder models. Some are completely distinct from administrative career paths (clinical ladders). Others allow for branching off from a clinical ladder into an administrative path after a certain point. Some clinical ladders simply require on-the-job experience for promotions, whereas others require additional education, including advanced degrees. In some models, moving up the ladder requires community or professional service and publication. Another distinction among models is the amount of additional responsibility that must be assumed as one moves up the ladder.

There is a widespread belief that clinical ladders do improve nurse retention. At the very least, they have the potential to help a facility retain its best and brightest nurses. Such an approach improves the professional identity of the nurse and generates loyalty. Another perspective is that if nurses with more experience in a given institution earn substantially more than those with fewer years at the specific organization, it becomes more costly to move. It becomes expensive to give up seniority. If this is the case, retention of the more experienced (and expensive) personnel becomes easier, but higher turnover rates may occur among the nurses at the lower (and less expensive) rungs of the ladder. Over time, this may lead to an organization with a large proportion of its staff near the higher compensation end of the career ladder.

The Hawthorne Effect

With all attempts to improve retention, it is necessary to be wary of the *Hawthorne Effect*, which is widely discussed in the general management literature. The Hawthorne Effect is based on a study in which a number of changes were made in a factory to examine their impact on worker productivity. With each change, productivity improved. However, it turned out that the specific changes were not directly responsible for the improvement. Improvement occurred as a result of the attention the workers were receiving.

Consider researchers' making factory lighting brighter to see whether more light improves worker productivity. Productivity, in fact, increases after the lighting is changed. Then the researchers add music, and productivity goes up again. If the lighting and music are responsible, then taking them away should reduce productivity to the earlier levels. However, removing the better lighting and the music causes productivity to go up even further. It is the **attention**, rather than the lighting or the music, that makes productivity improve.

All the efforts to improve nurse retention risk falling subject to the Hawthorne Effect. Put a career ladder in place and turnover decreases. Have joint awareness seminars with nurses, administrators, and physicians. Institute a bonus system. Have performance evaluations twice a year. Declare a new era of nursing autonomy. The one thing not known about any of the changes is whether it is the specific nature of the change that is significant or simply the response of nurses' recognizing the fact that the organization finally seems to care about them.

This does not mean that the changes in themselves have no impact. There has been enough literature reporting results to indicate that certain factors are in fact likely to improve nurse satisfaction and, it is hoped, retention. Open communication, greater participation in decision making, being salaried, and career ladders probably do make a difference. However, the element of change itself should not be underplayed.

Putting a career ladder in place and then assuming retention will take care of itself is not likely to work satisfactorily in the long run. The organization must adopt an attitude of continuous improvement—making changes each year to improve the lot of its nurses. It may well not be possible to improve all areas that affect nurse satisfaction in any one year, but a constant attitude of working toward improvement is needed. This may mean new major innovations each year, or it may mean modifications of past innovations. Some years, changes may be financial; other years, changes may relate to nursing image. A constant approach that looks each year to see what improvements can be added is more likely to have a lasting positive impact than a dramatic, one-shot change. Nursing staff should be able to see that the organization has a commitment to the improvement of the lot of nurses each and every year.

Determining the Cost

What does it cost to retain staff? As with any decision in a health organization, the cost-benefit ratio of a retention program should be estimated in advance and also evaluated after the program has been implemented. Having accurate data on current retention patterns and knowing the organization's goals provide the first step in determining the costs of the program. Although it is often difficult to associate a particular retention program with overall retention, some estimates can be made. If a new program such as free parking is instituted, the cost of that can be determined easily. Often, however, new programs have several goals and potential benefits. A hand-held computer system for nursing home visits may be intended to retain nurses who want to work in a high-tech environment where charting is easier. However, the computer system is also expected to improve the quality of patient care and to decrease the time nurses spend on documentation. Other programs aimed at improving retention may have additional benefits as well. Shared governance may be instituted to improve retention, but it may improve patient care and produce that benefit as well. Increasing salaries may retain staff in the short run, but as soon as the competitor across town increases its salaries, the benefits of such a program may disappear.

Determining the costs of turnover, and therefore the benefits of decreasing turnover, is more straightforward. What is important to remember is that the costs of turnover do not include just the costs of advertising for staff and the nurse recruiter's salary. Costs include the effect short staffing has on the remaining staff and the decreased productivity of new staff. Jones (2005) describes a detailed approach to determining the costs of turnover. She suggests that the following costs be included:

- Advertising/recruiting
- Costs of unfilled positions
- Hiring costs
- Termination costs
- Orientation/training
- Decreased new RN productivity[2]

For the hospitals studied by Jones, the mean cost per RN turnover was in the neighborhood of $64,000 (the range was $62,100 to $67,100). This was a huge increase over the $10,198 Jones reported in her 1988 study. The increase due to inflation, all other factors being equal, should have been to only about $12,000. However, the cost of having a vacancy and filling it with extremely expensive agency nurses, whom many hospitals are now forced to rely upon, had driven the cost of replacing a nurse to a bit more than the total cost of a nurse for one year. This is interesting because many personnel reports in business estimate that the cost of replacing a professional is approximately equal one year of salary for that professional.

Blaufuss, Maynard, and Schollars present an alternative approach to evaluating turnover costs in response to a specific incentive. They do not include general advertising and recruiting costs in their calculations because, they argue, hospitals must advertise regardless of turnover rates; there will naturally be some turnover in all organizations.[3]

They include interviewing, preparing for orientation, the orientation itself, and a learning period. They identify the individual cost of hiring each new staff member. In addition, they include estimated revenue enhancements as an offset to

[2] See Cheryl Bland Jones, "The Costs of Nursing Turnover: Part II, Measurements and Results," *Journal of Nursing Administration*, Vol.35, No. 1, January 2005, pp. 41-49, for a complete description of this approach.

[3] Judy Blaufuss, Jan Maynard, and Gail Schollars, "Methods of Evaluating Turnover Costs," *Nursing Management*, Vol.23, No. 5, May 1992, pp. 52–61.

the recruiting cost. This is particularly important when increasing staff can lead to raising the number of patients cared for. Essentially, if you look at the cost of attracting new staff, you must also consider the extra revenue the organization will earn if it has those new staff members.

Their formulation assumes that there will always be sufficient turnover to require constant advertising and recruitment of personnel. In that case, recruitment and advertising are essentially fixed costs. Clearly there is much truth to this view—especially in large urban hospitals and clinics. However, some nursing units and whole clinic facilities have gone for years with little turnover except for retirements. Another viewpoint is that if a facility can keep its turnover low, the resources that are spent on training new hires (not to mention the advertising costs) can be spent on other valuable work for the organization. In fact, many clinical educators express frustration about all the upgrading of skills and teaching established staff that they cannot accomplish because they have to spend so much of their time orienting and teaching new recruits.

■ RECRUITING STAFF

No matter how effectively an organization works to retain its existing staff, some turnover must be expected. Some staff members will retire; others will move to different parts of the country; still others may return to school for advanced degrees. Some replacement of staff will always be occurring. Such replacement is inherently costly. The costs of replacing staff include overtime and agency nurse costs while the position is vacant, advertising, interviewing potential employees, travel costs for recruiters, entertainment costs, moving costs, administrative processing costs, and new employee training.

Depending on the specific institution, these costs may be shared by the unit with the vacancy and the personnel department or they may all be borne by the unit with the vacancy. For example, if ads are run to replace a staff member for one unit, the cost of the ad may be charged back directly to the unit with the vacancy. If ads are run to attract candidates for a number of different units, the cost of the ad may be divided, and a share of the cost may be allocated among the various units. Alternatively, the price of advertisements may be borne solely by a department responsible for recruiting, such as the personnel or nurse recruitment departments. If units share the cost of advertising, then the operating budget should contain an estimate of the number of vacancies and the cost of advertisements for the year.

Other costs related to the replacement of personnel should also be budgeted. The average length of the vacancies should be anticipated, and the extra cost of overtime and agency nurses should be included in the coming year's operating budget. Newly hired employees are often less productive than experienced staff. This may require extra hours of nursing care per patient day, often in the form of overtime. An effort should be made to anticipate turnover and the costs related to turnover. Sufficient nursing care hours should be budgeted to allow for the lower productivity of new staff. If relocation costs are charged directly to the unit, those costs should be included in the budget as well.

Marketing

One of the key elements of recruiting is an effective marketing strategy. As long as an overall shortage of talented nurses exists, there will be winners and losers in the effort to recruit qualified personnel. Therefore, a plan must be developed for addressing the recruiting issue.

The essence of marketing is that, based on market research, the needs and desires of a group are determined, and then an effort is made to satisfy those needs and desires. Notice that this definition does not revolve around advertising, which may or may not be part of a marketing effort. The first step is to find out what nurses want from their employment. Next, efforts must be made to ensure that the hospital meets those needs to the greatest extent possible. Finally, it is necessary to be able to convey the fact that the needs have been met. Word-of-mouth is an important way nurses form opinions about a potential place of employment. If the facility's staff is well satisfied, they will spread the word to other nurses that their facility is a good place to work. That is one valuable recruiting mechanism—especially in populated areas where nurses have a selection of several places to work.

In performing market research, a decision should first be made concerning who it is that the organization wants to recruit. Is it new nurses, right out of school? Is it experienced nurses? Nurse managers? Specialists? Local nurses? Out-of-state nurses? In trying to determine what the potential employee wants and needs, it is of critical importance to evaluate correctly the group that is to be the target of the marketing effort.

Most health care organizations already have some staff, so there must be some attractive characteristics of the organization. In relative terms, all existing organizations have some strengths. Therefore, there should not be a hopeless attitude that says, "How can we compete with the rich, research-oriented medical center in town?" Perhaps many nurses would prefer to provide care in a patient-oriented rather than a research-oriented setting. It is important to identify the existing strengths of the organization so that the information can be conveyed to a target group.

At the same time, weaknesses must be identified and a long-term plan must be designed to overcome as many of those weaknesses as possible. Perhaps lack of convenient parking is the one overwhelming negative the organization has. In this case, replacing expensive advertising with a major fund-raising campaign to allow for the building of an enclosed parking garage may be an appropriate marketing strategy. This is an example of a one-shot, expensive solution of a recruiting problem.

In other cases, solutions may be less expensive but require ongoing efforts. For example, a hospital could distinguish itself through a concerted effort to develop a system of shared governance. Such efforts are not necessarily expensive. They do, however, require tremendous cooperation and commitment. The potential result is that expensive newspaper ads can be replaced by free news stories about the changes at the hospital. Nursing schools can be encouraged to have the organization's staff give lectures about the shared-governance approach employed by the organization. If the new system really provides something that nurses value, the word will eventually get out, even without advertising. Advertising may be employed to speed the communication process, if desired.

Note, however, that marketing does not start with advertising. It starts with the identification (or creation) of a need or desire and the filling of that need or desire. These elements must precede the advertising. Only then can a specific plan be developed regarding the communication of the strengths the organization has to offer. Advertising in newspapers, on television or radio, or by direct mail is one approach to that communication. College visits are another. Bonuses to existing employees who bring in new employees are yet another.

Each of these approaches often results in inquiries by potential employees. The package of material that the organization develops to respond to those inquiries is a critical element of the overall marketing strategy. The marketing strategy should take into account all the steps in the recruiting process. Generating inquiries without a strategy to follow-up effectively is one critical mistake often made by those who view marketing only in terms of advertising. If a strategy is likely to generate inquiries, the organization should not appear unorganized or uncaring when it receives those inquiries. This is the point at which the organization has the chance to reaffirm the feeling that caused the nurse to inquire about the position.

Suppose a hospital runs a newspaper ad that says, "Join the nursing staff at ABC Hospital, where nurses work in an environment of shared governance and shared commitment to the highest level of patient care." Some carefully planned literature must be available for the person who asks for more information about the shared-governance program. Its history, how it works, and the hospital's commitment should be included.

If the response to the inquiry leads to an interview, the interviewer should be aware that the candidate has inquired about the hospital's shared-governance program. The interview should include at least some specific discussion that emphasizes or highlights the shared-governance system.

Marketing is a critical element of recruiting. This does not mean that the organization has to sell people something that they don't want or need. Rather, having researched the wants and needs of a targeted nursing group, marketing should allow the organization to convey effectively to the target group the extent to which the organization has made efforts to meet those desires and needs.

Although advertising is not the first part of a marketing plan, in many instances it is an effective mechanism for speeding the word-of-mouth process. Targeted advertising can reach a potential group of employees effectively. This is particularly important in a competitive marketplace. If competing organizations are effectively communicating what they have to offer, your organization must be prepared to get its message to that group of potential employees as well.

One important element of advertising is that only a part of current advertising should be aimed at current recruitment. Another part, equally substantial, should be aimed at long-term image building. Often people associate with an organization because of its "well-known" reputation. Such reputations are built over a period of years. They are built through the effort of getting the message out year after year. When there is a staffing shortage, the institution advertises why it is a good place to work. It should also do so when there is no shortage of personnel. Image building is not a short-term response to shortages. By laying the groundwork over a long period of time, when the need for personnel occurs, the organization will have a head start over its competition.

In budgeting for a marketing plan, it is necessary to include the costs of advertising. However, any other costs related to the overall marketing plan should also be included in the budget. These might include consulting costs and the costs of doing market research.

Determining the Cost

Recruitment and replacement of staff is inherently costly. The costs of replacing staff include:

- Overtime and agency nurse costs while the position is vacant
- Advertising
- Interviewing potential employees

- Travel for recruiters
- Entertainment
- Moving
- Signing bonuses
- Administrative processing
- New employee orientation and training

■ USING ALTERNATIVE HEALTH CARE EMPLOYEES

Despite the efforts of organizations to retain nurses, nurse retention will be unable to solve all of a health care organization's nursing needs. And recruitment more often results in shifting the shortage from one organization to another, rather than eliminating the shortage. Thus, despite the best efforts to retain and recruit nurses, there will probably be at least some organizations with inadequate staffing. One suggested approach to solving this shortage is the use of alternative health care employees.

A variety of alternative health care employees are sometimes used. One approach is to use foreign nurses. This approach attempts to retain the concept of using RNs to the greatest extent possible. It comes to grips with a national nursing shortage by looking outside the United States. A different approach is to use non-RNs to perform activities that in the past had been performed by RNs.

Foreign Nurse Recruitment

Using foreign nurses is one possible alternative for staffing a health care institution. However, it involves a number of difficulties, ranging from regulatory problems to language barriers. On the other hand, many foreign nurses welcome the chance to come to the United States on either a temporary or a permanent basis, and this approach can be used to fill a large gap in the nursing staff.

Because of language problems, most foreign recruitment takes place in countries that are English-speaking, such as Canada, the British Isles, Australia, the Philippines, and India. Northern states may be able to recruit in Canada relatively easily, compared to other alternatives. For recruiting outside the continent, the expenses of travel and relocation can become substantial. An alternative to an organization's doing it all by itself is to use an agency and pay a flat fee for each nurse hired. The more nurses there are to be hired, the more likely it is to be cost-effective to undertake the entire recruiting project yourself.

If a strategy of foreign recruiting is chosen, the need for careful budgeting becomes essential. The choice between using a recruiting agency versus doing it yourself can have a dramatic financial impact. By developing a budget, the costs of each alternative can be considered. For example, suppose that an agency charges one month's salary for recruiting an individual plus one month's salary for relocation expenses. Recruitment agency charges could easily add an additional $10,000 to $20,000 to the cost of recruiting a nurse.

There may be additional recruiting costs. Some countries provide for emigrant nurses to have taken the language tests and State Board of Nursing examinations prior to emigration to the United States. If this is not the case, a significant cost of recruiting foreign nurses will be the time between their arrival and the time when they have completed all examinations and other requirements necessary to practice as an RN. During this period, they are being paid but are not fully productive because they may not work as RNs. Typically, they may work only as nursing assistants until they receive their U.S. license. Other costs include providing convenient housing and helping the nurses to settle in. Another cost is related to loss of recruits between their recruitment and when they can start work as RNs. A fairly lengthy period is required to meet various visa and other requirements, so there is a drop-out rate at that end. And if some of the nurses are unable to pass the NCLEX exam, the entire investment (plus their transportation back to their native countries) is lost.

A final issue with recruitment of foreign nurses is ethical. When the United States recruits nurses from foreign countries to fill our shortage, is there a serious loss of care for the citizens of the country from which the nurse came? Nurse education is expensive in any country. A few countries (such as the Philippines) have deliberately created nursing schools on the U.S. model explicitly to facilitate emigration of some of their people. But that is unusual. Most countries invest in nursing education to provide nurses to meet their own people's needs. And when the United States recruits from other countries to meet its own needs, the people of the country from which the nurses are recruited may be left with precious little health care available to them. This has been a very serious problem in Africa. Given that nursing pay in Africa is extremely low and that nursing pay in the developed countries is much higher, some countries in Africa have been left with so few nurses that large portions of their populations have been effectively left with no health care. At the writing of this book, the biggest problem has been the emigration of African nurses to Britain and other European countries. There have been discussions of the ethics of denuding Africa of health care workers for the benefit of Europeans. This concern can be avoided if the United States finds a way to fund nursing education so that adequate numbers of Americans can fill the nursing positions that will be needed over the next 30 years.

Alternative Care Givers

A drastically different approach to using foreign nurses is the alteration of the pattern of care within a health care organization such that more activities are assigned to non-RNs. There are many types of alternative care givers. They include, but are not limited to, the traditional alternative care givers: LPNs/LVNs and unlicensed assistive personnel (UAP) such as nurses' aides. Various new positions such as hosts or hostesses are also being developed to help organizations cope. Such a person would introduce patients to the unit and respond to many of the nonclinical needs and questions of patients and their families.

In terms of clinical assistive personnel, many approaches are being tried at different health care organizations around the country. In some cases, the RN is placed in a position of greater direct supervision of other types of staff who provide more of the care. In other cases, partnerships are developed between nursing and UAP. In many cases, the ultimate impact of using alternative care givers is less bedside time for the RN and more supervisory responsibility.

At the time of the writing of this book, no single approach has emerged as the dominant path for providing nursing care in the future. The main conflict seems to be between a model that would have RNs serving as supervisors of non-RNs versus a model in which nursing activities are divided into an RN subset and a non-RN subset. In the case of the former, RNs have a decreasing bedside role but greater authority and responsibility for patient care. In the latter alternative, RNs may spend as much time in bedside care but performing only activities that require the sophistication of an RN.

There is no question that throughout the first decades of the 21st century we will see a great deal of experimentation in search of a model that works well. The result may be several different models, each of which works well and attracts nurses with a preference for one approach versus another. There is little question, however, that the organization of nursing services in the year 2020 will be substantially different from that observed as of the writing of this book.

■ USING COMPUTERS

Changing the way nursing care is provided on the basis of staff shortages is a less than ideal way to let a profession evolve. The changes are not the result primarily of an impetus to find better ways to give care. Rather, they are the recognition of constraints in personnel availability. If nursing shortages could be permanently eliminated, the approach to delivering nursing care might be substantially different. The computerization of nursing units has been put forth as a potential solution to that dilemma.

Some claims have been made that as much as half of all nursing time is spent on documentation and that bedside computer terminals could save half of that time. If true, this would mean that up to one quarter of all required nursing time could be eliminated without taking away any time from nursing care provided to patients.

Although highly touted for their timesaving potential throughout the 1990s, computer systems have yet to live up to that glowing potential. The *hardware* (equipment) capacity exists. Technological advances have reached a point where terminals by each bedside are feasible. In fact, it would be surprising to see a new building for a health care organization that did not include computer access in every room as part of the building design. Gaining nurse acceptance of the use of unit or bedside computers has not turned out to be the problem that many predicted it would be. On the other hand, developing the *software* (computer programs) has been a complicated process.

Each health care institution tends to be unique in its procedures. This lack of industry standardization creates difficulties in developing software. Furthermore, the process of recording the activities surrounding patient care and integrating patients' clinical and financial information with those activities is a highly complicated task.

Whether the claims of 25% savings in staff time will ever be realized is uncertain. It is likely, however, that computer software advances will be made and that computer usage by staff nurses will become standard in most health care organizations. In the long run, this will be likely to increase the quality of patient care because of more accurate and timely information, while at the same time creating at least some efficiency in the use of nursing time. This should allow more RN time to be available for patient care. To the extent that computers reduce time spent on documentation relative to time spent in providing patient care, computerization should work both to reduce nursing shortages and to increase nursing satisfaction.

Summary and Implications for Nurse Managers

Nationwide shortages of nurses have occurred periodically. Having an understanding of approaches to deal with such shortages as they occur is essential for nurse managers. These approaches include attempts to retain existing nurses, recruit additional nurses, and find ways to provide quality nursing care with fewer RN hours, whether through the use of computers, alternative care givers, or some other means.

Summary and Implications for Nurse Managers—cont'd

From a budgeting perspective, the issue of retention and recruitment of staff members, whether RNs, LPNs/LVNs, aides, or other staff, is a significant one. There must be careful enumeration of all costs related to recruitment and retention. These costs include marketing research, consulting, advertising, travel, and relocation. They also include the costs necessary to make an organization attractive, such as training costs related to implementing a system of shared governance.

In some cases, decisions must be made regarding which budget will include the various costs related to these efforts. If alternative care providers are used, the change in staffing will clearly take place within each of the various nursing units. Computerization costs are also likely to be included in the specific capital and operating budgets of the various units. On the other hand, relocation costs for new staff are less obvious. Should they be included in the costs of the unit that will employ the staff member or in some other budget? The critical factor is that such costs must be anticipated and included in some budget, and there should be a clearly communicated understanding of whose budget that is.

One fundamental point in this process is the fact that in order for a specific organization to have an adequate staff, it must recognize a need to change over time. The environment in which health care organizations exist is in a constant state of change. Other career opportunities exist for potential staff. If a hospital job is not adequately attractive, a nurse can go into home health care or work in a physician's office. It is important to remain current in understanding what nurses desire from their employment in addition to a salary.

The successful organizations will be those that are aware of the desires of the workforce, respond to those desires, and effectively communicate to potential employees the ways in which they meet those needs and desires.

References and Suggested Readings

American Association of Colleges of Nursing (AACN). (2006). Nursing Faculty Shortage Fact Sheet. Downloaded April 20, 2006 from http://www.aacn.nche.edu/Media/Backgrounders/facultyshortage.htm

AACN. (2007). Preliminary Findings: 2004 National Sample Survey of Registered Nurses. Downloaded March 15, 2007 from http://bhpr.hrsa.gov/healthworkforce/reports/rnpopulation/preliminaryfindings.htm

American Nurses Credentialing Center (ANCC). (2005). *Magnet Recognition Program Application Manual.* Washington, D.C.: American Nurses Association.

ANCC. (2006). Magnet Program informational video (untitled). Downloaded April 18, 2006 from http://www.nursingworld.org/ancc/magnet/siteevals.html.

Badovinac, C.C., Wilson, S., and Woodhouse, D. (1999, July/August). The use of unlicensed assistive personnel and selected outcome indications. *Nursing Economic$* 17(4), 194-200.

Blaufuss, J., Maynard, J., and Schollars, G. (1992). Methods of Evaluating Turnover Costs, *Nursing Management* 23(5), 52-61.

Buerhaus, P. (2000). Implications of an aging registered nurse workforce. *Journal of the American Medical Association* 283(22), 2948-2954.

Cox, H.C. (1987). Verbal abuse in nursing: Report of a study. *Nursing Management* 21(11), 47-50.

Duncan, S.M., Hyndman, K., Estabrooks, C.A. Hesketh, K., Humphrey, C.K., Wong, J.S., Acorn S., and Giovannetti, P. (2001). Nurses' experience of violence in Alberta and British Columbia hospitals. *Canadian Journal of Nursing Research* 32(4), 57-78.

Dunn, S., Wilson, B., and Esterman, A. (2005). Perceptions of working as a nurse in an acute care setting. *Journal Of Nursing Administration* 13(1), 22-31.

Huston, C.L. (1996). Unlicensed assistive personnel: A solution to dwindling health care resources or the precursor to the apocalypse of registered nursing. *Nursing Outlook* 44(2), 67-73.

Jones, C.B. (2005) The Costs of Nursing Turnover, Part II, Measurements and Results. *Journal of Nursing Administration* 35(1), 41-49.

Knaus, W.A., Draper, E.A., Wagner, D.P., and Zimmerman, J.E. (1986). An evaluation of outcome from intensive care in major medical Centers. *Annals of Internal Medicine* 104(3), 410-418.

McClure, M.L., Poulin, M.A., Sovie, M.D., and Wandelt, M.A. (1983). *Magnet Hospitals: Attraction and Retention of Professional Nurses.* Kansas City, MO: American Academy of Nursing.

Nachreiner, N.M., Gerberich, S G., McGovern, P.M., Church, T.R., Hansen, H.E., Geisser, M.S., and Ryan, A.D. (2005). Relation between policies and work-related assault: Minnesota Nurses' Study. *Occupational and Environmental Medicine* 62, 675-681.

Nevidjon, B., and Erickson, J. (2001). The nursing shortage: solutions for the short and long term. *Online Journal of Issues in Nursing* 6(1). http://www.nursingworld.org/ojin/topic14/tpc14_4.htm

Sofield, L., and Salmond, S. (2003). Workplace violence: A focus on verbal abuse and intent to leave the organization. *Orthopaedic Nursing* 22(4), 274-283.

Forecasting

■ INTRODUCTION

Preparing budgets requires a number of preliminary steps, including forecasting. The importance of making an environmental review was discussed earlier (Chapter 2). A budget cannot be prepared without knowing the types of patients the organization is likely to treat. Nor can a budget be prepared without being aware of the competition and the actions competitors are likely to take. Similarly, a budget cannot be prepared without knowing such information as how many patients are likely to be treated and how sick they are likely to be. This is where forecasting comes in.

Forecasting techniques allow for predicting how many patients or patient days the organization or a particular unit or department will treat. Forecasting allows the manager to predict how sick the unit's patients will be. If a nurse manager were to attempt to prepare an operating budget without some prediction of these elements, there would be no way of determining how many staff members are needed. Forecasting can help to estimate how many chest tubes the intensive care unit will need and how many heparin locks a medical/surgical unit will consume. This will enable the nurse manager to plan the supplies portion of the unit's budget.

Forecasting is a tool that helps in preparing not only the operating budget but other budgets as well. If trends in the demographics of the community can be forecast, it is possible to prepare better long-range and program budgets. If it is forecast that a growing portion of the patient population will be Medicare patients, it can be determined what impact this will have on how quickly the organization gets paid. This will help in preparing the cash budget.

The range of items that can be forecast is relatively unlimited. It is possible to predict numbers of patients needing specific types of services, patient days, various supply items, the percentage of total operations performed by a specific surgeon, and so on. Generally, forecasting focuses on items that the manager must respond to rather than items that can be controlled. For example, a nursing unit may forecast how sick the patients will be. It cannot control severity of illness, but its budget must be a plan that responds to how sick the patient population is expected to be.

Forecasting should be undertaken as an early step in the budget preparation process. Virtually all managers forecast in some manner. Unsophisticated managers may forecast simply by using their best judgment or by basing the next year's costs on the current year's costs. It has been found that more formalized analysis of historical data can yield more accurate predictions than less sophisticated approaches. These predictions, in turn, form the basis of many decisions made in the planning process.

A formalized forecasting process can be divided into several steps. The first step is collecting historical data. The next step is graphing the data. The third step is analyzing the data to reveal trends or seasonal patterns. The fourth and final step is developing and using formulas to project the item being forecast into the future.

Before these steps are considered, there is one point that must be stressed. When a forecast is made, it is just an estimate of the future. Sophisticated approaches to forecasting allow the projection to be an educated estimate, but it is still an estimate. An intuitive hunch or gut feeling should **not** be ignored. The most sophisticated methods lack the feel for the organization that a manager develops over time. A forecast should never be accepted on the blind faith that if it is mathematical or computerized, it must be superior.

Quantitative forecasts are merely aids or supplements that managers should take into consideration along with a number of other factors, some of which often cannot be quantified and entered into formalized predictive models. The best forecasts result neither from naïve guessing, nor from advanced mathematics, but from an integration of quantitative methods with the experience and judgments of managers.

■ DATA COLLECTION

The first step in formalized forecasting is collecting historical data. Consider several examples. If a nurse manager wishes to make the most basic of projections—workload—she or he will first have to decide on a workload measure, such as number of patients or patient days. Then it is necessary to determine what the workload was in the past so that it can be projected into the future. This is referred to as a *time-series* approach to forecasting. Historical changes over time are used to help anticipate the likely results in a coming time period.

The methodology that is discussed in this section is broadly applicable. If one wanted to predict diaper usage in the maternity unit, one could use historical data based on the number of diapers used. Once the number of diapers needed is predicted, it would probably be necessary to focus on the expected cost per box of diapers. If the purchasing department has a good degree of certainty about the price of diapers for next year (such as a purchase contract specifying a price), this would be a pretty accurate approach. On the other hand, to predict the total cost for diapers directly rather than focusing first on the expected number of diapers, it would be possible to gather information on what total amount was spent on diapers in the past and use that to make a direct cost estimate.

In other words, it is possible first to forecast diaper usage and then to calculate the projected cost or to forecast diaper cost directly. The preferred choice would depend partly on whether information about the number of diapers to be used in the coming period is considered to be valuable information. Similarly, both the number of patient days and the severity of patients' illness can be predicted; then those data can be used to project the number of nursing hours needed, or historical information about the number of nursing hours consumed can be used to forecast nursing hours directly.

Appropriate Data Time Periods

There is often a tendency to try to make do with annual data. In fact, many operating budgets are annual budgets, specifying the total amounts to be spent on each line item for the coming year. However, when a manager is preparing an operating budget, it makes a lot of sense to use monthly rather than annual predictions of costs.

The easiest way to make monthly predictions is to take annual budget information and divide it by 12. In many industries it would be possible to use such a simple approach; production in one month may be much the same as it is in any other month. In the health care sector, such an expectation is not reasonable. The weather alone is likely to cause busy and slow periods. Winters are often busier times for health care organizations than summers are. Health care organizations must be prepared to have more staff available in busier periods. It is desirable to plan more vacations in slow periods and fewer during peak periods. Thus, it is important to be concerned with month-to-month variations within each year, as well as with the predictions for the year as a whole.

Furthermore, the number of days in a month will affect monthly costs. Many health care organizations, such as clinics, labs, and radiologists' offices, might be open only on weekdays. Some months have as many as 23 weekdays, whereas other months have as few as 20 weekdays. A 3-day difference on a 20-day base represents a 15% difference. Clearly, a difference that large would have a significant impact on the resources required for the month. Similarly, for a hospital, it is quite likely that the number of weekdays will have an influence because there are some days of the week when admissions and discharges tend to be higher than other days.

Monthly budgets are also important because they can be compared to the actual results as they occur. If there is a difference *(variance)* between the plan and the actual results, the cause can be investigated and perhaps a problem can be corrected immediately. Such variance analysis is the topic of Chapters 13 and 14. Without monthly subdivisions of the budget, it might be necessary to wait until the end of the year to find out if things were going according to plan. By then, of course, it would be too late to do anything about it for that year.

Thus, it is important for most health care institutions to have their costs broken down on a monthly basis and to do so in some manner that is more sophisticated than dividing the year's expected cost or volume by 12. Therefore, the data collected should generally be historical monthly data. For each type of item to be forecast (patients, chest tubes, diapers, costs), 12 individual data points are needed per year, representing values for the item being forecast for each month.

How far back should the data go? One year seems convenient, and it provides 12 data points. However, 1 year's worth of data provides only one piece of information about January, not 12. If this January was unusual (either very costly or unusually low in cost), that would not be readily apparent. It is likely that the next year would be predicted to be like this year. Therefore, more than 1 year's data are needed.

The use of 10 years' worth of data is often suggested for forecasting, although that has weaknesses as well. It is possible that so much has changed over the past 10 years that the data are no longer relevant. For example, over a 10-year span in a hospital, many types of supply items will be needed in later years that did not even exist during the earlier years. For that reason, it would seem that 5 years of data (or a total of 60 months) are a more reasonable heuristic (rule of thumb). If a nurse manager knows that things have not changed much on the unit in a long time, using more years of data will make the estimate a better predictor. If there have been drastic changes recently, then 5 years might be too long. Judgment is needed. One of the most important things a manager does is exercise judgment. Throughout the budgeting process, as in the other managerial functions undertaken, a manager can never escape from the fact that thoughtful judgment is vital to the process of effective management.

What Data Should Be Collected?

The fact that it is necessary to collect historical data concerning the item to be forecast has already been discussed. Too often, managers stop at that point because those data are sufficient to make a forecast. However, those data points are not all the data needed to make a **good** forecast.

Forecasting techniques mindlessly predict the future as an extension of the past, even though there are many things that change over time. Whenever forecasting is done, the manager should question whether there are factors that might have changed that will make the future different from the past. Are there in fact things that are changing? For instance, are demographics shifting? When it is predicted that the next January will be like the previous five Januarys, is the fact that last July there was a large influx of refugees into the community being ignored? Is a sudden shift in population caused by the closing of the town's auto plant being ignored? Is there a large new, moderately priced housing development being built that will mean more babies being born and more school children needing pediatricians in the community? The forecasting formulas to be developed will not take these recent factors into consideration. Forecasting formulas are based solely on historical information. The manager should collect additional data to use in making adjustments to the forecast results, based on her or his judgment.

For example, the availability of personnel can have a dramatic impact. For years, many health care organizations suffered from a shortage of available nurses. The result was high overtime payments to staff nurses and high agency charges for per diem nurses. If there has been a noticeable increase in the number of nurses available, then a manager should realize that the average hourly cost for nursing can now be decreased because of the elimination of much overtime and agency costs. A quantitative model for forecasting will not take this into account. Information about nurse availability must be collected, and the manager should give specific consideration to this information.

Note that a unit manager does not have to be a one-person information service. The personnel department can be asked about the outlook for hiring additional staff nurses. Administrators can be asked whether changes in third-party coverage are likely to have any impact. It is unreasonable to expect a home health agency's director of nursing to budget correctly for the coming year without knowing that the number of allowable Medicare-reimbursable visits has changed. Most home health agency financial officers would quickly be aware of such a change. This information should be communicated promptly to the Chief Nursing Officer. It is vital to open communication links with other managers throughout the organization to ensure receipt of necessary information that could help in the budget process.

It will not be easy to get information about some changes. For instance, there may be no central clearing person to provide an update on changing technology that will dramatically shift the demand for nursing personnel. Nevertheless, a unit manager must try to get that information and consider its likely impact on the unit. To some extent, nurse managers may have better information about changing technology than the organization's administrators have. First, nurse managers have clinical knowledge superior to that of non-clinical administrators. Second, nurse managers are likely to know what kinds of changes physicians in their clinical area are planning to implement.

It is also important for nurse managers to be aware of the organization's long-range plan, program budgets, and capital budgets. Many hospitals tend to guard budget data closely, with an "eyes-only" attitude. Only people with an immediate need are allowed to see any budget other than their own. It is important that administrators begin to understand that managers do have a need to see any budget that might even indirectly impact their own units or departments. For example, if a new clinical service winds up consuming a significant amount of nursing time that had not been planned for, much of it will likely be at overtime rates or will result in overtime elsewhere in the hospital. Had the impact of the service on the nursing department been planned for, overtime premiums might have been avoided. A manager who is to be held responsible for this overtime is entitled to have the information needed to anticipate demands on the unit and to plan for adequate staffing.

■ GRAPHING HISTORICAL DATA

Having collected all the relevant data that might help to predict the future, the next step is to lay out the historical data on a graph. In the forecasting approach discussed here, time is plotted on the horizontal axis. For instance, suppose that the unit manager wants to predict the next year's total nursing hours starting with January. Assume that it is currently October 2007 and that historical data from the past 5 years will be used. Data for October through December of 2007 are not yet available. Therefore, the horizontal axis begins in October 2002 and goes through September 2007 (Figure 6-1).

The vertical axis provides information about the item to be forecast. In Figure 6-1, it is nursing hours. The forecasting methodologies discussed later in this chapter allow a manager to predict workload estimates for the future, such as the number of patients or the number of patient days, the actual amounts of resource consumption (e.g., the number of nursing hours or the number of rolls of bandage tape), or costs. Depending on the procedures of your specific institution, some of these forecasts may be made by the accounting department rather than by nurse managers.

If costs or some other financial measures expressed in dollars are being predicted directly, the impact of inflation must be considered. If inflation is ignored as forecasting is done, the forecast becomes more complicated because it must predict not only a workload measure, such as the number of diapers for the coming year, but also the rate of inflation for the coming year. The problem of inflation and adjustments that can be made to allow for inflation are discussed in Chapter 4.

If a prediction is being made for next year's nursing hours (see Figure 6-1), the first point graphed would be the number of nursing hours worked in October 2002. The next point would be the number of nursing hours in November 2002, and so on.

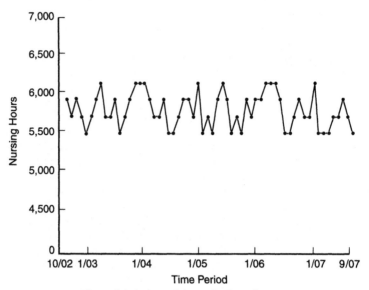

Figure 6-1 Basic graph for nursing hours forecast.

It is important to keep in mind that this forecasting approach is a time-series analysis—that is, the variable on the horizontal axis is always time. In time-series analysis, whether the manager is trying to predict workload, resources, or cost, the basic process is to look at how much of that item there was in the past and project that into the future. In order to make such predictions, the manager will have to be able to analyze the underlying cause of the variations in the data that have been graphed.

■ ANALYSIS OF GRAPHED DATA

Before any predictions can be made, it is necessary to assess the basic characteristics of the data that have been graphed. For instance, do the data exhibit *seasonality*? Is there a particular *trend*? Do variations from month to month and year to year appear to be simply random fluctuations? There may be patterns related to the passage of time that can be uncovered.

A visual inspection can usually provide a good picture of the type of pattern that exists. Here it is important to focus on a reasonably long time period, at least several years, as opposed to several months. By just looking at the past few months, it is possible to get a distorted impression of what is occurring. For instance, consider Figure 6-2. (Note that these are not the same data shown in Figure 6-1.) It appears that the number of nursing hours has a definite downward trend, but this graph covers a period of only 6 months.

Figure 6-3 shows the pattern for the full year. Now the graph gives a totally different impression. The number of nursing hours has not been steadily decreasing over time. For the first half of the year it was decreasing, and for the second half it was increasing. The pattern being observed is not likely to be indicative of a long-term decline. It is still not possible to tell, however, whether some basic change has occurred that caused a downward trend to reverse or whether the pattern is seasonal behavior. Next year, will the number of nursing hours continue to rise, as it appears to be doing

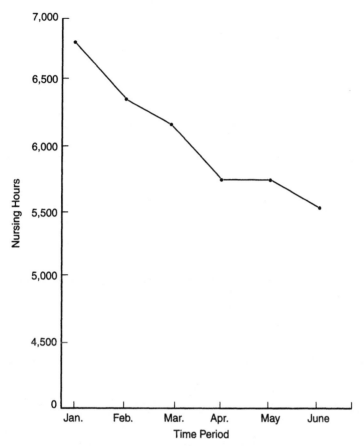

Figure 6-2 Six months' data for nursing hours forecast.

near the end of the year, or will it turn downward, as it did at the beginning of the graphed year? To answer this question, it is vital that data for at least several years be graphed.

Now look at Figure 6-4, which covers a period of 5 years. A pattern of falling and then rising hours occurs each year. This is clearly a seasonal pattern rather than a trend. Each year, the same pattern repeats itself.

When data for a sufficient number of years are graphed, the pattern that becomes apparent will generally fall into one of four categories. They are random fluctuations, trend, seasonality, and seasonality and trend together. Each of these patterns is discussed.

Random Fluctuation

It would be surprising if a unit or department consumed exactly the same amount of any resource 2 months or 2 years in a row. One year the winter will be a little colder than another and more people will get pneumonia. Another year prices will rise a little faster. One year some staff members will take more sick days than another. Yet these

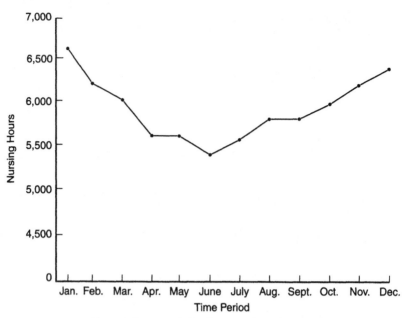

Figure 6-3 One year's data for nursing hours forecast.

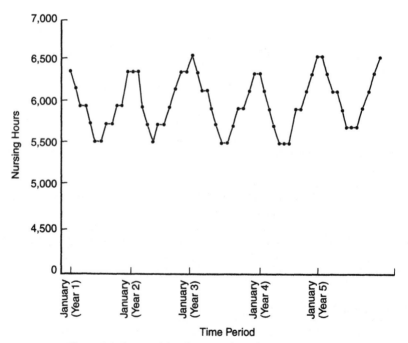

Figure 6-4 Five years' data for nursing hours forecast: seasonality.

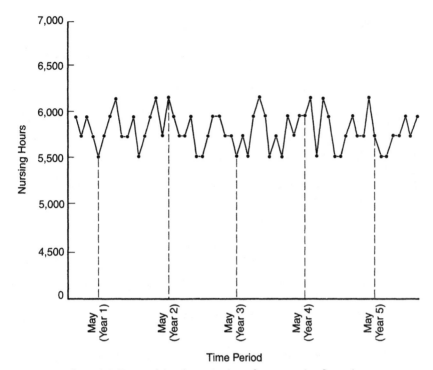

Figure 6-5 Five years' data for nursing hours forecast: random fluctuations.

events are not likely to be trends—it does not get colder and colder year after year. Nor are they seasonal. They are just random, unpredictable events.

When a graph exhibiting only random patterns is viewed, it should look something like Figure 6-5. As can be seen, there is no clear upward or downward trend. You will notice, for example, that each year the month of May is neither consistently higher nor consistently lower than it was the previous year. There is also no discernible seasonal pattern. May is not usually particularly busy nor particularly slow. May is a low month in the first year and a high month in the next year, relative to the values for the other months in those years.

Trend

In Figure 6-6, it should be noted that although the graph has its ups and downs, there is a clear upward trend. Because nursing hours rather than dollars are being considered here, this trend is not caused by inflation. Rather, it is probably caused either by an increased number of patient days or else by an increase in the amount of nursing time provided per patient day.

The underlying causes of observed patterns will not be determined in the forecasting process described here. The focus is strictly on projections of past items into the future. Whatever the cause, it appears that a definite trend exists. Unless there is information about expected patient days or a new policy regarding the relative ratio of nurses to patients, it would have to be assumed that this trend will continue.

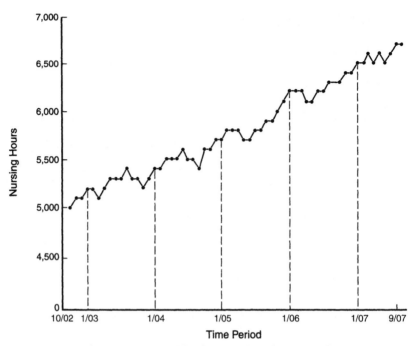

Figure 6-6 Five years' data for nursing hours forecast: trend.

However, managers should try to understand the underlying causes of patterns such as trends. This will better enable them to forecast correctly if something does change the underlying cause of the pattern.

Note further in Figure 6-6 that although the overall trend is upward, there is no discernible seasonal pattern. For example, January does not appear to be consistently high or low each year relative to the other months of those years.

Seasonality

Seasonal patterns are sometimes visible to the eye, as was the case in Figure 6-4. In health care, one is especially likely to see seasonal patterns because of seasonal disease patterns and as a result of the weather. Winter months bring with them ailments different from those that occur in the summer. For hospitals and home health agencies, these variations affect overall patient volume. On the other hand, nursing homes may be running at full occupancy all year round. Therefore, the number of patient days at a nursing home might not show any seasonality, although the specific care needs of the patients in a nursing home are likely to vary with the different seasons of the year.

Seasonality may not always be easy to spot. Therefore, it might be a worthwhile exercise to examine certain months that are known as peak or slow periods. Suppose that January is compared to June for each of the past 5 years and it is found that January almost always has higher levels of the item being forecast than June does. In that case, seasonality does exist, even though it is not readily apparent when the graph is inspected visually.

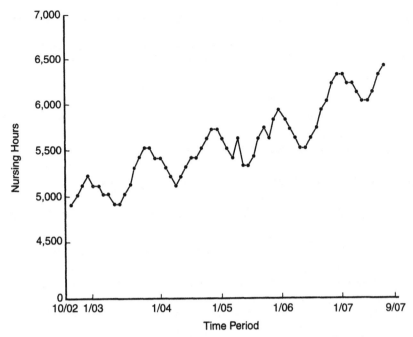

Figure 6-7 Five years' data for nursing hours forecast: seasonality with trend.

Seasonality and Trend

It is common for health care organizations to experience at least some seasonality. At the same time, due to increasing patient volume or the effects of inflation, upward trends are common as well. Downward trends may also occur. It is not at all unusual, therefore, for the organization to experience both seasonal influences and trends at the same time. Figure 6-7 shows an example of a historical pattern exhibiting both seasonality and trend.

Often the trend is more obvious than the seasonality in patterns that contain both. In these cases, it becomes especially useful to make several comparisons to see if certain months are always higher or lower than other months. Valid forecasts require an awareness of seasonal patterns if they exist.

■ FORECASTING FORMULAS

At this point, historical data have been gathered and graphed, and there has been a visual inspection of the graphs for apparent trends or seasonal patterns. It is finally time to begin using the information to make forecasts for the coming year. The approach taken for forecasting depends to a great degree on whether seasonal patterns, trends, both, or none are present.

An approach to forecasting each of these patterns is discussed later. First, however, it should be noted that the formulas below assume limited use of computer technology in performing the forecasting function. Much of the tedium and difficulty of the forecasting process is avoided if a sophisticated computer forecasting program is used.

Although the formulas discussed are valuable in situations in which a computer approach is unavailable, a computer solution is preferable. It takes less management time and can produce superior results. The costs of appropriate software are readily offset by the saved managerial time. A computer approach to forecasting is presented later in this chapter.

Random Fluctuations

The easiest forecasting occurs when there is no seasonal pattern or trend. For example, consider the budget for office supplies for the office of the Chief Nurse Executive. The need for these supplies may not vary much over time or with the particular workload level faced by the clinical nurses.

The most obvious approach in this case would be simply to add up the 60 monthly data points for the past 5 years and divide by 60. This will provide a monthly average. If every month is like every other month in terms of the item being forecast, this would be a reasonable approximation.

Caution must be exercised, however. Different months have different numbers of days. Even if there is no strong seasonal influence or trend, longer months may consume more of a resource. Months that have more weekdays may consume more of a resource. It may be necessary to adjust for factors such as days in a month or week-days in a month. For example, if weekdays use much more of a resource than weekends, rather than dividing the total for the past 60 months by 60, the total could be divided by the number of weekdays in the past 60 months. The result would be a predicted value per weekday. This value would be multiplied by the specific number of weekdays in each month in the coming year to get the appropriate forecast for each month.

Seasonality

If seasonality exists in the item being forecast, it means that some months are typically low and other months are typically high. If all 60 months for the past 5 years are averaged together, the seasonality becomes lost in the broad average. An approach is needed that is more sensitive to fluctuations within each year. The most obvious approach is to add together the values for a given month for several years and divide to get an average just for that month. For example, the past five February values can be totalled and then divided by five. This provides a February average for the past 5 years that can be used as a prediction for the next February.

This approach is not always acceptable. Suppose that seasonal variations do not repeat in the exact same month each year. For instance, suppose that February is usually the coldest month, causing patient days to peak because of many flu cases. Sometimes, however, January or March might be colder. Because of this variation in seasonality from year to year, a better prediction may result from adding January plus February plus March for the past 5 years. Thus, February is being based on January, February, and March. This total should be divided by 15 to get a prediction for the February of next year. Then March is estimated by adding February plus March plus April for each of the past 5 years and dividing by 15.

The key to this *moving-average* approach is to add up not only the month in question for the past 5 years but also the month preceding and the month following the month being predicted. This formula often gives a good prediction. However, there are also problems with this approach. Peaks and valleys in activity will be understated.

For instance, what if January were typically the busiest month of the year, with both December and February being less busy? Then, by averaging December and February with January, the slower December and February will cause the busier January to be understated in the forecast.

How can a nurse manager determine whether predictions will be improved by using calculations such as this one? Should the manager simply take an average of five Februarys or use January, February, and March information for 5 years to predict next February? One good way to make this determination is to try to use historical data (excluding data from the most recent past year) to predict the results of the past year. For instance, if 2007 has just ended, take data from 2002 through 2006 and use it to predict 2007. The actual results for 2007 are already known, so the prediction can immediately be compared to the actual results. This is a good way to test any formula to see if it is a reasonable predictor.

Keep in mind two things, however. First, no forecast will predict the future perfectly. The future is uncertain, and all the specific events that will occur can never be fully anticipated. Therefore, the prediction should not be expected to match the actual results precisely. Second, the predictions or forecasts using formulas must be adjusted based on the manager's own knowledge about the future. The formulas just use information about the past. If a manager has some information about the future that suggests that the future will not follow the patterns of the past, this information must be used to adjust the predictions of the formulas. The role of an intelligent manager should never be relinquished to the mathematical precision of a formula.

When a formula is tested by seeing how well it can predict what actually happened last year, there should be a determination of whether the predictions based on the formula are closer to what actually happened than the predictions that would have been used in the absence of the formula. If so, then it is a useful tool. Otherwise, the formula should be either modified or discarded.

Trend

If a trend is observed, it is desirable to project that trend into the future. Trends are usually represented by a straight line. However, trends tend to have some random elements within them. If one were to draw a straight line, it would not generally go through each historical point. Some points would be above the line and some would be below the line. A manager could just eyeball the points on the graph and try to draw a line that is as close as possible to all the points and that extends into the future. However, such manual attempts are likely to be inaccurate.

If the line is drawn too high or too low, the estimates for the future will also be too high or too low. Even worse, if the slope of the line is too high or too low, the error will be magnified, as seen in Figure 6-8. In this figure, the first month is assigned a value of 1 on the horizontal axis; the second month is 2, and so on. The solid line represents the best straight line that uses the known data to forecast the future. The dashed line represents a judgmental, eyeball estimate. Note that near the center of the graph, the two lines are relatively close. However, on the right side of the graph in the area of the forecast for the coming year, the two lines have diverged to the point where the number of nursing hours predicted differs a great deal, depending on which line is used.

One solution to this problem is to use a statistical technique called *regression analysis*. The goal of regression analysis is to find the unique straight line that comes

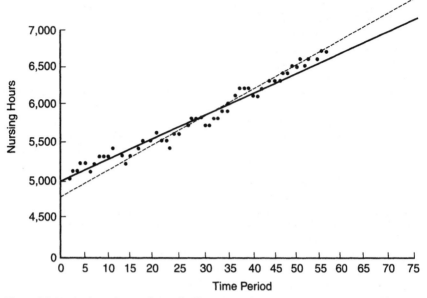

Figure 6-8 Nursing hours forecast for trend with no seasonality: regression versus judgmental forecast.

closest to all the historical data points. Regression analysis can be easily performed by a nurse manager using many types of hand-held calculators or on a computer using statistical software packages, such as the Statistical Package for Social Sciences (SPSS), spreadsheet packages such as Microsoft's Excel or LOTUS 1-2-3, or forecasting packages such as SmartForecasts.

Regression analysis is a technique that applies mathematical precision to a scatter diagram. The scatter diagram used in regression analysis is a graph that plots points of information. Each data point represents a dependent variable and one or more independent variables. The independent variable is sometimes referred to as the causal variable. It is responsible for causing variations in the dependent variable.

In forecasting, time is considered to be an independent variable, and a second variable is considered to be a dependent variable. For example, the dependent variable could be the number of patients treated by the organization. As time passes, the organization may have more or fewer patients. The change in the number of patients over time may reflect a random pattern, seasonal effect, trend, or seasonality and trend, as discussed in this chapter. If a trend exists, regression analysis will generate a line that is a good predictor of the future.

Regression is a tool that can help managers to manage better. The major difficulty in using regression is simply a fear of the process (and this relates not only to nurse managers but to all managers). However, when using a computer program, regression analysis does not require the user to do extensive mathematical computation. The computer carries out all the calculations.[1]

---

[1] Although regression is easy to perform using a computer, the user should have some familiarity with regression to interpret the regression results and their significance. See the regression discussion in Chapter 4 or in a statistics text.

Because regression analysis requires the manager to provide numerical values, months and years cannot be used by their names for the independent variables. An independent variable cannot be referred to as January 2002. Instead, the month names can be replaced by assigning numerical values. The historical months used for the analysis can be numbered 1 through 60 instead of using October 2002, November 2002, and so forth, to September 2007. Table 6-1 presents the data. After feeding the information into a calculator or computer (e.g., in month 1, there were 5,000 nursing hours; in month 2, there were 5,100 nursing hours; and so on through month 60, with 6,700 nursing hours), the calculator or computer is instructed to

TABLE 6-1 Nursing Hours—Historical Data for Trend with No Seasonality

Data Point	Date		Nursing Hours
1	October	2002	5,000
2	November		5,100
3	December		5,100
4	January	2003	5,200
5	February		5,200
6	March		5,100
7	April		5,200
8	May		5,300
9	June		5,300
10	July		5,300
11	August		5,400
12	September		5,300
13	October		5,300
14	November		5,200
15	December		5,300
16	January	2004	5,400
17	February		5,400
18	March		5,500
19	April		5,500
20	May		5,500
21	June		5,600
22	July		5,500
23	August		5,500
24	September		5,400
25	October		5,600
26	November		5,600
27	December		5,700
28	January	2005	5,700
29	February		5,800
30	March		5,800
31	April		5,800

Continued

TABLE 6-1 Nursing Hours—Historical Data for Trend with No Seasonality—cont'd

Data Point	Date		Nursing Hours
32	May		5,700
33	June		5,700
34	July		5,800
35	August		5,800
36	September		5,900
37	October		5,900
38	November		6,000
39	December		6,100
40	January	2006	6,200
41	February		6,200
42	March		6,200
43	April		6,100
44	May		6,100
45	June		6,200
46	July		6,200
47	August		6,300
48	September		6,300
49	October		6,300
50	November		6,400
51	December		6,400
52	January	2007	6,500
53	February		6,500
54	March		6,600
55	April		6,500
56	May		6,600
57	June		6,500
58	July		6,600
59	August		6,700
60	September		6,700

"run" (compute) the regression. When the computation is complete, it is possible to determine how many nursing hours would be expected in months 64 through 75, which represent the 12 months of next year. Note that months 61 through 63 have been intentionally skipped over. There are neither historical data points nor forecast points plotted for those 3 months. This is because those months represent the remaining months of the current year, for which data is not yet available. The goal is to develop predictions for the months in the coming year.

The results are shown in the scatter diagram in Figure 6-9. The regression results are plotted as a solid line for 2008 and are extended back from 2007 to 2002 with a

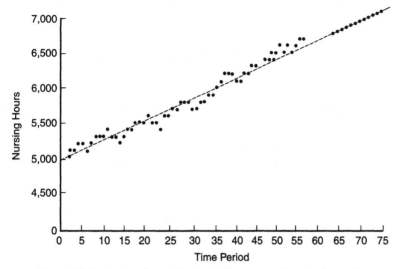

Figure 6-9 Nursing hours forecast for trend with no seasonality: regression results.

dashed line. The specific predictions of nursing-hour requirements for 2008, by month, are as follows:

January	6,772
February	6,800
March	6,828
April	6,856
May	6,884
June	6,911
July	6,939
August	6,967
September	6,995
October	7,023
November	7,051
December	7,079

Note that in Figure 6-9, the projections for the next year all fall on the trend line, even though in the past many points are not on the extended (dashed) trend line. Actual results for the coming year are not expected to fall right on the line; however, in the absence of any other information, the points on the trend line are the best prediction that can be made for the actual uncertain outcome. To guess higher than the trend line value would probably be too high. To guess lower than the trend line value would probably be too low.

Seasonality and Trend

Seasonality together with trend pose a more complex problem; yet it is likely to be a common occurrence, so the reader should pay special attention to the approach discussed here. This example will use the data provided in Table 6-2. The first step is to

TABLE 6-2 Nursing Hours—Historical Data for Trend with Seasonality

Data Point	Date		Nursing Hours
1	October	2002	4,900
2	November		5,000
3	December		5,100
4	January	2003	5,200
5	February		5,100
6	March		5,100
7	April		5,000
8	May		5,000
9	June		4,900
10	July		4,900
11	August		5,000
12	September		5,100
13	October		5,300
14	November		5,400
15	December		5,500
16	January	2004	5,500
17	February		5,400
18	March		5,400
19	April		5,300
20	May		5,200
21	June		5,100
22	July		5,200
23	August		5,300
24	September		5,400
25	October		5,400
26	November		5,500
27	December		5,600
28	January	2005	5,700
29	February		5,700
30	March		5,600
31	April		5,500
32	May		5,400
33	June		5,600
34	July		5,300
35	August		5,300
36	September		5,400
37	October		5,600
38	November		5,700
39	December		5,600
40	January	2006	5,800
41	February		5,900

TABLE 6-2 Nursing Hours—Historical Data for Trend with Seasonality—cont'd

Data Point	Date		Nursing Hours
42	March		5,800
43	April		5,700
44	May		5,600
45	June		5,500
46	July		5,500
47	August		5,600
48	September		5,700
49	October		5,900
50	November		6,000
51	December		6,200
52	January	2007	6,300
53	February		6,300
54	March		6,200
55	April		6,200
56	May		6,100
57	June		6,000
58	July		6,000
59	August		6,100
60	September		6,300

use a regression to predict a trend line for the coming year. Once a set of results for the regression has been plotted for each month in the coming year (January 2008 through December 2008), it should be noted that there is no seasonal appearance on the line predicting the next year. It is simply an upward-trending line (Figure 6-10) for 2008.

The next step is to extend the trend backwards into the 5 years for which there are historical data. This is fairly straightforward because it simply requires extending backward a straight line that has been already located for the coming year (see the dashed line in Figure 6-11).

Once the line has been extended backward, the manager must calculate how much above or below the line the actual value was for each month of the past 5 years. These amounts must then be converted into a percentage. For example, in January 2003 in Figure 6-11, there were 5,200 nursing hours, but the trend line was at a vertical height of 5,000. The actual value was 200 hours above the trend. Because it is a trend, however, it is necessary to convert it to a percentage. In this case, it is a positive 4%, because 5,200 is 4% above the trend-line point of 5,000.

Now simply revert to the seasonal approach. Add together the percentages that December, January, and February are over and under the trend line for the past 5 years and divide by 15. The result is a prediction of the percentage above or below the trend line January will be next year. Find the point on the trend line next year for January and multiply it by the moving-average percent to find how much above or

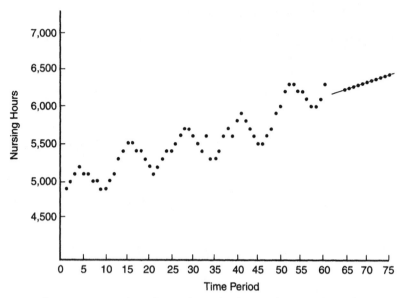

Figure 6-10 Nursing hours forecast for trend with seasonality: regression results.

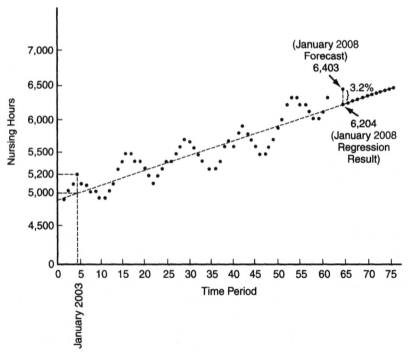

Figure 6-11 Nursing hours forecast for trend with seasonality: regression results extended back into historical data.

TABLE 6-3 Calculation of Moving Average Percent for January 2008

Month		Actual	Trend Line	Difference	Difference as a Percentage of Trend Line
December	2002	5,100	4,980	120	2.4%
January	2003	5,200	5,000	200	4.0
February	2003	5,100	5,020	80	1.6
December	2003	5,500	5,221	279	5.3
January	2004	5,500	5,241	259	4.9
February	2004	5,400	5,261	139	2.6
December	2004	5,600	5,461	139	2.5
January	2005	5,700	5,482	218	4.0
February	2005	5,700	5,502	198	3.6
December	2005	5,600	5,702	(102)*	(1.8)*
January	2006	5,800	5,723	77	1.3
February	2006	5,900	5,743	157	2.7
December	2006	6,200	5,943	257	4.3
January	2007	6,300	5,963	337	5.7
February	2007	6,300	5,983	317	5.3
				Total	48.4%
				Divided by 15 =	3.2%

*Figures in parentheses indicate negative amounts.

below the trend line the predicted point is. This process can be repeated for each month of the coming year.

For example, Table 6-3 shows the actual number of nursing hours incurred and the extended trend-line information for December, January, and February for 5 years.

The trend-line prediction for January 2008 from Figure 6-11 is 6,204. This is before adjustment for seasonality. In the calculation shown in Table 6-3, it was determined that for January the moving-average percentage is a positive 3.2% of 6,204. By adding 3.2% of 6,204 to the trend line value of 6,204, the resulting prediction adjusted for seasonality is 6,403. That point has been plotted for January 2008 in Figure 6-11. Similarly, to get the 2008 forecast for the entire year, this process should be repeated on a moving-average basis for each month in turn.

■ USING COMPUTERS FOR FORECASTING

The previous section on forecasting formulas demonstrates how complicated forecasting can become when historical data are influenced by both trend and seasonality. However, health care organizations frequently do have at least seasonality; both trend and seasonality are not uncommon. In recent years, nurse managers' ability to deal with such patterns has improved dramatically as a result of personal computers and specially designed computer software. These computer programs make the work of forecasting easier and the results more accurate.

A number of forecasting programs are available. This section discusses forecasting using one such program, SmartForecasts.[2] This program is an example of computer forecasting software that is not limited to linear forecasting. Regression analysis produces a straight-line forecast. When there is seasonality, certain months are always above the regression line and others are always below it. Software such as SmartForecasts can generate *curvilinear* (curved line) forecasts. That means that the forecast line generated will come closer to the historical points, and therefore its projections are likely to be closer to the results that will actually occur.

SmartForecasts provides a data entry format similar to that of an electronic spreadsheet (e.g., LOTUS 1-2-3 or Excel), with columns and rows. Each column represents a time period, and each row represents a variable to be forecast, such as patients or nursing hours.

Reconsider the forecast for the data from Table 6-2 using SmartForecasts. After the data are entered, one of the first steps is to print a time plot graph to get a visual sense of the data. Examination of the time plot in Figure 6-12 quickly alerts the user to the upward trend. Closer inspection reveals the seasonal nature of the data.

A number of different forecasting models are available within the software program. SmartForecasts allows the user to forecast nursing hours using regression analysis. However, if regression analysis is used, given the seasonality observed in the time plot, the same problem will occur as existed in Figure 6-10, requiring the same manual adjustments shown in Figure 6-11 and Table 6-3.

The key advantage of this software and other programs like it is that it allows the use of a curved line for forecasting. This removes the necessity of adjusting the trend line for seasonality. However, which forecasting approach should be used? Available methods include exponential smoothing, moving average, multiseries analysis, and so on.

Moving average approaches were used in the earlier section on forecasting formulas in this chapter. However, will that approach give the best result if other advanced statistical techniques are available? The best approach, until one is very familiar with forecasting, is to use automatic forecasting, which lets the computer choose the best approach. With the automatic approach the computer will calculate the forecast using a number of different methods to see which predicts best.

Figure 6-13 is the forecast graph generated by the software program. What does the graph consist of? The historical data points are connected by a solid line. The forecast during the historical (past) periods is dotted. Compare this dotted line with the regression line shown in Figure 6-11. During the first 5 years in Figure 6-11 the actual points are usually substantially above or below the regression line. Therefore, it is reasonable to assume that as the line is used to project the next year, each month's actual result is likely to be substantially above or below the forecast trend line.

Although the statistical theory is complex, effectively, the closer the forecast line comes to the actual results in the past, the more likely the forecast line is to come close to the actual results in the future. When the computer performs forecasting automatically, it examines how close the forecast line is to the historical actual points for each of a series of different forecasting methods. The computer can be given a command

---

[2] SmartForecasts is a trademark of Smart Software, Inc., 4 Hill Road, Belmont, MA 02178; telephone (617) 489-2743. Version 4.16 was used for Figures 6-12 and 6-13, and Tables 6-4 and 6-5 in this chapter. This chapter does not attempt to demonstrate all the capabilities of this software. The software program is used simply as an example of the use of computer forecasting. The use of the examples in this chapter does not represent a formal endorsement of the product.

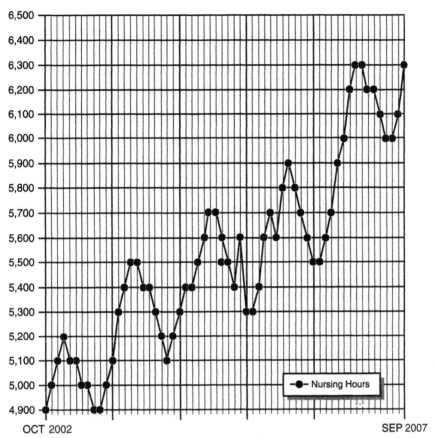

Figure 6-12 SmartForecasts time plot graph of historical data.

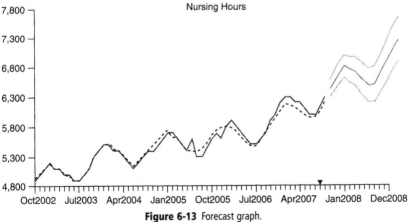

Figure 6-13 Forecast graph.

to examine the relative accuracy of the various forecasting methods examined. Table 6-4 shows the results of the competition among forecasting methods for this example. The best technique is Winters' multiplicative method. Winters' is a curvilinear approach that works extremely well for seasonal data. The data points are only 1.3% farther away from the forecast line for the next best method, another form of Winters' forecasting. However, using alternatives to the Winters' approaches generates much less accurate results.

In Figure 6-13 it is evident that the dotted forecast line for the first 5 years follows the actual results extremely closely. In some cases the solid and dotted lines are so close that they cannot be distinguished from each other. Therefore, the forecast line, when projected through 2008, is likely to give a fairly accurate estimate.

In the graph shown in Figure 6-13 there are solid lines above and below (bracketing) the forecast line projected into the future. These lines represent a margin-of-error interval. Forecasts can never be expected to be exactly correct. It is possible, however, to use statistics to get some idea of how large the difference might be between the forecast and the actual result. In this case, based on the statistical analysis there is a 90% likelihood that the actual result will fall somewhere between these solid lines. But graphs, although visually informative, are hard to read when it is time to write the actual forecast. Another computer command provides a numerical table of the forecast results. Table 6-5 shows the forecast results.

This table shows not only the forecast but also the margin of error or confidence interval above and below the forecast. If desired, that interval can easily be changed so that there is 95% or 99% confidence that the actual result will fall within the range of values between the lower limit and upper limit estimates. If the percentage is raised to a higher confidence level, the interval around the forecast line becomes wider. For example, for January 2008 the prediction is 6,821 nursing hours, and there is 90% confidence that the actual nursing hours will not be fewer than 6,622 or more than 7,020. If a manager wants to be 99% confident that the actual results will not exceed the boundaries of the projection, the lower limit value becomes lower and the upper limit higher.

In practice it is rarely necessary to be so precise. Although 95% or 99% confidence may be important for academic research studies, in practice, managers tend to have a greater degree of latitude. In fact, the SmartForecasts software program is preset by the manufacturer to give a 90% confidence. It is simple for the user to change that confidence level, given the way the software is set up, but one must question whether it is desirable. Essentially, a 90% confidence interval implies that nine times out of ten the actual result will fall within the bounds of the interval. That is an extremely good result for most managers' forecasts.

TABLE 6-4 Tournament Rankings for AUTOMATIC Forecasts of V1 Nursing Hours

Rank	Method	% Worse than Winner
1	Winters' multiplicative, weights = 22%, 22%, 22%	(winner)
2	Winters' additive, weights = 20%, 20%, 20%	1.3
3	Double exponential smoothing, weight = 8%	57.2
4	Linear moving average of 12 periods	65.0
5	Simple moving average of 1 period	118.3
6	Single exponential smoothing, weight = 59%	118.9

TABLE 6-5 Forecasts of V1 NURSING HOURS Using Multiplicative WINTERS' METHOD

Time Period		Approximate 90% Forecast Interval		
		Lower Limit	Forecast	Upper Limit
October	2007	6,284	6,434	6,584
November	2007	6,405	6,572	6,740
December	2007	6,520	6,704	6,888
January	2008	6,622	6,821	7,020
February	2008	6,549	6,766	6,983
March	2008	6,502	6,737	6,973
April	2008	6,391	6,641	6,891
May	2008	6,306	6,570	6,834
June	2008	6,210	6,493	6,775
July	2008	6,205	6,507	6,809
August	2008	6,311	6,633	6,956
September	2008	6,449	6,788	7,126
October	2008	6,634	6,996	7,358
November	2008	6,769	7,143	7,516
December	2008	6,897	7,282	7,666

Compare the results obtained by using Winters' multiplicative method (see Table 6-5, Figure 6-13) with the earlier result obtained by using the combined regression-analysis/moving-average approach (see January 2008 in Figure 6-11). As can be seen, the results differ. This is because the approach used earlier is less accurate than the Winters' method. Earlier, the January 2008 number of nursing hours was projected to be 6,403, whereas the Winters' method predicts it to be approximately 6,821. In fact, the earlier estimate is below the lower limit value of the 90% confidence interval. It is clear that using more sophisticated techniques can generate results that differ markedly from the manual approaches used before computer software was readily available. It is probable that the manual moving-average calculation will be more accurate than simply a judgmental guess. However, the computer-based Winters' solution is likely to be even more accurate.

It is also possible to refine the Winters' method even further. The computer makes some general assumptions when it performs forecasts using the automatic approach. If the Winters' method were immediately selected as the forecasting method instead of selecting automatic, some additional options would be provided to improve the forecast further. Specifically, the SmartForecasts software can be informed of the relative importance of the most recent level, trend, and seasonal factors. If the user knows that the trend is changing because of shifts in the underlying demographics of the community's population, it is possible to give more weight to the most recent trend than to the trend in the earlier years.

Not only can information be supplied to enable the computer to be more accurate, such as the relative importance of the recent trend, but it is also possible to modify the results of the computer analysis. Results can be adjusted directly on the forecast graph, or historical data points can be modified on the basis of some judgment or knowledge the user has that is not reflected in the historical information.

This is especially helpful when there is an outlier data point. For example, suppose that a rare event caused data for 1 month to be atypical. That data point can cause the forecast to be thrown off substantially. A better forecast may be obtained by judgmentally adjusting that data point's value. Judgmental adjustments are also needed because computer-generated forecasts assume that factors that affected nursing hours remain the same in the future as they were in the past. That may not be the case.

Initially, a manager is likely to use a forecasting program only to forecast one item at a time. However, as one becomes more adept at using computer-based forecasting, the program would probably be used to generate forecasts of a number of different variables. The user will also want to be able to save the data file to avoid having to re-enter data each time an analysis is to be performed. The SmartForecasts program has its own data files, and the data can also be stored in a wide variety of formats for future use, including Microsoft Excel spreadsheet files, ASCII (generic) files, or DIF files. By the same token, data in another format such as Excel, ASCII, or DIF can be read into SmartForecasts.

SmartForecasts is one of a number of forecasting programs that can be used in a personal computer. The most significant aspect of using sophisticated software programs is that they can generate a substantially improved result. The ability of the forecast line to curve in synchronization with the actual historical seasonal pattern decreases the required effort by the manager substantially, while enhancing the result.

■ DELPHI AND NOMINAL GROUP FORECASTING

The discussions in this chapter have assumed that reasonably reliable historical data are available. However, there will be many instances, especially in the case of new ventures, in which a forecast will be needed for a budget even though there are no reliable historical data. Subjective estimates will be required. In such cases, regression analysis and even computerized curvilinear forecasting will be inadequate to provide a solution. Two approaches commonly used to aid in making reasonable subjective forecasts are the *Delphi* and *Nominal Group* techniques.

In both approaches, a team or panel must be selected; it is composed of people who are likely to have reasoned insights with respect to the item being forecast. Although no one may have direct knowledge or experience, an attempt should be made to select a qualified group. Industrial experience has shown that by arriving at a consensus among a team of experts, subjective forecasts can be reasonably accurate.

The Nominal Group technique is one in which the individuals are brought together in a structured meeting. Each member writes down a forecast. Then all the written forecasts are presented to the group by a leader, without discussion. Once all of the forecasts have been revealed, the reasoning behind each one is discussed. After the discussions, each member again makes a forecast in writing. Through a repetitive process, eventually a group decision is made.

Obviously, there are weaknesses in the Nominal Group technique. One problem concerns lack of information. If different forecasts are made based on different assumptions, it may be impossible to reach consensus. Another problem concerns politics and personalities. As members of the group defend their forecasts, extraneous issues having to do with whose idea it is may bias the group's decision.

With the Delphi technique, the group never meets. All forecasts are presented in writing to the leader, who provides summaries to all group members. When a forecast differs substantially from the forecasts of the majority—either high or low—a request is made for the reasoning behind the forecast. This information is shared with all group members. Then a new round of forecasts is made. This process is repeated several times, and then a decision is made based on the collective responses.

Delphi has several particular advantages. By avoiding a face-to-face meeting, confrontation is avoided. Decisions are based more on logic than on personality or position. The dissemination of the respondent's underlying reasoning allows erroneous facts or assumptions to be eliminated.

These two methods both make use of the fact that individual managers cannot be expected to think of everything. Different individuals, bringing different expertise and different points of view to bear on the same problem, can create an outcome that is superior to the results any one of them could have produced individually. It is a cliché to say that two minds are better than one. Nevertheless, it is true that in many forecasting instances, the Delphi and Nominal Group approaches can substantially improve results.

Summary and Implications for Nurse Managers

Forecasting is an essential part of the budgeting process. Many elements, such as number of patients, lengths of stay, and levels of acuity, are essential ingredients of an operating budget. Preparing an operating budget cannot begin without some prediction of the values for these variables. The same holds true for other types of budgets.

Managers have great flexibility in selecting the variables that they choose to forecast. They can forecast the number of patients, the number of patient days, the quantity of a resource that will be consumed (e.g., the number of chest tubes needed or the number of nursing care hours), the amount that will be spent on supplies or personnel, or the acuity level of patients. Any variable for which historical data are available can be forecast using the methods discussed in this chapter.

The forecasting process consists of collecting data, graphing the data, analyzing the graphed data, and preparing prediction formulas. Care must be exercised regarding consideration of factors that are changing and that will prevent the future from being like the past. For example, a change in federal regulations concerning types of treatments covered by Medicare might have a dramatic impact on volume. Managers are aware of such changes, but computerized formulas are unlikely to take discrete, recent changes into account. The human role in the forecasting process is critical to generating accurate forecasts.

Analysis of the graphed data will help a manager determine whether the item to be forecast has been exhibiting seasonal or trend behavior, or both, or neither. Formulas can then be used to make predictions of the future.

It is important for managers not only to use common techniques of management but also to be prepared to be leaders in developing new techniques. The first decade of the 21st century is likely to see a rapid increase in the use of computers by health care managers. The first wave of microcomputer use saw widespread introduction of personal computers in situations where the same rote function had to be performed over and over. Computers clearly increase productivity by being faster at performing a calculation currently done many times. The next wave of computer use often represented a novelty. Computers were widely introduced but in many cases were used only as sophisticated typewriters (word processors).

Now, however, the average manager will start to use personal computers to manage better—not just to do an existing calculation faster or to type nice-looking letters. Forecasting is one area where the results of a manager's efforts will be superior because the use of a computer can allow a greater degree of sophistication to be merged with the already existing judgment and experience of the manager.

At the same time, one must always bear in mind that the sophisticated techniques of forecasting lack the judgment and experience of managers. Therefore, whether one is using a subjective Delphi technique or an objective computer program, the role of the manager in making the final forecast should never be understated.

References and Suggested Readings

Finarelli, H.J., and Johnson, T. (2004). Effective demand forecasting in 9 steps. *Healthcare Financial Management* 58(11), 52-56, 58.

Finkler, S.A., and Kovner, C.T. (2000). *Financial Management for Nurse Managers and Executives*, ed 2. Philadelphia: W.B. Saunders.

Finkler, S.A., and Ward, D.R. (1999). *Cost Accounting for Health Care Organizations: Concepts and Applications*, ed 2. Gaithersburg, MD: Aspen.

Horngren, C.T., Foster, G., and Datar, S.M. (1999). *Cost Accounting: A Managerial Emphasis*, ed 10. Englewood Cliffs, NJ: Prentice-Hall.

Lakdawalla, D., Goldman, D., Bhattacharya, J., Hurd, M.D., Joyce, G.F., and Panis, C.W. (2003).

Forecasting the Nursing Home Population. *Medical Care* 41(1), 8-20.

Wilkinson, P., Chalabi, Z., Raine, R., and Stevens, M. (2005). Evaluation of a pilot health forecasting system for England. *Epidemiology* 16(5), 93.

Williamson, J.D. (2003). Forecasting health service needs for older adults: Some sun, some clouds. *Medical Care* 41(1), 25-27.

Zimmerman, S. (1996). Forecasting and its importance to health managers in the ever-changing health care industry. *Hospital Cost Management & Accounting* 7(12), 1-8.

Strategic Planning and Business Plans

LEARNING OBJECTIVES
The goals of this chapter are to:

- Define strategic planning and management, their importance to health care organizations, and the benefits of the strategic planning process
- Describe the evolution of strategic management from long-range planning to strategic planning to strategic management
- Distinguish between broad, long-term goals and time-oriented, specific, measurable objectives
- Develop concepts of quality improvement in health care

- Discuss each element of a strategic plan
- Stress the importance of strategic thought by all managers in carrying out the operating budget
- Explain the role of the long-range budget and strategic plan in the planning process
- Define program budgeting and discuss the zero-base budgeting technique, stressing the importance of examining alternatives
- Outline the uses and elements of a business plan

■ INTRODUCTION

Strategic planning is the systematic process by which an organization determines its mission and the goals and objectives necessary to achieve that mission (Camillus, 1986; Allison et al., 2005). In a rapidly changing environment, this may require the leaders of the organization to specifically and regularly redefine the mission of the organization and its goals and objectives. *Strategic management* involves the process of evaluating the internal and external environment of the organization in order to acquire and allocate the resources necessary to achieve the organization's mission, (Hunger & Wheelen, 2006). This process includes an environmental assessment and depends heavily on data concerning the organization's external environment. The effectiveness of these strategic processes is critical to the organization's success. Managers and their staffs must not only do the things they do well, but must also carefully decide what actions to take to achieve their goals, and the priority for each activity. The strategic planning and management processes are time consuming, but without them, people in an organization may end up so busy accomplishing tasks that they don't take the time to ensure that the tasks they are doing help the organization to succeed.

Henry David Thoreau provides us with something to think about when we are too "busy" to develop plans for our work: "It is not enough to be busy—the question is, what are we busy about?" (Ellis and Pekar, 1980). This simple question should cause nurse managers to pause and consider their role in the budget process. Day-to-day routine activities often cause nurse managers to become overloaded.

Managers become so busy that they have little time to plan for the future or to introduce innovations. Then it becomes entirely possible for the organization's nursing service to become obsolete in its structure and how it functions within the organization. It is important for all managers to structure their jobs so that planning does not become pushed aside by the pressing day-in and day-out issues.

The application of strategy to managing organizations is still a developing field. In the middle of the 20th century, businesses began to place a growing reliance on *long-range planning*. Long-range plans focus on general objectives to be achieved by the organization over a period of typically 3 to 5 years. By the 1960s the term *strategy* had become commonplace, and long-range planning had started being referred to as *strategic planning*. It was contrasted with operational planning—the development of a detailed plan for the coming year.

When strategic planning was introduced, the concept of strategy was that operational planning is tactical, whereas long-range planning is strategic. Under strategic or long-range planning, an organization prepares a set of goals, and then a strategy is developed for accomplishing them. That strategy is formalized into a plan of action generally covering a horizon of 3 to 5 years.

In the late 1980s and the 1990s experts in the area started to use the more generic term strategic management to define better the role of strategic thought in organizations (Koteen, 1989). Such experts argue for a broad view of strategic planning. Into the 21st century, the primary focus remains the identification of broad, long-term goals and the creation of plans to achieve them. However, the current view of strategic management or strategic planning relies on the use of strategic thought in guiding the plans and actions of the entire organization (McNamara, 2006). This relates to short-term operational plans as well as long-range plans. In fact, the rapidly changing environment has dramatically reduced the time span for which strategic plans are developed. The planners may originally identify a 3 to 5 year time span for the plan, but review and revision of strategic plans on a yearly basis are common. Today, a strategic plan may even be considered to be a guide for only the coming year (McNamara, 2006). What has not changed, however, is that the strategic plan determines the organization's direction and priorities for at least the coming year. Thus the operating budget discussed in the next chapter must always be viewed in its context within the strategic plan of the organization.

Strategic planning is no longer simply long-range planning with a new name, as it was in the 1970s, 1980s, and 1990s. Strategic management "stresses three points: that the strategic planner is clearly the advisor and facilitator to line management decision-makers; that the program executive, not the strategic planner, is the key strategist; and that strategic planning is always integrated with other functions of the program management process—program design, organizing, budgeting, staffing, controlling, and evaluating" (Koteen, 1997, p. 21). Long-range planning may still be a part of strategic planning, but it is no longer the only feature.

The current philosophy is that thinking strategically should not be the sole domain of the strategic planners of the organization. Planning by professional planners is important but insufficient. Strategic thought should be an element of the job description of all managers throughout the organization because it is they who will be responsible for implementing the plan (McNamara, 2006). Nurse managers have a central role in strategic planning in this new philosophical approach. The way a nursing unit is organized to provide care, the way it establishes patterns of staff to provide care, and the financial budgets it develops to gain authorization of needed resources to provide care should all be outcomes of a strategic process managed at the unit level. The principal change from earlier views of strategic planning is the emphasis on bringing all managers into the direct process of working to achieve the organization's primary goals instead of focusing narrowly on specific short-term or departmental objectives.

This chapter first discusses the definition, aims, and benefits of strategic planning and strategic thought. It then focuses on several specific aspects of strategic management, namely, long-range plans, program budgets, and business plans.

■ PROCESS IMPROVEMENT

A theme for the provision of health services in the 21st century is improved quality of care at decreased cost. During the 1980s and 1990s, process improvement focused on reengineering, total quality management (TQM), and *continuous quality improvement (CQI)*. However, cost reduction was still the main priority during those decades. Shortly after the turn of the century (1999 to 2000), quality of care became a national focus and priority. This emphasis was the result of the Institute of Medicine's publication of *To Err Is Human: Building a Safer Health System* in 1999. This publication reported that at least 100,000 hospital deaths every year in the United States are caused by medical errors.

The attention of the federal government, American hospitals, health insurance companies, and health care practitioners was captured by this report. It caused a major shift in attention from cost reduction to quality of care. Although cost control was certainly not abandoned, virtually all key players in the American health care system understood the report's point that providing care that was error prone, providing the wrong care, or providing unnecessary care was enormously expensive, wasteful of precious health care dollars, and very often damaging to the patient. Society in general and patients in particular could not be well served by providing care that was unnecessary at best or harmful at worst. Therefore, a major shift in priorities took place among all institutional constituents of American health care: insurers, care providers, and the government.

The quality management approach adopted by The Joint Commission[1] and most health care facilities is based on the original work done by Deming and Juran. The key principle of their approach to quality was to reduce errors in production before they occurred. This was quite different from the approach prior to their major contributions; the earlier approach to quality had been to discover errors and then try to fix whatever had caused the errors. Deming introduced the concept of CQI, which many workers at the time converted into the slogan "If it ain't broke, fix it anyway," a play on the cliché "If it ain't broke, don't fix it." The Juran Institute has been a leader in assisting American businesses to develop and implement successful quality-improvement programs since 1979. The thinking and concepts of these two men formed the foundation for the Six Sigma approach to quality improvement (developed at Motorola company), which is one of the most respected quality-improvement programs in use today (Motorola University, 2006; Six Sigma Academy, 2006). Six Sigma is an approach in which the error rate is driven down to almost no errors—statistically defined as the likelihood of an error's occurring being at least six standard

---

[1] Formerly known as The Joint Commission on Accreditation of Healthcare Organizations (JCAHO). The organization has changed its name to simply, The Joint Commission. See http://www.jointcommission.org/ for more information.

deviations from the mean. That translates into an error rate limit of fewer than 3.4 errors per million opportunities for error. Each business must define what an opportunity for error would be in the context of its work or production processes. Six Sigma is a rigorous statistical approach to measuring quality and the work processes that produce quality by taking a preventive approach to errors (iSixSigma, 2006). This approach to quality improvement was founded by Deming and Juran, who helped Japanese businesses to base production quality control on a preventive approach to quality problems. All quality programs based on the work of Deming and Juran, including Six Sigma, use systematic, well-defined strategies to address continuous improvement in work processes and to diagnose and treat any problems concerning quality that do arise.

The U.S. business community did not initially accept the theories related to quality put forth by these two U.S.-educated scientists. From a strategic management perspective, production in America had been dominated by an attitude of getting it done and then fixing it if necessary. However, during the late 1940s, Japan made a commitment to developing their businesses for a worldwide customer base.

To accomplish that, Japan had to overcome the image that Japanese manufactured goods had extremely poor quality. In fact, during the 1940s and 1950s in the United States, the phrase, "made in Japan" was used as a joking way to describe cheap, poorly made products. However, shortly after World War II, both Deming and Juran were hired by business associations in Japan to bring their expertise in quality improvement to that culture. Their ideas of process improvement using statistical process control and various techniques of motivating workers by using their knowledge of manufacturing problems in the process of improving quality were widely adopted in Japan. As a result, Japanese-made goods became a world standard for quality. In America, however, the old methods were not working. The quality of American goods, once the benchmark of quality worldwide, deteriorated until, in the 1980s, "made in America" began to sound like the old joke "made in Japan."

As a result, American-made goods began to suffer serious sales losses, and not only in the world market; even in the United States, people began to seek out Japanese-made goods and eschew American-made goods—especially automobiles. There were many business reports and even news reports of the reasons for Japan's success and American businesses' failures in the marketplace. But in the end, all reports emphasized the poor quality and poor customer service offered by American businesses. As a result, most major American businesses adopted the Japanese quality-improvement techniques. Health care organizations were much slower to follow the trend, however.

There is a basic difference between quality problems in manufacturing and quality problems in health care. In manufacturing, quality problems generally produce scrap. Scrap is any part or product manufactured that cannot be sold because of errors in production. Scrap is obvious, and the cost of the wastage can be fairly easily calculated. A defective part often cannot be installed in a product, or if it is possible to install it, the bad part may well make the entire product nonfunctional and unable to be sold. The customer has no relationship with the product until it leaves the factory and is sold. And the customer is the person who purchases the product for use and is the individual to complain if the product's quality is problematic. Quality is not difficult to evaluate. A few simple questions can be asked: Does the product work as it should when first purchased? Does it continue to work as if still new for a reasonable amount of time after purchase? Does its usable life last a reasonable amount of time?

Does the product look good or has it been cosmetically damaged when purchased? The answers to these questions can give the product's producer a good idea of whether the organization is producing quality goods and services.

In health care, the situation is entirely different. The "product" might be defined as the services delivered to patients. But patients don't always know whether they are getting good-quality care. If medication errors are made, patients may know they are not getting better, but they may not know that it is because they received poor-quality care. Furthermore, patients are seldom the payers for the care received. Patients' insurance companies pay for the care, so even if patients complain about poor-quality services, the insurance companies may not complain; and it is those who pay for the services who are in the best position to demand improvement.

Ultimately, that meant that nobody with any power was forcing those who provided health care to monitor quality adequately or to take action to improve the quality of health care services. There was no national agreement that the outcomes of health care should be monitored and no national data to use as a quality index against which health care outcomes in individual facilities or practices could be compared.

Additionally, the fact that individual patients are part of the process increases the reluctance of health care providers to be held accountable for the outcomes of the care they provide. For example, most preventive health care recommendations require that patients carry out changes in their lifestyles. The provider has no control over patients' follow-through on prevention activities. Even treatment interventions that the provider does have control over, such as surgical procedures, may have results that are not entirely within the control of the provider. Different people have different body chemistries and health profiles. So people may have very different reactions to the same intervention. One patient may do extremely well after major surgery whereas a patient of similar age and health status may suffer serious complications or even die after the same surgery. Sometimes these aspects are not within the control of the care provider, even under the best of circumstances. What the provider can control is the care-delivery process.

As a result, most quality-monitoring practices in health care facilities and practices focused on monitoring the process of care—not on the outcomes. Nurses often monitored things like how many admission assessment documents and care plans were completed within 8 hours of admission to a hospital, whether the drugs in the drug cabinet and crash cart were all current (not expired), and whether the correct medications and supplies were on hand in the care unit. The process of care is extremely important, but a problem occurs when processes are monitored, rather than outcomes. How will anybody know whether the processes being carried out are likely to produce good outcomes if the outcomes are not measured?

During the 1980s and 1990s, the focus on the process of care began to be criticized as being inadequate after the publication of several studies by the National Medicare Database that showed wide variations in mortality rates among patients with the same illnesses who were being cared for in different hospitals and in different regions of the United States. In 1994, Dr. Linda Aiken and her research team published the results of a study that reported lower mortality rates in hospitals where the nursing care was considered to be of especially high quality (Aiken et al., 1994). Then in 1999, the Institute of Medicine published its landmark work, which reported that as many as 100,000 hospital deaths per year were caused by medical errors (IOM, 1999). The entire health care industry responded to this confirmation that varying personnel constellations and differing clinical practices had significant effects on the mortality rates of hospitalized patients. In particular, the Joint Commission stepped up its requirements for quality monitoring and for using the results of quality monitoring to improve care in the facilities they accredited (Luquire and Houston, 1998).

A new focus on "doing the right thing" came about. The old focus had been on "doing things right," but as the research demonstrated, the things providers in the health care system were doing were, in some important instances, not the right things to do. Several reviews of the National Medicare Database and the Agency for Healthcare Research and Quality (AHRQ) National Hospital Discharge Summary database revealed that medical protocols—and thus costs of care—as well as patient outcomes for the same medical problem varied widely by institution and region of the U.S. Measurement of patient care outcomes gained a great deal of attention. Hospitals with the best outcomes for each of a variety of medical problems treated were identified and became the *benchmarks* for other facilities. "Benchmark" means an indicator against which something else can be evaluated or measured; a standard. As used in health care, it typically means the facility or clinician with the best known performance in a particular area. Another clinician or facility can compare its performance against the benchmark to measure how well it is performing as compared with the best known performance. Benchmarking is discussed at greater length in Chapter 17.

The best performance may be in one of three areas, according to the theory of Donabedian, who identified the three components of care quality: the structure of care, the process of care, and the outcomes of care (Pronovost et al., 2006). When quality in health care is addressed, it is important to understand whether the author is talking about structure, process, or outcomes. And when outcomes are addressed, it is critical to know whether the author is talking about nursing outcomes (e.g., nursing satisfaction, nursing turnover, etc.) or about patient outcomes (e.g., cure rates, nosocomial infections, mortality, etc.).

In manufacturing, quality is almost entirely focused on product quality. However, in health care, the structure and process of care must also be measured and improved as ways of producing higher quality patient outcomes. Quality management in the health care arena today focuses far more on patient outcomes than was the case in the 1980s and 1990s. As a result of the Institute of Medicine's report on medical errors in hospitals, there is now a strong focus on the cost of problems related to clinical errors. A major source of clinical errors involves poor system structures and processes that make clinical errors almost inevitable. Much work must be done to address the design of care-delivery systems so as to determine which structures and processes predispose nurses to make clinical errors. This type of work is called reengineering. Quality theory tells us that it is important to involve the people providing care in the process of analyzing the system and designing and implementing improvements in the system because they are the people closest to the problem and are likely to know where some of the system's problems lie. In many cases, these types of efforts to plan and change benefit from the services of an expert in clinical systems design. Once a system's problems are identified, care structures and processes can be redesigned so that clinicians have systems that support instead of interfere with their efforts to deliver high-quality, error-free care. Unfortunately, managers complain that there is no time for planning, so errors continue to occur. This is a false savings. The costs of the ongoing errors can far exceed the planning and implementation costs. Observations of the Japanese production process have taught us that if more time is spent on planning, less will be done wrong and less will have to be fixed.

Many American corporations learned this lesson during the 1980s and 1990s as they lost some of their competitive edge. To regain that edge, corporations have adopted procedures that focus on avoiding the costs associated with poor quality. Examples of the change in attitude are apparent in the slogans adopted by corporations. For example, Ethicon, a manufacturer of sutures, adopted the policy "Get it right the first time, every time."

It costs money to produce quality. However, problems in quality also cost money, and sometimes a lot of money. TQM focuses on the issue of being responsive to the needs of customers, while at the same time reducing waste. Kirk notes in examinations of Japanese firms: "The most significant discovery was related to their determination to **build quality into the product (or service)** rather than to inspect for errors after the fact and assume that error removal would lead to quality. Many Japanese managers bought into the concept of planning and followed through on it—unlike many American managers who use the ready-fire-aim approach. 'We don't have time to plan,' some American managers say. Contrarily, many Japanese businessmen say, 'We don't have time **not** to plan'" (Kirk, 1992, 24). Nurse managers would do well to consider the costs of not taking time to plan. With more planning, fewer "things" might get done. But the things that are done are more likely to be the right things. And the things that don't get done may well be counterproductive—they are deliberately not done because planning has revealed those things to be detrimental to achievement of the organization's mission.

Various authors have identified different elements of TQM and CQI. Deming established 14 points related to TQM (Walker, 2005). They include such factors as a focus on the education and training of employees, viewing employees not only as providers but also as customers, quality insurance, and a constant focus on finding ways to improve quality.

TQM and CQI are not financial management tools per se, and a detailed analysis of the methods is not appropriate here.[2] However, TQM and CQI have tremendous financial implications. Historically, health care organizations have minimized planning and maximized control over day-to-day operations. The lesson of TQM and CQI is that managers will be more likely to achieve their objectives if they can redesign their work to allow much more time for planning and innovating. Such activities are not occasional but rather should be viewed as a major element of the management function. It is important to learn to focus on improving the service provided rather than simply making sure that it is provided.

In the first decade of the 21st century, the focus has shifted from concerns only about the cost of care to concerns that the best possible quality be provided at reasonable costs. This has forced a shift away from strictly TQM and CQI toward value-added analysis, which requires measurement of the value of health care services—that is, the outcomes of care. We must spend money only on activities that add value. All non-value-added functions represent wasted resources. And ineffective care protocols that produce suboptimal patient outcomes are wasteful. The key focus, however, should not be on reengineering, TQM, CQI, or value-added functions. The important focus for the manager should be on process improvement. Managers must find out which processes produce the best patient care outcomes and nursing outcomes;

[2] The interested reader is referred to the readings on the topic listed at the end of this chapter.

then they must manage clinical operations so that the best processes are applied consistently. This is the best approach for ensuring that society receives the best value for its health care dollars. In the long run, increased focus on the improvement of quality will lead to higher satisfaction among staff and patients, to lower costs, and to better patient outcomes.

■ STRATEGIC PLANNING

As noted earlier, strategic management calls for setting objectives, allocating resources, and establishing policies concerning those resources. Under this strategic-planning approach, all managers become involved in the process.

To establish and achieve goals, strategic planners have found it useful for the managers of an organization to focus on a series of key questions. The following questions are the most essential an organization must consider:

- Why does the organization exist?
- What is the organization currently?
- What would it like to be?
- How can we make the transformation to what it wants to be?
- How will it know when that has been accomplished?

These questions, in turn, lead to a large number of other questions. What are the organization's strengths? Its weaknesses? Its opportunities? Its threats? Who are the organization's primary customers? Are they being well served? Does the organization learn from its mistakes? Does the organization have a vision for the future? These questions are related to the organization as a whole, but they also relate to each department and unit within the organization.

Managers need to step aside from the current day-to-day activities and assess the nature of the existing organization. Has the organization over the years lost track of its reason for existence? Have environmental conditions, including the political, financial, and medical situations changed so that the organization needs to realign its mission? Is the current status of the organization the desired one? If not, the organization needs to address formally the issue of how it can change things to become the type of organization it believes it should be. Again, this is true for departments and units as well as for entire organizations.

Strategic planning asserts that the way for an organization to become the type of organization its leaders want it to be is to establish clear goals and objectives and a plan for achieving them. Goals are defined as the broad aims of the organization; objectives are specific targets to be achieved to attain those goals.[3]

Once goals and objectives have been identified, specific tactics can be designed to move the organization toward those goals. Tactical plans require resources. When managers prepare operating budgets they often fail to include the resources necessary to achieve the goals of the strategic plan. That is one reason strategic management now takes a more global perspective.

In developing a short-term operating budget for the coming year, the unit manager must decide whether to place more emphasis on short-run profits or long-term growth. Spending extra money on quality improvements now will generate immediate

---

[3] The planning literature is inconsistent in the definition of goals and objectives. In some instances the definition used here for goals is assigned to objectives, and vice versa.

expenses that will not necessarily be offset by current revenues. But the reputation for quality will generate more revenues in the future. If strategic plans and operating budgets are treated as being separate, it forces managers with responsibility for operating expenses to focus on reducing short-run expenses. That tends to be exactly the opposite of the long-run strategic goals of the organization as designed by those who develop the strategic plan. Therefore managers must balance the short-term objectives of their units or departments with the long-range vision for the organization. Developing and carrying out the operating budget should not be done without knowledge of the organization's strategic plan.

It is not clear whether any organization will ever get where it wants to be. The target goals tend to be modified over time in reaction to changes both within and outside of the organization. However, to make progress toward the goals, the organization should constantly be attempting to answer the various questions stated earlier and to take necessary actions based on the answers to those questions.

The Elements of a Strategic Plan

Strategic plans must be adapted to specific situations. The elements of a plan for one organization may not be perfectly suited to another. Flexibility is a positive attribute in the strategic planning process. For most organizations, however, the basic elements of a strategic plan include a:

- Mission statement or philosophy
- Statement of long-term goals
- Statement of competitive strategy
- Statement of organizational policies
- Statement of needed resources
- Statement of key assumptions

The Mission Statement or Philosophy

The first step in strategic management is the development of a *mission statement* for the organization, department, or unit. What is the purpose of the organization or unit? An organization cannot begin to plan goals effectively and allocate resources sensibly until it first clearly determines its reason for existence. Strategic planners refer to an organization-wide statement of purpose or focus as the mission statement. In the department of nursing this is often referred to as the philosophical statement.

A great deal of care should be taken in developing a mission statement. The mission statement of the organization should focus the organization by defining what it does. Some health care organizations set their mission statement either too broadly or too narrowly. At one extreme they wind up running restaurants or other non-health facilities that sap time and energy and often fail because the organization lacks expertise in that area. At the other extreme, growth and change are not encouraged by the statement, and the organization stagnates.

Some degree of limitation in the mission statement is beneficial; it forces the organization to concentrate on what it knows how to do. At the same time, the mission statement should allow for growth and intelligent diversification. The mission statement should be defined in such a way as to prevent the organization from exceeding its manageable boundaries but encourage exploration within those boundaries. Camillus, the noted author on strategic planning, writes that a health care organization engaged in providing eye-care services can describe itself as fulfilling the mission of examining eyes and writing prescriptions for corrective lenses or the mission of protecting and improving human vision. The first statement is essentially a description of activities in which the organization is engaged. The second statement, in contrast, identifies consequences rather than activities and thus leads to the identification of such possibilities as opening clinics where eye surgery is carried out, engaging in the development and possibly the manufacture of devices for rectifying faulty vision, and running programs for educating the public about the proper care of eyes (Camillus, 1980, p. 47).

The key to designing the mission statement is not to focus on what the organization does right now but to think about the range of possible types of activities that could be seen as a logical extension for the organization over time.

Statement of Long-Term Goals
Goal setting is the organization's attempt to set the direction for itself as it tries to meet its mission. Often an organization will have both quantitative and qualitative goals. Quantitative goals may relate to financial outcomes, such as rates of growth in the number of patients served and in revenues. Qualitative goals may relate to patient satisfaction and general reputation.

In developing the long-term goals of the organization, their timeless nature should be kept in mind. Objectives are intended to be attained within a specific time frame. Goals tend to stay in force over long periods. Providing the health care needs of an increasing percentage of the community's citizens is a long-term goal. Increasing the number of patients by 8% in the coming year is a specific, measurable objective.

Although statements of objectives are necessary, the statement of goals is of greater concern in strategic management. As managers attempt to respond in their operations to specific, time-oriented objectives, they should bear in mind the overriding goals that the organization wants to achieve. Innovations that allow the organization to take major steps forward toward achieving its long-run goals should constantly be sought by all managers.

Statement of Competitive Strategy
The organization's competitive strategy is its plan for achieving its goals—specifically, what services will be provided and to whom. The development of this strategy relies to a great extent on a thorough internal and external review. What are the organization's strengths and weaknesses, its opportunities and threats?

Competitive strategy is the planning of what care will be provided and to whom, in the context of other providers in the organization's service area. To develop such a plan, the organization must consider what competitors are or are not doing and what expertise the organization does or does not possess. Based on that information, the organization can decide where it should expand and perhaps where it should contract.

Essentially the organization must evaluate its mission and goals in light of its particular strengths and weaknesses and in light of the demand for services and competition in the external environment. Based on that evaluation, it can make a plan that will take advantage of opportunities that present themselves and plan a reaction to the threats that exist.

Statement of Organizational Policies
The role of policies is to specify what are and are not acceptable practices by the organization. The establishment of the mission and goals incorporates a set of values.

It integrates the values of the organization's founders, the values of its management and staff, and the values of the community. Those values should be incorporated in the decisions made by the leadership of the organization.

In most organizations no single person can review each and every decision and decide if it is appropriate. A set of policies that clearly indicates what actions are appropriate and what actions are not removes an unreasonable burden from managers throughout the organization. It removes the necessity for guesswork by individual managers in many specific situations.

Policy statements are substantially different from mission statements, statements of goals, and statements of competitive strategy. In each of the earlier statements there is a need to encourage creativity. Each one leaves room for the organization to innovate or grow. In contrast, policy statements are generally limiting. They provide the constraints that the organization wants to place on managerial discretion.

It is surprising to note that such constraints can ultimately enhance an organization's growth. If there are no specific policies, managers may find that they are chastised for specific actions without any rhyme or reason. They become uncertain as to when it is okay to take initiative and make changes and when higher levels of management want things done just the way they always have been done. This high degree of uncertainty eventually leads managers to become reluctant to innovate in any respect. The availability of specific procedures clearly delineates where innovation is not allowed. However, that also provides the manager a sense of where innovation is allowed and welcomed.

Statement of Needed Resources

Strategic planning cannot be held apart from the reality of the resources needed to carry out the plan. These include resources in terms of personnel, the facilities for the personnel to work in and with, and the other requirements for accomplishing the goals of the organization. Without linkage between the plan and the resources to carry it out, there can be little hope of achieving the organization's goals.

Statement of Key Assumptions

Part of the planning process is the development of a statement of key assumptions. Strategic management calls for decentralization of the planning process, so there must be a set of common guidelines that all managers use. If management expects to increase the number of its contracts with managed care organizations over time, that will affect the entire organization. The same assumption about such contracts should be used consistently by all managers. This allows for plans to be consistent and also improves the coordination of plans throughout the organization. It also helps to determine whether variations from the plan are the result of how the plan is being carried out or are related to the accuracy of the underlying assumptions.

Benefits of the Strategic Planning Process

A number of benefits result from having a strategic planning system. One of the predominant benefits is that it forces the organization to determine its long-term goals and come up with an approach to accomplishing them. Establishing long-term goals forces managers to decide what the organization's purpose is and to formalize that purpose. Many health care organizations were established long before any of the current employees worked for the organization. The original goals of the organization can easily become lost among the personal needs and desires of the current management and staff.

The process of establishing a formalized mission and goals gives a sense of direction to the organization.

A strategic planning system also promotes efficiency. Managers working toward clear goals are less likely to be inefficient. When everyone knows exactly what the organization is trying to achieve, there is a likelihood that less effort will be spent on unnecessary activities. A specific mission and stated goal also decrease the likelihood that some managers or departments will be working at cross-purposes with the organization as a whole.

The strategic planning process provides a means of communication among the various hierarchical levels of the organization. In large organizations (and sometimes even in relatively small ones) communication among organizational levels becomes difficult. The managers on the lower rungs may know that things are not being done efficiently. The managers at the upper rungs may believe that the systems they have in place are producing efficiency. Inadequate channels exist for moving information up or down through the ranks. Innovation in such cases is expected to be dictated by the higher levels of the organization. In fact, often the need for and opportunities for improvements are most visible at the lower levels. A strategic management process should allow new ideas to flow smoothly down and up.

Lower-level managers will learn more about why changes are taking place if they share the strategic plan and can see how changes relate to achieving the plan's goals. Higher-level managers will receive better information if lower-level managers focus some of their attention on factors that affect the organization's long-term goals.

The strategic planning process provides managers with an improved sense of the needs of the organization and of its environmental constraints. It has often been found that a partnership approach to management works better than a dictatorial approach. Managers who are told that they must live within constraints resist them. Managers who are asked to become part of a team to solve the problem of constraints learn to understand the difficulties involved with the constraints and are more willing to work cooperatively instead of adversarially.

The strategic planning process increases the level of organizational creativity in addressing problems. Successful organizations encourage rather than resist change. Managers should constantly be scanning their environments for approaching changes so they can be ready to act (Kerfoot, 2006). The world is always different from the way it was 20 years before. Organizations must change and adapt to survive. Change, however, doesn't occur at some arbitrary point every 20 years. It occurs gradually, in an evolutionary process. The fact that most organizations do things in a certain way now and did not do those things in that way 20 years ago indicates that someone tried a new approach and found it superior. Who was that someone? Was it the lucky one who accidentally fell upon an improved approach?

Generally, this is one area where organizations make their own luck. Creativity cannot be forced upon people. One cannot tell employees to be creative and to develop innovative improvements. However, creativity is natural to human beings, and it can be either fostered or stifled. An organizational milieu that is phobic to change or that tolerates suggestions for change only from a privileged few is highly vulnerable to competition. A key tenant of the Quality Improvement theory is that the organization that invites and respectfully considers the creative ideas of all members of the organization is more likely to succeed in its efforts to provide a high-quality product or service. But change must be judicious and must lead to improved ability to respond not only to the immediate changes in the health care environment that are usually occasioned by changes in medical technology and governmental or third-party payer rules and regulations. It must also position the organization to be responsive to pervasive, long-term trends in society (Kerfoot, 2006). A strong commitment to strategic management throughout the organization will convey the organization's view of creativity as a positive rather than a negative element.

Implementing a Strategic Management Process

In this chapter there is alternating reference to the strategic plan and to the strategic planning or management process.

The specific development of a strategic plan is discussed in the next section of this chapter. However, strategic management relies not just on a plan but also on a broad planning process. That process is one of making managers aware of the need to think strategically as they carry out all their management activities. In developing the long-range plan, managers must relate the plan to the mission. In designing specific program budgets or business plans, the manager must consider how the program will help the organization achieve its goals. In developing the specific details of the operating budget, again the manager should be trying to link the details with how they help the organization reach its long-term aims.

The remainder of this chapter focuses on several of the long-range elements of strategic planning. Specifically, long-range planning, program budgets, and business plans are addressed. As the reader proceeds to Chapters 8 through 12, which discuss operating, revenue, capital, performance, and cash budgets, the notion of trying to link operational activities with strategic thought should be kept in mind.

■ LONG-RANGE PLANNING

In developing the long-range budget, the organization begins the process of translating its general goals and objectives into a specific action plan. Long-range budgets and long-range plans are often referred to as the organization's strategic plan. Such plans generally cover a period of 3 to 5 years.

Given a strategic management process that calls upon managers to focus on the organization's goals, is a strategic plan essential? The answer is emphatically, "Yes!" Long-range planning is critical to the vitality of an organization. For organizations to thrive, they must move forward rather than remaining stagnant. The staff of an organization should be able to look back and see the progress that has been made over an extended period. Budgeting for 1 year at a time does not allow for the major types of changes that would take years to plan and implement. Yet that lengthy process is needed for the efforts that will substantially move the organization forward.

For example, suppose that one goal of the organization is to move from being a primary care community hospital to a regional tertiary care center. This cannot be accomplished by having each department attempt to modify its operating budget. An overall organizational plan is needed. Which of the new tertiary services can or should be added in the next 5 years? Which programs already exist but need to be expanded in the next 5 years to accommodate the changing role of the organization? These questions are specifically addressed in the strategic plan or long-range budget.

Nursing should be involved in this planning process. The success of the plan will depend on how well it is carried out. If the plan does not have adequate nursing input when it is prepared, it is unlikely that the nursing staff will support it fully.

Nurses must push their organizations to incorporate nursing leadership into the planning process not only for the good of nurses and nursing but also for the ultimate success of the organization.

The strategic plan may lay the groundwork for a fund-raising campaign to precede and parallel expansion of services. Or the plan may indicate that each year for 5 years, growth in specified existing profitable areas must be undertaken to offset the start-up losses that are likely to occur with the introduction of major new programs. Specific dollar amounts of additional revenue and new program costs may be projected only in terms of an extremely rough estimate. Although quite general, such a plan does give the organization enough specific information about the implications and requirements for the expansion into a tertiary care center to allow for the development of specific programs to move the organization toward that ultimate goal.

The strategic plan may be somewhat more detailed, showing projections of the dollar amounts expected to be available (and their sources) as well as which specific programs will be adopted and what their approximate costs will be. Because a strategic or long-range plan projects at least 3 and up to 10 years into the future, it is unlikely that revenue and cost estimates will be highly accurate. Therefore, although rough estimates are often included in such plans, they are generally not overly detailed or refined.

The plan should not focus only on major program additions. The services and programs that already exist are equally important to an organization. Expanding a service, contracting one, or even deleting a program or service requires the same consideration and planning as the addition of a program or service. A part of the planning process should be to address explicitly whether the services and programs that make up the majority of operations of the organization are to be retained at a steady-state level or whether they are to be contracted or expanded in scope.

One serious potential problem arises if this issue is ignored in preparing strategic plans. If existing programs are implicitly assumed to continue unchanged, a plan that includes a number of new programs may appear feasible. However, it may not be feasible when technological and other elements of change are considered explicitly as they relate to the ongoing operations of the organization. As an example, consider a dietary department that efficiently handles the current 500-bed hospital but is at its maximum capacity. It will require a major investment in new space and equipment to be able to handle a 100-bed addition. In an example closer to nursing, consider a clinic that would like to respond to a change in the local housing supply that will increase the number of children in the service area. If additional obstetric, gynecological, and pediatric services are to be added, the clinic will have to be able to recruit new physicians and nurses to provide those services. In an era of nursing shortages, the nursing department may not be able to recruit those additional nurses without significant changes in recruitment policies and funding. Therefore, expectations regarding existing programs should be reviewed explicitly and included as part of the plan.

Once the plan has been finalized and formalized, it serves as a guide for a number of years. Long-range plans are typically prepared only once every 3 or 5 years. Creating a new plan each year would only lead to constant changes in the organization's direction. This would result in wasted efforts and frustrated managers. However, such plans should be reviewed each year. Assumptions may turn out to be wrong. A cure for cancer could change patient volume. The external environment can change dramatically. An influx of refugees could change the demand for services.

Annual reviews allow the organization to adjust its strategic plan so that it is aligned with current events.

Each year, elements of the plan are brought into the current activities of the organization. The operating budget should be prepared on the basis of an understanding of the strategic plan. It should be designed to assist the organization in achieving the goals and objectives of that strategic plan. To make the transition from plan to operation, many of the proposed additions or changes will require a thorough evaluation. This may be accomplished through the development of a program budget.

■ PROGRAM BUDGETING AND ZERO-BASE BUDGETING

Program budgeting is the part of the overall strategic planning process that focuses on all the costs and benefits associated with a specific program. The program may be an existing one that the organization is considering expanding, contracting, or eliminating, or it may be a new program that the organization is thinking of adding. Program budgeting examines alternative programs to meet the organization's objectives and examines feasible alternative ways to accomplish each given program.

Some program budgeting is done within a nursing unit or department. Often, however, the program changes generated by a strategic plan have interdepartmental impacts. Such program changes are much more complicated because of the need for coordination among departments. It is vital that nursing participate fully in such interdepartmental planning. Working on key committees is essential not only to protect the interests of nursing but also, as noted earlier, to ensure that any plans developed make sense from a nursing perspective and can be supported by the nursing staff.

In most cases program budgets relate directly to the strategic planning of the organization. The projects being evaluated should be under consideration because they relate directly to moving the organization toward the achievement of its long-term goals. It is cause for concern when projects are being promoted by factions within the organization or by a particular powerful individual, but many others cannot understand how the project relates to the organization's mission and goals. In that case, the program budget is also a source of vulnerability for the organization. It may be unlikely that the program will succeed because of lack of adequate managerial support, or its potential benefits may be artificially inflated by its powerful supporters. This is a situation in which the organization's board of directors might be helpful. Because their regular jobs are external to the organization, they are likely to be more objective in evaluating the contribution of a particular program to the achievement of the organization's mission and goals. They can assist in determining both the value of the proposed endeavor to the organization and the appropriateness of its program budget.

Program budgets are substantially different from other types of budgets. Long-range budgets or strategic plans look in general terms at the entire organization over a period of years. The information in them is based on rough approximations rather than being highly detailed. Operating and cash budgets are detailed but only for the coming year. A program budget combines a great amount of detailed information relating to a long period for one specific program. Further, whereas most budgets focus on a given department's revenues and costs, program budgets compare revenues and expenses for an entire program, cutting across departments or cost centers.

A program budget compares all its costs and benefits to evaluate the entire program's effect on the organization over its lifetime. In doing this, the program's budgeting methods identify the costs and benefits of various programs aimed at the same goal or of differing approaches to one program. Because resources are limited, program budgeting often focuses on trade-offs. That is, program budgeting considers the extra benefit to be gained by spending additional money on a program. Alternatively, program budgeting considers how much of the benefit of a program would be lost if less money were spent on the program.

Zero-Base Budgeting

Zero-base budgeting (ZBB) is a popular budgeting technique that gained fame for its strong push toward analyzing all costs. Every expense from a base of zero must be justified. Until the introduction of ZBB, it was common for budget negotiations to revolve around appropriate amounts of increase in a budget: how much more should be spent next year than was spent in the current year? Implicitly, such an approach assumes that all current-year spending continues to be reasonable and justified for the next year. Only the amount of the increment is subject to examination and discussion.

In reality, as technology, diseases, and protocols change, some departments have growing financial needs, whereas other departments could get by with decreasing resources. The concept of requiring a zero-base evaluation is attractive because it means that budgets would not be allowed to become "fat" over time. Many organizations use ZBB analysis to see exactly how money is being spent within a unit or department. Such an approach requires existing programs to justify their continued existence (LaFaive, 2003). Rather than basing the future budget on the past budget, all expenditures in the proposed budget must be demonstrated to be necessary.

Additionally, the ZBB approach pays attention to alternative ways a given program could be offered. ZBB collects information regarding a program into a *decision package*. A decision package contains documentation in support of the program and summaries of the analyses performed. In that sense, the decision package is just a mechanism to ensure a formal, systematic review of each budget.

Each package contains a statement of the purpose of the program, the consequences of not performing the program, and the ways in which the costs and benefits of the program can be measured. More interesting, the package also includes statements of alternatives. These statements are the heart of ZBB.

ZBB provides a great degree of sophistication in the analysis of alternatives. Not only may different programs with separate decision packages be compared, but ZBB also compares three major types of alternatives within the decision package for each individual program. The first alternative involves ways to produce the treatment, service, or other output. The second set of alternatives relates to the quantity of treatments, service, or output to be provided. The third set of alternatives considers varying levels of quality.

For many nurses, considering trade-offs such as these is counter to their traditional education. Nurses, as health care professionals, are trained to provide the best possible care to each patient. At the higher level of organizational planning, however, it must be acknowledged that no health care provider can provide everything to everyone. The simple fact is, resources are limited. ZBB forces recognition of the need to determine the greatest overall good that can be provided to the entire population served by an organization, in contrast to the view of providing perfect care to each specific individual.

Perhaps the best way to understand how these alternatives are examined is to work through a potential program budget problem.

ZBB Case Study: Hemodialysis

Suppose that the hypothetical Wagner Hospital has decided, on the basis of its environmental review, that there is a pressing need for additional hemodialysis services in the community. In Wagner's long-range plan, the introduction of a hemodialysis program has been included, although the plan does not include much in the way of specifics other than to note that within the next 5 years some form of hemodialysis program should be instituted. This program was highly placed when priorities were established, even though it would have to vie for funds with several other important new programs that were also included in the long-range plan, such as a new primary care center.

Wagner has compiled a decision package for the hemodialysis program. The formal documentation in the package first notes the name of the program (hemodialysis) and the sponsoring department within the hospital (internal medicine). The stated purpose of the program is to reduce the levels of mortality and morbidity currently experienced in the community because of insufficient hemodialysis facilities. The resources needed for the program are stated in general terms. They include dialysis machines, physicians, nurses, technicians, supplies, and overhead items such as electrical power and physical space.

If Wagner were not a user of ZBB, it is likely that the renal specialists in the hospital would have designed a first-class hemodialysis center, perhaps as a new hospital wing, with five machines to satisfy all community needs. The proposal would have been a take-it-or-leave-it package, with strong political emphasis on its acceptance.

There is nothing wrong with wanting everything to be first class. It is not wasteful to provide top-quality care. However, that does not mean that an organization can afford to provide that care. Having a first-class hemodialysis center may mean that there will not be enough resources left for adequate cancer treatment.

Because Wagner Hospital uses ZBB, the hemodialysis plan cannot be approved until the performance of an analysis that examines a number of alternatives. The first issue concerns the level of output. How much treatment will be provided? Suppose that five machines would take care of the entire community demand now and for the foreseeable future. Suppose that the estimated annual cost of this alternative were $2 million, including depreciation, supplies, personnel, overhead, maintenance, and so on. A second alternative may be to purchase only four machines. Suppose that at this level it would still be possible to eliminate all mortality and morbidity, but some of the machines might have to operate two or three shifts per day, causing some inconvenience for nurses and physicians.

Four machines might cost a total of $1,700,000. Note that the number of machines would fall 20%, from five to four, but the costs would fall only 15%. That would be possible because some costs associated with the program are likely to be fixed. As discussed in Chapter 4, fixed costs do not change in total as the output level increases. Does this mean that five machines would be better than four because the hospital would get 20% more machinery for only 15% more cost? Not necessarily. That is the wrong comparison. The goal is to provide cost-effective, high-quality health care to the community. The goal is to avoid buying unnecessary equipment, thereby minimizing total costs rather than trying to minimize the cost per machine.

The alternative of four machines instead of five would save $300,000. Although there would be some inconvenience, the reduced cost would not result in any extra mortality or morbidity. The extra convenience gained by having five machines must be compared to the benefits available by spending $300,000 on some other program. Also, one must determine whether the extra machine generates any additional revenue or solely affects scheduling.

Other alternative levels of output might be the use of three machines, which would eliminate all mortality and 50% of the morbidity for a cost of $1,400,000; two machines, which would eliminate only 80% of the mortality at a cost of $1,100,000; and one machine, which would eliminate only 40% of the mortality at a cost of $800,000.

Itemizing the costs and benefits of the alternative output levels is informative. Unlike the usual all-or-nothing presentation for a new program, either five machines or no program at all ("We don't practice second-class medicine here!"), the choice is not that dramatic. In fact, in a constrained environment it may well be that upon seeing all the alternatives, the choice will come down to either three machines or four machines. Fewer than three may be considered inadequate to accomplish the long-run objectives; more than four may raise questions about priorities.

It is not only the amount of output that is a question here. The ZBB system requires that alternative ways to produce the output also be considered. Is there a choice? Isn't it hemodialysis machines or nothing? Perhaps the answer is yes, but one of the major roles of ZBB is to ask questions such as these.

Other alternative options must also be considered. Can patients be on the machine for a shorter time, thus increasing the number of people who have access to it? Can money be saved by buying machines with fewer accessories? Is there nursing support for a night shift in the hemodialysis clinic such that the machines are either in service or in the cleaning-disinfecting process between uses? Such questions almost certainly hit upon issues of quality. However, the trade-offs between quality and cost must be examined.

Trade-offs are always made, and they sometimes impact the quality of care. If one person dies of heart disease, it may be because not enough resources were devoted to having the latest open-heart surgery equipment. That person suffered from a lack of high-quality care. More resources devoted to heart surgery equipment might have saved that individual. Perhaps the hospital should cut back in another area and pursue the very best heart surgery. In the vast majority of cases, that would simply mean that people in the other area would die. The budgeting system must attempt to select projects that are carried out in a way that minimizes the overall negative impact on quality. That may mean undertaking two new services, each at less than the optimal level of care, rather than totally sacrificing the existence of either service so the remaining one could be run on an optimal basis. Table 7-1 provides a summary of the hemodialysis decision package and its focus on trade-offs in this hypothetical example.

In Table 7-1, line 6 raises the issue of whether all hemodialysis has to be performed in the hospital. One alternative might be to perform all hemodialysis in the hospital, but another alternative would be to perform hemodialysis in an outpatient dialysis clinic. The department could also offer in-home hemodialysis support services. Still another possibility might be to have a series of external locations spread throughout the community, one location for each machine. Or to best serve the community's population, planners might consider the use of one mobile van for each

TABLE 7-1 ZBB Decision Package—Hemodialysis

1. Name of program: Hemodialysis
2. Department: Internal Medicine
3. Purpose: Reduce mortality and morbidity due to lack of hemodialysis facilities
4. Resources required: Dialysis machines, physicians, nurses, technicians, supplies, overhead, home health services availability
5. Quantity or level of output alternatives:

Program and Level	Medical Implications	Cost
Five machines	Eliminates all mortality and morbidity; no inconvenience to staff	$2,000,000
Four machines	Eliminates all mortality and morbidity; some inconvenience to staff	1,700,000
Three machines	Eliminates all mortality and 50% of morbidity	1,400,000
Two machines	Eliminates 80% of mortality	1,100,000
One machine	Eliminates 40% of mortality	800,000

6. Alternative ways to produce the output: This section should consider the various approaches to providing the product and the cost of each. For instance, it should consider providing the care in the hospital, in clinics, in mobile vans, and in the home. For each way of providing the output, each output level (i.e., one machine, two machines, etc.) should be considered.
7. Alternative levels of quality of care: This should consider the cost of using different types of machines, changing the clinical options for providing the service, or changing the amount of time each patient is on the machine for each way of producing the output and for each level of output in terms of numbers of machines.

machine, allowing dialysis to be performed at many locations. This option might be especially effective in sparsely populated parts of Western states such as New Mexico, Wyoming, Montana, and the Dakotas.

The difficult part of the analysis is explicitly and creatively to seek and examine trade-offs. Specifically, it is necessary to ask whether more lives could be saved by the organization if it spent $300,000 less on hemodialysis and bought four machines instead of five. Could even more lives be saved in some other program if dialysis were cut to three machines and $600,000 less were spent on them? Three machines might mean less care and lower quality care—less time on the machine for each noncritical patient. What could $600,000 do elsewhere in the organization? Would $600,000 spent elsewhere provide enough benefit to justify less care and lower quality care in this area?

Suppose that in addition to hemodialysis, a primary care center has also been proposed. A first-class primary care center might cost $1 million per year (the numbers here are hypothetical). This primary care center would provide access to care for 50,000 visits per year (or about 12,000 people). However, a ZBB review of primary care indicates that for $600,000 a total of 35,000 visits could be handled. All children in the community could get immunizations, but some older patients would have to travel to an existing clinic.

Because of the large capital investment, the Wagner Hospital does not have sufficient cash to establish both a primary care center and a hemodialysis service at the ideal first-class levels. It is highly likely that without a zero-base review, the hospital might well select either hemodialysis or primary care—and the choice would probably depend largely on politics. The well-being of the community can get lost in the struggles among vested-interest groups within an organization.

TABLE 7-2 ZBB Cost Matrix—Hemodialysis

| | Alternative Quality Levels | | | | | | | | |
| | Quality of Machine/Patient Time on Machines | | | | | | | | |
Alternative Ways to Produce and Alternative Quantities	Best/Best	Best/Moderate	Best/Minimum	Moderate/Best	Moderate/Moderate	Moderate/Minimum	Minimum/Best	Minimum/Moderate	Minimum/Minimum
IN HOSPITAL									
5 machines	$2,000,000	$1,750,000	$1,500,000	$1,750,000	$1,500,000	$1,250,000	$1,625,000	$1,375,000	$1,125,000
4 machines	1,700,000	1,500,000	1,300,000	1,500,000	1,300,000	1,100,000	1,400,000	1,200,000	1,000,000
3 machines	1,400,000	1,250,000	1,100,000	1,250,000	1,100,000	950,000	1,175,000	1,025,000	875,000
2 machines	1,100,000	1,000,000	900,000	1,000,000	900,000	800,000	950,000	850,000	750,000
1 machine	800,000	750,000	700,000	750,000	700,000	650,000	725,000	675,000	625,000
IN ONE CLINIC									
5 machines	1,800,000	1,550,000	1,300,000	1,550,000	1,300,000	1,050,000	1,425,000	1,175,000	925,000
4 machines	1,500,000	1,300,000	1,100,000	1,300,000	1,100,000	900,000	1,200,000	1,000,000	800,000
3 machines	1,200,000	1,050,000	900,000	1,050,000	900,000	750,000	975,000	825,000	675,000
2 machines	900,000	800,000	700,000	800,000	700,000	600,000	750,000	650,000	550,000
1 machine	700,000	650,000	600,000	650,000	600,000	550,000	625,000	575,000	525,000

Alternative Ways to Produce and Alternative Quantities	Alternative Quality Levels								
	Quality of Machine/Patient Time on Machines								
	Best/Best	Best/Moderate	Best/Minimum	Moderate/Best	Moderate/Moderate	Moderate/Minimum	Minimum/Best	Minimum/Moderate	Minimum/Minimum
MULTIPLE CLINICS									
5 machines	1,950,000	1,700,000	1,450,000	1,700,000	1,450,000	1,200,000	1,575,000	1,325,000	1,075,000
4 machines	1,650,000	1,450,000	1,250,000	1,450,000	1,250,000	1,050,000	1,350,000	1,150,000	950,000
3 machines	1,350,000	1,200,000	1,050,000	1,200,000	1,050,000	900,000	1,125,000	975,000	825,000
2 machines	1,050,000	950,000	850,000	950,000	850,000	750,000	900,000	800,000	700,000
1 machine	750,000	700,000	650,000	700,000	650,000	600,000	675,000	625,000	575,000
MOBILE VAN									
5 machines	1,650,000	1,400,000	1,150,000	1,400,000	1,150,000	900,000	1,275,000	1,025,000	775,000
4 machines	1,400,000	1,200,000	1,000,000	1,200,000	1,000,000	800,000	1,100,000	900,000	700,000
3 machines	1,150,000	1,000,000	850,000	1,000,000	850,000	700,000	925,000	775,000	625,000
2 machines	900,000	800,000	700,000	800,000	700,000	600,000	750,000	650,000	550,000
1 machine	650,000	600,000	550,000	600,000	550,000	500,000	575,000	525,000	475,000

There might, however, be enough resources to provide both hemodialysis and primary care at slightly reduced levels of care. The hospital could add three dialysis machines and a primary care unit.

The zero-base review forces the examination of alternatives. It forces recognition of the fact that more lives would be saved by scaling back the size of hemodialysis and primary care and then providing both services. Given the explicit information contained in the ZBB reviews, both vested interest groups are likely to be more willing to accept the resulting compromise.

The ZBB Cost Matrix

Looking at the descriptions of alternatives in Table 7-1, it becomes apparent that presenting various possible alternatives can become complex. To help with this logistical problem, the ZBB decision package for each program can be summarized in the form of a matrix (Table 7-2). Each cell in the matrix shows the cost of providing a certain level of care, produced in a particular way and with a particular approach to quality. This makes all trade-offs explicit. In picking a particular cell from the matrix, the organization knows exactly what it is getting and at what cost. All cells meeting minimum requirements should be calculated.

In Table 7-2, the rows represent the cost of various numbers of machines placed in a variety of types of locations, such as all machines in the hospital or all machines in one clinic. All possible locations and all quantities of machines are included. The columns present the various possible types of machines. They are referred to as the best, moderate, and minimum. Alternatively, specific types of machines could be listed in the various columns. Similarly, assuming that the length of time a patient is on a dialysis machine is variable, one could think of the best, moderate, or minimal amounts of time.

Notice that the columns in Table 7-2 combine all quality-of-care possibilities. It is possible to have the best machine and the best amount of time on the machine. Or the hospital might have the best machine with a minimal amount of time, or the minimum acceptable machine with the best amount of time, and so on.

For any given cell in the matrix, the cost of a particular type of machine and the length of treatment time for each patient, as well as the number of machines and their locations, are calculated. It is possible that some cells are not feasible and will not have a value. For instance, if only two machines are purchased, it might not be possible for patients to have the longest (and best) amount of time on a machine.

If the hospital were to decide to spend $600,000 on primary care and $1,400,000 on hemodialysis, all cells on this hemodialysis matrix that have a cost over $1,400,000 could be eliminated. Then the organization could focus on the various combinations of quantity of care, quality of care, and ways to produce hemodialysis care that cost $1,400,000 or less. The most preferred alternative among those that are feasible for $1,400,000 or less could then be selected.

Table 7-1 is a relatively simple table, but in the real world, there are usually more complex alternatives. A more realistic alternative might ask, "Could the population be better served by a dialysis department that offers a continuous ambulatory peritoneal dialysis program as well as hospital-based hemodialysis services?" For example, see the expanded set of alternatives presented in Table 7-3. The dialysis department might have to offer support for all these ways of delivering dialysis services. Each of these new alternatives would be added into the cost matrix in Table 7-2. Although these services add only a few lines to the ZBB decision package in Table 7-3 as compared

TABLE 7-3 Expanded ZBB Dialysis Service Decision Package

Program and Level	Medical Implications	Cost
ALL HEMODIALYSIS		
Five machines	Eliminates all mortality and morbidity; no inconvenience to staff	$2,000,000
Four machines	Eliminates all mortality and morbidity; some inconvenience to staff	1,700,000
Three machines	Eliminates all mortality and 50% of morbidity	1,400,000
Two machines	Eliminates 80% of mortality	1,100,000
One machine	Eliminates 40% of mortality	800,000
Three machines and CAPD*	Eliminates all mortality and morbidity; no inconvenience to staff	1,600,000
Two machines, CAPD, and home hemodialysis program	Eliminates all mortality and morbidity; some inconvenience to staff	1,300,000
One machine, CAPD, and home hemodialysis program	Eliminates 95% of mortality, 80% of morbidity; some inconvenience to staff	1,000,000

*CAPD: continuous ambulatory peritoneal dialysis.

to Table 7-1, they significantly increase the complexity of the ZBB cost matrix presented in Table 7-2. We do not present an expanded cost matrix here.

Ranking Decision Packages

The resources of an organization are always limited, so it is rare that all proposed packages can be accepted. Therefore ZBB requires each manager to rank the alternative decision packages. The best alternative would be ranked number 1.

During the process of budget review and negotiation, managers at the higher levels of the organization will receive ranked decision packages from a number of subordinate managers. For example, a nurse manager with responsibility for a number of units might receive packages from each unit nurse manager. The packages from all these different units must be ranked in order of importance by the manager responsible for the group of units. Then the packages will continue up through the organization. The CNE and her or his administrative staff will rank all the packages received from all the different nursing areas.

In large organizations, the ranking process can become quite tedious. However, it is a necessary evil if the goal of the program budgeting process is to compare all the alternatives available to the organization and ultimately to allocate the organization's resources to those projects that best lead to attainment of the organization's goals.

■ BUSINESS PLANS

One approach to program budgeting that first became widely used in the latter part of the 20th century is the business plan. This technique, long used in industry, became popular in health care as it became clear that health care organizations would have to take a more businesslike approach to providing their services in an ever more difficult financial environment. It is a method that is still gaining support in all types of health care organizations.

What Is a Business Plan?

A *business plan* is a detailed plan for a proposed program, project, or service that includes information to be used to assess the venture's financial feasibility. Business plans are used by nurse managers to assess the likelihood of success of a wide variety of ventures. Nurse entrepreneurs should certainly prepare a business plan before starting a new venture. In addition, nurse managers working for an organization should prepare business plans for new programs or services to be offered by the organization. Often the plan is used as a sales document that makes the case for undertaking a new project. However, despite its advocacy role, the plan should provide an honest appraisal of the project. If, in fact, the proposed project is not good for the organization, that should be determined at the planning stage rather than after a large financial investment has been made to implement it.

The first step in planning a new program should be to understand which goals of the organization the program promotes. Does the proposed project fit with the organization's mission statement? In developing the plan, sufficient information must be gathered to indicate whether the proposed program will move the organization closer to its goals. In evaluating the plan, it is important not to lose sight of the original organizational goal to which the project relates.

For example, one business plan might relate to the development of a community education program for diabetics, whereas another plan might focus on providing home health care, and yet a third might focus on developing a new women's health clinic. All of these new programs might fit nicely within a mission of providing health care services to the community. It is possible, however, that some proposed new programs would not be expected to be profitable or even financially self-sufficient. The home health program, although breaking even, may not be profitable. However, it might be a necessary program that enables the organization to provide a complete care package to the various insurers with whom the medical center negotiates for business contracts. The program for community education might lose money. It might, however, fit into the element of mission that concerns providing important services on a charitable basis. On the other hand, the establishment of a women's health clinic may be based on the notion of earning profits to be used to subsidize the charitable elements of the organization's mission. The organization cannot provide some services at a loss unless it provides some at a profit or receives donations to offset the loss.

Even a new program aimed at a charitable mission requires a business plan. The fact that it is not expected to earn a profit does not remove the need to understand just how much of a subsidy it might require. At the same time, if the women's health clinic is being proposed to earn profits to subsidize the other operations of the organization, that should not be lost sight of during the planning process.

The plan should define the steps that are being taken to accomplish the organization's goal. It should clearly state the objectives of the proposed project and provide a linkage that shows how the plan's objectives will lead to the accomplishment of the organization's goal.

The plan must clearly communicate the concept of the project. It must also communicate the organization's ability to carry out the project. One can think of a business plan as a document that answers the questions one should ask before investing money in a project:

- What exactly is the proposed project?
- To what extent does the organization have the capabilities to undertake the project?

- Where will the organization acquire the capabilities that it lacks?
- Will the project make or lose money?
- How much?
- Does the organization have the financial resources to undertake the project?
- If not, where can those resources be obtained?
- How will the new product or service be marketed?
- What alternative approaches have been considered?
- Why is the proposed approach considered better than the alternatives?

The Components of a Business Plan

A business plan is a substantial document because it addresses all the key factors that contribute to the success of a new business. There are between 10 and 20 parts to a business plan, depending on the nature of the product or service and the business-planning model followed. All standard business plans include information about the product or service, the market for the new business, the ownership structure and organizational structure, a financial plan, and an implementation plan and schedule. The plan should have a section concerning the critical risks and problems the new business is likely to face and, ideally, an exit plan if the business is not a success (Pinson, 2004). The remainder of this section describes the elements of a business plan.

Description of Products or Services

The first step in developing a business plan is to specify precisely the new product or service to be offered or the nature of the expansion of an existing product or service. Nursing is often involved in new products and services, either in a support role or as the principal proponent. For example, the addition of a new type of laser surgery would clearly have implications for nursing. Changes would be likely to occur in the operating room as well as in the medical and surgery units. The project might be proposed by the surgeons, with the nursing department providing valuable assistance in developing the business plan. On the other hand, the decision to add an outpatient surgery unit might be suggested by the nursing director of the operating room. As such, it would be primarily a nursing business plan. Nurses can become involved in developing a variety of different programs and innovative services. Nurse entrepreneurs developing a new home care agency or additional home care services for an existing agency, a nurse staffing agency, an educational service business or a clinic managed by a nurse practitioner are just a few examples of projects that should have business plans.

Business plans can be developed for new ventures or ongoing organizations. When planning a new venture, it is important to consider market opportunities, resource needs, resource sources, and risks. Market opportunities are the identification of unfilled needs. The entire venture rests on this issue. What do people need that is not being provided or that is being provided in a less than optimal way? If a need does not exist, the venture is not likely to succeed. If the need does exist, what resources will be required to meet that need? How might the resources be obtained? What could go wrong? Finally, if the business isn't successful, how will those involved know when to cut their losses and dissolve the business? No one should ever enter a new venture without giving careful thought to the possible risks involved.

Existing organizations should consider strengths and weaknesses, opportunities and threats. New initiatives or programs can be developed to enhance an area in which the organization is already strong or to offset a weakness. At times the primary goal is to enhance a strength to make it even more difficult for competitors to challenge that strength. At other times the goal is to shore up a weakness. Existing organizations should also be on the lookout for opportunities and threats. At times a new program may be developed to ward off potential competition. At other times, competition falters and a temporary opportunity exists. Successful organizations try to anticipate or at least identify opportunities and threats and to respond to them on a timely basis.

Product Definition

Once a program has been proposed, the product or service must be carefully defined and the business setting analyzed. What is the specific product; what are the ways it can be provided; what are the resources needed to provide it? Are the patients homogeneous or mixed in terms of diagnoses? In terms of acuity? Are the required resources limited to labor and other operating items, or are capital investments needed as well? How long will it take to get the program up and running? Are there economic or technological trends that could impact patient demand in the future?

Business and Industry

Once the product or service has been fully described, planners should carefully consider the type of business they are getting into and the nature of the industry within which the endeavor will reside. Typically, the planner will have to acquire funding to start up the new business. A description of the proposed business is necessary. It should include facts about the customer base; the name, location, and size of the proposed business; the service area, growth potential, and capacity of the business; and any other identifiers that are important to specify to plan for the new business.

Planners must understand the industry of which the business will be a part. They need to know whether it is a new and growing industry, a mature industry, or an industry in decline. For industry information, planners should seek data concerning local, regional, and national gross receipts and potential growth or potential decline. Sources of data include consultants, the Federal Trade Commission, the Small Business Administration, the Bureau of Labor Statistics, and trade organizations and journals, among others.

Market Analysis

Having defined the product, the next step is a market analysis. This section describes critical aspects of the market for the product or service. Planners ask questions such as: Are there people who want this product or service and are willing to pay for it? Are any new medical technologies or medical procedures emerging that might affect demand for this product or service? How many potential buyers are there now, and how will that change over the next 5 to 10 years? How many other organizations offer the product or service? What are the market trends for this product or service? What *market share* can this organization get? Market share refers to a percentage of the total demand or volume for the product or service. For example, if there are 10,000 patients in the community who will be treated, and your organization gains a 10% market share, it will expect to treat 1,000 patients. The organization must be convinced that there will be sufficient demand to justify the investment in this project as opposed to some other project. Planners also must consider pricing. How should this product or service be priced? Can the product or service be priced below the competition's prices? Does the product or service have name recognition that might be used in promotions and advertising to enhance its market position?

The market analysis must consider who the patients will be and who the payers will be. Is the population largely insured or largely uninsured? If uninsured, are they eligible for Medicaid or another payment source? Having enough patients who can pay for the products and services is the first step. Equally important, however, is knowing the mix of patients.

The term "mix of patients" refers to the various types of ailments and the various types of payers. The types of ailments must be known so that the expected costs can be calculated. The types of payers is also important. What percentage are patients with Medicare, Medicaid, an HMO, or other insurance? What percentage has no coverage, so their bills will be likely to end up as either charity care or bad debts? The program's revenue can vary dramatically according to who will ultimately be responsible for paying the organization's charges. The charges represent gross revenues. Generally, however, only a portion of the total charges is collected because of government-mandated rates or special discount arrangements or because the patients are uninsured and unable to pay. The ultimate cash receipts must be known in addition to the volume of patients.

If the market analysis shows little demand or excessive competition, the planning process for this specific program may be discontinued. If it appears that there is demand for the product or service and a reasonable potential market share for the organization, the planning can continue. Understanding the nature and intensity of the potential competition is a key component of business planning. That part of business planning is addressed by a competitive analysis.

Competitive Analysis

The purpose of the competitive analysis is to describe the nature of the competition to be faced in the marketplace and to explain in detail how the start-up's strengths will be used to prevail against the competition in the effort to build market share. This section starts with a profile of the competitors. Who are they? What are their market share and competitive advantages? What weaknesses do they have that can be exploited to advantage? How do their products and services compare with those of the planners in terms of quality, price, and ease of use? The answer to these questions helps the planners to define their market niche. To be successful, every business has to fill a niche in the market. This is how a business is distinguished from that of the competition.

This section of the business plan should also address the current distribution of market share and how the new business will break into this industry and take a piece of market share for itself. Too often, planners think only of expected costs, revenues, and profits. But that is far too narrow a view of the business impact in the marketplace. Market share is equally important. Japanese business leaders have long recognized the importance of market share. At times, they have chosen to sell certain automobile products at a loss in order to build market share. Once they had market share—and customer awareness of their product and customer loyalty—they were able to raise prices to a profitable level. Questions to answer while developing this section of a business plan include: How much market share can you expect to start out with, and what market share is it reasonable for you to expect to get during the first 1, 3, and 5 years? How you acquire that share is your marketing strategy, which is addressed in the next section.

Understanding your competitors and how the competition might change in the foreseeable future is critical if you are to be able to plan for market penetration of your products and services. Planners need to know if there will be an increasing number of providers moving into their service area and competing for the same patients. If so, will this organization's market share fall?

The issue of competition is critical. Is there competition at present? If not, what is the potential for competition to develop? What will the competition do when it sees this organization's new program or project? What are the strengths and weaknesses of the competition? Once the market and competitive analyses are complete, the planners can prepare a marketing strategy.

Marketing Strategy

The purpose of a marketing strategy is to explain specifically how you will enter the market, obtain a niche, maintain a market share, and thereby achieve your stated financial goals. There are three steps to developing a marketing strategy. The first step is to define your market penetration goals. The next step is to delineate the factors that give your products and services an edge over those of the competition. The third step is developing a plan to market your products to your customers.

The market penetration goals will depend upon how new your product is and therefore on whether you are trying to break into an existing market or stepping into a brand new area. It is important to specifically determine market penetration goals in advance so that you will have a yardstick by which to measure your progress and success.

The factors that give new products and services an edge over those of the competition constitute your competitive advantage. These advantages will ultimately define the product's position in the marketplace. These are the features you want to advertise. An important part of product positioning is pricing. Obviously, pricing has to support the costs of providing the goods and services. But pricing also has to be done with awareness of what competitors are charging. Most people have a strong preference for the product with the lowest price. If you can't market your products and services at an attractive price and still make a profit, it is not worth starting the business. On the other hand, health care services are often very insensitive to price. Patients want the best care and don't care about price, especially if their insurance is paying for the care. So focusing on high quality, even if you have to charge more, may be a reasonable business strategy.

Then it is necessary to consider how you will make your products and services available to your prospective customers. There must be adequate supplies of your products and services, and they must be distributed to places where customers can find and purchase them. Demand won't help you much if your customers can't locate you and your product. How will you make your products visible and available to your customers? How will you "provide service after the sale"? People expect you to stand behind the products and services you offer. Who is authorized to handle customer complaints? What will you do about dissatisfied customers?

Next, decide how to advertise the product to the customer base. The goals here are to get the word out to people who would be interested in your product and to avoid wasting money on advertising that reaches people who are never going to buy your product (i.e., who are not part of your potential customer base). As an example, consider the futility of using a community-wide house-to-house mailer to market new-hire orientation services to hospitals and medical clinics. Advertising lets potential customers know that the new product is available. Promotional activities focus on persuading them to try your products in lieu of staying with your competition's products.

Finally, public relations are always a part of marketing. Your organization's reputation in the community is an important part of the attractiveness of the product to potential customers. Then when they see that the product is offered by a reputable company such as yours, they will be more willing to buy your products and services.

Organizational Structure and Ownership

The purpose of this section is to delineate the legal structure of a new business and to identify its owners. If the business is a new enterprise within an existing organization, the structure of the new business will most likely follow the existing structure. But for a new business, the structure must be defined. For example, will the business be structured as a sole proprietorship? Or will it be established as a corporation? If the business will have a single owner, will that owner take the personal risk of allowing the business to be a sole proprietorship or will the owner establish a limited liability company (usually called by its initials, LLC) in the state in which business is conducted in order to limit personal liability? Or will another business structure be selected? In some cases, the business will have to be licensed by the state. In that case, the ownership, legal structure of the business, and if required, officers of the company must usually be listed in an application for the business to be licensed in the state.

Management and Key Personnel

The purpose of this section is to demonstrate that the administration responsible for day-to-day operation of the business is capable, fairly compensated, and given every incentive to be successful. Members of the management team should be listed by name. Critical information should include their résumés (in the appendix) and a short narrative outlining the education, experience, special expertise, and business track record of each member of the management team. Funding agencies will want to be sure that the people operating the business have the knowledge and skills to do the job.

The planned management structure should be explained, and an organizational chart should be included. The most common management structure of middle-sized and large organizations is a bureaucratic structure, and that is almost certainly the structure that the parent organization will exhibit if the new business is a service department created within an existing organization. However, a very small new business is more likely to have a simple structure. One person is the owner-manager and any employees report directly to the owner, who has final say over all business decisions. A variety of other structures may be selected, but bureaucracies and simple structures are the most common management structures.

Finally, the key personnel who will work in the business should be identified. In this section, it is important to identify key employees who have important skills needed for the business to operate. When the new business is to have a board of directors, this section is where the planners list the members of the board and the skills and support they bring to the business. Many businesses appoint a small group of highly knowledgeable or influential people to guide the direction of the new organization and help to determine its mission and business strategies. Members are chosen on the basis of their expertise in the business (often retired executives), for their ability to ensure good publicity (often newspaper publishers and local TV news station executives), or for their political power (sometimes these people are former elected officials or a mayor, governor or legislator).

Rough Financial Plan

After the market analysis has been completed, and assuming that it indicates that a demand exists for the product, a rough financial plan can be developed. The purpose of this rough plan is to determine whether the project warrants further attention. The rough financial plan revolves around an operating budget.

The operating budget includes rough estimates of both revenues and expenses. The revenues can be calculated based on the demand projections derived from the market analysis. The expenses can be based on rough approximations of the types and amounts of the various resources needed.

The results of a rough financial plan are imprecise. The purpose of the plan is to arrive at one of three findings. The first possible finding is that the cost of the program will far exceed the revenues under any reasonable set of assumptions. In that case, managers should save their time by discontinuing the planning process if the project is being evaluated solely on financial merit. The second finding is that the program looks as though it will definitely be profitable. In that case, the manager can proceed with the substantial investment of time required to develop a fully detailed plan. The third finding is that it is unclear whether the project will be profitable.

The third result creates some difficulty for managers. A major potential danger in program planning is that the more time the manager working on the data collection has invested in the analysis, the harder she or he will push for adoption of the project. The more time managers invest, the greater their psychological need to justify that investment by having the plan indicate that the project is favorable. This could result in a bias in the collection and interpretation of data concerning project feasibility.

Given the unknowns that one encounters in putting any new program into place, there should be a healthy degree of skepticism about any new project. "If it's such a good project, why isn't someone else already doing it?" is a reasonable question. Therefore, one should always continue with analysis cautiously. There may be a good answer to the question of why someone isn't already doing it. But the issue should be considered. Generally, if the rough analysis indicates just borderline profitability, then plans should be discontinued unless factors lead the manager to believe that a more detailed analysis might in fact produce information in the project's favor. More often than not, there are unanticipated problems that reduce profitability as a project progresses. If the project was borderline in the beginning, losses may well result. It is better to discontinue work on such projects sooner rather than later. If, however, the rough financial plan suggests that the business will be sufficiently profitable that it is worth proceeding with, a detailed financial plan should be prepared.

Detailed Operations Plan

Assuming that planning for the project is still continuing after the rough financial plan, the next step would be to develop a detailed operations plan, including an implementation schedule. The essence of this plan is to consider the entire impact that the new project will have on the existing operations of the organization.

The first element of the plan is to consider the physical location and structure required by the program or project. Next one must consider the specific human resources required. Equipment and supplies must also be taken into account. These are all direct costs of the project. It is possible, however, that the project will also cause indirect costs to vary. For instance, the admitting department may need more personnel. The marketing department may have to make a substantial effort to get the new service off the ground. The engineering department may have to devote many personnel hours to the project. It is necessary to account for the impact of the program on all of the organization's overhead components.

Having determined the steps in implementing the new business, planners should identify major milestones for the project. They must know the start-up events that have to occur for the business or program. If selling a service (such as an educational or consulting program), they need to line up some customers and have them sign contracts. They must acquire office space, furniture, computers, and other necessary equipment. They must hire staff, create the programs and products, develop policies, and see to all the other elements the business or program will need to get off the ground.

A particularly good graphic approach for displaying milestones and when they are to be achieved is use of a Gantt chart (Figure 7-1). Note that items are ordered in temporal sequence (things that will be done first are listed first, regardless of importance). A Gantt chart is visually easy to interpret and shows when the planners expect to accomplish certain milestones. The chart can be created in most word processing programs or on a spreadsheet or through specialized business software that supports the creation of Gantt charts.

Finally, the operational plan should include an Exit Plan section that deals with dissolving the business if it is not successful. This is where planners provide a formal plan for determining the point at which the endeavor will be abandoned and articulate a systematic plan for closing down the business should it prove unsuccessful. They must decide what indicators of success or failure to measure and how those indicators will be interpreted in terms of business performance. Specifically, they specify what performance levels will indicate that the business is not meeting its goals and should be disbanded. Planners should set up specific times during the first 2 to 3 years to meet with the board, consultants, or other advisors to discuss the progress of the business. If it is as good as or better than expected, the decision will probably be to continue the business. However, a decision should be made in advance about how much worse than expected performance has to be to make the decision to shut down the operation. The reason this decision should be made during business planning is that once people have invested time, energy, and commitment to an endeavor, it is very difficult for them to be objective about poor performance. Many people have continued to "throw good money after bad" long after objective observers could see

Milestone	Oct	Nov	Dec	Jan	Feb	Mar	Apr
Secure initial contracts	■						
Search for adequate office space	■	■					
Order letterhead and other office supplies	■	■					
Order office furniture	■	■	■				
Hire personnel	■	■	■				
Begin work on first contracts	■	■	■	■			
Sign a minimum of two new customers	■	■	■	■	■		
Sign three additional customers	■	■	■	■	■	■	
Performance review and continuation decision	■	■	■	■	■	■	■

Figure 7-1 Example of a Gantt chart.

that the business was failing and that it was more likely to continue to fail than to recover. If the project planners do not have a reasonable exit plan, people can act like gambling addicts, forever expecting the big break and never knowing when to quit. An exit plan is a tool to help people avoid the mistake of continuing a failing business long after it should have been dissolved.

At what time point should this review be conducted? In the Gantt chart, the company performance review is scheduled for April. This review was scheduled so as to force the founders, managers, and other reviewers to take time to formally review the business at a point when it has operated long enough that it is possible to assess its likelihood of success or failure.

Detailed Financial Plan

Once a thorough analysis has been made concerning the various impacts of the proposed plan on the operations of the organization, a detailed and thorough financial plan can be developed. This financial plan incorporates all the information from the operations plan, considering the financial impact of the resources to be used. This information will ultimately be used to determine whether it is possible to go ahead with the new program.

The financial plan has three critical elements: a break-even analysis, preparation of budgets, and the development of a set of *pro forma* financial statements. Pro forma financial statements present a prediction of what the financial statements for the project or program will look like in the future.

The break-even analysis provides information about the minimum volume of patients that must be achieved for the new program to avoid losing money. Many new programs or projects start with low volume and gradually attract more patients. The pattern of growth in the volume of patients is predicted as part of the market analysis. Break-even analysis is valuable because, combined with the volume projection, it can help give the organization a sense of how long it will take before the new program stops losing money. The techniques of break-even analysis are discussed in Chapter 4.

Budget preparation includes the development of an operating budget, a cash budget, and a capital budget. These budgets are prepared for 3 to 5 years into the future, starting at the initiation of the venture. The cash and operating budgets are commonly prepared on a monthly basis over that time. Many new ventures take several years to become operational. If budgets were prepared for just 1 year into the future, they would not present a full sense of the mature entity. Often there are few patients when a venture first starts. Legal or policy requirements for minimal staffing levels may cause losses in the first quarter or half year for even the most successful initiatives. Longer range, more detailed budgets can provide a better picture of what is likely to happen once the organization is fully operational and has a stable (or preferably growing) patient population.

Although many nurse managers in large organizations are responsible only for the expenses of their units, that is rarely the case in new ventures. The developers of the business plan must consider the revenue flow critically. The revenue budget must include estimates of patient demand, broken down by type of care or services to be consumed. The payer mix must be estimated as well. In other words, the developers must determine what percentage of the patients will receive each type of treatment offered and what percentage of patients' care will be paid for by Medicare, Medicaid, and so on. The amount to be charged for each service must be decided, and the expected amount to be collected by payer for each service must be forecast. All this information is used to estimate the amount of revenue to be earned. See the discussion of revenue budgets in Chapter 9.

Various expenses also have to be planned according to the same estimates of patient demand used to predict revenue. Preparation of the expense budget requires that decisions be made concerning how large a facility is needed to house the service at the start and later as it grows. Will the venture start with a small amount of space and add additional space as required? Or will it open with enough space to handle expected patient volume for at least several years into the future? Will all the equipment be purchased at the start, or will it be acquired in phases? How much staff is needed when the venture opens for business, and at what volume levels will additional staff be hired? Clearly, business-plan budgets must address many questions about the timing and amount of expenses that do not come up in running an ongoing department of an existing organization.

The capital budget considers the acquisitions the organization will have to make for buildings and equipment that have multiyear lives. Unlike ongoing departments that focus capital budgets on additions or replacements, new ventures are faced with evaluating many capital acquisitions all at once. However, it is important to give each acquisition the same careful consideration one would if only a few capital assets were being acquired. Capital acquisition errors made by a start-up venture can be costly. If it turns out that a $500,000 piece of equipment is really not adequate and has to be replaced with a $600,000 alternative that was considered but rejected as being too expensive, the attempt to "save" $100,000 on the initial purchase can be devastating to the financial success of the start-up venture.

The *cash-flow budget* provides information on how much cash the program or project will spend each year and how much cash will be received. This information is not available from the operating budget for the program. That budget focuses on revenues and expenses. However, revenues are generally received some time after the patients are treated. In many cases it takes payers (including Medicare, Medicaid, HMOs, and others) weeks or months to pay for the services provided. On the other hand, cash outlays at the beginning of the project may be substantial. In addition to paying salaries on a current basis, the organization will have to acquire supplies, equipment and, in some cases, buildings.

In the case of salaries and supplies, the time between cash payment and ultimate cash receipt may be a matter of months. In the case of buildings and equipment, substantial amounts of money may be needed to start the program, whereas the receipt of cash from the use of the buildings and equipment may stretch out over a period of years. Therefore, it is important for the organization to know the amount of cash required. That information will allow the organization to decide whether it has sufficient cash available to undertake the project. Cash budgeting is discussed further in Chapter 12.

Pro forma financial statements present a more comprehensive summary of the financial implications of the plan than is provided by the budgets developed as part of the rough financial plan.

Pro Forma Financial Statements

Every organization has a set of financial statements that are summaries used to indicate the financial position of the organization at a point in time, as well as the financial results of its activities for a period of time. Often financial statements are used to indicate the organization's financial position at the end of its fiscal year and its revenues, expenses, cash receipts, and payments for an entire fiscal year. The most typically used financial statements are the *balance sheet* (also called the statement of financial position), the *operating statement* (also called the activity statement or the income statement), and the *statement of cash flows* (or the cash flow statement).

The balance sheet provides a listing of all the resources and obligations of the organization. The resources owned by the organization are called *assets*. The obligations of the organization are called *liabilities*. If the assets exceed the liabilities, the difference is called *net assets* or *owners' equity*. The assets always equal the total of the liabilities plus the net assets or owners' equity. Therefore the balance sheet will always be "in balance."

The operating statement is a listing of all the revenues, less all the expenses. The difference is sometimes referred to as the net income. Many health care organizations refer to the difference as the excess of revenues over expenses or the change in unrestricted net assets. This is the primary measure of an organization's profitability.

The statement of cash flows is a categorized listing of all the organization's cash receipts and cash payments.

Using the budgets and the various projections and assumptions about the proposed program or project, the key financial statements are projected for each year into the future, usually for a period of 3 to 5 years. Any predictions beyond 5 years are generally considered unreliable. Any predictions for fewer than 3 years fail to provide a picture of what the financial impact of the program is likely to be once it is fully up and running.

Pro forma statements allow the user to determine some basic financial information about the proposed program or project. The pro forma balance sheet indicates for each future year what the year-end obligations are likely to be relative to the resources. One would always want to have sufficient resources to be able to pay obligations as they become due. The pro forma operating statement indicates the project's expected profitability for each future year. The pro forma cash flow statement provides a summary of the information from the cash-flow analysis discussed earlier.

Forecasting

The detailed financial plan, as noted previously, includes a break-even analysis, budgets, and a set of pro forma financial statements. To get the information needed for these elements, the business plan relies heavily on forecasts.

To prepare a cash-flow analysis and to generate pro forma financial statements, a great number of items must be forecast. These include, but are not limited to, inflation, regulation, revenues, wage rates, availability of personnel, detailed expenses, cash flows, and patient volumes. To make these forecasts, the techniques discussed in Chapter 6 are employed.

Sensitivity Analysis

In developing the detailed financial plan, a helpful technique is *sensitivity analysis*. Sensitivity analysis is concerned with the fact that often a number of assumptions and predictions are made in calculating the financial aspects of a business plan. The number of expected patients used to develop pro forma financial statements is the result of a forecast, which may not be exactly correct. The revenues are based on a stated average charge, which is an assumption. The actual rates charged may be higher or lower. Sensitivity analysis is a process whereby the financial results are recalculated under a series of varying assumptions and predictions. This is often referred to as "what-if" analysis.

Suppose that the pro forma financial statements lead one to believe that the proposed project will be a reasonable financial success. Using sensitivity analysis, one could then say, "What if there are 5% fewer patients than expected? Or 10% fewer? What if there are 5% more patients than expected? Or 10% more? What if the average amount charged is raised by 10%? What if the number of staff nurses needed is three FTEs greater than anticipated? What if the construction costs are $30,000 more than expected?

Essentially, sensitivity analysis provides recognition of uncertainty. Uncertainty creates risk. Before a final business plan is put together and accepted, it is important to have some idea of the magnitude of risk involved. By going through the what-if analysis, one can get a sense of how unfavorable the financial results would be if some things do not occur exactly as hoped or expected. If a project can show an expected favorable financial result over a range of what-if questions, it can provide an extra degree of assurance. If that is not the case, then one must carefully question whether the potential benefits are worth the risks that must be undertaken.

Examination of Alternatives

A final consideration in the development of a detailed financial plan is the examination of alternatives. There is often more than one way to execute a new program. The alternatives relate to factors such as the capacity of the program, the approach to providing the service, and the quality of the program. The business plan should be based on having selected one specific approach after having considered a wide variety of potential alternatives. Calculations regarding the costs and benefits of the various alternatives that have been considered become part of the final business plan package.

The Elements of a Business Plan Package

With business plans, as with great cooking, presentation of the finished product is an essential component of the process. Business plan development requires a significant amount of time and effort. The finished result is often a long document. Unless carefully presented in a final package, many of the benefits of the work may be lost.

The first and most critical element is a concise executive summary. The executive summary should be brief. Ideally, it is no more than one page. It may be two or three pages if absolutely necessary. The summary should convey what the project is, why it is being proposed, and what the most likely projected results are. This should be able to be stated in just a few brief sentences. If the information in the summary indicates that the project is worth pursuing, the reader will read further.

The next part of a business plan should be the detailed plan with the sections described earlier. Such a plan is generally about 20 or 30 pages long. This should provide a much greater amount of detail than the executive summary. It includes all the specific documentation for the calculations that underlie the plan in either the body of the plan or in an appendix.

The business plan should describe the mission of the organization and the way in which the proposed program fits in with the mission. It should provide a description of both the product or service and its potential consumers. The plan should explain how the new product fits in with the organization's existing services. It should explain why there is a belief that the organization has a competitive edge in offering this product or service that will allow it to gain and maintain a certain level of market share. The profitability of the program should be discussed in greater detail than that provided in the executive summary. The pro forma financial statements should be included.

It is essential that the business plan discuss potential risks. Regulation and other elements that would impede the project should be discussed as well. Finally, the plan should include some estimate of the requirement of management time needed to implement the program and a statement of commitment by the manager who will bear primary responsibility for the implementation of the program.

Within the body of the business plan package are the detailed analyses of each element. Included are detailed descriptions or schematics of the product and service, results of the market research indicating market potential and competition, a detailed time line for implementation of the plan, a detailed marketing plan for attracting patients, and a detailed financial plan that includes the analysis used to develop the pro forma statements. Some of the data may be organized into appendices to the business plan.

By dividing the business plan into these three sections—executive summary, full detailed analysis and appendices—the manager allows other managers less familiar with the project to understand it. This will allow the project to get a fair examination and should lead to a reasoned final decision about whether to implement the proposed program.

Readers who plan to prepare a business plan should read one of several books on the topic listed in the section at the end of this chapter.

Summary and Implications for Nurse Managers

Nurse managers at all levels of the organization have insights that can result in significant operational changes that will move the organization closer to its strategic goals. That is why strategic management takes the view that strategic planning is not limited to the development of the long-range plan and program budgets. Strategic management must exhibit itself through strategic thought by managers throughout the organization. All nurse managers should make themselves aware of their organization's mission and goals as well as its specific objectives and policies. Knowing only the philosophical statement of the nursing department alone is too narrow a view.

The organization-wide goals developed in the strategic management process are used as a point of reference when assessing where the organization has been, where it is going, and what it hopes to accomplish in the coming years.

Strategic management requires a significant effort from managers at all levels. However, that effort is rewarded. Careful planning reduces the extent to which managers move from crisis to crisis. It promotes the efficient use of resources and the financial health of the organization. It results in goal setting and the establishment of a vision for the organization. Strategic planning helps ensure that managers will identify opportunities and take reasonable risks to take advantage of those opportunities. Strategic management promotes organizational change within a stable framework of constant mission and goals.

The strategic plan or long-range budget indicates which programs are to remain at a steady state, which are to be reduced in size or eliminated entirely, which are to be expanded, and which are to be added. This gives impetus to specific program budgets in which a unit, department, or program undergoes a complete assessment.

Summary and Implications for Nurse Managers—cont'd

Using a method such as ZBB, the organization's managers can systematically examine all the implications of a program over its lifetime. The program can be compared to others that would achieve the same end. The program can also be assessed in terms of alternative ways to produce the output, alternative levels of quality, and alternative levels of quantity of output.

Program budget analyses can uncover unneeded costs in existing programs. There is waste in health care organizations as in virtually all organizations. Further, program budgeting can help the organization to make effective choices of how to best use limited resources. Trade-offs among various alternatives can be more clearly assessed with the increased information provided by program budgets about the impact of different available options.

The organization can settle for a less-than-first-class bedside computer system but can also have new unit-based DVD players for patient education. Alternatively, it can have a new first-rate bedside computer system and forgo having unit-based DVD players. It is impossible, in this book, to say which of the choices would be better. However, there should be an awareness that the alternatives do exist. The organization should not blindly get a first-rate bedside computer system because of internal political pressure and then simply accede to the fact that there is no money for DVD players. The alternatives should be considered and an explicit choice made.

Program budgeting techniques are as effective for reviewing the operations of an ongoing unit as they are for evaluating a new program. The way a nursing unit performs its tasks may go unchanged from year to year. A ZBB review, however, can force the manager to consider whether there are alternative ways or levels of effort that could be used to accomplish the unit's goals.

Performing a zero-base review for a nursing unit, department, or organization is expensive. It takes a substantial amount of time to evaluate all the cost elements of a budget. It is much simpler to indicate that the next year's operating budget will be 2% more than the current year's. However, the chances of making a significant positive gain for the organization are much higher when a thorough justification of each and every expenditure is undertaken. Managers tend to accept the status quo. Instead, managers should spend less time on day-in, day-out routine activities and more time on being innovative. Examining all aspects of a unit's operations can result in significant and lasting benefits for the unit and the entire organization.

Business plans are documents that are becoming essential for the introduction of new programs. Such plans help managers to complete a comprehensive examination of a proposed program. By making such a thorough review, the manager and the organization gain an in-depth understanding of the program as well as its financial implications for the organization.

Strategic management has broader implications than simply use in specific areas, such as zero-base reviews or business plans. Managers should be creative in their applications. For example, there are many models for the delivery of nursing services. Each one has financial, quality, and other implications. A nurse manager who understands strategic management can apply its principles when the organization makes choices among alternative delivery care models. In this way the choice made will reflect consideration of the wide range of factors that relate to that decision.

References and Suggested Readings

Aiken, L., Smith, H., & Lake, E. (1994). Lower Medicare mortality among a set of hospitals known for good nursing care. *Medical Care* 32(8), 771-787.

Allison, M., and Kaye, J. (2005). *Strategic Planning for Nonprofit Organizations*, ed 2. Hoboken, NJ: Wiley Publishing.

Anvari, A., ed. Wisdom Quotes: Quotations to Inspire and Challenge. http://www.anvari.org/fortune/Quotations_UA/53.html; downloaded July 15, 2006.

Berwick, D., Godfrey, A., and Roessner, J. (2002). *Curing Healthcare: New Strategies for Quality Improvement.* Hoboken, NJ: Jossey-Bass/Wiley Publishing.

Camillus, J.C. (1980). *Strategic Planning and Management Control.* Lexington, MA: Lexington Books. p. 18.

Camillus, J.C. (1986). *Practice of Strategic Planning.* New York: National League for Nursing.

Cortes, T.A. (1996). Zero-based budgeting for a radiology service: A case study in outsourcing.

Hospital Cost Management & Accounting 8(2), 1-6.

Ellis, D., and Pekar, P. Jr. (1980) *Planning for Nonplanners,* New York: Amacom. p. 24.

Faugier, J. (2005). Developing a new generation of nurse entrepreneurs. *Nursing Standards* 19(30), 49-53.

Finkler, S.A., Ward, D.R., and Baker, J. (2007). *Essentials of Cost Accounting for Health Care Organizations,* ed 3. Boston: Jones and Bartlett.

Hunger, J.D., and Wheelen, T. (2006). *Essentials of Strategic Management,* ed 4. Upper Saddle River, NJ: Prentice Hall.

Institute of Medicine (IOM). (1999). *To Err Is Human: Building a Safer Health System.* Washington, D.C.: Institute of Medicine.

iSixSigma. (2006). New to Six Sigma: A Six Sigma Guide for Both Novice and Experienced Quality Practitioners: iSixSigma. http://www.isixsigma.com/library/content/six-sigma-newbie.asp; downloaded July 20, 2006.

James, C. (2005). Manufacturing's prescription for improving healthcare quality. *Hospital Topics: Research and Perspectives on Healthcare* 83(1):2-8.

Jeffs, L., Merkley, J., Jeffrey, J., Ferris, E., Dusek, J., and Hunter, C. (2006). Case study: Reconciling the quality and safety gap through strategic planning. *Canadian Journal of Nursing Leadership* 19(2), 32-40.

Kerfoot, K. (2006). Megatrends, the annual report, possibilities. *Nursing Economic$* 24(1), 47-49.

Kirk, R. (1992). The big picture: Total quality management and continuous quality improvement. *Journal of Nursing Administration* 22(4), 24.

Koteen, J. (1997). *Strategic Management in Public and Nonprofit Organizations,* ed 2. New York: Praeger, 19-21.

LaFaive, M. (2003). *The Pros and Cons of Zero-based Budgeting.* Testimony before the House Appropriations Subcommittee on General Government. Macinack Center for Public Policy. http://www.mackinac.org/article.aspx?ID=5928; downloaded March 24, 2007.

Lighter, D., and Fair, D. (2004). *Quality Management in Healthcare: Principles and Methods,* ed 2. Boston: Jones and Bartlett.

McNamara, C. Strategic Planning (in nonprofit or for-profit organizations). http://www.managementhelp.org/plan_dec/str_plan/str_plan.htm; downloaded July 20, 2006.

Motorola University. (2006). About Motorola University. http://www.motorola.com/content.jsp?globalObjectId=3071-5801; downloaded May 12, 2006.

Pinson, L. (2004). *Anatomy of a Business Plan: A Step-by-Step Guide to Building a Business and Securing your Future,* ed 6. Chicago: Dearborn Trade Publications.

Pronovost, P., Holzmueller, C., Needham, D., Sexton, J., Miller, M., Berenholtz, S., Wu, A., Perl, T., Davis, R., Baker, D., Winner, L., and Morlock, L. (2006). How will we know patients are safer? An organization-wide approach to measuring and improving safety. *Critical Care Medicine* 34(7), 1988-1995.

Six Sigma Academy. (2006). Delivering Results: Quantify, Execute, Sustain. http://www.6-sigma.com/; downloaded May 10, 2006.

Twenhafel, R. (2005). How to start an independent practice: The nurse practitioner's guide to success. *Journal of Pediatric Nursing* 20(1), 52.

The Operating Budget

by Christina M. Graf,
with contributions by
Steven A. Finkler and Mary McHugh

LEARNING OBJECTIVES
The goals of this chapter are to:

- Explain the various factors in preparing an operating budget
- Describe the financial structure of health care organizations
- Review the planning elements of an operating budget
- Discuss the elements of an activity budget
- Explain the types of patient classification systems and the related issues of reliability and validity
- Provide a detailed approach to developing an operating budget, including determining unit workload, other units of service, the revenue budget, staffing requirements, the personnel budget, the positions/hours budget, the salary budget, and the nonsalary budget

- Define FTEs and variations in definitions of FTEs
- Discuss the impact of alternative coverage patterns on the preparation of the operating budget
- Describe the role of productive and nonproductive time
- Explain calculations of differentials, premiums, and overtime
- Create an awareness of the need to account for float, on-call, call-back, and agency nurse time
- Describe the rationale for and approach to budget negotiation
- Discuss the elements of budget finalization
- Discuss budget implementation

■ INTRODUCTION

The operating budget is a plan that projects the health care organization's anticipated activity, required resources, and associated revenues and expenses for a specified period of time—generally 1 year. The framework for the operating budget is reflected in the financial structure and reporting system of the organization. An operating budget supports the day-to-day work of the organization and its financial subunits and is the budget used by department managers on a monthly basis to determine the financial performance of their departments.

■ FINANCIAL STRUCTURE

Most health care organizations follow the same general format in financial structures and systems, with some variation in specifics. The format for the financial structure is the organization's *chart of accounts*. The chart of accounts gives structure to the recording and reporting of a firm's transactions. It organizes these data to make them useful and meaningful for management of the enterprise. The chart of accounts identifies the areas of responsibility that constitute the work of the organization and the categorization of transactions occurring within these areas. It is specific to an organization and reflects that organization's unique reporting needs.

The financial structure is based on the *responsibility center*, a program or area of activity within the organization. This term emphasizes the concept of the manager's control of and accountability for a defined area of activity. These centers may be either *revenue-producing*, such as pharmacy and laboratory, or *non-revenue-producing*, such as housekeeping and administration. On this basis, the chart of accounts may term these areas *revenue centers* or *cost centers*. Individual departments may be single cost centers or may be composed of several cost centers.

Typically, nursing departments are made up of multiple cost centers that describe discrete physical locations or operational areas: individual patient care units, operating rooms (ORs), postanesthesia recovery, ambulatory clinics, emergency department, administration, and so on. In many settings, particularly inpatient settings, nursing is not directly reimbursed for its services in the same way that, for example, pharmacy is reimbursed according to the type and amount of drugs provided. Nursing services are included in overall routine charges for room and board, procedures, or visits, as are services such as housekeeping and dietary. If these routine charges appear on nursing cost center reports, the cost centers may be designated as revenue producing for accounting purposes. Operationally, however, nursing in these organizations is not seen as being revenue producing. In some hospitals, nursing costs have been accurately described, separated from the routine charges, and used as the basis for determining nursing charges. In these circumstances, nursing's contribution to revenue generation for the organization is defined explicitly. The revenue generated by nursing is clearly delineated in some other settings as well. Visits by nurse clinicians in the home care setting or by nurse practitioners in the ambulatory setting, for example, directly generate revenue for the organization. (See Chapters 9 and 18 for further discussion.)

The financial reporting system for the responsibility center and the department identifies the revenue generated and expenses incurred for each accounting cycle (generally 1 calendar month or one 28-day period). Cumulative totals for the fiscal year-to-date (YTD) are also reported, as are totals (both for the month and the YTD) for departments and for the total organization. The organization's revenue is based initially on *charges*, or the prices that it sets for specific services. The sum of these charges is described as gross *patient revenue*. However, not everyone pays the full charge for the services provided. Under the federal Diagnosis-Related Group (DRG) system, for example, Medicare pays a fixed amount per inpatient admission based on the patient's discharge diagnosis, which may or may not cover the charges generated during that admission. Medicaid systems vary from state to state, but they usually pay an amount less than the charges. Other third-party payers, such as Blue Cross and managed care organizations, commonly negotiate a discounted payment rate that is less than charges. The difference between the charge and the discounted rate is referred to as a *contractual allowance*. Typically, health care organizations also provide some level of *free care* or *charity care*, which also reduces the amount the organization expects to be paid. These allowances are identified as *deductions from revenue*, and the gross revenue less deductions from revenue is called *net revenue*. (Note that *bad debt*, bills that non-charity care patients do not pay, are considered a business expense and not a deduction from revenue.) Revenue reported in the individual responsibility center, however, generally reflects only the charges for specific services provided for that area of activity.

Expenses reported in the responsibility centers are generally limited to *direct expenses*, those expenses that can be specifically and exclusively related to the activity within that area. Note that direct expenses can be further subdivided into direct and indirect patient care costs. This subdivision differentiates the unit costs that can be specifically related to providing care for individual patients (direct) from those that support the overall operation of the unit (indirect). In this differentiation, salaries paid to staff nurses for hours spent providing care to patients would be considered direct care costs, whereas the salaries paid for hours devoted to orientation or continuing education would be considered indirect care costs. Similarly, dressing supplies or IV fluids would be identified as direct care costs, whereas notepads and similar office supplies would be identified as indirect. Both direct and indirect patient care costs, however, would be classified as direct unit expenses. *Indirect expenses*, such as administrative and personnel costs or heating and lighting expenses, are shared by all departments. These expenses are usually not allocated to individual cost centers in the revenue and expense report or are allocated according to standard costing methodologies and are referred to as *overhead*.

Within the monthly financial report, individual revenue and expense items are sorted into like groupings and reported by account. For example, expenses incurred within a given time period are separated into two major categories: employment costs and nonsalary expenses. Within these two categories, expenses may be further subdivided. Employment costs can be reported according to types of employees (RN, non-RN), types of hours (straight time, overtime, vacation, sick), types of differentials (evening, night, on-call), and categories of fringe benefits (Federal Insurance Contributions Act [FICA], health insurance). Nonsalary categories could include subgroupings such as patient care supplies, instruments, office supplies, equipment, and subscriptions. Supply expenses identified as interdepartmental refer to those expenses initially incurred by one department and later charged to the end-user department. For example, pharmacy may purchase bulk supplies of stock drugs, then charge them to the individual patient care units as unit stock supplies are replaced. Telephone bills may initially be charged to a central communications office, then allocated to individual areas based on actual utilization of services. Although these expenses are not purchased directly from the vendor by the end-users, they are real expenses to the responsibility center and require the same level of management as other supply expenses. The chart of accounts provides the identifying numbers and descriptions of these accounts.

Figure 8-1 is a sample revenue and expense report for one cost center. This report lists both actual and budgeted revenues and expenses for the month and YTD, as well as a variance (budget minus actual). The expenses in this example are listed as positive numbers, and the revenues are listed as negative numbers. Some organizations would show revenues as positive and expenses as negative. In the variance column the mathematical sign indicates actual performance against budget. In our example, negative variance (parentheses) for either revenues or expenses means that the unit did not do as well as projected; positive variance (no parentheses) means that the unit did better than projected. Some organizations may reverse this, using a positive variance as unfavorable. Other organizations eliminate variance signs altogether and designate variances as favorable to budget or unfavorable to budget. As long as the reporting is consistent within the organization, it does not matter which approach is used.

It is, however, very important to understand exactly how to read each of the figures. The column labeled Budget lists the amount of money in each category that the unit

| | | | RESPONSIBILITY CENTER: 611 GENERAL SURGERY | | REPORT FOR: JANUARY, 2008 | | |

THIS MONTH			ACCOUNT	YEAR-TO-DATE		
Actual	**Budget**	**Variance**	**NUMBER/DESCRIPTION**	**Actual**	**Budget**	**Variance**
311. Revenue						
($371,026)	($365,800)	$5,226	010 Routine	($3,244,410)	($3,221,400)	$23,010
(2,987)	(3,153)	(166)	020 Other	(27,590)	(27,768)	(178)
($374,013)	($368,953)	$5,060	Total Operating Revenue	($3,272,000)	($3,249,168)	$ 22,832
411. Salary Expense						
$85,115	$85,127	$12	010 Salaries—Regular	$730,881	$749,665	$18,784
2,758	0	(2,758)	020 Salaries—Per Diem	2,758	0	(2,758)
3,209	4,101	892	030 Salaries—Overtime	40,128	36,115	(4,013)
10,885	11,220	335	040 Salaries—Differential	97,995	98,810	815
7,168	7,066	(103)	050 FICA	61,285	62,222	937
7,235	7,363	129	060 Health Insurance	62,125	64,846	2,721
2,212	2,358	146	070 Pension	19,855	20,766	911
1,896	1,915	19	090 Other	17,228	16,868	(360)
$120,478	$119,150	($1,328)	Total Salary Expense	$1,032,255	$1,049,292	$ 17,037
611. Supply Expense						
$4,976	$4,084	($892)	010 Patient Care Supplies	$41,692	$35,961	($5,731)
118	202	84	020 Office Supplies	1,097	1,780	683
371	366	(5)	030 Forms	3,111	3,224	113
0	127	127	040 Supplies Purchased	1,210	1,122	(88)
250	191	(59)	050 Equipment	1,553	1,683	130
125	149	24	060 Seminars/Meetings	1,163	1,309	146
25	17	(8)	070 Books	145	150	5
0	112	112	080 Equipment Rental	385	987	602
31	64	33	090 Miscellaneous	388	561	173
$ 5,896	$ 5,312	($ 584)	Total Supply Expense	$ 50,744	$ 46,777	($ 3,967)
911. Interdepartment Expense						
$934	$921	($13)	010 Central Supply	$7,828	$8,114	$286
1,137	1,121	(16)	020 Pharmacy	9,527	9,868	341
1,915	1,888	(27)	030 Linen/Laundry	16,046	16,628	582
105	297	192	040 Maintenance	977	2,618	1,641
211	212	1	060 Telephone	1,962	1,870	(92)
0	21	21	070 Photocopy	124	187	63
0	13	13	090 Miscellaneous	165	112	(53)
$ 4,302	$ 4,473	$ 171	Total Interdepartment Expense	$ 36,629	$ 39,397	$ 2,768
$130,676	$128,935	($1,741)	Total Operating Expense	$1,119,628	$1,135,466	$ 15,838

Figure 8-1 Sample revenue and expense report.

expected to receive in revenues or spend on expenses. The left side of the table shows this month's revenues and expenses. The columns on the right side show all the revenues and expenses for this year so far. Recognizing that revenues are listed as negative numbers, consider the first line under "311. Revenue." This is the item listed under Number/Description as 010 Routine. Consider the Year-to-Date figures. Note that actual and budget revenues are in parentheses. The budgeted amount, that is, the amount that the planners expected to receive, was $3,221,400. But what they actually received was $3,244,410. The amount they received was $23,010 more than they expected when they prepared the budget. That is why this amount is listed in the last column as a variance. And because revenues were higher than expected, there are no parentheses around the number $23,010.

Now look at the first line under "611.Supply Expense." Again looking at the right-hand Year-to-Date columns, consider the line for 010 Patient Care Supplies. The planners expected to generate $35,961 in expenses, but instead higher costs of $41,692 were incurred. The difference is $5,731. Because higher-than-expected expenses are unfavorable, the variance column shows that $5,731 in parentheses. However, it would be a mistake to assume automatically that the unit had been carelessly with supplies. Certainly, supply usage and especially supply wastage is a very important issue in managing a nursing unit, and the manager must constantly be concerned with encouraging the staff to be thrifty in their use of supplies. But the reality is that revenues were also higher than expected, and the extra supply usage might well have been a function of a higher number of patient days. The extra patients required more supplies but also generated more revenue. This illustrates one of the problems of having fixed rather than variable budgets.

In any operation in which activity changes on a day–to-day or month-to-month basis, it is important to recognize that revenues and expenses must reflect that variable activity. This issue is explored further in Chapter 13, but for now, it is important to recognize that having some expenses higher than budgeted might be good in some instances, and having revenues higher than expected might or might not be good, depending on the relationship between patient workload and supplies usage.

■ COMPUTERIZING THE BUDGET PROCESS

It is appropriate at this point to discuss the value of computerizing the budget process. For the nurse manager, the most important aspects of preparing the budget are those that involve creativity and critical thinking—analyzing data, setting goals, projecting resource needs, determining effective mix, allocations of shifts to staff, and the like. Throughout the budget process, the manager will identify or be asked to consider variations in the budget assumptions, operational goals, or unit plan. These variations will require recalculation of the impact of potential changes on the proposed budget. Unless technologic support is available throughout this process, the manager is likely to spend time doing endless mathematical calculations rather than analyzing the effect of the variations on the operations of the patient care area.

Ideally, with an integrated, computerized management information system, the manager accesses the existing workload and personnel databases and describes options for the unit's workload and resource requirements. The system calculates the impact of various options, including revenues, personnel costs, and supply expenses, according to the methodologies and formulas established for the organization and for the individual responsibility center. The manager then reviews and evaluates the operational impact of the various options and uses this information during the budgeting process. When the final budget is approved, the system is programmed to produce a budget that is seasonalized according to defined parameters, relevant targets, and comparisons of actual experience to both fixed and variable budgets.

Most health care organizations provide some level of computer support for the budget process, for example, determining annual salary and differential costs, calculating fringe benefit expenses, producing a seasonalized budget, and comparing actual experience to fixed budgets. This level of support is helpful in eliminating the repetitive, tedious work of calculation. When this support is available, it is extremely important that the manager understand the methodology of producing budgetary data in order to ensure that it is being analyzed and utilized appropriately.

However, the level of sophistication that provides integrated computerized support for unit-and discipline-specific analyses of workload data and projection of required resources is commonly unavailable to the nurses managing the units. In the absence of that level of technological support, it is still possible for the manager to simplify budget calculations using software available for microcomputers. Spreadsheets can be developed for calculations related to all the budget components and can be customized to reflect the specific approaches of the institution and the requirements of the individual unit. The advantages in simplifying the process and promoting accuracy in calculation more than justify the time taken to create budget spreadsheets. To the extent that these spreadsheets are consistent across units, summarization by department and division is also facilitated.

There are several key elements in developing a spreadsheet:

1. Describe the mathematical processes. What are the variables involved? How are they related? What are the calculations or formulas used to express those relationships?
2. Limit data entry and maximize computer calculation. Set up the spreadsheet to enter data only once. Reference the initial entry cell for additional uses of the same data element. Create calculations using cell references, even if a number in a formula is unlikely to change.
3. Test the spreadsheet against a known entity to ensure accuracy of calculations.

Relatively simple and useful spreadsheets can be developed with some basic computer skills. For the more experienced computer user, the ability to link spreadsheets, create macros, and utilize database programs can be valuable assets in developing an operating budget. All the examples in this chapter and the sample budget forms in the Appendix can be converted into spreadsheets.

In our experience, many nurses are unfamiliar with the capabilities and uses of electronic spreadsheets. They are an invaluable tool for managers, and nurse managers who aren't familiar with their use should avail themselves of one of the many modes for learning them. There are adult education classes in high schools, community colleges, and many universities that teach spreadsheet use. Sometimes such classes are available through local community recreation centers. In addition, several companies place advertisements on television and the radio for their self-learning CDs that help people learn various Microsoft Office tools, including Excel. Finally, there are several free sites on the Internet—including one sponsored by the Microsoft Company—that provide free tutorials on the use of Excel. A selection of these is listed at the end of this chapter.

■ PLANNING FOR THE OPERATING BUDGET

Executive management is charged with the overall responsibility for the operating budget of the organization, and the fiscal staff provides support and direction throughout the budgeting process. However, effective administration of the operating budget requires the active primary involvement of the responsibility center manager in planning, preparing, and implementing the budget.

Planning for the individual responsibility center takes place within the context of the total organization and department. The nurse manager must identify and consider those factors that affect the activity of the area and therefore affect the operating budget. Obviously, the overall goals and objectives of the organization, as defined in the programming process, are an essential element. Definitions of the philosophy and objectives of nursing consistent with those of the larger organization are also necessary. The organizational structure and nursing care delivery system must be clearly defined because they will affect the level and mix of nursing personnel required. In addition, analysis and planning, occurring on all levels, will generate specific budget assumptions and operational goals.

The budget assumptions incorporate those more global projections that are not the responsibility of any single department but that affect all—or most—areas of the organization. Much of the data needed is obtained from forecasting, as described in Chapter 6. Assumptions may include (a) significant activity projections, such as total admissions, length of stay, patient distribution by DRG, and patient day distribution or occupancy by unit, visits, or procedures; (b) revenue projections, such as rate changes or payer mix changes; (c) wage and salary decisions, such as general and merit increase rates or changes in fringe benefit levels; and (d) factors to be used for projecting supply expense, such as inflation rates. The budget assumptions may also describe overall parameters or targets for total revenue, expense, or profit margin.

Operational goals include organization, department, and unit plans and may be related to patients, staff, or systems. Patient-related goals may involve a change in service, such as developing a multiple trauma area within an orthopedic specialty unit; expanding an existing service, such as increasing the number of telemetry monitors on a medical unit; or adding to available services, such as implementing a pediatric play therapy program. Staff-related goals may include planning changes in staffing mix, implementing a clinical ladder program, or defining expanded continuing education requirements. System-related goals address such aspects as implementing computerized documentation or expanding the quality assessment program. Once these goals are established and defined, they must be prioritized.

In addition to the goals for the organization and the nursing department and unit, the nurse manager must also be aware of projections or changes within other departments that will affect nursing. If the pharmacy department plans to implement a computerized medication administration system or the communications department changes its method of allocating telephone charges, the operating budget for the nursing department could be affected significantly.

The nurse manager's unit plan addresses both unit goals and the context, as described earlier, in which these goals will be implemented. The format for presenting the plan is determined both by the manager's need for clarity and in consideration of the environment in which the budget will be reviewed. That the budget is a logical representation of the unit plan may not be apparent to others. If the plan is described in clear and concise language, with accurate and pertinent documentation, the manager can effectively explain and defend specific components of the budget.

ACTIVITY BUDGET

The *unit of service* is a measurement that describes the activity of the organization or a part of the organization. It is the basis for determining revenue generation and for describing resource requirements.

At its most basic level, an activity report simply totals the number of times a particular activity occurred within a given time period. It may identify patient days, discharges, procedures, or visits as the units of service for this purpose. In the inpatient setting, the *census* is the most frequently reported activity measurement. Within this report, several consistent definitions are used:

Beds: number of beds available for occupancy

Census: number of patients occupying a bed at a specific time of day (usually midnight)

Percent occupancy: census ÷ beds available × 100

Patient day: one patient occupying one bed for one day

Average daily census (ADC): patient days in a given time period ÷ number of days in the time period

Average length of stay (ALOS): patient days in a given time period ÷ number of discharges or admissions in the time period

In ambulatory settings, the units of measurement are quite different. There are no beds as such, so patient days and beds are not part of the activity level measurement. Their activity variables typically include such elements as the following:

Appointments: total number of appointment slots available

Appointments kept: allocated appointment times when a patient appeared for a visit

Appointments not kept: allocated appointment times when a patient was absent

Average time for an appointment kept: the number of minutes of provider time (physician, physician's assistant, nurse practitioner) per visit

Average minutes of wait time to room: the number of minutes from appointment time to the time the patient was taken to an examination room

Average minutes of wait time to provider visit: the average number of minutes from appointment time until the provider actually contacted the patient in the examination room

Nursing time per appointment kept: average number of minutes of nursing time provided to a patient per clinic visit

Lab tests per visit: average number of laboratory tests provided to patients per clinic visit

Radiology tests per visit: average number of tests or procedures provided in the radiology area per clinic visit

The activity measures most commonly used in health care are often inadequate for measuring nursing activity and workload. In the OR, for example, activity can be described as the number of operative procedures performed. But a dilation and curettage (D & C) that takes 30 minutes and an exploratory laparotomy that takes 2 hours will generate different personnel requirements, supply needs, and charges. Measuring OR activity in terms of time provides a clearer picture of the workload. If the unit of measurement—the unit of service—is 30 minutes of operating time, then the D & C will consume 1 time unit and the exploratory laparotomy will consume 4 time units of service and together, the two procedures consume 5 time units of service. This is a more precise measure than simply reporting 2 procedure units. This system still does not completely describe the workload, however. Depending on the nature of the surgery and the condition of the patient, the exploratory laparotomy may require that only two nurses be present, or it may require three or four. The D & C requiring two nurses utilizes two resource units (30 minutes of nursing time), whereas the exploratory laparotomy requiring three nurses still consumes only 4 resource units. Thus, the time measure does not reflect the actual level of nursing resources required.

The ability to describe workload accurately in terms of required resources, particularly personnel resources, becomes even more difficult on the inpatient care units. As a measure of activity, the census assumes that all patients are equal and have the same nursing care needs. In fact, patients' needs vary significantly not only as a result of their medical conditions but also of their ages, economic conditions, psychological statuses, family situations, and other factors. It is because of this diversity of patients' needs for nursing care that many organizations have now implemented some form of patient classification system (PCS).

Patient Classification System

Patient classification is a process of grouping patients into homogeneous, mutually exclusive groups. The DRG system, for example, is one method of patient classification. For nursing, patient classification groups patients according to their requirements for nursing care.

The two approaches to PCSs most commonly used are prototype and factor evaluation. The *prototype instruments* describe the characteristics of patients in each category. Individual patients are then assigned to the category that most closely reflects their nursing care requirements. The *factor evaluation instruments* identify selected elements of care—critical indicators—that are the most likely predictors of nursing care needs. Individual patients are then assessed for the presence or absence of these critical indicators and, based on this, assigned to a category. Other approaches to patient classification, using frameworks based on nursing diagnosis or measures of nursing intensity, have also been developed. Particular systems may classify patients **retrospectively,** identifying what nursing care needs were met, or **prospectively,** anticipating what the nursing care requirements will be.

In addition to grouping patients into similar categories based on nursing care needs, the PCS also quantifies the workload within the categories by assigning a *relative value* to each category. The system describes the resources required for each category as either ranges or averages of nursing care time and, based on these times, assigns relative weights to each of the categories. Thus, a classification system with four categories might identify relative values as follows:

Patient Type	Care Hours in 24 Hours		Relative Value
	Range	*Average*	
1	0.5– 2.9	2.0	0.4
2	3.0– 6.9	5.0	1.0
3	7.0–15.4	10.0	2.0
4	15.5–24.0	22.0	4.4

Note that the numbers under Patient Type have no real value but are simply descriptors. They could as easily be labeled A,B,C,D. The indication of nursing resources required is in the column labeled Care Hours in 24 Hours. To determine the Relative Value, one category is assigned arbitrarily the value of 1.0, and all other categories are assigned values in relation to it. In this example, the type 2 patient, with average care hours of 5.0 has been assigned the 1.0 value. Because the type 3 patient requires an average of 10 hours of care, or twice as much as the type 2 patient, the relative value for this category is 2.0. Similarly, the type 1 patient requires an average of only 2 care hours, or 40% of the hours required by the type 2 patient, and therefore has a relative value of 0.4.

The relative value scale can then be used to describe workload for a given unit or organization. Within each category or type, the number of patients is multiplied by the relative value for that type, and the resultant category workloads are added for a total workload. The actual census is thus weighted to reflect the acuity of the patients.

Patient Type	Number of Patients	Relative Value	Workload
1	4	0.4	1.6
2	8	1.0	8.0
3	5	2.0	10.0
4	1	4.4	4.4
Total	18		24.0

In this example, the unit census of 18 generated a workload of 24.0. The average relative value or average acuity for this patient group is:

$$\text{Workload} \div \text{Census} = \text{Acuity}$$
$$24.0 \div 18 = 1.33$$

Using this workload, it is possible to describe the differences among units with the same census but with dissimilar patient populations and to identify trends in patient populations.

In some organizations, the average Care Hours in 24 Hours, also referred to as *hours per patient day (HPPD)*, is used instead of the relative value scale. In order to be meaningful, the appropriate HPPD must be identified for each category, as it is with the relative value unit (RVU) methodology. The calculation of workload then applies the average HPPD identified for each patient category to the number of patients in that category.

Patient Type	Care Hours in 24 Hours *Range*	*Average*	Number of Patients	Workload
1	0.5– 2.9	2.0	4	8.0
2	3.0– 6.9	5.0	8	40.0
3	7.0–15.4	10.0	5	50.0
4	15.5–24.0	22.0	1	22.0
Total			18	120.0

In this approach, the average hours become the expression of the relative values for each of the categories. The description of average acuity for this population could be expressed as:

$$\text{Workload} \div \text{Census} = \text{Acuity}$$
$$120.0 \div 18 = 6.67$$

It is important to understand that this process of patient classification identifies only workload or units of service, a measurement of the activity that generates the need for resources. The advantage of the relative value scale over the average required hours scale is that the former clearly describes the patient population, whereas the latter may be confused with a calculation of resources to be allocated. The determination of the actual resources required for a particular unit or organization is a separate process that is discussed later in this chapter.

In order to be useful, the PCS must be credible both to the nursing staff and to those outside nursing—administrators, financial officers, and others—who will be exposed to the PCS data. Both the validity and reliability of the system must therefore be clearly established.

A PCS is developed using a specific framework that defines the elements of workload to be measured. The *validity* of the tool is the degree to which it actually measures what it intends to measure. Validity testing should occur as the tool is being developed, and results of that testing should be made available to users and prospective users. The validity of a tool may be compromised, however, if significant definitions are changed or if the tool is otherwise adapted to reflect the idiosyncrasies of a particular organization. Also at issue may be the currency of the framework and the definition of the elements of workload. This is of particular concern if a PCS tool is not updated and revalidated periodically. Tools that were developed in the 1980s may still measure what they were originally intended to measure. However, these tools may not be valid now if they have not been updated to reflect the significant changes that have occurred in health care, nursing practice, and patient requirements for care.

One small example of a significant change that impacts workload is the use of intravenous fluids (IVs). In the early 1980s, many hospitalized patients were treated with oral and intramuscular medications, rather than IVs. And when IVs were used, they were typically manually controlled by nurses who counted drops per minute. Today, the vast majority of hospitalized patients have IVs and it would be impossible for nurses to control all those IVs manually. So virtually all IVs used in hospitals are now controlled by volumetric pumps. The amount of time allocated to nurses to (manually) manage one IV was not insignificant. Today, the amount of time required to manage one IV (on a volumetric pump) is much less because the machine does all the regulating of the drip rate. Nurses do not have to calculate drops per minute required to administer the ordered fluid volume, nor do they need to check the IVs as often. Not only does this change save nurses much time, it is also safer for the patients. Therefore, the workload for managing IVs should have been updated from the 1980s.

The *reliability* of the PCS tool addresses the consistency of rating. Different observers assessing the same patient at the same time should generate the same rating. The prototype tools are more subjective, making this degree of reliability more difficult to achieve. The factor evaluation tools are more objective, but their reliability depends on clear definition and consistent interpretation of the critical indicators. Although initial reliability testing is part of the development of the system, continuous measurement of reliability must be the responsibility of the users. Ongoing reliability testing generally involves two or more raters independently assessing a defined percentage of classified patients at specified intervals. Reliability scores of 100% (no discrepancies in ratings) are always the target. With the prototype tools, reliability addresses only agreement of type. With the factor evaluation tools, reliability will be demonstrated, ideally, by agreement on both patient type and individual critical indicators.

Skepticism about PCS on the part of the nursing staff commonly relates to questions of validity—does this tool really measure our workload? Extensive discussion of the framework and methodology of the system may be needed in order to generate acceptance by and support of the staff. Skepticism about PCS on the part of those outside of nursing may relate to questions of validity but more frequently focus on issues of reliability. The PCS is usually administered by the nursing department and involves the unit staff members who will be affected by the outcome. This may lead to questions about the possibility of manipulating the data to the advantage of nursing, particularly if the data demonstrate increased workload and increased need for resources. These are pertinent and legitimate questions, and nursing must be prepared to respond by demonstrating system reliability.

Alternative Systems of Workload Measurement

Most patient classification systems focus on the patient in the acute care inpatient setting. Less numerous but equally necessary are systems that describe nursing workload in other clinical settings. In the OR, for example, workload is driven by the number and types of cases and the length of time they require. In postanesthesia recovery, the number of patients, length of time necessary for recovery, and variable intensity of care needed over the course of the recovery period determine workload. Workload in home care and ambulatory settings reflects number of visits, visit length, and care rendered during the visit. The primary indicator of workload in nursing homes may be the level of independence of residents related to activities of daily living. This may also be an indicator in rehabilitation facilities. With the decreasing length of stay in acute care facilities, however, rehabilitation hospitals are seeing more acutely ill patients whose rehabilitation needs are complicated by medical needs formerly not seen. These organizations may find that a PCS similar to that used in an acute care setting is appropriate for describing workload.

Workload measurement systems for these various settings may be available via either commercially produced programs or established organizational systems. In the absence of adequate workload measurement systems, it is possible for a manager to develop a measurement system that provides more complete information on nursing workload. One approach that has been used successfully in a variety of situations is to differentiate the existing, less precise measures according to resource requirements generated, aggregate those with similar resource requirements, and weight them in relationship to one another. This approach, using a RVU, creates a representative and consistent measure of workload that can be valuable in projecting, measuring, and evaluating performance. Although the RVU methodology does not provide an absolutely precise level of measurement of inputs, its advantage is that it adjusts for variations among patients and their needs without excessively complicating the data collection process.

Construction of a relative value scale is conceptually simple. Different activities (outputs) are described according to the standard, expected, or target resources (inputs) they require. The required resources are measured in a consistent unit, such as dollars or staff hours or minutes. The activities are then aggregated into categories based on similarity of required resources. One of the categories is selected as the benchmark, with a value of 1, and all other categories are given relative values based on the relationship of their required resources to those of the benchmark category. For example, if the benchmark category requires resources amounting to $500, a category with required resources of $750 will have a relative value of 1.5, and a category with required resources of $400 will have a relative value of 0.8.

The methodology for developing a relative value scale is as follows:

1. Identify resource drivers. What are the significant activities that generate resource utilization?

2. Specify significant elements of these resource drivers. Among these drivers, what accounts for variations in resource utilization (e.g., length of procedure or visit, number of staff required)?
3. Determine which activities or elements are being measured and reported and can be accessed easily. These may include only volume statistics or another descriptor of complexity such as visit or case length. The relative value scale will be developed for the elements already being reported.
4. Measure or quantify resource utilization for unreported elements related to reported elements using the desired unit of measurement, such as minutes or hours or dollars. The unreported elements can be quantified using focused audit; that is, measuring the real time or dollars for a representative number of each of the drivers and calculating the average. Existing standards or targets can also be used to quantify the elements.
5. Calculate total resource requirement for the reported activities. For each reported driver, sum the total resource requirement using the actual average or the standard or target measurements.
6. Determine the benchmark that will constitute a relative value of 1. This can be a unit of measurement (for example, 1 RVU = 1 hour of staff time or 1 RVU = $100 of expense), or it can be the average resource utilization for one driver (e.g., the most frequently occurring procedure). Selection of the benchmark is up to the discretion of the developer of the RVU scale and is whatever works best in the situation.
7. Calculate relative values for all reported drivers. Calculation divides the resource requirement for each driver by the resource requirement for the measure identified as having a relative value of 1.

For example, a home visit program may identify visits as the primary resource driver. Variations in resource utilization result from the length of the visit (typically 15, 30, or 45 minutes) and the time required for the associated documentation (usually 5 minutes, except for initial visits, which are generally 30 minutes in length but require 15 minutes for documentation). This results in four visit categories. Category I is selected as the benchmark, and 1 RVU equals 20 minutes of staff time.

Type	Visit Time	Documentation	Total Time	RVU
I	15	5	20	1.00
II	30	5	35	1.75
III	45	5	50	2.50
IV	30	15	45	2.25

If the developer selected category III as the benchmark instead, then 1 RVU equals 50 minutes of staff time, and a category I visit has an RVU of 0.40.

Type	Visit Time	Documentation	Total Time	RVU
I	15	5	20	0.40
II	30	5	35	0.70
III	45	5	50	1.00
IV	30	15	45	0.90

The value of the benchmark changes in each of these examples, but the relative value of each procedure to the other remains the same. Category III has 2.5 times the resource requirement of category I in each situation.

PERIOD 1				PERIOD 2			
PROCEDURE	N	RVU	WORKLOAD	PROCEDURE	N	RVU	WORKLOAD
I	28	1.00	28.0	I	10	1.00	10.0
II	55	1.75	96.3	II	53	1.75	92.8
III	37	2.50	92.5	III	46	2.50	115.0
IV	11	2.25	24.8	IV	18	2.25	40.5
Total	131		241.5	Total	127		258.3

Figure 8-2 Calculating workload for home visits.

For subsequent workload measurement, the reported procedures can be weighted using the RVU to identify changes in total resource requirements and compare and contrast them over time. For example, Figure 8-2 contrasts the number of procedures and the RVU-based workload for two time periods. Although the volume in period 2 has decreased by 3% over period 1, from 131 units of service to 127 units, the workload has increased by almost 7% from 241.5 RVUs to 258.3 RVUs.

With the conversion of 1 RVU = 20 minutes of staff time, it is easy to quantify the difference in staff time required in period 2 compared to period 1:

Period 1: 241.5 RVUs × 20 minutes = 4,830 minutes/60 minutes = 80.5 hours
Period 2: 258.3 RVUs × 20 minutes = 5,166 minutes/60 minutes = 86.1 hours

Instead of requiring fewer staff hours in period 2, as the number of procedures suggests, the RVU-based workload calculation demonstrates that, because of the change in mix of procedures, more staff hours were required.

In the process of budgeting or of measuring performance, the relative value-based workload volume measure is the basis for determining resource requirements. It quantifies the need for direct nursing care, to which will be added the calculation of other resource needs, such as coverage for indirect time, benefit time, and down time.

Developing a relative value scale can be a time-consuming process. It is certainly not needed if existing reported volume measures accurately reflect variations in nursing care requirements. However, if reported volume statistics do not differentiate among activities requiring more or less nursing care time, the time and energy expended in developing an RVU scale may be justified because it will provide a more accurate and realistic quantification of care requirements. As new procedures are added, RVUs can be incorporated using the same methodology. It is also useful periodically to review and update the calculation of the RVUs. This can be done by repeating the focus audits and reevaluating the standards and targets, an activity that is a logical companion to the annual budget planning process.

■ DETERMINING UNIT WORKLOAD

The individual inpatient nurse manager is generally not involved in projecting patient admissions, mix, and length of stay, and only infrequently is involved in allocating patient days to individual patient care units. Once this determination has been made, however, the manager identifies the projected workload for the unit. Using current and historical data available from the PCS, average acuity is determined. Current actual acuity may be the most reasonable predictor for budgeting purposes unless the patient population is expected to change significantly.

Assume, for example, that a 35-bed general surgical unit has a YTD average census of 28.7 and an average workload of 34.7. The unit is budgeted for 11,133 patient days in the coming fiscal year, and the proportionate distributions among patient type, and therefore average acuity, are expected to remain the same. Calculating the projected average workload becomes relatively simple, as demonstrated in Figure 8-3. The projected workload is increased solely because of the increase in projected census from an ADC of 28.7 to an ADC of 30.5.

If, however, there is a projected change in the patient population, the calculation becomes more complex. Given the same current PCS data for this unit, assume that the projections for the coming fiscal year predict the following:

- 1,533 days (4.2 ADC) of current type 1 patient days will be lost to expanded outpatient services.
- 2,190 days (6.0 ADC) will be added because of the relocation of subspecialty patients from another unit.
- The relocated patients currently generate two thirds of the days as type 2 and one third of the days as type 3.

FY _08_

RESPONSIBILITY CENTER: _611 - GENERAL SURGERY_

CURRENT PCS ACTIVITY:

PATIENT TYPE	AVERAGE DAILY CENSUS	RELATIVE VALUE	AVERAGE WORKLOAD
1	6.3	0.4	2.5
2	15.0	1.0	15.0
3	6.4	2.0	12.8
4	1.0	4.4	4.4
Total	28.7		34.7

Workload _34.7_ ÷ ADC _28.7_ = Average Acuity _1.21_

Projected Workload:

Patient Days _11,133_ ÷ 365 = Average Daily Census _30.5_

ADC _30.5_ × Average Acuity _1.21_ = Workload _36.9_

Figure 8-3 Workload/units of service budget.

FY _08_

RESPONSIBILITY CENTER: _611 - General Surgery_

PATIENT TYPE	CURRENT ADC	PROJECTED CHANGE	REVISED ADC	RELATIVE VALUE	PROJECTED WORKLOAD
1	6.3	-4.2	2.1	0.4	0.8
2	15.0	+4.0	19.0	1.0	19.0
3	6.4	+2.0	8.4	2.0	16.8
4	1.0	—	1.0	4.4	4.4
Total	28.7	+1.8	30.5		41.0

Workload _41.0_ + ADC _30.5_ = Average Acuity _1.34_

Figure 8-4 Workload/units of service budget.

The projected workload in this example (Figure 8-4) has increased not only because of the increase in projected census but also because of the change in the mix of patients and their average levels of acuity. Obviously, the workload can be very different for the same number of patients when identifiable changes in patient population are factored into the calculations.

■ DETERMINING OTHER UNITS OF SERVICE

Often nurse managers may need to project units of service other than patient days and related workload: clinic visits, surgical procedures, deliveries, hemodialysis procedures, and the like. To do this, the manager identifies the most representative and discrete units of service for which data are available. These data will be used for determining revenue as well as for describing resources required, so the units of service should also reflect the charging structure. For example, if clinic visits are categorized by time (e.g., 15 minutes, 30 minutes, 45 minutes) or by type (e.g., screening, limited, intermediate, extended, comprehensive), the units of service should be projected in each of the categories. The forecasting methods described in Chapter 6 can be used in predicting these units of service. With a workload measurement system and historical data about volume of units of service and distribution across workload categories, the manager can then calculate the workload in the same manner as that described for the inpatient care units.

A clinic may have to use a different method of calculating staffing needs and work hours. A clinic is not a 24-hour-a-day, 7-day-a-week operation, so the planner must determine the number of staff needed to serve the clinic's patients so as to keep operations moving smoothly. One goal is to minimize the time physicians are idle, waiting for patients to be moved into and out of the examination and treatment rooms. Staffing may have to be planned on the basis of the number and different kinds of staff needed to achieve that goal. Box 8-1 on p. 197 represents the staff needed to keep an orthopedic surgery clinic operating smoothly. Note that a typical orthopedic clinic has several surgeons, each of whom will have his or her OR days and clinic days.

■ REVENUE BUDGET

The actual calculation of revenue for specific units of service is straightforward: units of service multiplied by the price per unit. Obviously, if similar activities or procedures are priced differently, each price type must be projected and calculated individually. For example, if the room charges vary for private and semiprivate rooms, the revenue projections must be based on the number of patient days projected for each type of room.

However, with the advent of the DRG-based prospective payment system for Medicare patients and the proliferation of alternative reimbursement systems and managed care programs in the private sector, calculating revenue has become increasingly complex. Distribution of patients by DRG, special discounts or allowances, and projections for free care must all be factored when determining revenue. In addition, individual state regulations may affect the revenue that an organization will be able to generate. These calculations are generally done by the finance department for the total hospital.

At the same time, individual responsibility centers may still calculate revenue based on charges and units of service, although this does not represent the actual revenue of the organization. It does, however, provide useful data to the organization in projecting total revenue and determining changes in pricing structures and reimbursement formulas. The decision about whether to project revenue based on charges for units of service or on contractual reimbursements and free care delivered is an important one. The unit is not in control of the number of admissions or of the type of payer (if any) that will cover the services. Yet recognizing how much care is being provided to self-pay, indigent, and contractually covered patients is important information when projecting whether the unit will lose money or provide an excess of revenues over expenses. In an era when some hospitals have been forced to close their doors because of a large volume of unpaid care, this matter is a critical survival issue in some health care facilities.

Bedside nurses typically want to provide the very best services, supplies, and equipment to every patient. They may become dissatisfied and morale may suffer if management cannot provide the same level of care to all patients, regardless of the payment the organization will receive for the patients. This is an issue the unit manager must consider carefully. Most nurses will do their best to help self-pay patients minimize costs by safely minimizing the use of supplies and charge services if they understand the cost of care. However, most bedside nurses do not have information on the costs of services, supplies, and equipment. When the staff are informed and included in decisions about resource allocation and utilization, a surprising amount of cooperation in the conservation of resources is typically obtained. However, staff that are left out of decision making that directly affects them and the care they provide may well end up resenting management.

The calculation of revenues and expenses serves to quantify the relationship of particular services to total revenue generation. For this reason, it is vital that nursing, which has traditionally been considered to be non-revenue-producing, design methodologies to cost nursing services and to identify nursing's contribution to revenue generation and expense control. Where nursing has been able to separate itself from umbrella service charges, this contribution is readily apparent. (Revenue budgeting is discussed more extensively in Chapter 9; costing nursing services is discussed in Chapter 18.)

■ PERSONNEL BUDGET

The personnel budget generally represents the greatest expenditure for the nursing cost center and is also the part of the budget over which the nurse manager has the most control. It is therefore the most time-consuming portion of budget preparation. Within the personnel budget, the nurse manager must identify full-time equivalents, positions, and employment costs.

Full-Time Equivalents and Positions

To prepare and manage the personnel budget, it is important to understand the concept of *full-time equivalent* (FTE) and to differentiate between that and *position*.

A position is one job for one person; regardless of the number of hours that person works. Personnel reports generally describe positions by job category and regularly worked hours (full time, part time, or per diem) and identify the number of people by cost center and department. Position control, vacancy, and turnover reports are also generated using positions.

An FTE is based on the concept of an employee working for a full year. If one assumes that an organization has an 8-hour shift for a typical worker, over the course of a full year, that worker would be paid for 2,080 hours. This calculation is fairly simple:

$$8 \text{ hours a day} \times 5 \text{ days a week} = 40 \text{ hours per week}$$
$$40 \text{ hours per week} \times 52 \text{ weeks per year} = 2,080 \text{ hours per year}$$

If all employees were full-time workers, working exactly 2,080 hours, the number of positions and FTEs would be identical. However, health care provider organizations often have part-time workers. To prepare a budget, it is necessary to focus on the total cost of labor. Knowing the number of positions is not sufficient if the workers are not all paid for the same number of hours. How is it possible to determine total labor needs if one worker is a full-time employee and another is a half-time employee? This is a situation of apples and oranges, and it is necessary to have some common denominator that will convert all the positions into a common measure so that it is possible to determine the amount of labor that will have to be paid for. That common denominator is the FTE.

One full-time employee could be hired and paid for 2,080 hours. That would constitute 1 FTE. Or two individuals who work half time could be hired, each working 20 hours a week. Together, they would provide the same amount of work and earn the same total amount of pay as one full-time worker, so they too are considered to constitute 1 FTE. Or four quarter-time employees could be hired, and their hours would add up to 1 FTE. Or one half-time and two quarter-time positions could be created. That would also add up to 1 FTE.

One can think about the number of hours per year, month, week, or payroll period or about the number of shifts per time period that would constitute 1 FTE as follows:

	Total Hours	8-Hour Shifts
Per year	2,080	260
Per month[1]	173.3333 …	21.6666 …
Per 4-week payroll period	160	20
Per 2-week payroll period	80	10
Per week	40	5

The value of FTE conversion becomes readily apparent when reviewing payroll reports, which describe the employee population in terms of hours paid. In analyzing these reports, it is useful to identify trends and to compare current levels of utilization with previous levels. Paid time reported in total hours is cumbersome and inefficient for management purposes. If, for example, a manager has paid 15,892 hours in the first quarter (13 weeks) of the fiscal year and 4,992 hours in the next 4 weeks, are the paid hours increasing or decreasing? And if this week's paid hours total 1,185, how does this relate to previous experience? The application of the FTE standard enables the manager to compare and analyze these hours. Simply take the number of paid hours in each time period and divide by the number of hours that the standard full-time employee would be paid during the same time period. A full-time employee would be paid for 520 hours in 13 weeks (13 weeks × 40 hours per week), 160 hours in 4 weeks, and 40 hours in 1 week. Figure 8-5 demonstrates the results of the FTE calculations.

The most recent week's experience thus demonstrates a decrease from previous reporting. The manager may then question whether this represents a decrease in available care hours. It will be helpful, therefore, to determine whether the variation is related to productive or nonproductive time. *Productive* (worked) *time* includes straight time and overtime. *Nonproductive* (benefit) *time* includes paid sick, vacation, holiday, and other paid nonworked time. These can be calculated using the same methodology (Figure 8-6).

This demonstrates for the manager that, although there is a slight change in productive time, the most significant factor influencing paid FTEs is the fluctuation

---

[1] Per-month bases are rarely used in FTE calculations because the conversion is not in whole numbers.

NUMBER OF WEEKS REPORTED (A)	TOTAL HOURS PAID (B)	TOTAL HOURS PER FTE (C)	TOTAL FTEs PAID (D) = (B) ÷ (C)
13	15,892	520	30.56
4	4,992	160	31.20
1	1,185	40	29.63

Figure 8-5 Calculating FTEs from total paid hours.

NUMBER OF WEEKS REPORTED	TOTAL HOURS PAID		TOTAL HOURS PER FTE	TOTAL FTEs PAID	
	PROD (B)	NONPROD		PROD (E) = (B) ÷ (D)	NONPROD (F) = (C) ÷ (D)
13	13,244	2,648	520	25.47	5.09
4	4,082	910	160	25.51	5.69
1	1,030	155	40	25.75	3.88

Figure 8-6 Calculating productive and nonproductive FTEs.

in nonproductive time. The same methodology can be used to determine whether the variations are related to changes in use of full-time versus part-time staff or of professional versus nonprofessional staff. These conclusions are not readily apparent by simply looking at the total hours.

Variations in the Definition of FTE

In some institutions, the standard work week has been determined to be something other than 40 hours, or the equivalent of five 8-hour days. For example, in an increasing number of hospitals, the standard work week is three 12-hour shifts a week. For the 12-hour shifts that are so common today, in which nurses work three 12-hour shifts per week for full-time pay, the FTE base is as follows:

	Total Hours	12-Hour Shifts
Per year	1,872	156
Per month	156	13
Per 4-week payroll period	144	12
Per 2-week payroll period	72	6
Per week	36	3

In a number of other hospitals, the standard work week is $37\frac{1}{2}$ hours, or five $7\frac{1}{2}$-hour days. If full-time employment is considered to be based on this standard work week, the calculations for FTE are as follows:

	Total Hours	$7\frac{1}{2}$-Hour Shifts
Per year	1,950	260
Per month	162.5	21.6666 ...
Per 4-week payroll period	150	20
Per 2-week payroll period	75	10
Per week	37.5	5

Note that the difference from the description of FTEs for traditional 8-hour shifts is a result of the decrease in the number of hours per shift. Therefore, the total hours are fewer, although the total number of shifts remains the same.

Another scheduling variation that may affect the definition of FTE is the employee who works and is paid for seven 10-hour days in a 2-week period. This would total

70 hours in 2 weeks, or an average of 35 hours per week. If this is considered the standard for a full-time employee, the calculations for FTE would be:

	Total Hours	10-Hour Shifts
Per year	1,820	182
Per month	151.6666 ...	15.6666 ...
Per 4-week payroll period	140	14
Per 2-week payroll period	70	7
Per week	35	3.5

In this example, both the number of shifts and the total hours are affected by the variations in the definition of the standard.

A common pattern used in ambulatory facilities is to schedule employees to work four 10-hour shifts per week. The breakdown of shifts and hours for that plan is:

	Total Hours	10-Hour Shifts
Per year	2,080	208
Per month	173.333 ...	17.333 ...
Per 4-week payroll period	160	16
Per 2-week payroll period	80	8
Per week	40	4

This plan works particularly well for clinics because toward the end of the day, appointments can easily extend well beyond the usual 5 or 6 pm closing time. This schedule permits the manager to schedule nurses to come in at 8:30 am to prepare for the clinic's opening time at 9 am, and the nurses stay until 7 pm to handle late patients and to clean up, restock, and get ready for the next day. In this example, although the number of work hours per week and per year do not vary from those associated with a standard 8-hour day, the number of shifts is affected by the variation from the definition of the standard.

In identifying the appropriate calculations for FTEs in a given organization, it is important to describe the full-time employee in terms of total hours paid. In the example given in Figure 8-6, for instance, the full-time employee who works 70 hours in a 2-week period may, in fact, be paid for 80 hours in that same 2-week period, with the additional 10 hours considered to be paid nonproductive time. In this case, the FTE equivalent in paid hours would be 2,080—the same total hours as the FTE in the original example. The definition of an FTE will be determined by the personnel and payroll policies of the organization. If the manager clearly understands the definition appropriate to that organization, the formulas and calculations described throughout this chapter can easily be adapted to any particular situation.

In designing an FTE plan, it is important that the organization take into account not only the convenience for the organization in getting the hours covered, but also the characteristics of the workforce. A 12-hour work shift 3 days a week may be very attractive to some nurses, but others may be unable or unwilling to handle those long hours. As of 2000, the average age of the nursing workforce was over 50 (Bowles & Candela, 2005; Halm, et al., 2005). Older nurses are at much higher risk for on-the-job injuries (Guthrie et al., 2004). Employers must view and treat all employees equally for legal and moral reasons. However, the reality is that people lose strength and endurance after the age of 40. A tired nurse (whatever the age) is much more likely to suffer an on-the-job injury and to make clinical errors than is a rested nurse. And older nurses are more likely to become exhausted during an extended shift.

The manager must consider well whether older nurses will leave rather than remain in a job that overtaxes their physical abilities. This phenomenon is very likely to affect perioperative areas because the American Organization of Perioperative Nurses (AORN) reports that the average age of OR nurses in the U.S. is now above 55 (Bacon, 2005). This obviously means that there are a sizable number of nurses in their 60s and perhaps even 70s still working in the OR. The ability of people of that age to carry out the physical labor involved in moving patients onto and off of an OR table and in positioning them for surgery may be compromised in general, particularly after working many hours at a stretch. In an era of severe nursing shortages, however, it is usually impossible to replace these older nurses. Rather, the OR director is likely to be asking them to stay past retirement age because they cannot be replaced. And this situation is highly likely to become more problematic as the baby boom generation ages and as the age for Social Security eligibility is raised.

The wise manager will consider carefully the wants and needs of the nurses available to work, and will plan work shifts and schedules that are attractive and suitable to the characteristics of the labor pool available. It may be most advantageous to consider making a variety of different work schedules available to the staff, so nurses can have some (albeit limited) choice in the schedules they work. People who are happy with their hours and who are assigned work consistent with their physical abilities are more likely to remain in the workforce longer. And in an environment in which retirees cannot be replaced easily, retaining the workers one has may be the only way to keep the facility operating fully.

Statistical Relationships

Analysis of historical and current paid FTE and hours data relates paid hours to activity and workload using a variety of statistical ratios. Hospitals commonly use the following statistical relationships:

EPOB (employee per occupied bed)   = paid FTEs ÷ ADC
HPPD (hours per patient day)   = paid hours ÷ patient days

Obviously, the elements of the equations (FTEs, ADC, hours, and days) must cover the same time period. Also, the formulas may use either **total** paid FTEs or hours, or **productive** (worked) FTEs or hours. This must be clarified in the description of the data. Similar formulas can be developed for other areas (paid hours per OR case hour, for example, or total paid FTEs per 100 clinic visits), provided that the formulas express logical relationships.

For individual managers, the most useful staffing reports relate workload to the hours available to manage that workload. Thus, nonproductive (benefit) time is not included in this reporting, and productive time is reported as hours per unit of service. In some systems, this productive time can be further subdivided so that the **direct** hours, which vary based on workload, are separated from the **indirect** hours, which may be fixed (such as a nurse manager's hours) or may vary by number of staff (such as educational or meeting hours).

Determining Staffing Requirements

The most critical step in preparing the personnel budget is to determine the staffing required for the projected activity. Where a PCS is being used to calculate workload, this requirement can be described as hours per workload unit (HPW).

It is important to remember that the determination of care hours in the PCS framework is used primarily as a means to establish relative values for the various classification categories. In the system example described earlier in this chapter, the requirement of 5 hours of care in 24 hours for a type 2 patient may or may not fit a specific institution or unit situation. Staffing requirements are influenced not only by patients' needs for nursing care but also by the nursing care delivery system in place, nursing and physician practice patterns, physical environment, staffing mix, level of support services, and degree of computerization, among other factors. These are rarely the same from one organization to another and can even vary among units within one organization. Each organization, therefore, must determine its own target HPW unit. This can be done in several ways.

One approach is to employ the techniques of management engineering, such as time and motion or work sampling studies. These studies quantify actual time spent in caring for patients of various types and can yield valid projections of work hour requirements. However, this approach assumes that what is currently being done is what should be done, and this underlying assumption may not be accurate. In addition, the studies can be time-consuming and expensive and should be repeated periodically to determine the impact of changes in practice or other factors.

Probably the simplest but also the least appropriate approach is to adopt some local, regional, or national standard of required hours. Frequently, this is the basis for comparison among nursing departments using the HPPD measurement. It assumes that organizations can be—and should be—similar in their requirements for nursing hours. As we have seen, however, requirements can vary widely from one setting to another as a result of multiple factors other than patient type. Targets for nursing care hours, therefore, cannot be transferred from one organization to another, nor can one standard be applied equally to all institutions.

Arriving at target nursing care hours by a process of analysis and negotiation may be a less formally structured approach but can ultimately be more appropriate and effective. This approach assumes that the manager, using professional management judgment, can describe nursing staffing requirements based on analysis of staffing and outcome data specific to that unit, on an understanding of the environment in which care is given, and on a realistic assessment of what is possible within that environment. In some organizations, a single target may be determined for all units with exceptions identified for individual unit situations. In others, each unit may develop a target, with the overall organizational target derived from the cumulative unit totals.

Target Hours per Workload Unit (HPW)

The HPW target reflects the nursing care hours required in 24 hours for each unit of work. It is important to clarify what is and is not included in that target. The HPW target includes only productive or worked time. Within this time, however, the manager must account for:

- Direct patient care—time actually spent with patients.
- Indirect patient care—activities related to individual patients' care but performed away from the patient, such as preparing medications.
- Unit activity—activities not related to a specific patient, such as report, rounds, and stocking supplies.
- Other support activities—meetings, educational programs, and orientation, for example.
- Personal time—paid only; excludes unpaid meal breaks.

The manager must understand which of these activities is included in the ongoing reporting of the HPW. The calculation of the projected HPW will be assumed to contain the same elements. Any elements not reflected in the HPW must be budgeted separately.

The HPW target reflects variable staff (i.e., those whose numbers tend to fluctuate based on workload). The requirements for fixed staff, such as the nurse manager or secretary, are not driven by workload and are budgeted in addition to the variable staff.

The HPW target identifies only the total hours required for the workload described. It does not describe either the type of hours (i.e., mix of staff) or the distribution of hours by time of day or day of week. These elements are generally expressed as percentages that are applied after the total required hours per 24 hours is calculated. Together with the total required hours, they will be used to determine the daily staffing pattern.

Calculating Total Hours Required

For the general surgical patient care unit described earlier, using the workload calculated in Figure 8-4, assume that the target set for the budgeting process is:

$$HPW = 3.5$$

This target includes all the categories of worked hours described, with the exception of orientation time. The average workload multiplied by the target hours for each unit of workload will give the total hours of nursing care required in 24 hours for the unit. Figure 8-4 shows that a total of 41.0 workload units is expected, so the hours of care required can be calculated as follows:

$$\text{Workload} \times \text{HPW} = \text{Hours/24 hours}$$
$$41.0 \times 3.5 = 144$$

Using a basic 8-hour shift, the number of staff needed during the 24-hour day can then be determined:

$$\text{Hours/24 hours} \div 8 = \text{Shifts/24 hours}$$
$$144 \div 8 = 18.0$$

Thus, 18 nurses, each working an 8-hour shift, will be needed to cover the 144 hours of work.

Impact of Required Minimum Staffing

In many inpatient settings, the minimum staffing for a patient care area, if there are any patients on the unit, is two. And often—especially in intensive care units and small emergency departments, there must be minimum of two RNs on duty at all times, regardless of the number of other personnel present. In other areas, the definition of required minimum staffing may be driven by a commitment to availability of services. In the OR, for example, the requirement may be that a specified number of rooms be available for a specified period of time. In the ambulatory setting, this may translate into having the capability of some set number of visits per day. Minimum staffing requirements lead to productivity inefficiencies whenever the level of required nursing care is lower than the level of care that could be provided during the work hours filled by the minimum staffing requirement. However, the benefits of the minimum staffing requirements may outweigh the costs of productivity inefficiency. For example, the requirement of two staff on a hospital unit provides a safety factor in the event of medical or environmental emergencies. In other areas, the ability to schedule procedures or visits without extensive delays may have significant implications for patient care or patient and physician satisfaction or may have marketing effects that will lead to increased volume and thus increased productivity.

Whatever the rationale, minimum required staffing must be factored into the calculation of FTEs. On inpatient units the total number of staff in 24 hours calculated using workload may be greater than the minimum required. However, when the shifts are distributed throughout the day on the basis of the distribution of care, it may be evident that during the night shift, fewer than two staff will be routinely assigned. In this situation, the manager will adjust the staffing pattern for nights to match the minimum (without altering the day and evening allocations because those are necessary to meet patient care needs). This adjusted staffing pattern will be used as the basis for determining other worked time, benefit time, and total FTEs. Generally, in areas like the OR, the required staffing levels for the number of rooms available at different times of the day and on different days of the week are the basis for determining staffing. Analyzing activity and calculating workload is done in conjunction with these figures not only to address productivity but also to identify times when the usual activity surpasses these minimums and requires additional staffing. Whatever the situation, it is important in the budgeting process to look at minimum staffing issues together with staffing required by workload in order to present a true picture of resource requirements.

Distribution by Mix and Shift

The next step in the process is to design a daily staffing pattern that distributes the staff according to mix and shift. Distribution by skill mix varies significantly from one organization to another as well as within one organization. It is driven not only by patient acuity but also by organizational and departmental goals and by availability of particular categories of personnel. Distribution by shift exhibits more similarities than dissimilarities for patient populations with similar levels of acuity. In general, the more acute the patient population, the closer the distribution comes to equal numbers of staff on all shifts.

Distribution by mix and shift is initially calculated according to identified percentages and then adjusted based on the reasonableness of the projections and the unique needs of the unit. If the nurse manager initially projects a 70% staff nurse mix and anticipates needing a shift distribution of 40% on days, 35% on evenings, and 25% on nights, then the calculation for the number of staff nurses on days is:

$$\text{Total staff} \times \text{\% RN} \times \text{\% days} = \text{Staff nurse shifts on days}$$
$$18.0 \times 70\% \times 40\% = 5.04$$

The same distribution can be used for all other shifts and categories (Variable Staff [Preliminary] in Figure 8-7). The numbers are then adjusted to reflect the actual number of staff who will be scheduled each day. Based on the needs of the unit, the nurse manager may determine that four staff are sufficient on the night shift and redistribute the balance of the night shift coverage to days and evenings. In addition, the unit's needs may support only one nursing assistant on each shift. The balance of

FY _08_

RESPONSIBILITY CENTER: _611- GENERAL SURGERY_

Bed Complement _35_ Total Patient Days _11, 133_ % Occupancy _87.1%_

ADC _30.5_ × Average Acuity _1.34_ = Average Workload _41.0_

Average Workload _41.0_ × Target HPW _3.5_ = Hours/24 Hours _144_

Hours/24 Hours _144_ ÷ 8 = Shifts/24 Hours _18.0_

DAILY STAFFING PATTERN
Variable Staff (Preliminary):

SHIFT DISTRIBUTION		_40_ %	_35_ %	_25_ %	
Mix	Position	7–3	3–11	11–7	Total
70 %	Staff Nurse	5.04	4.41	3.15	12.6
10 %	LPN/LVN	0.72	0.63	0.45	1.8
20 %	Nursing Asst	1.44	1.26	0.90	3.6
	Total	7.20	6.30	4.50	18.0

Variable Staff (Adjusted):

SHIFT DISTRIBUTION		_42_ %	_36_ %	_22_ %	
Mix	Position	7–3	3–11	11–7	Total
72 %	Staff Nurse	5.5	4.5	3	13
11 %	LPN/LVN	1	1	0	2
17 %	Nursing Asst	1	1	1	3
	Total	7.5	6.5	4	18

Support Staff:

Position	7–3	3–11	11–7	Total
Secretary	1	1	1	3
Unit Aide (M–F)	1	1	—	2
Total	2	2	1	5

Fixed Staff: Nurse Manager _1.0_ Clinical Specialist _1.0_

Figure 8-7 Personnel budget worksheet.

the nursing assistant hours would then be redistributed to other categories. Fractions of shifts, if they occur at all, are generally rounded to one decimal place. This indicates that on a given percentage of days, an additional staff person may be scheduled.

The final staffing pattern (Variable Staff [Adjusted] in Figure 8-7) reflects these adjustments and will form the basis not only for calculating the total required FTEs but also for generating the unit work schedule. Mix and shift percentages can be recalculated based on the adjusted staffing pattern and used as targets against which performance will be measured.

Because both the workload and the required hours have been expressed as daily averages, the staffing pattern reflects this average and does not address variations based on the day of the week. If a particular unit experiences significant, consistent changes in workload based on the day of the week or on weekday and weekend variations, the total weekly workload can be calculated (average daily workload × 7) and redistributed using unit specific trend data. The staffing patterns for each day of the week, or for weekdays versus weekends, can then be calculated individually. Where variations are less dramatic, the average daily staffing pattern is usually sufficient for budgeting purposes, and the variations are managed in day-to-day scheduling and staffing.

The requirements for staffing a clinic are typically based on the need to have personnel available to take care of the patients coming in to see a particular primary care practitioner (whether that be a physician, nurse practitioner [NP], or physician's assistant [PA]). A typical plan for such a clinic is shown in Box 8-1.

The surgeons and PAs begin seeing patients at 9 am on regular clinic days, so nurses must be in by 8:30 am to check the appointment schedule, get charts ready, and ensure that the rooms are ready to receive patients by 9 am. Because it tends to be in the afternoons that clinics become busier due to back-ups and emergencies, an extra part-time Medical Assistant is needed from 3 to 7 pm. Note that for the surgery clinics, each surgeon has an assigned PA who serves as First Assistant in

BOX 8-1 Sample of a Typical Clinic Staffing Plan

Orthopedic Surgery Clinic Staffing Plan Monday, Wednesday through Friday		Orthopedic Surgery Clinic Tuesday	
		Dressing Change Clinic	
1. 8:30 am-7 pm	2 Nurses	8 am-6 pm	2 Nurses
2. 9 am-5:30 pm	2 Medical assistants	8 am-12 pm, 1 pm-5 pm	1 Receptionist
3. 3 pm-7 pm	1 Medical assistant	9 am-5 pm	1 NP
4. 10 am to 7 pm	4 PAs	**Operating Room**	
5. 8 am-12pm, 1 pm-5 pm	1 Receptionist	**Tuesday through Thursday**	
6. 8 am-7 pm	2 X-Ray techs	7 am-5 pm	4 PA-1st Assists
7. 8 am-7 pm	2 Lab techs		

Physician Clinic Schedule		Physician OR Schedule	
Mon:	Dr. Adams, Dr. Gumieny, Dr. Ortiz, Dr. Shureshi	Tues:	Dr. Andrews, Dr. Phillips, Dr. Trujillo, Dr. Teese
Wed:	Dr. Phillips, Dr. Trujillo, Dr. Teese, Dr. Adams	Wed:	Dr. Andrews, Dr. Gumieny, Dr. Shureshi, Dr. Ortiz
Thur:	Dr. Shureshi, Dr. Trujillo, Dr. Gumieny, Dr. Andrews	Thurs:	Dr. Ortiz, Dr. Teese, Dr. Phillips, Dr. Adams
Fri:	Dr. Ortiz, Dr. Teese, Dr. Phillips, Dr. Andrews	Fri:	Dr. Trujillo, Dr. Gumieny, Dr. Adams, Dr. Shureshi

Surgery and assists with seeing patients in the clinics. The surgeons and PAs work 10-hour shifts, so they are scheduled to work 4 days per week. The clinic is open the fifth day (Tuesday), but only for dressing changes. There is, of course, a surgeon on call but not regularly staffing the dressing-change clinic. In this clinic, the office manager has contracted with the hospital to pay for 1 day per week of the orthopedic nurse practitioner's time so she can staff the dressing-change clinic. The particular personnel and hours worked may be different from those seen in a hospital, but the principles of staff coverage are the same. However, the driving force for staffing requirements in such a clinic tends to be physicians' schedules instead of patient days or patient acuity.

■ CALCULATING COVERAGE FOR DAYS OFF AND NONPRODUCTIVE TIME

The average daily staffing pattern for this unit must be maintained 7 days a week. But the 18 staff identified in the variable staffing pattern will work only 5 days a week. In addition, they will sometimes be ill or on holiday—time for which they will be paid but during which they are not available for patient care. Therefore, these 18 FTEs must be supplemented by enough additional FTEs to maintain the daily staffing pattern.

Five shifts per week are equivalent to 1 FTE, so one 8-hour shift equals 0.2 FTE and the coverage for days off for 1 FTE equals 0.4 FTE, or 2 days off out of each 7-day week. For every shift required in 24 hours in the daily staffing pattern, 1.40 FTEs must be budgeted to account for weekday and weekend coverage.

$$\text{Shifts/24 hours} \times 1.4 = \text{FTE for 7-day week}$$
$$18 \qquad \times 1.4 = \qquad 25.2$$

Each of these 25.2 FTEs, however, will take paid nonproductive time, for which coverage must also be provided if the staffing pattern is to be maintained. To calculate the coverage required for paid nonproductive time, existing payroll data are used to identify the nonproductive time as a percentage of the productive time. In the example shown in Figure 8-8, nonproductive time is subtracted from total paid hours to identify productive hours. Nonproductive hours are then divided by productive hours to identify the nonproductive time as a percentage of the productive time. This unit is therefore paying productive time plus an additional 17.4% of productive time in nonproductive hours. (It is important to recognize that this is not equivalent to 17.4% of total paid time. The total paid time will include the productive time plus the nonproductive time. In this example, the nonproductive time represents 14.8% of the total paid time, or 6,368 nonproductive hours ÷ 43,008 total paid hours. However, at this point in the budget process, we have identified only productive time requirements, and using 14.8% as the nonproductive coverage requirement would understate the unit's needs.) By combining the above, we can determine a single factor:

$$\text{Shifts/24 hours} \times \text{Coverage for days off} \times$$
$$\text{Coverage for nonproductive time} = \text{Total FTEs required}$$
$$1 \times 1.4 \times 1.174 = 1.64$$

Therefore, for every person required in 24 hours, 1.64 FTEs must be budgeted to maintain the daily staffing pattern for a 7-day week and to cover for nonproductive time. Using this factor, the required FTEs can be identified by position and also

FY _08_

CALCULATION OF NONPRODUCTIVE TIME

Factor for days of nonproductive time:

YTD as of _Payroll period #20 ending 2/18/07_

(a) Total paid hours _43,008_

(b) Total paid nonproductive hours _6,368_ (sick + vacation + holiday + other paid nonworked)

(c) Total paid productive hours (a) – (b) _36,640_

(d) % paid nonproductive (b) + (c) _0.174_ (convert % to decimal)

(e) Factor = 1 × 1.4 × 1(d) = 1 × 1.4 × _1.174_ = _1.64_

CALCULATION OF TOTAL REQUIRED FTEs

CATEGORY	SHIFT/24 HOUR	FACTOR (e)	TOTAL FTEs REQUIRED	BUDGET FTE	
				ST	OT
Nurse Manager	1.0	—	1.0	1.0	—
Clinical Specialist	1.0	—	1.0	1.0	—
Staff Nurse	13.0	1.64	21.3	21.0	0.3
LPN/LVN	2.0	1.64	3.3	3.2	0.1
Nursing Assistant	3.0	1.64	4.9	4.6	0.3
Secretary	3.0	1.64	4.9	4.8	0.1
Unit Aide (M–F)	2.0	1.174	2.4	2.4	—
Total	25.0		38.8	38.0	0.8

Figure 8-8 Personnel budget worksheet.

by shift within position, if necessary, by simply applying the factor to each category of the daily staffing pattern. Note that in the example in Figure 8-8, the factor is not applied to the nurse manager or clinical specialist because their particular responsibilities are not assumed by someone else in their absence. Also, although a single nonproductive percent was calculated for the entire staff, it is possible with detailed personnel data to calculate nonproductive percentages for each role group separately. This may be advantageous if there is significant variation in the actual nonproductive time among those groups. Finally, in this example, coverage for the unit aide, scheduled only for Monday through Friday, is calculated only for nonproductive time. Coverage for days off is not included because the unit aide is not replaced on the weekend days off.

■ CALCULATION OF OTHER WORKED HOURS

In this example, the target HPW includes all activities related to the variable staff, with the exception of orientation. Suppose, however, that the reported actual HPW does not reflect off-unit activities for the variable staff, such as meetings, educational programs, and the like. The target HPW will reflect only those elements that are reflected in the reported HPW, and the manager will have to project other worked hours. Using the same approach as described in the calculations for nonproductive time, the other worked hours can be calculated as a percentage of the direct/indirect worked hours. If in 13 weeks the average HPW is 3.4 for an average workload of 34.7, then the total direct/indirect hours would be:

$$\text{Workload} \times \text{HPW} \times 7 \text{ days} \times 13 \text{ weeks} = \text{Total direct/indirect hours}$$
$$34.7 \times 3.4 \times 7 \times 13 = 10{,}763 \text{ hours}$$

If in that same 13 weeks, the manager paid 11,052 productive hours, then:

$$\text{Paid productive hours} - \text{Direct/indirect hours} = \text{Other worked hours}$$
$$11{,}052 - 10{,}736 = 316 \text{ hours}$$

$$\text{Other worked hours} \div \text{Direct/indirect hours} = \% \text{ Other worked hours}$$
$$316 \div 10{,}736 = 2.9\%$$

Thus, for every FTE budgeted for direct/indirect care, an additional 0.029 FTEs must be budgeted for other worked hours. A combined factor can then be derived:

$$\text{Shifts/24 hours} \times \text{Coverage for other worked hours} \times \text{Coverage for days off} \times$$
$$\text{Coverage for nonproductive time} = \text{Total FTEs}$$
$$1 \times 1.029 \times 1.4 \times 1.174 = 1.69$$

In this circumstance, for every shift required in 24 hours, 1.69 FTEs must be budgeted to provide complete coverage. Obviously, it is important that the nurse manager clearly understand what is included in the reported and target HPW in order to calculate accurately the FTEs that must be projected.

■ ALTERNATIVE COVERAGE PATTERNS

For those settings that do not require relatively consistent 7-day-a-week coverage, the approach to identifying both productive and nonproductive coverage requirements must be adapted. In ambulatory settings, for example, coverage is generally not required for weekends or scheduled holidays. In perioperative areas, staffing requirements are generally reduced significantly on the weekends. In these circumstances, it is more appropriate to identify the varying levels of coverage required and calculate annual requirements for productive time.

An ambulatory clinic, for example, might be covered from 8 am to 6 pm on weekdays, except for 9 scheduled weekday holidays. Coverage requirement is four staff nurses each day. Total productive hours required, therefore, will be:

$$52 \text{ weeks} \times 5 \text{ days} = 260 \text{ days} - 9 \text{ holidays} = 251 \text{ days}$$
$$251 \text{ days} \times 10 \text{ hours} \times 4 \text{ staff nurses} = 10{,}040 \text{ hours}$$

If the experience of this setting is that nonproductive time historically has accounted for 14.8% of total paid time, then on the average each full-time staff nurse's productive time is 85.2% (100% − 14.8%) of total paid time. This can be converted into hours:

$$2,080 \text{ hours (1 FTE)} \times 85.2\% = 1,772 \text{ productive hours}$$

If one FTE works a total of 1,772 productive hours in the year, and the ambulatory clinic requires 10,040 productive hours per year, then the total FTE requirement will be:

$$10,040 \text{ hours required} \div 1,772 \text{ worked hours per FTE} = 5.7 \text{ FTEs}$$

The same approach can be used for perioperative areas that function 7 days a week but are staffed differently on different days. Staffing patterns can be developed separately for weekdays and weekends or even for each day of the week if that more accurately reflects the needs of the unit. Total annual hours can then be calculated, and the total required FTEs identified using the same method as described for the ambulatory setting. For example, assume that the surgery suite is generally staffed by a total of 40 shifts of 8 hours on Mondays through Fridays. On Saturday, however, only 12 shifts are required, and on Sundays and scheduled holidays, only 6 shifts. Total annual productive hours required, therefore, are:

$$
\begin{aligned}
251 \text{ weekdays} \times 40 \text{ staff} \times 8 \text{ hours} &= 80,320 \text{ hours} \\
52 \text{ Saturdays} \times 12 \text{ staff} \times 8 \text{ hours} &= 4,992 \text{ hours} \\
61 \text{ Sundays/holidays} \times 6 \text{ staff} \times 8 \text{ hours} &= 2,928 \text{ hours} \\
\text{Total required} &= 88,240 \text{ hours}
\end{aligned}
$$

Again using the experience of 14.8% nonproductive time as a percentage of total paid time, the average productive hours for 1 FTE equals 1,772 hours per year. Therefore:

$$88,240 \text{ hours} \div 1,772 \text{ hours/FTE} = 49.8 \text{ FTEs required}$$

■ IMPACT OF FLEXIBLE STAFFING PATTERNS

In an effort to respond to the needs of their staff as well as those of their patients, many hospitals have instituted various forms of flexible scheduling, including shifts of varying lengths (4–, 6–, 8–, 10–, and 12–hour shifts are not uncommon) or varying weekly schedules (such as 7 days on and 7 days off or two 12-hour and two 8-hour shifts per week). In general, these different flexible staffing patterns have a greater impact on managing the budget, and particularly on the scheduling process, than they do on preparing the budget.

Provided that the flexible patterns result in the same average number of hours available for the workload of the unit, the approaches to budgeting already described are sufficient. For the general surgical unit described earlier, instead of having 18 staff scheduled for 8 hours each, the flexible schedule might result in 4 staff working 12 hours each and only 12 staff working 8-hour shifts.

$$
\begin{aligned}
4 \text{ staff} \times 12 \text{ hours} &= 48 \text{ hours} \\
12 \text{ staff} \times 8 \text{ hours} &= \underline{96} \text{ hours} \\
\overline{\underline{16}} \text{ staff} &\qquad \overline{\underline{144}} \text{ hours}
\end{aligned}
$$

This means that there are only 16 staff working that day, but the available hours remain the same (144 hours). The budget calculations therefore remain the same.

However, if the schedule variation leads to a change in the available hours, the budget can be affected. One example of this is the implementation of a 10-hour 4-day work week. Suppose that 4 of the 18 staff required for the unit's staffing pattern work 10-hour days. In fact, they are providing 40 hours of care during the 24-hour period, the equivalent of 5 staff working 8-hour shifts. In this situation, only 13 additional staff should be needed to meet the 144 hour total staffing requirement.

$$
\begin{array}{llll}
4 \text{ staff} & \times & 10 \text{ hours} & = & 40 \text{ hours} \\
13 \text{ staff} & \times & 8 \text{ hours} & = & 104 \text{ hours} \\
\overline{17} \text{ staff} & & & & \overline{144} \text{ hours}
\end{array}
$$

However, if the additional 2 hours of each of the 10-hour shifts are overlapping hours occurring at times when the workload does not support the additional hours, then problems can arise. Either the unit has fewer hours than needed at some other time during the 24 hours or the schedule provides for the original total of 18 staff, resulting in the scheduling of 8 hours more than workload supports.

$$
\begin{array}{llll}
4 \text{ staff} & \times & 10 \text{ hours} & = & 40 \text{ hours} \\
14 \text{ staff} & \times & 8 \text{ hours} & = & 112 \text{ hours} \\
\overline{18} \text{ staff} & & & & \overline{152} \text{ hours}
\end{array}
$$

Some flexible scheduling patterns will have a greater effect on nonproductive time. For example, if staff nurses working 32 hours per week on nights are paid for 40 hours for the week, the additional hours may in some organizations be considered paid nonproductive time. This will significantly affect the calculation of nonproductive time and may require a separate determination of the nonproductive factor for that category of staff. Other variations in scheduling may affect the total paid hours per FTE, as discussed earlier in this chapter. The formulas presented here for determining required FTEs will be applicable in those situations, provided the FTE hours represent the particular variation.

Impact of Alternative Sources of Coverage

In calculating the total FTEs required for the unit, the initial assumption is that all FTEs will reflect regular positions on the unit and that the unit staff will provide coverage for days off and nonproductive time. In most organizations, however, at least a part of this coverage is provided by overtime. This is particularly likely to occur when absences are unplanned. In other situations, centralized float staff, per diem staff, or agency staff may be used regularly to provide this coverage. All the hours provided by these alternative sources of coverage must be covered by the total hours allocated to the unit. Therefore, the nurse manager must identify those FTEs or portions of FTEs that will be needed to support this supplemental staff.

Using the current and historical unit data, the nurse manager can estimate the overtime, float, per diem, or agency hours that will be needed or are most likely to be used. These hours are converted to FTEs and deducted from the total FTE complement for the unit. (Allocation of overtime hours is shown in Figure 8-8.) The remaining hours and FTEs will be identified as specific positions for which the nurse manager is authorized to hire staff. If float, per diem, or agency staff are used only rarely to cover temporarily vacant positions, the dollars allocated to the vacant positions can be assumed to cover the alternative staff, and the nurse manager can be authorized to hire into all positions. Overtime, on the other hand, should always be budgeted, unless unit history indicates that it is not used, because it is generally paid at a much higher rate.

Impact of Vacancies

In some organizations, the nurse manager is asked to project a vacancy factor. This approach is based on the assumption that, particularly in larger departments such as nursing, there is always a certain amount of turnover and therefore always some vacancies and that the budget can be reduced on the strength of those vacant positions that do not generate salary costs. The flaw in this thinking is that, if the budget does in fact accurately reflect workload and the resources required for that workload, alternative sources of coverage for the vacant positions will be required, and the monies in fact will be used. In fact, temporary coverage may cost more than the budgeted salary costs during the time the positions are vacant. To the extent that it is possible, the nurse manager should attempt to estimate turnover and vacancy for the unit in order to plan for sources of coverage for vacancies and for orientation of replacement staff.

Call-Back Time

In some specialty areas (such as the OR), the staff may be subject to being called back in urgent situations to cover workload that has been unanticipated and not projected in the baseline budget. Generally, these hours are overtime hours for the regular staff; however, they are productive hours in addition to those already calculated (unless the workload-generated staffing patterns clearly incorporate call-back time) and must be added to the budget. The projection of call-back hours is usually based on analysis of historical data, and the hours are converted to FTEs.

Call-back time is becoming more controversial as more facilities change to 12-hour shifts. If a nurse is called back to the OR for an emergency procedure late at night after working a 12-hour shift and is still scheduled for another 12-hour shift the following day, the nurse may well end up working for 12 hours, going home and resting for a few hours, and being called back for a lengthy all-night procedure—and then being required to continue working right through the next 12-hour shift. Even young people have great difficulty handling what turns into essentially a 36-hour shift. Virtually nobody can safely practice during that kind of a work stretch. And nurses in their 50s or 60s or older may well suffer physical harm to their own bodies as the result of such demands. As Buerhaus et al. (2000) noted:

> The continued aging of the RN workforce has important implications for employers. Efforts to restructure patient care delivery must be more ergonomically sensitive to older RNs, who are more susceptible to neck, back, and feet injuries and have a reduced capacity to perform certain physical tasks compared with younger RNs who once dominated the workplace. (page 2,953).

Most physician practices recognize that older physicians simply cannot take night call. When younger physicians are brought into the practice, it is made clear to them that night call will not be shared equally. Relieving older nurses of call-back duty is not so easy. Younger nurses may complain that all work should be shared equally among the entire nursing staff, and concerns about age discrimination arise with employees. Some facilities have tried to make sure call-back is scheduled for a night when the nurse has had at least 24 hours off after the call period is over in case the nurse has to work for most of the call hours. That approach certainly provides recovery time for the nurse, but it does little to protect patients from the kinds of errors that exhausted staff called back after having already completed a 12-hour shift are likely to make. It is likely that a significant number of older nurses will retire or transfer to a less physically demanding job rather than accepting the burdens call-back schedules impose. But with a nursing shortage, replacing nurses who leave the perioperative area will be extremely difficult for some OR managers. This can be a very significant issue in rural hospitals where the opportunity to replace a vacant OR nurse position with another experienced perioperative nurse is limited or nonexistent. If nurses are called back very infrequently, call-back requirements are not likely to be a serious morale or safety problem. However, in some facilities, the nurses have to come in on many of their scheduled call-back nights. That kind of life disruption becomes a dissatisfier very quickly and can result in high turnover among the nurses in the unit.

Nursing management must carefully consider all the costs involved in requiring call-back duty. If it engenders turnover, the costs of having call-back duty may far exceed the costs of hiring one or two nurses for the night shift in the OR. Some personnel researchers have claimed that it costs the equivalent of 2 years' salary to replace an experienced nurse (Atencio et al., 2003; HSM Group, 2002). Another cost to consider is the need to relieve an exhausted nurse who was called back by replacing that nurse with a per diem nurse to protect patient safety. It is likely that the manager will have to pay very high hourly rates to secure a nurse from a per diem agency on short notice to cover the vacancy caused by the call-back. The costs of turnover and increased use of per diem nurses can very quickly exceed the cost of hiring one or two nurses to cover the night shift.

If night nurses are hired to enable the manager to eliminate call-back duty, the manager may want to consider assigning these nurses duties that would normally be performed on day shift so that the amount of idle time is minimized. For example, policy and procedure manuals need to be reviewed and updated on a regular basis, quality management data must be collected and analyzed, and in-service educational programs need to be developed. These are the types of activities that might be assigned to the night nurses during shifts when no emergency surgeries take place. A careful cost analysis might lead to the conclusion that it is less expensive to hire a night nurse than to assign call-back duties to the regular staff.

Orientation

A department of nursing normally experiences some turnover during the year and may also identify necessary staffing increases. This leads to the recruitment of new staff members, who will require some period of orientation. During the orientation period, new staff are not considered to be contributing to meeting the workload requirements of the unit. In some circumstances, they may be hired to replace staff who will leave but have not yet left. At other times, the staff vacancy may exist, but coverage will be needed for the unit until the orientee is able to assume full responsibility for patient care. In either case, the orientee's hours are in addition to the productive hours required for patient care. Based on analysis of turnover statistics and projections for future changes in staffing needs, it is possible to estimate the number of staff in various job categories who will be hired in the coming year.

Using the average number of weeks of orientation for each job category, the total annual orientation hours are calculated and converted to FTEs. This may be done on a departmental level, with all orientation expenses allocated to one cost center, or it may be determined by unit and added to each cost center budget. If orientation coverage has been included as part of the reported HPW or as part of the calculation for other worked hours, it will not have to be added separately.

■ POSITION/HOURS BUDGET

The next step in personnel budget preparation is to convert FTEs into positions and hours. By comparing the currently authorized position and FTE complement to the projections, the nurse manager can identify where additions and deletions need to be made.

The Position/Hours Budget (Figure 8-9) lists both the current authorized positions and the current authorized FTEs. Comparing this to the Personnel Budget Worksheet (see Figure 8-8), it may be seen that a net increase of 4.6 total FTEs, including overtime, has been requested in fiscal year 2008 (FY08) over those currently authorized. In addition, there will be a change in the distribution of these FTEs. Increases are projected for staff nurse full-time (FT) and part-time (PT), LPN/LVN[1] part-time, and nursing assistant full-time. A decrease is projected in the LPN/LVN full-time category. Although straight-time (ST) hours are increasing, overtime (OT) hours are projected to decrease.

Note that in the example, the part-time positions vary in the number of hours assigned. The 10 part-time staff nurse positions may reflect 10 half-time (0.5 FTE) positions. The three part-time nursing assistant positions, however, obviously cannot be half-time positions but more likely represent positions of 0.2 FTE (8 hours per week) each. The one part-time unit aide position covers an average of 16 hours per week (0.4 FTE), equivalent to two of the nursing-assistant positions.

Hours for full-time positions are calculated by multiplying the positions by the number of paid hours for one FTE, generally 2,080 hours. Hours for part-time positions are not calculated according to any standard but reflect the sum of the actual hours allocated to each individual position. Straight-time hours are divided by 2,080 to identify straight-time FTEs in each position category. Overtime hours are calculated by multiplying the overtime FTEs (from the personnel budget worksheet) by 2,080 hours. Overtime hours are listed with full-time FTEs because they address hours over the full-time complement. Straight-time and overtime hours can then be totaled and divided by 2,080 hours to identify total FTEs in each position category. The positions and hours are then added to determine totals for the cost center and the hours converted to FTEs.

If the nurse manager has identified FTEs and hours to be allocated for float, per diem, or agency staff not regularly assigned to the unit, the FTEs required to cover them should be identified clearly in the budget as positions not available for recruiting and hiring.

■ SALARY BUDGET

Having completed the FTE and position budget preparation, the nurse manager is now ready to convert them into dollars. The employment-cost budget includes several components: regular salaries, differentials and premiums, overtime, and fringe benefits. In calculating these elements, the costs associated with special programs

---

[1] In most states this position is licensed practical nurse, or LPN. In several states this position is referred to as licensed vocational nurse, or LVN.

designed as recruitment and retention incentives must also be considered. These programs can be costed-out and managed in a variety of ways, so it is imperative that the nurse manager become knowledgeable about the details of the organization's specific programs. Likewise, if all or part of the staff belongs to a collective bargaining unit, the requirements and limitations covered by the employment contract must be well understood and factored into the employment-cost calculations.

FY _08_

RESPONSIBILITY CENTER: 611 GENERAL SURGERY

CURR AUTH POSITIONS	POSITION TITLE	ST Hours	ST FTE	OT HOURS	OT FTE	TOTAL HOURS	TOTAL FTE
1	Nurse Manager	2,080	1.0	—	—	2,080	1.0
1	Clin Specialist	2,080	1.0	—	—	2,080	1.0
~~18~~ *16*	Staff Nurse FT	*33,280* ~~27,040~~	*16.0* ~~13.0~~	*624* ~~1,040~~	*0.3* ~~0.5~~	*33,904* ~~28,080~~	*16.3* ~~13.5~~
~~8~~ *10*	Staff Nurse PT	*10,400* ~~8,320~~	*5.0* ~~4.0~~	—	—	*10,400* ~~8,320~~	*5.0* ~~4.0~~
~~3~~ *2*	LPN/LVN FT	*4,160* ~~6,240~~	*2.0* ~~3.0~~	208	0.1	*4,368* ~~6,448~~	*2.1* ~~3.1~~
~~1~~ *2*	LPN/LVN PT	*2,496* ~~832~~	*1.2* ~~0.4~~	—	—	*2,496* ~~832~~	*1.2* ~~0.4~~
~~3~~ *4*	Nsg Asst FT	*8,320* ~~6,240~~	*4.0* ~~3.0~~	624	0.3	*8,944* ~~6,864~~	*4.3* ~~3.3~~
3	Nsg Asst PT	1,248	0.6	—	—	1,248	0.6
4	Secretary FT	8,320	4.0	208	0.1	8,528	4.1
2	Secretary PT	1,664	0.8	—	—	1,664	0.8
2	Unit Aide FT	4,160	2.0	—	—	4,160	2.0
1	Unit Aide PT	832	0.4	—	—	832	0.4
~~42~~ *48* Total		*79,040* ~~69,056~~	*38.0* ~~33.2~~	*1,664* ~~2,080~~	*0.8* ~~1.0~~	*80,704* ~~71,136~~	*38.8* ~~34.2~~

CURRENTLY AUTHORIZED

$$\text{ST FTE} = \frac{69,056}{2,080} = 33.2$$

$$\text{OT FTE} = \frac{2,080}{2,080} = 1.0$$

$$\text{TOTAL FTE} = \frac{71,136}{2,080} = 34.2$$

CURRENTLY PROJECTED

$$\text{ST FTE} = \frac{79,040}{2,080} = 38.0$$

$$\text{OT FTE} = \frac{1,664}{2,080} = 0.8$$

$$\text{TOTAL FTE} = \frac{80,704}{2,080} = 38.8$$

Figure 8-9 Position/hours budget worksheet.

Regular Salaries

In projecting regular salaries for the employment cost budget, the nurse manager begins with current staff salaries. In the example shown in Figure 8-10, the nurse manager has been provided with a salary budget worksheet, which lists, for the part-time staff nurse category, all employees currently in the cost center, their regular weekly hours expressed as FTEs, regular shifts, hourly rates, and regular annual salaries. The first step is to correct the information for each staff member to reflect what will be in effect at the beginning of the new fiscal year. Amy Coram, for example, will receive a merit increase before the beginning of the new fiscal year, and her salary

---

FY _08_

RESPONSIBILITY CENTER: 611 GENERAL SURGERY

JOB CATEGORY: STAFF NURSE PART TIME

NAME	FTE	SHIFT	BASE HOURLY RATE	BASE ANNUAL SALARY
Briggs, Martha	0.2	3–11	$23.03	$9,580
Coram, Amy	0.5	11–7	~~$22.69~~ _24.28_	~~$23,598~~ _25,253_
Douglas, Ida	0.5	7–3	$27.44	$28,538
Francis, Jamie	0.5	7–3	$19.47	$20,249
Howells, Robert	~~0.5~~ _0.8_	3–11	$24.79	~~$25,782~~ _41,250_
Martins, Mary	0.8	3–11	$29.25	$48,672
Ridley, George	0.5	7–3	$23.32	$24,253
~~Westbury, Vickie~~ _TERMINATE 4/15/07_	~~0.5~~	~~11–7~~	~~$20.79~~	~~$21,622~~
VACANT	0.2	7–3	22.28	9,270
VACANT	0.5	11–7	19.47	20,248
VACANT	0.5	11–7	22.28	23,176

Total This Job Class:

Positions ~~8~~ _10_

FTEs ~~4.0~~ _5.0_

Base Salary ~~$202,292~~ _250,489_

Figure 8-10 Salary budget worksheet.

is adjusted by the estimated amount of the increase. The revised annual salary is calculated simply as follows:

$$FTE \times 2080 \times Hourly\ rate = Annual\ salary$$
$$0.5 \times 2080 \times \$24.28 = \$25,253$$

Robert Howells will be increasing his regular hours in the new fiscal year, and this is also corrected in the FTE column. The same formula will be used to correct his salary. Vickie Westbury will be resigning before the end of the fiscal year and so is deleted from the worksheet.

Because only 3.8 FTEs are now represented on the worksheet, but 5.0 are projected for the new fiscal year, hours are identified and salaries estimated for the vacant positions. In estimating salaries for vacant positions, the nurse manager should estimate the probability of hiring new graduates versus experienced employees. In this cost center, the nurse manager is projecting that one of the three vacant positions will be filled by a new graduate at starting salary and two by experienced staff nurses. Again, the formula noted earlier is used to calculate the total annual salary. If FTEs have been budgeted for float, per diem, or agency staff, these costs are calculated separately because they are usually paid at rates different from those paid to regular staff.

When salary-budget worksheets have been completed for all categories of personnel, the results are added to obtain total straight-time salary expenses for the cost center.

Differentials and Premiums

Calculating the costs of differentials and premiums requires a clear understanding of the organizational policies that govern these additions to base salary. Differential and premium rates commonly vary among positions and therefore should be calculated individually for each job category.

Shift Differentials

Differentials are usually paid to staff who work the evening or night shift. These differentials may take the form of an hourly dollar amount, a percentage of base hourly pay for hours worked, or a monthly, quarterly, or annual lump sum. Calculating the impact of these differs but is simple.

If differentials are paid based on an hourly dollar amount, the calculation of the differential is made on the basis of the staffing pattern. Suppose, for example, that the staff nurse night differential is $2.50 per hour for all worked hours worked between 11 pm and 7 am. Based on the staffing pattern (see Figure 8-7), the manager has projected the scheduling of three staff nurses (24 hours) for coverage each night. The differential for staff nurses on the night shift can then be calculated as follows:

$$Hours/night \times 365 \times Hourly\ rate = Total\ annual\ night\ differential$$
$$24 \times 365 \times \$2.50 = \$21,900$$

If the policy calls for a percentage of base hourly pay for hours worked, the first step is to calculate the average hourly salary of the night staff nurses. If the night differential is 15% of the base hourly rate, and the average hourly rate of the night staff nurses is $20, the differential is $20 × 15% = $3 per hour. This rate can then be applied to the formula described above.

If the night premium is a lump sum—for example, $1,000 per quarter or $4,000 per year per FTE—the calculation takes the number of FTEs in the straight night shift position multiplied by the annual lump-sum premium.

Weekend Differentials and Premiums

In many organizations, staff receive a differential or premium for working the weekend shifts. If this is an hourly rate or an hourly percentage of base rate, the total expense for the cost center can be calculated in the same manner in which the shift differentials were calculated in the previous examples. Again, the staffing pattern is the basis for determining the number of weekend hours generating the premium. The definition of eligible weekend shifts may include only Saturday and Sunday hours or may include some parts of Friday and Monday hours. Organizational policies must be consulted to determine this definition.

Holiday Premiums

Staff may receive a premium for working on certain scheduled holidays—Christmas or Labor Day, for example. The policies of the organization govern the shifts for which the premium is paid as well as the rate at which it will be paid. The staffing pattern for the holiday is the basis for determining the number of hours of premium to be budgeted for the cost center. Multiplying total annual holiday hours by the holiday premium rate yields the total annual holiday premium expense.

On Call Premium

In areas that require staff to be available to return to work if needed, staff are usually paid a premium to restrict their activities and be available for call-back between scheduled shifts. This premium is usually some hourly amount, which is paid for any restricted hours excluding those during which the employee is called back to work. (If called back, the employee is paid regular or overtime hourly rates, with appropriate differentials and premiums for the hours related to the call-back. These hours were calculated earlier as part of the total FTE complement.) Calculation of the on-call premium involves determining the number of on-call hours required in a year, less the number of call-back hours. If an OR, for example, has two staff on call every night of the year on the 11 pm to 7 am shift and two staff on call on weekends and holidays from 7 am to 11 pm, the total number of on-call hours is:

$$
\begin{aligned}
2 \text{ staff} \times 365 \text{ days} \times 8 \text{ hours} &= 5{,}840 \text{ hours for 11--7 coverage} \\
2 \text{ staff} \times 104 \text{ days} \times 16 \text{ hours} &= 3{,}328 \text{ hours for weekend coverage} \\
2 \text{ staff} \times 9 \text{ days} \times 16 \text{ hours} &= \underline{288} \text{ hours for holiday coverage} \\
\text{Total} &= \overline{9{,}456} \text{ hours coverage}
\end{aligned}
$$

If, in addition, the manager has projected that the total call-back hours in the year will be 832 hours and has calculated them as overtime hours in completing the personnel budget, they can be deducted from the total coverage hours (9,456 hours coverage − 832 hours call-back = 8,624 hours on call). Calculation of the total expense is hours on call multiplied by the hourly on-call premium rate.

Overtime

Overtime payment practices are governed by the Fair Labor Standards Act (the federal wage and hour law). These are minimal regulations that may be enhanced by state law, organizational policy, or union contract. Therefore, overtime payment practices may vary among organizations. Minimally, overtime is paid to staff in eligible job categories for all hours worked beyond 40 hours in a week. Overtime for these staff is calculated at the actual average hourly rate for the period (including differentials and premiums) times 1.5 for all qualifying hours. Because it is difficult to predict which individual employees will in fact work the overtime hours budgeted for the cost center, the simpler method is to determine an average total hourly rate (including differentials and premiums) for the staff in a particular job category and use this rate to calculate the projected overtime expense.

Assume, for example, that the total straight-time annual salaries for the 4.0 FTEs of full-time secretaries identified in Figure 8-9 have been calculated at $79,040 and the annual differentials and premiums at $11,446. Overtime costs can be calculated as follows:

$$\text{Total annual salary} + \text{Total annual differentials/premiums} = \text{Total wages}$$
$$\$79,040 + \$11,446 = \$90,486$$

$$\text{Total wages} \div \text{Total FTEs} \div 2080 = \text{Average total hourly rate}$$
$$\$90,486 \div 4.0 \text{ FTEs} \div 2080 = \$10.88/\text{hour}$$

$$\text{Average total hourly rate} \times 1.5 \times \text{OT hours} = \text{OT costs}$$
$$\$10.88 \times 1.5 \times 208 = \$3,395$$

General and Merit Increases

Calculating salary expense for the new fiscal year has thus far been based only on current fiscal year salaries. The impact of projected general and merit increases must be identified too. The policies and practices of the organization will determine how these costs are to be included. Increases may be calculated on the total regular salary costs for the entire cost center, by job category, or even by individual.

General and merit increases affect only the base salary rate and are not applied to costs of differentials and premiums that are hourly dollar amounts or periodic lump-sum payments. However, the increases will affect premiums that are a percentage of base pay as well as overtime costs. These categories of expenses will have to be adjusted to reflect the anticipated increases.

Fringe Benefits

Fringe benefit expenses include the organization's share of the costs of FICA, health insurance, life insurance, workmen's compensation, unemployment insurance, any contributions the facility makes to the employees' retirement plans, and other benefits. These may be calculated as a percentage of the total employment costs, with the specific percentages identified for the manager in the budget assumptions. In some organizations, the various fringe benefit costs are calculated by the personnel, payroll, or finance department, rather than by the individual cost center manager. In others, the human resource department or the finance department provides the assumptions or factors to use in calculating fringe benefits.

A fairly simple personnel budget for a hospital Nursing Education Department is presented in Figure 8-11. In this department, the clinical nurse specialists (CNSs) who are employed primarily in specialty units are asked to develop and present an in-service education program. Their time for that work is covered by the Nursing Education Department budget. The number of hours budgeted for each CNS annually is determined, then that number of hours is divided by 2,080 to obtain a percentage of the CNS's FTE to be paid by the Nursing Education Department.

Clinical Education Department: 2008 Personnel Budget Detail							
Name	Position Title	FTE	Annual Hours	Hourly Rate	Annual Direct Cost	Indirect Costs[1]	Total Annual Budget
Banes, Martha	Department Director	1	2,080	$40.25	$83,720.00	$23,441.60	$107,161.60
Jones, Suzanne	Assistant Director	1	2,080	$32.45	$67,496.00	$18,898.88	$86,394.88
Martino, Maria	Educational Specialist	1	2,080	$26.50	$55,120.00	$15,433.60	$70,553.60
Jefferson, Candice	Secretary I	1	2,080	$12.50	$26,000.00	$7,280.00	$33,280.00
O'Brien, Erin	OB CNS	0.003	6	$33.60	$201.60	$56.45	$258.05
Corbin, Francis	Acute Care NP	0.01	21	$41.10	$863.10	$241.67	$1,104.77
Angelo, Angela	Cardiac CNS	0.01	21	$34.00	$714.00	$199.92	$913.92
Thomas, Mary	Pediatric CNS	0.005	10	$28.20	$282.00	$78.96	$360.96
Norman, Tom	Neonatal NP	0.0025	5	$42.25	$211.25	$59.15	$270.40
Sullivan, Michael	Orthopedic CNS	0.001	2	$31.50	$63.00	$17.64	$80.64
Roger, Alicia	Diabetes CNS	0.01	21	$30.46	$639.66	$179.10	$818.76
Kowalski, Gretchen	Women's Health CNS	0.005	10	$31.60	$316.00	$88.48	$404.48
Personnel		4.0465	8,416.72		$235,626.61	$65,975.45	$301,602.06

[1]The total indirect expenses have been calculated as an average of 28% of direct salary expenses by the Finance Department.

Figure 8-11 Sample personnel budget.

■ NONSALARY BUDGET

The nonsalary budget projects all direct expenses of the cost center other than employment expenses. Generally, these expenses include medical services, supplies, or activities not individually charged to the patient (e.g., routine patient care items, nourishment, office and paper supplies, noncapital equipment, education and consultation costs, maintenance). In some circumstances, patient-chargeable items—orthopedic implants, for example—may be initially charged to the cost center and then charged to the patient when used. In this case, the corresponding revenue is also reflected in the cost center's revenue budget.

Nonsalary expenses are allocated to individual accounts that group similar expenses within the cost center. In analyzing nonsalary expenses, it is important to identify specifically the costs included in each account. The chart of accounts will give a brief description of these costs, with more detail provided by reports generated through the finance department or through the department that provides the supplies or services (e.g., dietary, central supply, maintenance). These reports itemize the various components of the account expense, the volume or frequency of use, the cost per unit and extended cost (total units × cost per unit) for each component, and the total expense charged to the account.

The most useful reporting of nonsalary expenses relates both the volume or frequency of use and the expense to relevant indicators such as workload or number of staff. Statistical relationships frequently calculated for direct expenses related to patient care, for example, may describe cost per discharge, cost per patient day, or cost per workload unit. Education cost may be expressed as expense per FTE or expense per position. As with other formulas, these must express logical relationships within like time frames.

The simplest method of calculating nonsalary expenses—and also, unfortunately, the least accurate—is to identify a total cost per unit of activity (patient day, workload unit, procedure, visit), multiply by the projected units of activity, and adjust for inflation. As we have seen, however, not all nonsalary expenses are related directly to activity. Educational expenses, for example, are more directly related to the number and mix of personnel, and maintenance expenses to the amount of specialized equipment or to the age and condition of the physical facility. The wheelchair purchased under noncapital equipment during the current year should not have to be replaced in the coming year, but additional IV poles may be required instead.

The key to budgeting nonsalary expenses, therefore, is to identify the most reasonable predictor within each account and to make expense projections based on that predictor. In some cases, more than one predictor may be needed. For example, assume that the delivery room's disposable linen account includes linen packs for vaginal deliveries and cesarean sections and scrub clothes packs for fathers attending deliveries. The predictor for the linen packs is logically the number of vaginal deliveries and cesarean sections projected. The predictor for the scrub clothes packs, however, may be the attendance at prepared childbirth classes, if this correlates more closely with the number of fathers attending deliveries.

In determining predictors for expense accounts, the emphasis must be on reasonableness. Theoretically, it may be possible to identify and project the cost of each item within an account. Some accounts, such as patient care supplies or pharmacy stock supplies, can incorporate tens or hundreds of different items. It is more practical for these accounts to group items according to the most likely predictor and identify separately only those items, if any, that generate a significant proportion of the expense within the account and are related to a different predictor or price variation. If suture prices are anticipated to increase by 15% and other patient care items by 10%, the OR expenses will be significantly affected, and the cost of sutures must be predicted separately. On patient care units where sutures are only occasionally used, the effect will be relatively small and sutures can be grouped with other patient care items.

In projecting expenses for accounts such as noncapital equipment or educational programs, a more direct approach is possible. Planning for the unit will include identification of specific equipment items that will have to be purchased. The manager can determine which seminars or conferences will be of value, the number of staff that will attend each, and the extent to which their expenses will be reimbursed. Other expenses, such as leased equipment, subscriptions and books, consultation services, and maintenance contracts, are also budgeted using this more direct approach.

Obviously, the manager must incorporate into the expense budget projections and costs related to the changes identified in the planning stage of the budget preparation. If the number of telemetry monitors on a medical unit is going to be increased, the cost of the monitors themselves will be part of the capital budget, not the operational budget. The expense related to electrocardiogram paper, however, is an operational expense, and it is one that will increase with the addition of the new monitors. This cost must be calculated and added to the operational budget. It is equally important to describe changes that have the potential to reduce expenses because of a change in practices, procedures, or products. Expenses for IV therapy, for example, would be reduced if plans include reducing the frequency of tubing changes, simplifying the taping procedure, or utilizing a less expensive administration setup.

Communication and coordination with related departments is also important in preparing the nonsalary expense budget. These departments will not only have necessary information on the cost of various items and activities, but they will also be able to identify operational changes that will affect unit expenses. If the pharmacy plans to implement system changes that require replacing a single-page medication record with a multiple-copy form, the cost of each record will increase significantly. The budget projection for forms must therefore reflect not only volume but also the increased unit cost of the medication record.

This coordination is particularly important if certain departments' charges to other cost centers are based on interdepartmental transfer of expenses. The print shop, for example, may house the duplicating machine and incur costs for the machine, paper, ink, and related maintenance. These expenses are then transferred to cost centers based on the number of copy pages made. The net result of the transfer should be zero (i.e., the amount credited to the print shop and the amount charged to the cost centers should be the same). Unless there is communication between the print shop and the cost centers, either or both budgets are likely to be misstated.

Most nonsalary expenses are calculated at projected volume multiplied by current cost and then adjusted for inflation. The forecasting techniques discussed in Chapter 6 may be useful in projecting the volume of a number of nonsalary items. The inflation factors are generally identified by management for broad categories (e.g., medical supplies, food, linen, drugs), and the most appropriate factor is selected for each expense category. Some expenses may be calculated directly—for example, contract maintenance according to the terms of the contract or education funds based on known registration fees for meetings and seminars.

■ REVIEW AND SUBMISSION

The next step in the budget process is to summarize the projected activity and the resource requirements, revenues, and expenses for submission. At this point it is important to review them for accuracy, appropriateness, and consistency in the total budget package.

Accuracy relates to the correctness of mathematical calculations. It can be confirmed by reviewing each calculation. It is often helpful, however, to compare the results of the manager's calculations to a benchmark, such as the current budget or actual YTD figures, to determine whether they are reasonable. Apparent inconsistencies may have a logical basis or they may be the result of errors in mathematical calculations.

For this sample cost center's revenue and expense budget (Figure 8-12), the finance department has provided the YTD total of actual revenue and expenses and a 12-month projection for the current year. The projection is a straight-line projection, calculated by annualizing the YTD total actual (dividing the actual by the number of months represented—in this case, 9—to derive an average per month and then multiplying that average by 12 months). This calculation assumes that the averages of the actual YTD totals will continue through the end of the fiscal year. The assumption is questionable, but the 12-month projection provides a potentially helpful check against the budgeted figures. For example, consider the central supply expense in Figure 8-12. The budgeted expense is projected to be lower than the estimated annual expense for the current year. The unit activity—census, acuity, and workload—is projected to increase in the coming year, as shown in Figure 8-4, and the unit activity should be a reasonable predictor of the central supply expense. Unless the manager can explain why the expenses are anticipated to be lower than current projections, a detailed review of calculations should be done before the budget is submitted.

It is also important to review the budget plan once again in relationship to the budget assumptions, operational goals, and unit plan identified at the beginning of the process. The proposed budget should enable the manager and staff to implement the plan with a reasonable expectation of success. Budget plans that understate personnel requirements in relation to projected activity will not promote the accomplishment of the stated goals. The resources can be increased, the goals scaled back, or the systems and methods of implementation adapted so as to establish congruency. It is equally important for this review to identify any overstatement of requirements for resources. This may occur if operational efficiencies related, for example, to changes in systems of delivering medications or processing orders have not been incorporated into the budget plan. Submitting a budget plan that is intrinsically inconsistent or inappropriate for the expressed assumptions and goals creates significant difficulties in implementation. In addition, it leaves the manager's level of fiscal responsibility open to question.

■ NEGOTIATION AND FINALIZATION

When all cost center budgets have been submitted, they are totaled to make up the operating budget for the organization. This initial budget is reviewed in relation to the operational objectives identified in the initial planning stages. If the objectives

RESPONSIBILITY CENTER: 611 GENERAL SURGERY

ACCOUNT NUMBER/ DESCRIPTION	FY 07 JAN–SEPT YTD ACTUAL	FY 07 ANNUAL BUDGET	FY 07 PROJECTED ACTUAL	FY 08 BUDGET PROJECTION
311. Revenue				
010 Routine	($3,244,410)	($5,556,030)	($5,561,846)	($6,258,903)
020 Other	(27,590)	(47,893)	(47,297)	(45,832)
Total Operating Revenue	($3,272,000)	($5,603,923)	($5,609,143)	($6,304,736)
411. Salary Expense				
010 Salaries - Regular	$ 730,881	$1,292,966	$1,252,939	($1,503,349)
020 Salaries - Per Diem	2,758	0	4,728	0
030 Salaries - Overtime	40,128	62,288	68,791	48,565
040 Salaries - Differentials	97,995	170,419	167,991	188,606
050 FICA	61,285	107,316	105,060	124,778
060 Health Insurance	62,125	111,842	106,500	104,236
070 Pension	19,855	35,816	34,037	40,275
090 Other	17,228	29,092	29,534	33,806
Total Salary Expense	$ 1,032,255	$ 1,809,738	$ 1,769,580	$2,043,635
611. Supply Expense				
010 Patient Care Supplies	$ 41,692	$ 62,023	$ 71,472	$84,728
020 Office Supplies	1,907	3,070	3,269	3,225
030 Forms	3,111	5,560	5,333	5,041
040 Supplies Purchased	1,210	1,935	2,074	1,161
050 Equipment	1,553	2,903	2,662	3,548
060 Seminars/Meetings	1,163	2,258	1,994	2,580
070 Books	145	258	249	258
080 Equipment Rental	385	1,703	660	677
090 Miscellaneous	388	968	665	968
Total Supply Expense	$ 51,554	$ 80,677	$ 88,378	$ 102,186
911. Interdepartmental Expense				
010 Central Supply	$ 7,828	$ 13,995	$ 13,419	$13,327
020 Pharmacy	9,527	17,019	16,332	19,362
030 Linen/Laundry	16,046	28,678	27,507	29,331
040 Maintenance	977	4,515	1,675	1,935
060 Telephone	1,962	3,225	3,363	3,225
070 Photocopy	124	323	213	317
090 Miscellaneous	165	194	283	258
Total Interdepartmental Expense	$ 36,629	$ 67,948	$ 62,793	$ 67,824
Total Operating Expense	$ 1,120,438	$ 1,958,363	$ 1,920,751	$2,213,645

Figure 8-12 Sample revenue and expense budget worksheet.

cannot be met under the projected budget, then adjustments must be made to ensure operating effectiveness. It is at this point that the most difficult phase of budget preparation, the negotiation phase, occurs.

If the organizational objectives call for a greater profit margin than the proposed budget would yield, the projections must be adjusted to increase revenues, decrease expenses, or both. The degree to which operating revenue can be increased has usually been well defined by this point in the process. If operating revenue is increased as a result of increased volume, related increases in expense must also be identified. Frequently, however, the focus is directed toward reducing expenses. To accomplish this, decisions must be made about the relative priorities of programs, personnel projections, and equipment and supply needs in the various departments and cost centers. This negotiation takes place at all levels of the organization, and cost center managers as well as department directors must be prepared to participate in the process.

In negotiating the budget, the manager relates the projections to the plans and goals developed at the beginning of the budget process. The manager must be prepared to describe and justify the factors that determine the projections presented. The most effective justifications should be clear and concise and should include objective and reliable data. The level of understanding of the audience is also an important consideration: negotiation among nurse managers using the same PCS will require less explanation of activity projections than presentation to a budget committee whose members are unfamiliar with the concepts of acuity and workload. Because it may not be possible to implement all goals and projections, the manager must also be prepared to discuss the relative priority of these proposals and the potential impact of implementing or not implementing them. Finally, the manager must be able to evaluate the unit's goals and priorities in relation to those of other departments and the total organization. With limited resources available to the organization as a whole, staffing increases requested in support departments may have significant positive implications for the nursing staff and may justify modifying or deferring nursing proposals.

Although decisions and approvals on budget proposals are the responsibility of senior management, they are influenced by the information presented during the negotiation process. Provided that managers are able to articulate clearly their projections and requirements, decisions can be made that promote organizational goals and objectives and that generate commitment and support.

After decisions and approvals have been communicated, the manager will adjust the cost center's budget if necessary and prepare for its implementation. Because the budget has been calculated for the fiscal year, it will be necessary to determine the allocation of the annual figures by accounting periods, sometimes called seasonalization of the budget. It is useful for managers to project how the money in the budget will be divided up among the 12 months of the year. The 12-month budget will be what the unit or department manager will use to track the budgetary performance of the unit every month. An example of the 12-month budget for the Nursing Clinical Education Department is presented in Figure 8-13.

When the manager spreads the annual costs across the individual months, it is necessary to take issues such as the impact of seasonality into account. The simplest seasonalization method is to allocate units of service, hours, and dollars equally across all periods (i.e., divide the totals by 12 [or 13, if the organization has 28-day accounting cycles] and assume that the activity and resource utilization will be similar in each month). Notice that the department staff costs in Figure 8-13 are the same every month.

Most organizations and units, however, experience seasonal variations in activity and in resource utilization. Admissions and attendant workload may be noticeably lower from mid-November through the first week in January. Workload, and therefore productive time requirements, may be similar in March and in July. However, nonproductive time may be much greater in July because of vacation scheduling. In addition, numbers of orientees may be greater during the summer months if the nursing department employs a significant number of spring graduates.

It is possible to manage these seasonal variations, even if the budget is spread equally across all months, by using statistical relationships and historical trends. If the manager is scheduling staff to ensure consistent available hours per workload, then fewer direct care hours will be paid over the winter holiday weeks and at other periods of decreased workload. This will provide an offset for those times in which the workload is greater than average. Knowing from analysis of historical data that increased orientation and nonproductive hours will be required in the summer months, the manager may limit the use of alternative sources of coverage earlier in the year in order to have additional hours

Expense Item	Jan	Feb	Mar	Apr	May	Jun	Jul	Aug	Sep	Oct	Nov	Dec	Total
Clinical Education Department: 2008 Operating Budget by Month													
Personnel													
Department Staff	$15,153.49	$15,153.49	$15,153.49	$15,153.49	$15,153.49	$15,153.49	$15,153.49	$15,153.49	$15,153.49	$15,153.49	$15,153.49	$15,153.49	$181,842
CNS & NP Faculty	$540.00	$350.00	$250.00	$200.00	$200.00	$150.00	$175.00	$250.00	$360.00	$275.00	$250.00	$0.00	$3,000
Allocated Office Utility and Building Expenses													
Office Building Expense	2750.00	2750.00	2750.00	2750.00	2750.00	2750.00	2750.00	2750.00	2750.00	2750.00	2750.00	2750.00	$33,000
Heat & Air Conditioning	175.00	175.00	150.00	80.00	80.00	125.00	250.00	250.00	175.00	80.00	150.00	150.00	$1,840
Electric	50.00	50.00	50.00	50.00	50.00	50.00	50.00	50.00	50.00	50.00	50.00	50.00	$600
Water/Sewer	45.00	45.00	45.00	45.00	45.00	45.00	45.00	45.00	45.00	45.00	45.00	45.00	$540
Office & Printing Supplies													
Printer Cartridges	210.00	210.00	210.00	210.00	210.00	210.00	210.00	210.00	210.00	210.00	210.00	70.00	$2,380
Printer Paper	120.00	120.00	120.00	120.00	120.00	120.00	120.00	120.00	120.00	120.00	120.00	120.00	$1,440
Desk Supplies	100.00	100.00	100.00	100.00	100.00	100.00	100.00	100.00	100.00	100.00	100.00	100.00	$1,200
Minor Equipment	50.00	50.00	50.00	50.00	50.00	50.00	50.00	50.00	50.00	50.00	50.00	50.00	$600
Printing and Binding						6215.00						6215.00	$12,430
Photography						2360.00						2360.00	$4,720
Clinical Supplies													
IVs and IV tubing	1010.00	1010.00	275.00	275.00	982.00	1010.00	760.00	275.00	275.00	275.00	275.00	100.00	$6,522
Dressings	340.00	340.00	100.00	100.00	300.00	340.00	240.00	100.00	100.00	100.00	100.00	62.00	$2,222
Monitor paper	450.00	450.00	150.00	150.00	350.00	450.00	250.00	150.00	150.00	150.00	150.00	70.00	$2,920
Injectables	300.00	300.00	80.00	80.00	200.00	300.00	180.00	80.00	80.00	80.00	80.00	40.00	$1,800
Sterile Packs	535.00	535.00	170.00	170.00	375.00	535.00	250.00	120.00	120.00	120.00	120.00	35.00	$3,085
Misc. C;linical supplies	50.00	50.00	50.00	50.00	50.00	50.00	50.00	50.00	50.00	50.00	50.00	50.00	$600
Totals	$21,878.49	$21,688.49	$19,703.49	$19,583.49	$21,015.49	$30,013.49	$20,633.49	$19,753.49	$19,788.49	$19,608.49	$19,653.49	$27,420.49	$260,741

Figure 8-13 12-month budget for a Department of Nursing Education.

available to use at a later date. It may also be possible to limit the number of prescheduled nonproductive hours that will be approved in any particular time period in order to distribute the actual use of nonproductive time more evenly throughout the year.

A more useful approach for the manager is to describe the most likely distribution of activity and need for resources expected during the fiscal year and to seasonalize the budget accordingly. Frequently, this method of seasonalization is used for the entire hospital and is based primarily on anticipated fluctuations in admissions or patient days. This seasonalization usually approximates (although does not necessarily mirror) the fluctuation in workload and direct care hours. However, it may not relate as well to the utilization of nonproductive hours. Based on historical data and unit practices, it is possible to project the expected variations in use of nonproductive hours and to seasonalize the hours and salary budget using these projections. Simply calculate the percent of total annual nonproductive time used in each month (refer to the forecasting methods described in Chapter 6) and apply those percentages to the total nonproductive time budgeted for the coming fiscal year.

■ IMPLEMENTATION

At this point the manager must focus on the most important part of the process: implementing the budget plan. As a plan, the budget describes anticipated outcomes in the unit and organization for the fiscal year. It is the responsibility of the nurse manager to initiate the steps necessary to put the plan into effect and to provide leadership for the staff in achieving the goals articulated in the plan.

An important aspect of implementation relates to the management and utilization of the resources identified in the plan. For personnel, this means the translation of the annual FTE budget into short-range scheduling patterns that take into account variations around the averages identified in the budget; for example, weekday-to-weekend variations in workload or seasonal fluctuations in census or use of benefit time. It also applies to the day-to-day and shift-to-shift staffing adjustments needed to meet changing patient care needs. For nonsalary expenses, this means developing or streamlining systems for acquiring and maintaining supplies and equipment.

Implementation also incorporates systems for monitoring actual experiences and comparing them to projections. One method is based on fixed-budget analysis, which compares total actual FTEs and expenses to the fixed budget. However, this approach does not account for the fluctuations in workload that are likely to occur during the budget year. A more useful monitor is based on a flexible budget approach and looks at the resources utilized in comparison to the changing workload. For the manager who has developed a budget based on targets for HPW, the nonproductive factor, and staff mix, comparison of actual to expected experience in these parameters is more valuable. These targets are expressions of the relationship of resource utilization to workload. If the workload increases and the hours provided for each unit of work are constant, then the total care hours will increase but the HPW will remain the same. Similarly, if the workload decreases, the manager can be expected to adjust total care hours downward but still maintain the target HPW. To the extent that the identified relationships are maintained, the manager is following the budget plan and can explain and justify variances from the fixed budget. Monitoring actual performance against the budget can also identify trends or variations that, if they persist over time, may require midcourse corrections to the original budget. The systems used in analyzing, monitoring, and controlling the administration of the budget are discussed in Chapters 13 and 14.

Summary and Implications for Nurse Managers

To prepare an operational budget, a nurse manager must be familiar with the financial structure and reporting systems of the organization and with the data reported through these systems. These data are analyzed in conjunction with other known factors to define operational goals and to predict levels of activity and resource utilization. Nurse managers must understand the overall priorities and directions of the entire organization so that the budget plan is congruent with the organization's goals and objectives. They must also understand the characteristics of their current staff and of the labor pool from which they need to recruit additional staff and replacement staff due to turnover and retirements.

The actual preparation of the operational budget translates these goals and predictions into numbers. The activity budget identifies and quantifies the units of service or workload, which determine resource requirements. The revenue budget projects the income that will be generated by that activity.

The personnel budget identifies full time equivalents (FTEs) from the staffing plan and position control report. The workload is the basis for quantifying the productive hours needed, as well as allocating those hours by employee category and by shift. Calculating coverage required for nonproductive time is based on historical data and organizational policies. These hours are added to the productive hours to determine total FTEs, which are then described by hours and positions. The salary budget includes expenses for regular salaries, differentials and premiums, fringe benefits, and related employment costs.

Projections for the nonsalary budget are based on the most reasonable predictor for items or activities included in the different expense accounts and reflect the identified goals of the unit. Communication and coordination with related departments increase the accuracy of the budget projections.

Following negotiation and finalization, the nurse manager is responsible for the implementation and administration of the operating budget.

References and Suggested Readings

Arnold, L., Drenkard, K., Ela, S., Goedken, J., Hamilton, C., Harris, C., Holecek, N., White, M., (2006). Strategic positioning for nursing excellence in health systems: Insights from chief nursing executives. *Nursing Administration Quarterly.* 30(1), 11-20.

Atencio, B., Cohen, J., and Gorenberg, B. (2003). Nurse retention: Is it worth it? *Nursing Economic$.* 21(6), 262-268, 299.

Bacon, D. (2005). Results of the 2005 AORN Salary Survey Trends for Perioperative Nursing. *AORN Journal.* 82(6), 965-972.

Beglinger, J. (2006). Quantifying patient care intensity: An evidence-based approach to determining staffing requirements. *Nursing Administration Quarterly.* 30(3), 193-202.

Bleich, M., and Hewlett, P. (2004). Dissipating the "Perfect Storm": Responses from nursing and the health care industry to protect the public's health. *Online Journal of Issues in Nursing.* 9(2), 2. Available online through the Directory of Open Access Journals: http://www.doag.org

Bowles, C., and Candela, L. (2005). First job experiences of recent RN graduates: Improving the work environment. *Nevada RNformation.* 14(2), 16-19.

Buerhaus, P.I., Staiger D.O., Auerbach, D.I. (2000). Implications of an aging registered nurse workforce. *The Journal of the American Medical Association.* 283, 2948–2954.

Center for American Nurses. (2005). *Workforce for the Future: Spotlight on Mature Nurses.* Summary Report. Silver Spring, MD: Center for American Nurses.

De Silets, L. (2004). BUDGET$!!!! BUDGET$!!!! BUDGET$!! *Journal of Continuing Education in Nursing.* 35(2), 52-53.

Dunham-Taylor, J., Pinczuk, J. (2006). *Health Care Financial Management for Nurse Managers: Merging the Heart with the Dollar.* Sudbury, MA: Jones and Bartlett.

Finkler, S.A., Ward, D.R., and Baker, J. (2007). *Essentials of Cost Accounting for Health Care Organizations,* ed 3. Boston: Jones & Bartlett.

Forte, J. (2005). Tap techno-solutions to workload measurement. *Computers in Nursing, 23*(1), 56, 58-59.

Goodin, H. (2003). The nursing shortage in the United States of America: An integrative review of the literature. *Journal of Advanced Nursing. 43*(4), 335-343.

Guthrie, P., Westphal, L., Dahlman, B., Berg, M., Behnam, K., and Ferrell, D. (2004). A patient lifting intervention for preventing the work related injuries of nurses. *WORK: A Journal of Prevention, Assessment & Rehabilitation. 22*(2), 79-88

Halm, M., Peterson, M., Kandels, M., Sabo, J., Blalock, M., Braden, R., Gryczman, A., Krisko-Hagel, K., Larson, D., Lemay, D., Sisler, B., Strom, L., Topham, D. (2005). Hospital nurse staffing and patient mortality, emotional exhaustion, and job dissatisfaction. *Clinical Nurse Specialist. 19*(5), 241-251.

Heinrich, J. (2001). Nursing workforce: Emerging nurse shortages due to multiple factors. *GAO Report to Health Subcommittee on Health.* Washington, D.C.: U.S. General Accounting Office. 1-15.

HSM Group, Ltd. (2002). Acute care hospital survey of RN vacancy and turnover rates in 2000. *Journal of Nursing Administration. 32,* 437-439.

Letvak S. (2002). Retaining the older nurse. *Journal of Nursing Administration. 32*(7/8), 387-392.

Lipscomb, J., Trinkoff, A., Brady, B., and Geiger-Brown, J. (2004). Health care system changes and reported musculoskeletal disorders among registered nurses. *American Journal of Public Health.* 94(8), 1431-1435.

Miranda, D., Nap, R., de Rijk, A., Schaufeli, W., Iapichino, G. (2003). Nursing activities score. *Critical Care Medicine.* 31(2), 374-382.

Saba, V., and McCormick, K. (2005). *Essentials for Computers for Nurses,* ed 3. New York: McGraw-Hill.

Spence, K., Tarnow-Mordi, W., Duncan, G., Jayasuryia, N., Elliott, J., King, J., Kite, F. (2006). Measuring nursing workload in neonatal intensive care. *Journal of Nursing Management.* 14(3), 227-234.

Waters, V. (2003). Overcome hidden expenses, migrating staff. *Nursing Management.* 34(5), 20-24.

Online Microsoft Excel Tutorials: Annotated List

For Beginners

1. This is a good tutorial for beginners who have never used a spreadsheet. It contains a number of modules on different Excel functions: http://www.baycongroup.com/el0.htm *Note: To get to the tutorial materials, click on Lesson 1, Lesson 2, etc. They don't look like hyperlinks, but they are.*

2. This is a basic tutorial of Excel. Specific examples may refer to Excel (but most items discussed should work in other spreadsheets): http://www.usd.edu/trio/tut/excel/index.html

3. Another useful site is *MiStupid.com* which has a variety of tutorials on several Microsoft, Palm, Windows, Office, and other programs. The link to the Excel tutorial is: http://www.mistupid.com/tutorials/excel/index.htm

For Intermediate Users

The above "beginner" tutorials are best for beginners and visual learners. But some students may need tutorials that address some of the more advanced functions. Here are two slightly more advanced Excel tutorials:

1. This tutorial provides more depth with more complex functions: http://www.fgcu.edu/support/office2000/excel/index.html

2. This tutorial is directly from the Microsoft Company. It has a large number of mini-tutorials on both basic and fairly advanced functions of Excel. There are 38 tutorial modules on how to use Microsoft Excel on this site: http://office. microsoft.com/en-us/training/CR061831141033.aspx

Revenue Budgeting

LEARNING OBJECTIVES
The goals of this chapter are to:

- Discuss sources of revenues
- Explain the importance of prices and volume in revenue budgeting
- Clarify why revenues are often ignored in nursing budgets
- Discuss when revenues should be considered in nursing budgets
- Provide examples of revenue budget calculations
- Discuss revenues from managed care organizations
- Define capitation
- Explain the impact of capitation on risk
- Provide an example of how capitation rates can be calculated
- Define risk-sharing pools and discuss their use

■ INTRODUCTION

The last chapter discussed preparation of a nursing unit's operating budget. However, it focused primarily on the expense side of that budget. Operating budgets consist of both revenues and expenses. This chapter focuses on issues related to revenues. Revenues are the amount the organization earns in exchange for the services it provides. Revenues are critical for every organization.

Revenues must be adequate to cover all the costs of providing services during the current year. Additionally, revenues should be great enough to provide a profit. This is true whether the organization is a for-profit or not-for-profit organization. Profits are used to expand the type of services offered, to expand the volume of services offered, and to replace buildings and equipment. Both inflation and technological advances often cause new capital acquisitions (see Chapter 11 for a discussion of capital budgeting) to be more expensive than those they replace. Profits earned each year help the organization to have sufficient resources for replacements and expansion.

There are many different sources of revenues that are relevant to nurses. Typically one thinks of patient revenues. These are amounts that are received either directly from patients or from third parties such as insurance companies. They are payments for health care services provided. Buppert explains some of the mechanisms for getting reimbursement directly for nursing services.[1] However, in various nursing

---

[1] Buppert, C. (2005). Third-party reimbursement for nurse practitioners' services on trauma teams: Working through a maze of issues. *Journal of Trauma-Injury Infection & Critical Care.* 58(1), 206-212.

situations there are a wide variety of other revenue sources as well. Swansburg has listed some sources of nursing revenue as:

- grants
- continuing education
- private practice
- community visibility
- health care students and staff
- health maintenance organizations (HMOs)
- city health departments
- industry
- unions
- third-party payments
- professional corporations, and
- nurse-managed centers.[2]

This list is far from exhaustive. For example, specialty units like neonatal intensive care units, pediatric units, and burn units may have community sponsors that regularly carry on fundraising activities for these specialty units. An example is the relationship many burn units have with the local fire department. Many burn victims are indigent or uninsured, and without community support, the hospital would be unable to maintain burn care services. In many communities where there is a public hospital with a burn unit, the local fire department holds an annual fundraiser for the burn unit. This charitable program can raise significant amounts of money upon which the burn unit depends for equipment and supplies.

In a growing number of situations, nurse managers are required to prepare revenue budgets and are held accountable for revenue. This chapter begins with a discussion of some basic issues and addresses a number of questions related to revenues. What are they? How are they earned? Why are they often ignored in discussions about nursing budgets? When should they be considered? Next, the chapter moves on to a discussion of the calculations of revenues as it relates to nursing.

The chapter concludes with a discussion of issues related to managed care revenues, with a particular emphasis on issues related to revenues from capitation arrangements. That section provides an introduction to managed care concepts, including risk. The role of risk pools in revenue budgeting is also addressed. An example of how capitation rates can be determined is provided.

■ THE REVENUE BUDGET

The operating budget for any organization consists of a revenue budget and an expense budget. In many situations, nurses have been held accountable for revenues. For example, traditionally the director of the operating room (OR) has been charged with earning a profit on the basis of having revenues that exceed costs. Units or departments that have revenue budgets are called *revenue centers* in health care. They are often called *profit centers* in other industries. However, in most cases, nurse

---

[2] Swansburg, R.C. (1997). *Budgeting and Financial Management for Nurse Managers*. Boston: Jones and Bartlett.

managers are given authority over expenses only. Units or departments that do not have revenue budgets are called *cost centers* or *expense centers.*

Why Aren't All Nursing Units Revenue Centers?

In most industries, including health care, managers are generally responsible for expense centers. Imagine buying a car. Perhaps you go to a new car dealer and buy a car for $25,000. Suppose that the dealer in turns pays $23,000 to the manufacturer. How should the manufacturer view the $23,000 of revenue it received? In order to make the car, there was an engine department, a bumper department, a door department, a steering-wheel department, and other departments. Should each of those departments be revenue centers, assigned both revenues and expenses, or just expense centers? In your mind, how much of the $25,000 you paid for the car was for the engine? How much for the bumper? In turn, when the dealer bought the car, how much was it paying the manufacturer for each component?

In reality, as a buyer, you viewed the purchase as one lump sum. You probably did not divide the car into the pieces made by the various departments, assign a value to each piece, and make sure that the total value of the individual pieces plus the cost of the labor to put them together into a finished car came to exactly the $25,000 you were paying. Neither did the dealer when it paid $23,000. Therefore, it is difficult for the manufacturer to divide up its $23,000 of revenue into parts and assign them by department. The important issue for the manufacturer is to produce high-quality parts efficiently. Each department is given an expense budget based on what it should cost for efficient manufacture of the parts made by the department. As long as the total cost of all the parts, plus the labor to put them together, plus overhead are less than the $23,000 the dealer paid to the manufacturer, the manufacturer is making a profit. This is fairly typical of most organizations. Revenue is not generally assigned to individual managers, departments, or units.

In any health care organization that receives a lump-sum payment for each patient, it makes sense to avoid setting up revenue centers. In many health care organizations, nursing is like the engine department. It is critical to the final product. The car being manufactured cannot run without an engine. Many health care providers cannot provide treatment to patients without nurses. However, if patients pay on a flat basis, such as a fixed DRG payment regardless of resources consumed, it is difficult to decide how much of the total payment is for nursing as opposed to other services.

However, not all patients pay a flat amount for their care. There are still many situations in which patients are charged for radiographs, lab tests, and pharmaceuticals. Why not charge for nursing services as well? Historically, the division of health care organizations into revenue and expense centers was based on differential consumption. If all patients consumed exactly the same amount of a resource provided by a department, it was considered to be an expense center. If different patients consumed different amounts, the department was established as a revenue center. For example, some patients have operations and some do not. Of those who have operations, some have long, costly ones, while others have short, relatively inexpensive ones. As a result, the OR was established as a revenue center, charging a different amount to different patients.

In contrast, consider the security guard standing at the front door of the hospital. The guard protects the entire organization—its employees, its patients, and their visitors. It is difficult to argue that one patient consumes more benefit from the guard than another. The security guard will therefore be considered to be part of an expense center. All the costs of expense centers will be aggregated and charged to the patient in a lump sum, such as a daily room charge.

Some departments provide differential services, but it is just not worth the cost and effort of measuring and assigning those services. For example, different patients consume different amounts of laundry. But it would be expensive to track exactly how many sheets and towels are used by each patient. Instead, the laundry department is an expense center.

Nursing units were historically treated the same as the laundry! Yes, different patients do consume different amounts of nursing resources. However, it was costly to track that differential consumption. Exactly how much service is consumed by each specific patient? It would not be feasible to hire an accountant to follow each nurse and keep track of how much of the nurse's time was used to provide care to each patient. However, some hospitals have managed to use their patient classification system to charge separately for nursing services. In the early 1980s, there was considerable interest in cost accounting systems that facilitated charging separately for nursing services (Ballard et al., 1985; Edwardson & Giovannetti, 1987), and several hospitals managed to contract with their major third-party payers (notably Blue Cross Blue Shield in Arizona) to charge for nursing services based on the patient's classification or on a checklist of specific nursing services delivered to each patient. In the latter system, as part of their charting for each patient, nurses completed a one-page checklist on the nursing care delivered that shift. From those lists, the daily nursing charge was generated. There was a standard room charge that was equivalent to the price of a local motel room, but nursing care was not incorporated into the room charge.

Today the health care industry is making rapid progress in the area of computerization. Nurses could scan their ID cards whenever they provide care to a patient, and computers could track the varying amounts of nursing care received by various patients. So it is now becoming more feasible to charge different patients different amounts for the nursing services they receive. Nevertheless, movement toward making nursing a revenue center in hospitals has been slow. Finance officers have been resistant to change. However, there does finally seem to be some movement toward making the nursing portion of health care revenues more explicit. Both Maryland and Maine now have laws requiring separation of nursing on hospital bills.[3] This could be the beginning of a trend that would substantially extend the nurse manager's involvement and responsibility for revenues.

When Is a Nurse Manager Responsible for a Revenue Budget?

Despite the slow movement to nursing revenue centers in hospitals, there are many situations in which nurse managers are already responsible for developing revenue budgets, and these situations are likely to increase rapidly in the near future. In some cases these opportunities will occur in hospitals, where nurses are already responsible for revenue budgets for the OR, recovery room, labor and delivery, and some other departments. However, hospitals should not be the focus, because their role in

[3] Swansburg, p. 26.

providing health care services has been diminishing. The past several decades have seen a clear shift away from hospital inpatient care to provision of care on an outpatient basis. This shift has created growing opportunities for nursing to have revenue responsibility.

In outpatient settings, nurse managers are often responsible for the revenue budgets of outpatient surgery units, clinics, community health centers, public health services, hospices, and home care agencies. During the past 20 years, a number of nurse practitioner clinics have been established. Their mission is usually to provide care to underserved populations, such as people in rural and frontier areas of the nation and indigent populations in both rural and urban settings. Because primary care is the product provided, nurse practitioners in those clinics are solely responsible for revenue generation. Additionally, there have always been nurses who have established private businesses. Nurse entrepreneurs have been consultants in management, education, research, and clinical practice, and they have established private nursing care businesses that provided nursing care on a fee-for-service basis. (These are not nurse practitioners; they provide services that any RN might provide, such as diabetic teaching, private-duty nursing in the home, and other general nursing services). Many nurses have obtained education in nontraditional therapies and practices, such as massage therapy, therapeutic touch, electrolysis and laser hair removal, acupuncture, and other nontraditional health-related services. Some have opened private businesses providing these services to the public. These are just a few of the types of businesses nurse entrepreneurs have created, but this list is by no means comprehensive. In many cases, nurse entrepreneurs must prepare revenue budgets for their own clinical practices, consulting practices, or other types of ventures. Nurse educators may be responsible for tuition revenues. Nurse researchers are responsible for grant revenues. The situations in which nurses must prepare and manage revenue budgets are extensive and growing.

The Elements of a Revenue Budget

The basic elements of a revenue budget are simple—price and volume. The revenue budget essentially consists of the price charged for each service provided by the unit, department, or organization multiplied by the number of units of service provided. The complications involved in a revenue budget are estimating the volume of services to be provided, deciding on the prices to charge, and estimating how much of the total amount charged will actually be collected.

Consider a simple example. Suppose that Best Clinic treats patients on a cash basis. That is, patients pay for their treatment in cash as the treatment is provided by the clinic. If 10 patients are expected to be treated, the charge to each one is $100, and all amounts are collected, the revenue will be:

$100 per patient × 10 patients = $1,000 of revenue.

Even this simple first look at revenue is complicated. How did the organization decide to charge $100? How did it decide that 10 patients were likely?

Prices or Rates

A number of different types of prices are used in health care. Organizations set a price or charge for their services. However, some payers pay a percentage of the charge that is less than 100%, based on a contractual agreement. Other payers pay a flat amount per case, regardless of the amount charged. Hospitals are sometimes paid on a per diem basis or a per discharge basis. The per discharge payment may be adjusted for diagnosis or might be a broad average payment, regardless of patient type. Some payers just reimburse the organization for the costs that have been incurred in providing care. Home care can be reimbursed by a flat amount per visit or can be paid by a flat amount per patient, regardless of the number of visits required. Under *capitation*, discussed later, the health care provider is paid a flat amount per member, regardless of whether the member consumes any health care resources at all or consumes very large amounts of resources.

For ongoing organizations, the finance department may provide the nurse manager with information about the prices (often called rates) that will be charged for each service. In such cases, the manager is primarily responsible for estimating the future number of each type of patient to be treated and for multiplying the volume of each service by the given prices to arrive at the revenue budget. The main difference between this and the $1,000 of revenue for Best Clinic discussed earlier is the fact that typically there will be many different kinds of patients whose care require differing prices, and the manager must be as accurate as possible in estimating the future volume of each type of patient.

In some cases, however, the nurse manager is responsible for setting prices. This is often referred to as *rate setting*. Prices can be *market-based, cost-based, markup-based*, or negotiated. Market-based prices are those that are set based on a survey of what others in the community are charging for the same services. If you charge substantially more than others are charging, in some cases you may lose your customers. Some organizations intentionally set prices below the competition in an effort to stimulate business. The success of strategies to undercut the competition or to charge above the market (and make more profit per patient) depends largely on how sensitive buyers are to price.

Many individuals shop around to buy a car, seeking the lowest price for what is essentially the exact same commodity. For example, if a specific model car from a specific manufacturer is sold by three different dealers in the area, the customer may shop for the best price among the three dealers. What if a gall bladder operation can be obtained from three different surgeons at three different hospitals? The customer is less likely to view the operations as being identical. Shopping may be based more on the reputation of the surgeon or hospital than on the price.

Suppose that a nurse manager starts a home care agency in an area that already has two home care agencies. Will potential customers consider the service to be identical and therefore look for the lowest price? The nurse entrepreneur can decide to compete by charging less than the competition; or might decide to market the service directly to potential patients as being better in some way (higher-quality nurses, more caring attitude, and longer visits); or might decide simply to charge the market price and then focus marketing efforts on hospital discharge planners who are responsible for referring patients to home care agencies.

Alternatives to market-based prices are cost-based or markup-based prices. Cost-based refers to charging exactly your cost. The word "cost" typically means average cost. There are many instances in which law or regulation requires such prices. For example, a state might mandate that home care agencies charge Medicaid exactly the cost of providing care. Markup-based prices are those where the manager determines the cost of care and sets the price a certain percentage above cost. For example, if a visit costs $40 to provide, an organization with a 20% markup would charge $48 for the visit (i.e., $40 + [20% × $40]).

It is also becoming more common for health care providers to negotiate rates with insurance companies. The negotiation can result in a variety of payment approaches, such as flat fees, percent discounts, or payments per episode. Depending on the proportion of customers whose bills are paid through a contract with one or more insurance companies and depending on the nature of the contract with the insurance company, preparation of the revenue budget can range from being a simple task to being quite a complex task. When a clinic has multiple contracts with a variety of different insurance companies, combined with a population of uninsured (self-pay) patients and perhaps subcontracts from another health care organization, revenue projections can become complicated. Yet those are the situations in which careful revenue budgeting is most important; the profit margins will probably be narrow, and projecting revenues accurately may make the difference between the success and failure of the enterprise.

Suppose that Best Clinic, using a market-price strategy, sets its price at $100. Does that mean that the clinic will collect $100 for each patient? In reality, patients do not usually arrive with cash in hand. More often they have insurance. Some insurers will pay the full $100. But that is extremely rare. Many insurers pay only a specific amount for a particular service. Others demand a percentage discount. Often prices paid by insurers are the results of protracted negotiations. A complete revenue budget must take into account the fact that health care providers do not usually collect the full amount charged.

For example, Blue Cross might say it will pay only $60 for a clinic's service. If you want to accept a Blue Cross patient, you can charge $100, but then you must give a $40 contractual allowance (i.e., a discount based on your contract with Blue Cross). Your net charge, after subtracting the contractual allowance is therefore $60. So in preparing a revenue budget, it would be necessary to estimate the percentage of patients who are insured by Blue Cross and calculate their net revenues as being $60 rather than $100. Another insurer might negotiate a percentage discount rather than a specific price for each service. Suppose that some of the clinic's patients are insured by Aetna and that the clinic's agreement with that insurer calls for them to pay 80% of charges. Best Clinic's revenue budget might look like Table 9-1. Total net

TABLE 9-1 Best Clinic Revenue Budget for the Year Ending December 31, 2009

Patients by Payer	Gross Revenue	Contractual Allowances	Net Revenue
2 Blue Cross patients	$ 200	$ 80	$120
$100 × 2 = $200 gross revenue			
$100 − $60 = $40 allowance per patient			
$40 × 2 patients = $80 allowance			
3 Aetna patients	300	60	240
$100 × 3 = $300 gross revenue			
$100 × 20% = $20 allowance per patient			
$20 × 3 patients = $60 allowance			
5 Other patients	500	0	500
Total	$1,000	$140	$860

TABLE 9-2 Best Clinic Revenue Budget for the Year Ending December 31, 2009

Patients by Payer	Gross Revenue	Contractual Allowances	Net Revenue
2 Blue Cross patients	$ 200	$ 80	$ 120
$100 × 2 = $200 gross revenue			
$100 − $60 = $40 allowance per patient			
$40 × 2 patients = $80 allowance			
3 Aetna patients	300	60	240
$100 × 3 = $300 gross revenue			
$100 × 20% = $20 allowance per patient			
$20 × 3 patients = $60 allowance			
1 Medicaid patient	100	45	55
1 Medicare patient	100	30	70
3 Other patients	300	0	300
Total	$1,000	$215	$785

revenue is $860, rather than the $1,000 revenue originally calculated for the 10 patients.

Some of the clinic's patients might be Medicare or Medicaid patients. Assume that Best Clinic has one of each. Suppose that Medicaid regulations call for it to pay the cost of care and that the cost of each visit is $55. The allowance for the Medicaid patient is therefore $45. Suppose further that Medicare has a fee schedule that calls for it to pay $70 for this type of patient. The allowance for the Medicare patient is therefore $30. The revenue budget would now appear as seen in Table 9-2. Note that the total net revenue is $785.

At this point it is clear that health care organizations often collect substantially less than the amount they charge for services. One reason that health care providers charge so much for health care services is that so many customers receive discounts. This is exacerbated by the fact that some customers do not pay their charges at all. Some patients will not be able to pay for their care because they don't have the financial resources. Others may just not be willing to pay.

In the former case, the organization may decide to treat the patient as a charity case. In such instances the organization will charge a lower amount or nothing at all. Suppose that one of the patients treated has no insurance and is poor. Best Clinic decides to give the patient a 75% discount. In that case, if the patient actually pays the bill, the gross revenue from that patient will be only $25. However, many indigent patients do not provide accurate mailing addresses or simply ignore any bills that do arrive. Care that is being given as charity is not included as part of gross revenues. It is a gift, rather than a charge that is not collected. The cost of that care, however, will be included in the expense budget.

Some patients have the resources to pay for care but never pay. This occurs in two different ways. Some patients do not have insurance and simply fail to pay part or all of their bills. Many patients do have insurance but are required to pay a portion of the charge—perhaps 20% or 30%. That portion is called a *co-pay* or *co-payment*. If patients fail to pay the co-pay portions, the insurance company often will not pay

TABLE 9-3 Best Clinic Revenue Budget for the Year Ending December 31, 2009

Patients by Payer	Gross Revenue	Discounts and Contractual Allowances	Net Revenue
2 Blue Cross patients	$ 200	$ 80	$ 120
$100 × 2 = $200 gross revenue			
$100 − $60 = $40 allowance per patient			
$40 × 2 patients = $80 allowance			
3 Aetna patients	300	60	240
$100 × 3 = $300 gross revenue			
$100 × 20% = $20 allowance per patient			
$20 × 3 patients = $60 allowance			
1 Medicaid patient	100	45	55
1 Medicare patient	100	30	70
1 Charity self-pay patient (75% discount)	25	0	25
1 Bad debt self-pay patient	100	0	100
1 Other self-pay patient	100	0	100
Total	$ 925	$215	$710
Less bad debt expense			−100
Net revenue less bad debts			$610

those either. When patients do not pay amounts that have been charged to them, the amounts not paid are referred to as *bad debts*. Bad debts may arise from self-insured patients who do not pay their bills or from insured patients who do not pay their co-payments. Many health care organizations now collect co-pay charges at sign-in, before the patient has been seen by the health care provider. Organizations should bill promptly, send monthly statements, and use collection agencies, if necessary, to collect as much of the money owed to them as possible. Assume that Best Clinic has one *self-pay patient* whose bill is not paid.

Table 9-3 shows the net revenue for the clinic. Note that the bad debt is included in net revenue and then subtracted separately as an expense. Accounting rules for reporting the financial results of an organization require bad debts to be treated as expenses rather than revenue reductions. Bad debts are isolated in this way to highlight them. Some organizations do a better job and some a worse job of collecting amounts owed to them. Seeing the bad debts as a separate item helps the reader get a sense of how well a particular organization has done in this area.

It is important to note that Best Clinic expects to collect only $610 for providing care to the 10 patients (see Table 9-3). Even though there were 10 patients who received a $100 service each, only $925 was charged in total (because of the charity care), rather than $1,000. The final amount collected was $610 because of allowances and bad debts. Unless the manager is careful to go through this computation, there may be a mistaken assumption that the organization has much more money available to spend on providing care than is actually the case. It is critical to estimate the actual amounts that will be collected for each patient as carefully as possible. This means spending time trying to determine the likely rate of bad debts (often on the basis of historical experience), reviewing contracts with insurers to determine payment rates, and even considering such aspects as discounts given to credit card companies for patients who charge their bills.[4]

Bad-debt control is an important part of revenue management. No business can survive long if a substantial number of its bills are ignored by its customers. Given this fact, the wise organization—or nurse entrepreneur—will develop policies and procedures to ensure payment of the patients' portions of the bills. For example, many surgery departments now require that patients pay their portion of the expected surgery bill prior to or at the time the surgery is scheduled, at least for nonemergency surgeries. Nonemergency surgeries often will not be scheduled until patients have paid their portions of the bills—or if scheduled, the surgery will be cancelled if the patient does not pay on the day of surgery. Some facilities collect the co-pay when the patient checks in for the procedure, but that approach can lead to a serious problem of cancelled surgeries when the patient shows up without the required co-pay. It is not unusual for the patient's portion of a surgery bill to exceed $20,000. For example, the expected total bill for a joint replacement is typically more than $50,000. If the patient's insurance company pays only 60% of the bill, the patient's portion of the bill will be $20,000. Given that the bill has probably already been discounted through the contractual arrangement with the insurance company, failure to collect the patient's portion means that the hospital will suffer nearly a $20,000 loss on the procedure. Given the difficult finances faced by most hospitals, the surgery department must collect that co-pay in advance to avoid the high probability that it will not be paid at all if the patient is billed after the procedure.

Even if a health care provider does its best to collect co-pays from patients, that doesn't mean that bad debts can be avoided. For example, some health care insurance companies have run into financial difficulties and been unable to pay their bills to health care providers. Combined with the fact that according to the U.S. Census bureau in 2006, approximately 47 million Americans were uninsured (Hoover, 2006) and that there are millions of uninsured undocumented workers and their families not counted in that number, health care providers in hospitals, clinics, ambulatory care centers, and all other health care facilities are at high risk for failure due to bad debt if the financial and business managers do not develop procedures to minimize bad debt.

Volume Estimates

Even if the amount collected per patient is meticulously considered, the revenue budget still depends heavily on estimates of volume. Volume can be estimated using the forecasting techniques that are discussed in Chapter 6. Note that it is not sufficient to estimate total patient volume. The volume of each type of patient or procedure for which there is a different charge must be estimated. This may entail estimation of home care visits by nurses versus aides. Or perhaps a manager will have to estimate patients, patient days, treatments, hours, procedures, and tests. Some degree of flexibility is required to forecast on the basis of type of patient or type of procedure or test, depending on the specific requirements of a particular situation.

---

[4] If a patient charges a $100 bill for health care services on a credit card, the credit card company will typically pay the provider anywhere between $95 and $98. The difference between the $100 charge and the amount the credit card company pays is a fee to cover the costs and some of the profits of the credit card company.

TABLE 9-4 Surgery and Clinic Revenue Budget for the Year Ending June 30, 2010

Revenue Source	(A) Quantity	(B) Rate or Charge	(C = A × B) Gross Revenue	(D) Average Net Charge	(E = C × D) Revenue Net of Discounts and Allowances
Same-day surgery					
Private insurance	1,000	$1,500	$1,500,000	75%	$1,125,000
Medicare	600	1,500	900,000	80%	720,000
Medicaid	400	1,500	600,000	60%	360,000
Self-pay	500	1,500	750,000	70%	525,000
Clinic patients					
Private insurance	3,000	250	750,000	75%	562,500
Medicare	1,800	250	450,000	80%	360,000
Medicaid	1,200	250	300,000	60%	180,000
Self-pay	1,500	250	375,000	85%	318,750
Gift shop	7,000	17	119,000	99%	117,810
Donations	400	200	80,000	100%	80,000
Subtotal			$5,824,000		$4,349,060
Less bad debt expense					−112,500
Net revenue less bad debts					$4,236,560

In preparing the revenue budget, it is extremely important to consider all possible sources of revenue or support. In addition to patient charges for services, these sources might include ancillary activities, such as gift shops or restaurants, endowment income, gifts, and grants. Clearly, the final revenue budget will be more complex than that shown in Table 9-3 and will show revenues not only by type of payer but also by different types of patients or procedures and by including information about other types of revenue. Table 9-4 presents a somewhat more sophisticated example for an outpatient organization that provides both same-day surgery and a variety of clinic services. However, even this example is simplified because it breaks patients down only into same-day surgery versus clinic groups, as opposed to a more detailed breakdown by type of surgery, visit, procedure, or test.

In Table 9-4, the first column on the left indicates the various revenue sources, listing the different types of patients by payer and listing other revenue sources. The next column, column A, Quantity, indicates the forecast volume level for each revenue source. In this example, 1,000 same-day surgery patients with private insurance are expected. There are anticipated to be 7,000 purchases from the gift shop and 400 donations.

Moving to column B, Rate or Charge, the full charge, on average, for each type of service is indicated. For example, the average same-day surgery charge is expected to be $1,500. Obviously, a more realistic budget would show different types of surgery patients and different charges for each type. Column B also notes that the average purchase at the gift shop is $17 and the average donation to the organization is $200.

Column C, Gross Revenue, can be found by multiplying column A by column B. This represents the total of all charges by the organization to its patients, as well as gift shop charges and donations.

Column D, Average Net Charge, represents the average percentage of the full charge that is collected. For example, if private insurance payments typically average 75% of the full charge, column D shows 75%. Note that the percentage shown for self-pay patients in this column reflects contractual allowances but not bad debts, which appear later in the exhibit.

The percentage shown for the gift shop reflects the fact that the organization provides a 10% discount for purchases by employees. If employees account for 10% of all purchases from the gift shop, that would result in an average discount of 1% across all gift shop sales (i.e., a 10% discount to employees who make up 10% of all purchases = 10% × 10% = 1% discount on all sales, on average).

Column E is simply column C multiplied by column D. This represents the amount expected to be collected. At the bottom of this column, bad debts are shown to be $112,500. This represents 10% of all amounts charged to self-pay patients (i.e., [$750,000 same-day surgery + $375,000 clinic] × 10%). The 10% typically would be based on historical bad-debt experience. Note in Table 9-4 that although Surgery and Clinic expects to have gross charges of $5,824,000, it expects to collect only $4,236,560 for the services provided for the year.

Environmental Scan

In predicting revenue for the coming year, managers should consider many issues. Managers must be concerned not only with what they might want to do but also with other factors, such as the economy, inflation, growth, employment, interest rates, competition, and so on. Managers should undertake a common-sense review of the likely impact of the economic environment on the organization. Just as an environmental scan is essential for budgeting in general, the information from the scan should be applied to the revenue budget.

Even a change in the proportion of patients covered by each type of insurer is a significant event. Looking at Table 9-4, consider what would happen to Surgery and Clinic in if an economic downturn forced a number of patients with private insurance to shift to Medicaid. In the table, it is clear that Medicaid pays a much lower percentage of charges than private insurance pays. Such a shift could have a dramatic impact on the total revenues collected by the organization. Note that the number and type of patients would remain the same; therefore, the costs would remain the same. But a shift in payer mix can dramatically change both the revenues and the overall fortunes of the organization, and managers must anticipate and consider the impact of such changes.

■ REVENUES FROM MANAGED CARE

In an environment highly focused on controlling the costs of providing health care services, *managed care organizations* (MCOs) have flourished. A managed care organization is any organization that tries to control the use of health care services to provide cost-effective care. MCOs try to eliminate provision of care that is not needed or is not cost-effective. The debate that often surrounds managed care relates to how to define care that is not cost-effective.

Sometimes it is easy to spot cost-effective solutions. Suppose that a mother and newborn are physically well and could be discharged from the hospital after 2 days. However, it is desirable to check the infant for jaundice on the third day. Should the mother and infant be kept in the hospital for a third day, or should a nurse practitioner go to see the mother and infant in their home on the third day? The cost of the home visit is substantially less than the additional day in the hospital. Assuming that clinical outcomes are equally good if the mother and infant are discharged after the second day, if they are insured by an MCO they will probably be sent home after two days. The result is lower cost and no decline in outcomes.

However, there are many ethical problems that arise from the definitions of cost-effective care used by many MCOs. What if a screening test is needed to determine whether a patient has a problem that is serious but highly unlikely? Perhaps the test costs $5,000 and would produce a positive result in only 1 of 1,000 people screened. That means that if the test were performed on 1,000 people it would probably find one person with the illness. The thousand tests would cost a total of $5,000,000. Managed care would probably deem that screening test not to be cost-effective and would refuse to pay for it. In contrast, before the advent of managed care, if a physician ordered the test, many insurance companies would have paid for it. Is it right to deny payment for that screening test? It is particularly problematic that the unfortunate patient who develops the serious problem may blame the provider for not ordering the test early when the problem was treatable, rather than blaming the insurance company that refuses to pay for the test. Policies that benefit insurance companies financially and help to control total spending on health care may lead to very poor outcomes for a few individuals. There has been much discussion in the American media and governmental bodies about balancing the wish to provide all possible services to every individual that might benefit versus the vital need to control health care costs. That is a moral dilemma with no easy answer.

Capitation Versus Fee-for-Service

Prior to the use of managed care, almost all care was provided on a *fee-for-service* basis. Fee-for-service means that there is a charge for each type of service provided. Patients or their insurance companies paid according to the specific services they consumed. If patients had lab tests, they were charged for the lab tests. If patients had home care visits, they were charged for the visits. Patients consuming more services were therefore charged more than patients consuming fewer services. Managed care proponents argue that the fee-for-service system encouraged overprovision of services. If the health care provider earns more money as more services are provided, why not provide a lot of services, whether needed or not?

The last sentence might outrage some. How can some big insurance company decide what services are needed and what services are not? But the reality is that many abuses, especially Medicare fraud, have been found to exist. Some patients did receive lab tests, home visits, and even dangerous surgical procedures—that were unnecessary (Hazle, 2005; Russel et al., 2002). And to some extent it is hard to determine what really is necessary. Would patients who receive home care visits once a day benefit if there were two visits a day instead? In some cases, probably so. But how much would they benefit? Would the extra benefit be worth the extra cost of the additional visit? These are difficult questions to address. What can be said is that the assumption (correct or incorrect) that fee-for-service leads to some overprovision of services was one factor leading to the development of capitated payment.

Capitation is a flat payment per covered member (sometimes referred to as per covered life), regardless of the amount of care provided. Capitation agreements are contractual agreements between two parties for the provision of some defined set of health-related services in exchange for a flat periodic payment per patient. The purchaser of the services is the managed care company, and the seller is the health care provider. Although the most common capitated contracts are between MCOs and physicians or hospitals, such contracts can also be established with a variety of health care organizations run by nurses, such as home care agencies or community health centers. Dunham-Taylor and colleagues suggest that nurses can find opportunities in a capitated environment by marketing programs focused on prevention, safety, substance abuse, obesity and exercise, nutrition, family planning, independent clinics, home health care, and hospice care.[5]

A nurse could contract with an MCO to provide certain services to its members for a premium payment per member per month. The MCO would provide a list of covered members and would pay a flat monthly amount, regardless of how much care the members consume. In some months, the nurse will receive payment for some members who do not consume any care at all as well as for other patients that consume a lot of care. One should not look at the profit or loss for any specific member. It is necessary to consider the total of the capitated payments received for the month for all members, in contrast to the total amount of services provided to all covered members that month.

Although capitated payments to nurses may not yet be extremely common, they do exist. One example is the community nursing organization (CNO) demonstration project for managing care on a capitated basis. Under a Medicare demonstration project, four CNOs receive capitated Medicare payments to provide a range of services to approximately 10,000 frail elderly patients in their homes and communities. The CNOs, which are nurse-managed, provide home health care, physical therapy, occupational therapy, and speech-language therapy services as well as medical equipment and supplies and ambulance services, along with preventive services. Initial data suggest that the CNOs may provide an important means of reducing utilization of higher-cost services while providing a range of needed services to the frail elderly.[6]

Many MCOs do not use capitation for all their contracts. Instead they may negotiate a discount from normal fees. In those cases, revenue is still paid on a fee-for-service basis (although the fee may be discounted), and the discussion related to revenue earlier in the chapter applies. Capitation, however, is a dramatically different form of payment.

From the viewpoint of the MCO, capitation is beneficial because there is no incentive for providers to over serve patients. If a home care patient receives extra visits, no extra payment is received by the agency, so there is no reason to deliver unneeded care. From the perspective of the provider, capitation provides a predictable revenue stream. Daily ups and downs in the flow of patients do not impact the regular monthly receipt of capitation payments. The payments are received whether the managed care members get sick or not.

[5] Dunham-Taylor, J., Penny Marquette, R., Pinczuk, J.Z.(1996). Surviving capitation. *American Journal of Nursing*. 96(3), 28.
[6] Personal e-mail communication from David Keepnews, September 28, 1999.

It is also sometimes possible to negotiate payments in advance of the provision of services. A new nurse entrepreneur, just starting out and with many expenses, can work out an arrangement to receive capitated payments at the beginning of each month. That money can be used to pay rent and salaries. It provides some revenue stability to the practice.

Capitated payment also has the potential to simplify paperwork. Each month the provider gets a list of covered members. When a member comes for treatment, the provider often collects a minimal co-payment from the member (perhaps $10) on the spot. The only other payment is the monthly capitation.

The essence of the concept behind capitation is that it shifts risk to the provider of care. Under fee-for-service, the patient, employer, or insurance company is totally at risk. The more health care services the patient consumes, the more the patient or insurer pays. Capitation, however, puts the provider at risk. The more health care services consumed by a covered patient, the worse off the provider will be. This creates a situation in which the provider benefits from keeping the patient healthy. It also gives providers an incentive to restrict their services to procedures and medications that have a reasonable probability of benefitting the patient. Much has been written about the waste incurred by providing futile services, especially at the end of life. Futile services are procedures and medications that have virtually no chance of improving the patient's condition but are, for one reason or another, provided to (some might say inflicted on) terminal patients. Futile care is not only expensive, it may increase suffering. Capitated systems provide a real financial disincentive for futile care.

The great advantage of capitation is that it provides an incentive to primary care providers to focus effort on preventive services. It is obviously better for patients to stay healthy, and capitated systems make keeping people healthy financially better for providers. Preventive care is less costly to the provider than curative care, so providers are more likely to provide services that keep patients healthy. Also, all providers have an incentive to use the lowest cost-efficacious treatment. Rather than providing more care to the patients they have, the way to increase revenue moves to having more covered members.

The danger of the system, of course, is that providers have an incentive to deny services to patients. There is a danger in paying providers **not** to provide services. Most patients do not know about all the options that might benefit them. All the provider need do is simply avoid mentioning a potentially beneficial—but expensive—service. Even when the patient suggests a potentially beneficial service, the provider may tell the patient that the service would not be beneficial (or might even be harmful) in that patient's particular case. Although most providers have ethics that would prevent such behavior, the profit motive is such a large incentive that some abuse is to be expected.

There have been outcries against capitated systems because of patients' concerns that this system tends to pit the welfare of ill patients who need expensive treatments against the profit motive of the provider. This is of particular concern when the outcome is life-threatening to the patient, such as denying care that will result in expensive, life-long services such as solid organ transplants. In 2006, a scandal broke about an HMO's failure to provide kidney transplants to patients. The HMO managers even rejected kidneys that were nearly perfect matches for individual subscribers, over 100 of whom died while waiting for transplants (Ornstein & Weber, 2006). The HMO's explanation was that the problems were caused by their inexperience in running a transplant program and by paperwork problems involved in trying to implement a new transplant program. Others, however, have suggested that it is more profitable to let a chronically ill kidney-failure patient die than to provide the transplant.

The transplant case created headlines, lawsuits, and fines that have been damaging to the HMO. Thus, it may be said there is a disincentive for HMOs to deny care that may result in death or permanent disability—and bad publicity. But some forms of care denial are unlikely to carry those kinds of consequences. In cases in which death or observable injury to the patient is not at risk, the incentive to deny care may be much greater and much harder to document. Pain management is an area particularly vulnerable to abuse. For example, labor pain can generally be greatly relieved or eliminated by epidural anesthesia, but labor epidurals are expensive. If the provider can deny the patient a labor epidural, the patient suffers, but the provider makes more money. Capitated systems require additional controls related to ensuring that best practice care protocols are followed so as to reduce the provider's incentive to deny patients proper care.

Nurses who manage businesses that deal with capitated payment should set policies and procedures that ensure that all patients entrusted to the organization receive best practices care, including respectful, kind, and supportive providers. Best practices are care protocols that have been found to be effective. They can be found in evidence-based practice journals, in clinical research reports, through the Agency for Healthcare Research and Quality (AHRQ)'s evidence-based practice reports on the Internet (http://www.ahrq.gov/clinic/epcix.htm), and through reviews of clinical practice evidence in the Cochrane Library's database of systematic reviews. A reputation in the community for providing excellent care at a reasonable cost is the best marketing tool for convincing insurance companies to send their subscribers to your organization. Providing high-quality care is also associated with better financial performance (Jiang et al., 2006). In a capitated system, an organization increases revenue by increasing the number of subscribers who choose it for their care (Vonderheid et al., 2006). Subscribers are likely to demand access to facilities with a reputation for excellent care, and health insurance companies are more likely to desire a contract with a provider that provides excellent care while keeping costs highly competitive.

Money Flows Under Capitation

In most capitated systems the primary payment comes from the purchaser of health insurance. This is generally the employer and employee, who share the cost of the premium. The insurance company, often an HMO, keeps part of the premium and uses the rest to pay for health care services. The two largest groups to receive payments are hospitals and physicians.

The key to revenues under capitation are the capitation rate and the number of capitated members. Suppose that a home care agency contracts with an MCO to provide all home care visits needed for $12 per member per month (PMPM). If the MCO has 250 members who will be covered by the contract, the monthly revenue will be:

$$\$12 \text{ PMPM} \times 250 \text{ members} = \$3,000$$

and the annual revenue will be:

$$\$12 \text{ PMPM} \times 250 \text{ members} \times 12 \text{ months/year} = \$36,000$$

The key to increasing revenue in a capitated environment is to have more covered members. This could occur by gaining a greater share of the members signed with one MCO or by signing additional contracts with other MCOs. Bear in mind that fixed costs will not change (rent on physical facilities, salary for an office manager, etc.), so the volume of members (and therefore the total amount of capitated revenue) becomes critical to success. As long as the capitated payments exceed variable costs, having more members leads to better financial outcomes.

Developing Capitated Rates

As a provider of health care services, setting the capitation rate is critical. Often a contract is signed committing the provider to accept the agreed-upon rate for at least a year. If the rate is set too low, the organization will lose money on patients throughout the year. Setting capitated rates is much more complicated than ordinary price-setting because capitated rates depend critically on utilization.

In a fee-for-service payment situation, one tries to compare the price of a particular service to the cost of providing that service. For example, suppose that the average cost of providing a home care visit is $38 and the fee charged is $45. One can therefore anticipate a profit on each visit. However, in a capitated situation, the payment is the PMPM, regardless of the number of visits for each patient. In negotiating a capitated rate, it is critical to evaluate the population covered and the likely utilization rate by that population. For example, an elderly population will obviously have far more home care visits than a younger population.

The starting point in determining a capitation rate is identifying the exact services to be covered by the contract. Next, the provider must obtain estimates of the use of each service offered. Utilization rates should be adjusted for actual population demographics. Costs should be estimated and converted to PMPM equivalents. It is helpful to set the marginal cost (i.e., incremental or additional cost) for the services to be provided as the lower limit and the fee-for-service charges as the upper limit for rate negotiations. Calculating the PMPM cost of each component on a charge, average-cost, and marginal-cost basis provides the manager with solid information for negotiating. These elements of determining a capitation rate are discussed in the following paragraphs.

There is usually easy agreement about the services to be provided. The MCO wants to protect itself by having contracts to provide the services its members will need, so it will clearly specify what it wants to buy. In some cases, however, if there is great uncertainty about the cost of a service or the utilization of the service, there may be a *carve-out*. That is a service that would normally be provided but is excluded. For example, if liver and heart transplants are expected to be expensive and rare in a population, then a provider of surgical services (e.g., a hospital) might exclude, or carve-out, those two services from a contract to provide all hospital surgical care. If a patient needs a carved-out service, it would be provided on a fee-for-service basis.[7]

Determination of expected utilization is more complex. A good place to start is with historical demand data. For example, assuming that a home health agency

---

[7] *Note:* State and federal laws may impact which services can and cannot be carved-out of a coverage contract. For example, some states legislate that all health insurance policies must cover annual mammograms and Pap tests for women.

has already been providing services, it can use its own records to estimate the typical frequency of visits. Unfortunately, most providers can ascertain the visit frequency only for those patients who have at least one visit, treatment, admission, or other episode of care. What about all the members of the general population who do not seek any care during the year? Estimating utilization of capitated populations is difficult because the payment covers all members, whether they receive any care or not. Furthermore, the population covered by the managed care contract may be more or less likely to require care than the organization's historical patient base.

Although the MCO may offer its perspective on the amount of care that is needed for the population, one must consider that the managed care company has a vested interest in underestimating required care. The managed care company wants to pay the lowest rate it can. Often it is necessary to employ the services of an actuarial firm. Such a firm can examine the covered population, consider historical utilization rates for that population, adjust for utilization rates for the particular geographic region, and adjust for the genders and ages of the covered population.

Once the services to be provided have been determined and the utilization rates have been estimated, the next element in the process is for the provider to determine the fee-for-service charges, average costs, and marginal costs for the services to be provided under the managed care contract. The charges are needed because that is the amount that the provider would ideally like the MCO to pay. If the agreed-upon capitation rate provides as much money as charges would have provided, the contract is bringing in additional patients and additional revenue at prices as good as are currently being earned.

Average cost represents a middle ground. In the short run, a rate based on average costs would make the provider better off. If some costs are fixed, as they undoubtedly are, the additional patients would improve the short-term profits of the provider. Marginal costs represent the minimum that should be accepted. If the capitated price provides less than the marginal cost, the provider will actually be financially worse off because of the contract with the MCO. In that event, getting more subscribers onto the provider's role will result in even more losses.

MCOs will offer a price stated as a PMPM. This is because employers pay premiums on a monthly basis, based on the number of insured employees for the month. As job turnover occurs, employers eliminate some individuals from health insurance coverage and add others. The MCO will in turn eliminate some individuals from the payments made to the provider each month. Therefore, cost should be converted to PMPM equivalents.

Setting a Capitation Rate: An Example

Assume that you are the manager of a home care agency. You are currently negotiating a capitated rate with an MCO. Your charges for visits are currently $60 for a visit by an RN and $40 for a visit by an aide. Based on the history of the agency with noncapitated patients, plus information provided by an actuary, you have the following expectations regarding utilization by members of the MCO[8]:

1.2 RN visits per member per year and
3.0 aide visits per member per year.

---

[8] The data used in this example are hypothetical and do not reflect true utilization rates or costs for any home care agency.

To provide the visits, you will need additional nurses and aides. The number of nurses and aides depends on productivity levels. Suppose you expect the following number of visits per employee:

1,400 patient visits per RN per year and
1,000 patient visits per aide per year.

And suppose further that the annual salaries, including benefits, for nurses and aides are:

Annual compensation $50,000 per RN and
Annual compensation $15,000 per aide.

The direct labor cost for the visits can be calculated PMPM as follows:

RN Visits

Average cost per visit = $50,000/1,400 = $35.71 per visit
Per member per year   = $35.71 × 1.2 visits per year = $42.85
PMPM rate   = $42.85 ÷ 12 months
             = $3.57 PMPM

Aide Visits

Average cost per visit = $15,000/1,000 = $15.00 per visit
Per member per year   = $15.00 × 3 visits per year = $45.00
PMPM rate   = $45.00 ÷ 12 months
             = $3.75 PMPM

Each visit requires some supplies. Assume that the supply cost per visit is $5. This can be converted to a supply cost PMPM as follows:

Supplies
$5 per visit × 4.2 visits = $21.00
$21 ÷ 12 visits per year = $1.75 PMPM

In addition, support staff will be working for the agency. In some cases, such staff may be fixed, while in other cases it may be variable. For example, the cost of the office manager will not vary with the number of visits. But other staff members are needed to schedule patient visits. The more patients, the more staff hours needed for such activities. Assume that the agency has found that it needs one tenth of an FTE of a support staff member for each FTE nurse or aide, and that support staff members earn $20,000, on average. The number of such support staff is considered to vary with the number of nurses and aides and therefore with the number of members. The number of support staff that does not vary with the number of visits is included in other overhead, as shown below.

Number of RNs per member   = 3.0 visits/1,400 visits per RN = 0.00214
Number of aides per member   = 1.2 visits/1,000 visits per aide = 0.0012
Total nurses and aides per member = 0.00214 + 0.0012 = 0.00334
Support staff   = 0.00334 × 0.1 support staff per nurse
                 or aide
                 = 0.000334 support staff personnel per
                 member
Support staff cost   = 0.000334 × $20,000 = $6.68 per
                 member per year
Support staff cost PMPM   = $6.68 ÷ 12 months = $0.56 PMPM

Note how cumbersome the calculation becomes because of the small fractions. Utilization rates are often stated per thousand members to avoid dealing with small fractions.

Alternatively, if the support staff calculation had been done per thousand members, it would appear as follows:

Number of RNs per 1,000 members = 3.0 visits × 1,000 members ÷ 1,400 visits per RN
= 2.14 RNs per 1,000 members
Number of aides per 1,000 members = 1.2 visits × 1,000 members ÷ 1,000 visits per aide
= 1.2 aides per 1,000 members
Total nurses and aides = 2.14 + 1.2 = 3.34 nurses and aides per 1,000 members
Support staff = 3.34 × 0.1 support staff per nurse or aide
= 0.334 support staff personnel per 1,000 members
Support staff cost = 0.334 × $20,000 = $6,680 per 1,000 members per year
Support staff cost PMPM = $6,680 ÷ 1,000 members ÷ 12 months = $0.56 PMPM

Notice that whether the calculation is performed on a per member basis or per 1,000-member basis, the PMPM result is exactly the same. Assume that all other costs, such as fixed staff, rent, and electric work come out to $3 PMPM.

Based on the above information, a PMPM based on average costs can be calculated as follows:

	PMPM
RNs	$3.57
Aides	3.75
Supplies	1.75
Support staff	0.56
Other overhead	3.00
Average cost PMPM	$12.63

It was noted earlier that the manager should calculate rates based on charges, average cost, and marginal cost. We have just calculated the average cost as being $12.63. Earlier it was noted that the charges for the agency are $60 for an RN visit and $40 for an aide visit. This can be converted to a PMPM as follows:

1.2 RN visits per member × $60 per visit ÷ 12 months = $ 6.00 PMPM
3.0 aide visits per member × $40 per visit ÷ 12 months = $10.00 PMPM
Total charge for RN and aide visits   = $16.00 PMPM

The marginal cost of the visits can also be determined. The RNs, aides, supplies, and support staff will all increase if the contract is signed. The other overhead is fixed and will be incurred in any event. Therefore, the marginal cost of providing the additional visits is $9.63 per member per month (i.e., $12.63 average cost − $3.00 other overhead). We can now compare the three measures:

	Charge	Average Cost	Marginal Cost
Per member per month	$16.00	$12.63	$9.63

This comparison provides the manager with critical information needed to enter PMPM capitation rate negotiations. The goal is to negotiate revenue as close to the $16 PMPM charge as possible but in no case to lower than the $9.63 marginal cost. Once the rate has been agreed on, the revenue from the agreement is simply the capitation rate multiplied by the number of members covered by the agreement.

Incentive Risk Pools

Managed care contracts often also include incentive arrangements to minimize overall costs. For example, suppose that all providers are capitated, except for hospitals. Assume that hospitals are paid on a discounted fee-for-service basis by the MCO. How can the MCO encourage providers to avoid unnecessary patient hospitalizations? A common arrangement is the use of inpatient services *risk pools*. Risk pools consist of some money that has been withheld from each provider. The withheld amount is eventually paid to the provider if utilization achieves certain targets.

For example, suppose that the home care agency discussed earlier negotiates a $13 PMPM capitation rate from a managed care provider for 2,000 members. The agency is entitled to revenue of $26,000 per month ($13 PMPM × 2,000 members). However, the MCO is concerned about the incentives created by capitation. It worries that the agency might try to save money by not providing all the visits needed because the agency receives the same $13 PMPM regardless of the number of visits provided.

Failure to provide visits when they are needed might result in a patient's being rehospitalized. This is a poor outcome for the patient and costly for the MCO. To avoid this outcome, the MCO might withhold 10% of the capitated payments until a year-end reconciliation is performed. That amount is combined with money withheld from other providers to create a risk pool. The agency would receive only $23,400 each month ($26,000 × 90%). At the end of the year, the agency would get back part of the money or the entire amount, according to actual hospital utilization versus the expected level of hospital utilization. If hospital utilization is unexpectedly high, the risk pool is used to pay the hospital, and there may be nothing left in the pool to pay the agency. The agency can lose the entire 10% that had been withheld. But if hospital costs are very high, the MCO will be liable for any costs that the risk pool cannot cover. So both the providers and the MCO are at risk for losing some money if utilization is higher than expected. This is referred to as *risk-sharing*.

It should also be noted that in some cases withhold arrangements may lead to poorer care. For example, to keep hospital utilization low, physicians or nurse practitioners might fail to admit patients who actually need hospital care. Some would argue that MCOs are not really worried about quality of care at all. From that perspective, risk pools are established solely to save money for the MCO by discouraging patient admissions and other costly forms of care. Nurse managers involved in managed care negotiations must always consider the implications of the contract for the quality of care to be provided to their patients.

Summary and Implications for Nurse Managers

Revenues are the amount the organization earns in exchange for the services it provides. Revenues are critical for every organization. Revenues must be adequate to cover all costs of providing services during the current year. Additionally, revenues should be great enough to provide a profit. Profits are used to expand the type and volume of services offered and to replace capital equipment.

In some situations, nurses are not given revenue responsibility because their actions cannot affect the revenues of the organization. This would be the case in a situation in which all patients pay a fixed fee, regardless of services received. More commonly, however, nurses have not been given revenue responsibility because historically it was difficult to assess the amount of nursing resources consumed by various patients. Computer technology is removing this barrier, and it is becoming more feasible to charge different patients for the differing amounts of nursing services they receive. Nurse managers should continue to push for revenue responsibility.

Continued

Summary and Implications for Nurse Managers—cont'd

The basic elements of a revenue budget are simple—price and volume. The revenue budget essentially consists of the price charged for each service provided by the unit, department, or organization multiplied by the number of units of service provided. The complications involved in a revenue budget arise in estimating the volume of services to be provided, deciding on the prices to charge, and estimating how much of the total amount charged will actually be collected. Nurse managers who are responsible for the revenue of their unit, department, or organization should be actively involved in estimating or at least understanding these factors.

Managed care organizations (MCOs) require special attention because of the way they pay for services. An MCO is any organization that tries to control the use of health care services to provide cost-effective care. In some cases MCOs pay in much the same way as other payers, often negotiating a discount from standard fees or charges. In some cases, however, MCOs pay providers based on capitation.

Capitation refers to paying a set amount for each covered member, regardless of the amount of care consumed. From the viewpoint of the MCO, capitation is beneficial because there is no incentive for providers to overserve patients. From the perspective of the provider, capitation provides a predictable revenue stream. Nurse managers must understand their costs in order to negotiate effective capitation rates. They should also attempt to negotiate advance monthly payments if their organization frequently has trouble meeting its monthly expenses that must be paid in cash.

Nurse managers should always be cautious when working on capitated arrangements. In such arrangements, the MCO shifts risk to the provider. If, for whatever reason, patients consume more resources than expected, it is the provider who will lose money as a result. Many providers buy insurance called stop-loss protection to protect themselves from severe losses resulting from unexpectedly high patient utilization rates.

The capitation payment, called the PMPM rate, must cover all costs and profits for the organization related to the covered members. The starting point in determining a capitation rate is identification of the exact services that are to be covered by the contract. Next, the provider must obtain estimates of the utilization of each service covered. Utilization rates are generally stated per thousand members. Utilization rates must be adjusted for actual population demographics. Costs must be converted to PMPM equivalents. It is helpful to use the marginal cost for the covered services as the lower limit and to use the fee-for-service charges as the upper limit during rate negotiations.

Once the PMPM has been determined, it can be multiplied by the number of covered members to determine the organization's revenue from the MCO. The key to increasing revenue in a capitated environment is to get more covered members. Special care should also be paid in negotiating risk pools. Risk pools represent portions of the PMPM rate that are held back and may not be paid if utilization rates or costs for specific types of care exceed a set amount.

References and Suggested Readings

Ballard, D., Barach, K.B., Cullen, J. (1985). The variable nursing charge system at the hospital of Saint Raphael. In F.A. Shaffer (Ed.), *Costing Out Nursing; Pricing Our Product.* New York: National League for Nursing.

Buppert C. (2005). Third-party reimbursement for nurse practitioners' services on trauma teams: Working through a maze of issues. *Journal of Trauma-Injury Infection & Critical Care.* 58(1), 206-212.

Cleverley, W.O. (2005). *Essentials of Health Care Finance,* ed 5. Boston: Jones and Bartlett.

Dacso, S.T., Dacso, C.C., eds. (1999). *Risk Contracting and Capitation Answer Book.* Gaithersburg, MD: Aspen.

Dunham-Taylor, J., Marquette, R.P., Pinczuk, J.Z. (1996). Surviving capitation. *American Journal of Nursing.* 96(3), 26-30.

Edwardson, S., Giovannetti, P. (1987). A review of cost-accounting methods for nursing services. *Nursing Economic$.* 5(3), 107-117.

Gapenski, L.C. (2004). *Healthcare Finance: An Introduction to Accounting and Financial Management.* Chicago: AUPHA Press.

Hazle, M. (2005) Redding Medical Center criminal and civil cases settled. *Record Searchlight.* Downloaded April 6, 2007. http://www.geocities.com/three_strikes_legal/RMC_case_settled.html.

Hoover, K. (2006). Uninsured rate up as health coverage through work declines. *Austin Business Journal.* September 8, 2006. Downloaded from: http://austin.bizjournals.com/austin/stories/2006/09/11/story18.html.

Hunstock, L.M. (1996). Managed care and the world of capitated payment. In Flarey, D.L. and Blancett, S.S. *Handbook of Nursing Case Management: Health Care Delivery in a World of Managed Care.* Gaithersburg, MD: Aspen.

Jiang, H., Friedman, B., Begun, J. (2006). Sustaining and improving hospital performance: The effects of organizational and market factors. *Health Care Management Review.* 31(3), 188-196.

Leeth, L. (2004). Are you fiscally fit? Move your department from moneypit to moneymaker by creating new—and capturing hidden—revenue. *Nursing Management.* 35(4), 42-47.

McHugh, M., Dwyer, V. (1992). Measurement issues in patient acuity classification for prediction of hours in nursing care. *Nursing Administration Quarterly.* 16(4), 20-31.

Ornstein, C., Weber, T. Kaiser to pay record $2 million fine for kidney program. *Los Angeles Times,* August 10, 2006. Downloaded from http://www.latimes.com/news/local/la-me-kaiser10aug10,0,3276737.story?coll=la-home-headlines

Rapsilber, L.M., Anderson, E.H. (2000). Understanding the reimbursement process. *Nurse Practitioner.* 25(5), 36, 43, 46.

Russell, S., Fagan, K., Said, C. Unneeded open-heart surgeries, and complex, expensive diagnostic probes. *San Francisco Chronicle.* November 2, 2002.

Swansburg, R.C. (1997). *Budgeting and Financial Management for Nurse Managers.* Boston: Jones and Bartlett.

Tumolo J. (2005). Revving up revenue. *Advance for Nurse Practitioners.* 13(5), 14.

Vonderheid, S., Pohl, J., Schafer, P., Forrest, K., Poole, M., Barkauskas, V., Mackey, T. (2004). Using FTE and RVU performance measures to assess financial viability of nurse-managed centers. *Nursing Economic$.* 22(3), 124-134.

Wyld, D.C. (1996). The capitation revolution in health care: Implications for the field of nursing. *Nursing Administration Quarterly.* 20(2), 1-12.

Zaumeyer, C. (2004). Generating revenue. *Advance for Nurse Practitioners.* 12(12), 16.

Zelman, W.N., McCue, M.J., Milikan, A.R., Glick, N.D. (2003). *Financial Management of Health Care Organizations: An Introduction to Fundamental Tools, Concepts, and Applications.* Malden, MA: Blackwell.

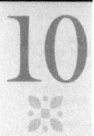

Capital Budgeting

LEARNING OBJECTIVES
The goals of this chapter are to:

- Define capital budgeting
- Explain why there is a separate accounting process for capital budgets
- Discuss the generation of capital budget proposals
- Describe capital budget justification and prioritization models
- Introduce the concept of the time value of money
- Explain the concept of relevant costs for capital budgeting

- Recognize the role of politics in capital budgeting decisions
- Generate an understanding of the benefits of formal decision models for capital project evaluation
- Explore the factors involved in evaluating capital budget items

■ INTRODUCTION

A capital budget consists of four basic components: capital item identification, item justification, item priority and, in most organizations, competitive bids for items with a cost exceeding a specific threshold. Sometimes, the organization has a form that presents on a single page each item, along with its price, justification, priority rating, and bids. That way, the decision makers can sort by item rather than by department in the capital budget review and approval meetings. Sometimes, building and renovation costs are included in the regular capital equipment budget process, and in other organizations a separate budget process is used for new buildings and renovation of existing space. If the latter is the approach, there is typically a special budget form to request new building projects and renovations. However, capital requests constitute a budget and budget process separate from the operating budget and budget process.

■ DEFINITION OF CAPITAL BUDGETING

Capital budgeting is the name commonly used for planning the acquisition of long-term investments. These investments can range from investments as small as the acquisition of a new IV pole to projects as large as the complete rebuilding of a hospital at a new location.

The key element in capital budgeting is that the building or piece of equipment being acquired has a lifetime that extends beyond the year of purchase. Anything that the organization builds or buys and starts to use in one year that will still be useful in future years is considered to be a capital item. Additionally, many organizations set a minimum dollar figure below which capital items are treated as part of the operating budget. (This issue is discussed in detail in the next section.)

Capital budget items are treated separately from the regular operating budget process. Every year, each unit or department lists all items with a multiyear life separately from operating budget expenses. These capital items go through a separate review and approval process. If approved, these capital acquisitions are accounted for separately from regular operating budget expenses.

Once the organization has completed its program budgeting process (see Chapter 7), any program changes such as the addition of a new service should be communicated to all departments that will be affected by that program change. This will allow the departments to consider the implications of the program change on both their capital and their operating costs. If the program change requires that a department provide services that require multiyear investments, those proposed acquisitions would become part of the department's capital budget. The capital budget also contains any other requests for purchases of multiyear items for the continued support of existing services.

Capital budget items are often referred to as *capital assets*. They are also referred to as *long-term investments, capital investments, capital acquisitions,* and *capital items.* In all cases, the word "capital" is used to signify the fact that the item's life extends beyond the year of purchase. Capital budget items generally are purchased to replace older items of a similar nature, to improve productivity (substituting equipment for more expensive labor), to improve quality of care (often adding newer technology), or to provide equipment for a new service or to expand an existing service. A variety of other reasons to acquire capital assets also arise from time to time such as for equipment that will improve employee safety or visitor comfort.

■ WHY HAVE CAPITAL BUDGETS?

Long-term investments are worthy of special attention for several reasons. First, capital items receive particular scrutiny because of their costs. Unlike day-to-day supplies that have relatively minor costs, capital investments commonly involve significant amounts of cash, all tied up in a single investment decision.

For example, heparin locks appear in the operating budget, and monitors for the intensive care unit (ICU) are part of the capital budget. Suppose that the nursing department purchases 50 heparin locks from a new supplier and is completely dissatisfied with their quality. Even if it has to throw the locks away, the loss is limited. On the other hand, if 10 new monitors are purchased for the ICU, at a price of $80,000 per monitor, there is an $800,000 investment. If it turns out that the monitors do not provide the information required and have to be replaced immediately, the financial loss is obviously much greater. The more expensive the acquisition, the more closely the proposed purchase needs to be examined.

Not only is it necessary to assess the immediate capabilities of capital acquisitions because of their large dollar cost, but it must also be recognized that their multiyear lives mean that the organization is committing to these items for a long time. For example, disposable gloves are part of the operating budget. Renovating space is part of the capital budget. If one brand of disposable gloves starts to decline in quality over time, the organization can shift to a different supplier. If the nurses' stations throughout a nursing home are totally renovated and it is then determined that there are quite a few inconvenient features about the new stations, the units will likely have to live with those inconveniences for 10 years or longer. The longer the commitment represented by an acquisition, the more carefully the decision to buy it must be scrutinized.

As a consequence of the high cost of and long-term commitment to many capital budget items, it is important to examine alternatives when developing capital budget proposals. Just as with zero-base budgeting for a complete program, reviewing alternatives is critical when evaluating capital assets. What will happen if an old piece of equipment is not replaced? Will it break down? If it does, what effect will that have on patient care? What if it is replaced with a cheaper model or one with less capacity? What benefits will there be if it is replaced with a model that has greater capacity? Reviewing a variety of alternatives will help to ensure that resources are not spent unnecessarily and that the unit or department does not regret its decision after a year or two.

In considering why the capital budget is distinct from the operating budget, however, the high cost and lengthy time commitment required by capital acquisitions are not in themselves sufficient reasons to justify the completely separate and duplicative budgeting process that capital budgeting represents. Alternative approaches could still be satisfactorily reviewed. If high cost and long-time commitment were the only issues, a manager would be justified in arguing that these items should be included in the operating budget but reviewed carefully. After all, nursing personnel are included in the operating budget and they represent millions upon millions of dollars of cost each year. Why create the whole separate process of capital budgeting?

The third and critical reason that a separate capital budgeting process exists relates to the multiyear nature of capital assets. They are only partly used up in any one year, and in any one year the organization earns only part of the revenues that the capital assets generate over their useful lifetimes.

The expenses included in an operating budget for a specific year represent the cost of the services the organization provides in that year. Operating budget revenues for any year are the amounts of money that the organization is entitled to receive in return for providing services in that year. In the case of capital assets, the amount spent to acquire the asset exceeds the amount used up in a single year because the asset lasts more than 1 year. Some of the capital asset remains available to provide services in the future. And the revenues that are received as a result of the investment will be earned over a number of years.

If capital items are included in the annual operating budget, substantial confusion will arise. The purpose of the operating budget is to compare the revenues and expenses for 1 year. Including the acquisition cost of multiyear assets in the operating expense budget would make the costs of providing services appear to be misleadingly high. It would cause the budget to convey a distorted picture of the organization's financial viability. By mixing expenses that are just costs of a single year with the acquisition costs of capital items, the receipts in the first year will often not cover the cash outlay, so few capital projects might seem affordable. Investments must be viewed over their entire lifetimes if fully informed decisions are to be made. There must be a way to show the carryover benefits of long-term investments into subsequent years. Capital budgets provide the means of accomplishing this.

In the capital budgeting process, a plan is made for acquiring capital assets. All, some, or none of the items requested by a department in its capital budget proposal will be approved and subsequently acquired. For those items that are approved, a depreciation schedule will be developed. Depreciation is a means of allocating a share of the capital item's cost over a period of years. Suppose that the organization buys an $80,000 monitor and that it is anticipated that the monitor will be used for 10 years before being replaced. The organization will allocate a part of the $80,000 cost into the each of the 10 years of the monitor's useful life by *depreciating* it at a rate of $8,000 per year for 10 years. The $80,000 cost of the capital item will be included in the capital budget once. Each year, $8,000 will be included in the operating budget as an expense. This reflects the fact that one tenth of the capital item is being used up each year to provide that year's services. Each year an appropriate share of the cost of the monitor becomes a part of the operating expense budget. Thus the capital budget is linked to the operating budget through the annual depreciation charges of the capital items that have been acquired.

■ HOW MUCH DO CAPITAL ASSETS COST?

Capital assets are often quite expensive, as was noted earlier. However, high cost is not a required element for an asset to be a capital asset. The only requirement is that the capital asset must be able to provide useful service beyond the year it is first put into use.

If a nursing unit acquires a ballpoint pen for $.89 and starts to use that pen 1 week before the end of the fiscal year, the pen is technically a capital asset if it is still functioning during the first week of the next fiscal year. From a theoretical point of view, the pen clearly meets the multiyear definition of a capital asset.

However, in order to keep accounting records accurate, the cost of capital assets must be depreciated, and a depreciation charge must be assigned to the operating budget for each year during the useful life of the asset. It does not seem practical to have a staff of accountants keeping track of each ballpoint pen purchased. The accounting cost would exceed any benefit gained.

As a result, most organizations set a minimum dollar limit on capital assets. Items of low cost are treated as part of the operating budget, even if they have a multiyear life. For instance, most health care organizations have a minimum cost requirement of anywhere from $500 to $2,500 in order for an item to be included in the capital budget. Anything below the cutoff is treated as a routine operating expense.

In fact, cutoffs of $500 or $1,000, seen in many hospitals, are far below the $3,000, $5,000, or $10,000 cutoffs that are observed in many other industries. Why do hospitals maintain fairly low dollar cutoffs for the items that will be treated as capital assets and those that will not? The answer has to do at least partly with government reimbursement. The Medicare system historically paid a flat DRG payment for each Medicare patient discharged. Thus, if a hospital provides a patient with extra lab tests or more hours of direct nursing care, no additional payment is provided for those extra resources.

However, that flat payment was for operating costs. Until recently, Medicare made an additional payment to hospitals to cover a portion of their capital costs. Suppose that a hospital has a $1,000 cutoff for capital assets. A $750 refrigerator for a nurses' station would be treated as an operating cost. No additional Medicare payment would be received to pay for the refrigerator. If the same hospital had maintained a $500 cutoff for capital items, the refrigerator would be over that threshold.

It would be considered a capital asset. In this case, in addition to the DRG operating payment, Medicare would pay the hospital an additional amount to cover a portion of the $750 cost of the refrigerator. This is referred to as a cost pass-through. Thus, hospitals had a definite financial incentive to keep their capital asset cutoff as low as possible. The result is that more of their acquisitions were categorized as being capital costs, and they received more total Medicare reimbursement for the same group of patients than would otherwise be the case. However, Medicare has phased out reimbursement based on the costs of capital equipment. Therefore, it would not be surprising to see hospitals raise their capital cutoff levels.

■ CAPITAL ITEM IDENTIFICATION

The starting point in the capital budgeting process is generating proposed investments. In the case of nursing, such proposals may occur either directly or indirectly. The manager of a nursing unit may desire some remodeling of the unit. The nurse manager in a home health agency may propose acquiring several company cars to reduce travel time to patient homes (assuming public transportation is currently being used). The nurse manager in the coronary care unit or the OR of a hospital may suggest acquiring a particular piece of equipment. These are examples of direct capital budgeting proposals. It will be up to the nurse manager, with the assistance of financial managers, to prepare the capital budget.

Many indirect proposals also affect nurse managers. For example, the pharmacy may suggest adding a new piece of equipment that will automate the reconstitution of a particular drug. Not only will there be a savings in the pharmacy in terms of reduced technician time required in preparing the drug for reconstitution, but there will also be a savings in nursing time and improved patient safety if the nurses currently do the reconstitution of the drug on the floor. In such cases, the pharmacy will be performing the majority of the analysis, but the nurse manager will be called upon to help determine the potential impact on the nursing budget.

Figure 10-1 presents an example of the type of worksheet a nurse manager would use to list capital proposals. (See the Appendix at the end of this book for an example of the specific instructions that a nurse manager might receive with a form of this type.) The first column represents the manager's priority ranking for the request. The most important acquisition would be ranked number 1. The second column indicates the types of capital items being requested. They include construction or remodeling (CR); replacing an existing item (RE); replacing and upgrading an existing item (RU); purchasing an item that is an addition to similar existing items and adds to their capacity (AS); and purchasing an additional item that is not currently available in the unit (AN).

Developing the list of proposals is the first step in the capital budgeting process. There are a variety of issues that will typically lead to proposals for capital budgeting. Some capital projects are obvious. When the roof starts to leak, it had better be repaired. It would be preferable, however, if the roof could be prevented from leaking. The long-range plan of the organization should require that capital expenditures be made on a systematic basis. Reroofing is one example. Replacing all the hospital beds is another. The maintenance department of the hospital is commonly the cost center that has to deal with such routine, although infrequent, capital expenditures. In many hospitals, bed replacement is a nursing department responsibility. Such replacement should not be done in a haphazard way.

CAPITAL BUDGET WORKSHEET

FY____

COST CENTER____

PRIOR. #	TYPE CR/RE/RU AS/AN	EQUIP. QTY	DESCRIPTION	UNIT COST	EXTENDED COST	COMMENTS

Figure 10-1 Capital budget worksheet.

The nursing department should take the approach of systematizing capital expenditures. For example, suppose that each nursing station has a refrigerator. The refrigerators can be added to the capital budget proposal (see Figure 10-1) when they break down. That is an unfortunate approach because it will result in a nursing station's being without a working refrigerator for a number of months or in an unexpected and unbudgeted expenditure for a new refrigerator. An alternative to this would be a formalized approach to generating capital budget proposals.

Basically, such a formalized approach requires managers to maintain a list of all capital items for which they are responsible. If a nurse manager is responsible for 15 refrigerators, among other capital items, a plan should be established. The plan may be to replace all 15 refrigerators every fifteenth year. If one assumes that most refrigerators will last between 14 and 18 years, this may be a reasonable approach. One problem with this approach is that it places the entire cash outflow in a single year. An alternative would be a staggered system, in which one refrigerator is replaced every year. The cash flow to buy refrigerators will remain pretty much the same each year, and equipment will not be getting very old because the organization is constantly replacing the older items. On the other hand, the organization will not get volume discount if it buys just one refrigerator each year.

Whichever approach is taken, listing all capital items will draw attention to the replacement of many routine items before they wear out and break down. To generate all appropriate capital proposals, managers should go beyond simply listing the items and showing their projected replacement date. Managers should think about and encourage all nurses in their departments to consider the following: Is the cost of care too high? Is there something we could do to reduce the cost of care? Is the quality of care acceptable? What could be done to improve the quality of care? Is the capacity adequate?

Many of the suggestions that result from those questions impact both the operating budget and the capital budget. There is a tendency for individuals to complain that things are not done the way they should be done. Having a mechanism for suggestions can result in benefits in several ways. First, it lets individuals get the complaints off their chests, which makes them feel better. Second, if changes are instituted, the nurses will be happier because they will not have to put up with whatever they were complaining about. Third, they will tend to be more motivated in their work if they are in a responsive environment. Finally, the suggestions will help the organization run more efficiently and provide higher quality, more cost-effective care.

A number of proposals will be generated through this overall process. For nonfinancial managers, the difficult issues of capital budgeting rarely concern the generation of capital investment proposals. Such proposals will be generated. The key issue is whether the proposals merit the investments. It is the evaluation of the proposals that poses the most difficult problems.

■ EVALUATION OF CAPITAL BUDGET PROPOSALS

The evaluation of capital budget proposals is commonly carried out by financial managers. However, it is useful for nurse managers to understand the elements of the evaluation process. Such an understanding provides the nurse manager with additional insights into the capital budget process. This in turn helps nurse managers prepare capital budget proposals, including strong supporting justifications for the expenditures.

Data Generation

The first step in the evaluation process is to collect data about the project. Specifically, information must be collected about how much cash will be spent or received each year over the life of the investment or project. The difference between the cash received and the cash spent in any given year will be referred to as the *net cash flow* for that year.

The typical capital investment has a negative net cash flow in the first year or several years because more money is spent on the acquisition than is being received from its use. The cash flow often becomes positive in subsequent years.

Nurse managers can generally seek the aid of financial managers of the organization for the specific estimates of cash inflows and outflows. Cash inflows can be particularly difficult because the entire billing process is normally handled outside of the control of nurse managers. On the other hand, with respect to estimating costs, a nurse manager is more likely than any financial manager to be able to estimate what resources will be needed and when. The payroll and purchasing departments are great aids in converting the raw resource information into dollars based on projected salaries and prices. This estimating process should be done separately for each year in which the capital asset is expected to provide useful service.

It is not adequate simply to estimate the total amount to be spent and the total receipts over the lifetime of the investment. This ignores something called the *time value of money*. The time at which cash is received or spent is just as important as how much is received or spent. For example, suppose that the organization is considering two alternative investments in photocopy equipment for the Department of Nursing Services. Both projects require a total cost of $10,000 for the machine, and both will have identical copying capabilities. It seems that the two offers are identical.

Suppose, however, that the organization has to pay $10,000 for one machine at the time of purchase, but the other offer is an installment purchase requiring five annual installments of $2,000 each. If the organization were to accept the first alternative, its expenditure would be $10,000, all in the first year. If the machine has a 5-year life expectancy, then the operating budget for each of the next 5 years would include a prorated depreciation cost of $2,000. If it goes with the second alternative, paying installments of $2,000 per year, the operating budget will again show a $2,000 cost for each of the next 5 years. Are the alternatives equal?

The answer is definitely and emphatically no! In the case of the first project, all $10,000 is paid at the start. In the second project, only $2,000 is paid immediately, allowing the organization to hold onto the other $8,000. This $8,000 can be invested in interest-bearing savings accounts. Each year when it's time for the next payment, the organization will be able to keep the interest earned. This interest can be spent on more capital assets or perhaps on nursing staff increases. Clearly, the organization is better off if it can hold onto most of the $10,000 and pay for the photocopy machine gradually over time. This is a carryover from the philosophy of program budgeting—capital budgets should examine alternatives and their trade-offs. It is not enough simply to evaluate whether the department can afford a photocopy machine. Capital budgeting should examine alternative machines and alternative payment plans, such as buying outright versus installment purchase. When the payments occur is critical to the outcome of the analysis.

In estimating the cash flows, care must also be taken to include relevant and exclude irrelevant cash flows. For example, if the organization is a *proprietary* (for-profit) concern, it should consider the impact of any investment on income taxes. It may well be that two different investments, both providing the same health care services, will have totally different tax implications. In the photocopy machine example, suppose that there were a third alternative: to lease the machine for 5 years. There are a number of tax laws aimed specifically at the issue of leasing. It may well turn out that, depending on the organization's specific situation, there are significant tax benefits when the equipment is leased rather than purchased, or vice versa. If the tax consequences of a capital investment are ignored, the manager might select the wrong alternative.

It is important to note that the relevant cash flows concerning a project are the *incremental* cash flows. "Incremental" refers to the amount by which the organization's cash flow would change if the project is undertaken versus if it is not undertaken. The incremental flows are the changes in the total amounts received and the changes in the total amounts spent because of the acquisition of the capital asset.

If the manager is trying to determine the cost of adding a new piece of equipment, it is necessary to include in the incremental costs the purchase cost of the equipment and of any additional supplies and labor needed. If the equipment uses a lot of electricity, that cost should be included as well. Suppose, however, that if the equipment is acquired, administrative overhead will be assigned to that equipment through the cost allocation process. For example, a portion of the salary of the organization's chief executive officer might be allocated to the unit. This is an irrelevant cost in deciding whether to purchase the equipment. This cost will be incurred by the organization whether it buys the equipment or not. Even though the organization's accountants may assign some of that administrative cost to the unit using the equipment, the cost should not be included when determining whether the organization should acquire the equipment. The manager must be able to determine whether the added costs of having the new equipment can be covered by the added revenues. The organization will incur the administrator's salary cost in any case; it should not require the new equipment to bear a share of that cost as a prerequisite for approving the acquisition.

The other side of the coin is that all incremental costs should be considered. For instance, suppose that several nurses will be needed to care for patients treated by the equipment. Suppose further that the equipment is used only during the day and that the nurses using the equipment are paid regular daytime wages. Because of shortages of available nurses, however, assigning nurses to work with patients using this equipment results in an increase in overtime for nurses elsewhere in the hospital. Without the machine, the hospital would not have had to pay those overtime costs. In this case, even though the nurses directly working with the equipment are not collecting overtime, the additional overtime costs incurred by the hospital should be considered a part of the operating costs of the proposed investment in the machine.

Sometimes the incremental costs may be indirect. Consider the home health agency that wants to buy cars for several of its nurse employees so that time spent waiting for public transit can be spent on more visits to patients. Politically, the purchase of cars for some of the nurses may mean that an agency car will have to be acquired for at least the chief executive officer of the agency and perhaps several other top-level managers as well. If so, the decision of whether to acquire cars for the nurses or home aides must include all the cars that otherwise would not have been purchased, even those that are not directly used to improve service to the patients.

Choosing Among Capital Assets

Item Justification

A justification must clearly state the reasons the manager wishes to acquire the item. It should identify the benefits the organization will realize from the purchase, and it should also identify consequences of failure to purchase the equipment. Finally, if the manager recommends purchasing from a supplier whose bid was not the lowest, there should be a justification for selecting that vendor over the vendor who submitted the lowest bid.

A justification should explain clearly and concisely why the item is needed. A justification specifies the benefits to the organization from acquisition of the item and consequences for the organization if the item is not acquired. For example, the average age of nurses was 38 in 1985. In 2010 it will be 45 (Bliss, 2005). This means many working nurses are in their 50s and 60s. Therefore, lifting patients carries a much higher risk for injury to employees today than it did when the average age of hospital nurses was much younger. Furthermore, the cost of treating an on-the-job injury is much greater than it used to be. Therefore, the justification for acquiring lifting equipment will be to avoid injuries to employees and the costs related to such injuries.

Sufficient resources are not usually available to allow an organization to acquire all the items it desires. The capital budget facilitates choices that have to be made in the allocation of the organization's resources. It is appropriate to justify each requested purchase by giving a description of the item, its cost, its impact on operating expenses and revenues, and the justification for acquiring it. Figure 10-2 provides an example of a justification for a capital asset acquisition.

The justification should be thorough and should specifically indicate the consequences if funding for the item is not made available. Equipment costs include not only purchase price but also shipping, installation, and employee training. Construction costs should be reviewed by the planning and engineering departments. In all cases, vendor estimates or proposals should be included if possible. The impact on operating costs should include salaries, fringe benefit costs, maintenance costs or maintenance contracts, utilities, supplies, and any interdepartmental impacts. Incremental revenue to be generated by the capital asset, if any, should be described and estimated to the greatest extent possible.

The capital budgets for all departments are evaluated in light of available cash. An investment that seems to make a lot of sense to a clinical department manager may have to be deferred for a year or indefinitely, simply because the organization does not have enough cash to make the purchase. Cash budgeting is discussed in Chapter 12.

In choosing among alternative capital proposals or even in evaluating just one proposed item, managers need to determine whether the amount of money to be spent is justified by the anticipated economic return. Decision making can be substantially improved by having a system for evaluating capital acquisitions that considers the economic ramifications of the decision. Rational decision making calls for formalized, systematic, quantifiable evaluation. Such evaluation must consider not only the financial impact of decisions but also the clinical impact. The overall goals of providing medical services call for providing high-quality care; this must be a critical element in the manager's thinking. Unfortunately, quality of health care is not easily measured.

Priority Rating_____

CAPITAL EQUIPMENT BUDGET ITEM JUSTIFICATION FORM

Department_____ Date_____

Requesting Dept. Manager_____ Extension_____

Equipment or Construction Requested (Name & Description):_____

Vendor List:_____

Need/Justification Category:

☐ *Equipment Request*	☐ *Construction Request*
☐ Routine Replacement	☐ Upgrade in Styling/Comfort of Patient Care Area
☐ Non-Routine Replacement	☐ Needed to Improve Patient Safety
☐ New Standard of Care Requirement	☐ Needed to Improve Patient Care Quality
☐ Required to Implement New Program	☐ Needed to Improve Employee Comfort
☐ Will Increase Profits from Service	☐ Needed to Improve Employee Safety
☐ Upgrade in Styling/Comfort of staff, Patient or Visitor Area	☐ Upgrade in Employee Work or Break Area
☐ Upgrade Safety of Visitor Area	☐ Physician Recruitment Agreement Item
☐ Regulatory Requirement	☐ Additional Patient Care Services Request
☐ New inventory (reg. req.)	☐ New Clinical Service
☐ Additional inventory (reg. req.)	☐ Expanded Clinical Service
☐ Replacement Inventory (reg. req.)	
☐ Other (please explain)	☐ Other (please explain)

Need Justification Narrative:

_____
_____
_____
_____
_____

Purchase Cost Information	Performance Cost Information (Annual)
Equipment Purchase Cost:	Personnel Cost:
Number of Units:	Supplies Cost:
Delivery/Installation Costs:	Service Contract:
Training Costs:	Utilities Cost:
Other Acquisition Costs:	Annual Lease Cost:
OR Construction Contract/ Fees Amount:	Other Annual Costs:
Total Start–Up Costs:	Total Annual Performance Cost:

Acquisition Recommendation	☐ Purchase	☐ Lease

Figure 10-2 Capital justification form.

The dilemma of achieving high quality at low cost is not one that can be solved easily. Neither economists and accountants nor health care providers have found a way to reconcile completely the costs of investments with both the dollar revenues the investments generate and the improved quality benefits. Certainly, if an investment will improve quality and generate adequate revenues to cover its cost, there is no problem. Difficulty arises if the costs of an investment exceed the potential dollar revenues, but there are quality-of-care issues that make the investment desirable. Does the organization go ahead with the investment or not?

There is no easy answer to this question. One thing became clear in the 1980s; the tremendous growth of the health care sector put serious strains on the national economy. As a result, throughout the 1990s, more and more pressure was put on the health care sector to slow its cost increases. This pressure continues today. Therefore, it is likely that there are going to be severe limits on the total revenues available to health care organizations. Health care organizations will not be able to afford to make investment decisions based solely on the informal knowledge that the investment will improve quality. That approach, which has been a common one in the health sector, will start to threaten the survival of many health care institutions. The increasing prominence of managed care will exacerbate this situation.

At the other extreme, it must be recognized that traditionally, organizational politics has had a great deal to do with acquiring capital assets. Often, the decisions have not been made on the basis of economic analysis, financial return on money invested, or even the impact on quality care. Decisions have been made on the basis of political clout. This can be a significant factor in the perioperative area where politically powerful surgeons may influence capital budget decisions. Although it is true that some capital items are necessary because they allow for less invasive surgery or have other benefits that make their use the new standard of care, occasionally surgeons will want items listed as first priority that should be lower on the priority list. This is where the justification for the purchase becomes helpful. It may assist decision makers to differentiate between "I want this very badly" and "We cannot continue doing business without this item." It will be impossible to remove politics entirely from the process. However, requiring the person requesting the item to provide clear justification for its purchase is the first step toward controlling inappropriate political influence. Decision makers can use the justifications as the foundation of a more formal evaluative process for capital budget expenditures.

Item Prioritization

The organization's capital expense request form should offer the manager a way to prioritize equipment requests. The best way to accomplish this is to have a standardized priority rating system so that the administration knows which equipment is wanted the most. Obviously, if a manager marks all requests with the highest priority, the manager's failure to discriminate in importance among the requests may affect that manager's annual evaluation and may result in administrators' selecting a dollar amount and approving the largest number of requests that fit the limit, rather than choosing the items the manager wants most. This is not an optimal way to make capital equipment purchase decisions.

There are two types of prioritization schemes. The first simply asks the manager to prioritize the budget requests for the department from 1 to n, with n representing the total number of budget items requested by the department. The advantage of this system is that it makes clear the ordering of items' importance to the department. Also, if one department has a particularly high contribution to the organization's financial well being, that department can easily be prioritized, and more of its capital requests may be approved than another department's. Because the ratings are local to the department and not standardized across the organization, this system tends to generate somewhat less controversy when one department's requests must be favored over other departments' requests. The three disadvantages of this scheme are that: (1) it provides little or no information about how critical each item is to the operation of the department or to the organization as a whole; (2) it provides no information to guide decision makers in deciding which items across all departments to approve; and (3) it is somewhat more subject to institutional politics than the second rating system.

The second scheme provides a standardized priority rating system, and the manager rates each item according to that system. Because the rating system is used throughout the organization, all items' ratings are relevant to a single standard, and the importance of items requested by different departments can be directly compared. In addition, the priority rating system forces the manager to use a relatively objective standard for prioritizing capital budget items. And this system is somewhat less vulnerable to politics than the first system. The disadvantage is that decision makers may have to approve requests by departments that make abundant contributions to the financial well-being of the organization rather than approving higher priority items requested by departments that make less of a financial contribution to the organization, and this system may make that reality more politically difficult to deal with. Given the tight budgets of most health care organizations, decision makers often need to prioritize capital budget requests, at least to some degree, according to how critical the requesting department is to the organization's financial well-being. Another disadvantage to this system is that it does not provide information about which item is most important to the department if there are two or more items with the same priority rating. Finally, because this system is somewhat less vulnerable to political pressures (although no system is free from those influences), failure to approve requests of politically powerful individuals can cause other problems in the organization.

Prioritization schemes usually list issues that are most important to the organization such as those shown in Table 10-1. Managers should be provided with training or a manual on how to apply the definitions.

This is just one example of a possible priority rating scale. Many others with different numbers of priority ratings and different definitions exist. It is important that the ratings clearly differentiate among the importance levels of the requests, and that clear definitions and examples be provided to the managers who generate the capital requests. The managers will still have to exercise judgment in selecting a priority rating for a request; however, the organization should provide explanations and examples that assist the managers in appropriately prioritizing each request.

Obtain Competitive Bids

If a manager orders supplies, it is assumed that the manager of the purchasing department "shops around" and finds the best price. In many larger facilities, the purchasing department manager has contracted with a single business-supply company. The facility agrees to use only that supplier in exchange for discounted prices on supplies, office equipment, and/or furniture. Many capital equipment items are covered under that contract, so bids are unnecessary because only that supplier may be used to purchase the items. Other types of capital acquisitions are not available from the contract supplier, and still others cannot be purchased off-the-shelf. New clinical information systems, buildings, and remodeling projects are among the types of capital purchases that are unique and so cannot be bought off-the-shelf. How can one be sure to get the best price for these unique items? Generally, it will be necessary to get multiple bids for these types of capital items.

The organization might have a policy that any item that will last more than 1 year and cost more than $1,000 must be included in the capital budget. The item

TABLE 10-1 Example of a Priority Rating Scale

Priority Rating	Rating Definition
1	Requested item is essential to continued operation of department.
2	Requested item has potential for high return on investment.
3	Requested item will significantly increase efficiency, safety, and/or profitability of department operations.
4	Requested item will improve quality of environment or employee morale or will pay for itself within 2 to 3 years and has an expected service life of 5 years or more.
5	Requested item will replace or upgrade existing equipment or décor, including scheduled replacement program items.

Instructions for Use of Priority Ratings

1. Use this priority rating only for equipment or construction mandated by regulatory or accreditation agencies, and without which the department or an essential service in the department will have to be shut down. For example, the justification for this priority rating would be of the following nature: "The physiologic monitors in SICU need frequent repair and the service person tells us that parts will no longer be available after this year; so he will not be able to maintain their operability after this year. An SICU cannot legally be operated without physiologic monitors at every bed."

2. Use this priority rating for items that will generate sufficient revenue to pay for themselves within 1 year and will continue to generate revenues for at least 4 more years. Profits generated must be in excess of $1,000 per month after the item has paid for itself. For example, the justification for using this priority rating would be of the following nature: "Demand for MRI services has reached the point at which some less urgent scans are being sent to another facility, thus losing profits. A second MRI scanner will generate sufficient profits to pay the purchase price in 8 months, after which it will generate excess revenue over expenses of approximately $18,500 per month." Or, "The new patient lift will reduce the incidence of employee back injuries. The average workmen's compensation cost for one back injury is now $20,000, and the department averages three back injuries a year. The lift costs $22,000 and has an expected life of 10 years. Thus, it is expected to pay for itself the first year by resulting in 3 fewer back injuries."

3. Use this priority rating for items that are designed to improve employee safety, or will significantly improve the quality of the environment for employees and/or visitors, or will generate sufficient revenue to pay for themselves within 2 to 3 years, and are both unlikely to become obsolete in less than 5 years, and have an expected service life of at least 5 years so that they will eventually provide a positive return on investment. For example, the justification for using this priority rating would be of the following nature: "Purchase of this item will allow the cosmetic surgeon to start providing face-lift surgery at this hospital instead of taking his patients to a competing hospital 40 miles away. Start-up expenses will be recovered in the first year. In subsequent years, the average profit to the hospital for this prepaid elective procedure will be $5,000 per case." Or "Purchase of this bed will reduce the development of pressure ulcers in comatose patients by 90%. The reduction in prolonged length of stay due to decubitus formation will produce savings that will pay for the bed in 3 years. Because the expected life of the bed is 5 years, this item will not only produce greater patient safety but should also provide a small return on investment in the fourth and fifth years."

4. Use this priority rating for items that will improve the attractiveness of the facility to patients and visitors or will permit the department to offer a new service that will provide limited return on investment or that will positively impact employee morale. For example, the justification for using this priority rating would be of the following nature: "This renovation of the ICU family waiting area will significantly improve the comfort of the area by providing space for amenities such as couches, free coffee, a TV and a magazine rack, and will provide a small side room for vending machines for soft drinks, sandwiches, and fruit. These items will greatly improve visitor comfort, especially at times the cafeteria is closed. Additionally, it will add a small conference room where families can have privacy during consultations about the patient with physicians and nurses."

5. Use this priority rating for planned replacement of major items that are currently functioning, but that should be replaced on a regular basis to prevent downtime resulting from sudden failure due to age. Also use this category for upgrading equipment and for renovations that will improve the appearance of the facility in the eyes of patients and visitors and thus make the facility more attractive to customers. For example, the justification for using this priority rating would be of the following nature: "The chairs in the Obstetric Department waiting room have generated complaints by visitors who have indicated that the chairs are uncomfortable. Because the current trend is toward more family members coming to the hospital during labor and delivery, and only two family members or labor coaches are permitted in the room at a time, the waiting room is experiencing more use and is being used for longer periods of time by family members. More comfortable chairs are expected to reduce complaints generated by the discomfort of those in the waiting area."

must be justified and prioritized. Will it be necessary to get multiple bids for each item? No. It is time-consuming and costly to obtain bids. Generally, bids are obtained only for particularly expensive items.

For example, the organization's policy may be that any acquisition with a cost greater than $5,000 requires bids if its acquisition is not governed by a prior institutional purchase contract. That will ensure that the best price is obtained, all things considered. "All things considered" means that the lowest bid is not always selected. There may be other factors, such as better quality of care, a supplier's better service record, a more stable supplier company, or other considerations that will influence the ultimate decision.

The process of obtaining bids may be simple, as with the purchase of refrigerators or other items that the contracted business-supply company does not carry. Or it may be a very complex process requiring specification of the item's functionality or design, as with construction projects and major information system purchases. In most cases, the manager—together with staff and perhaps consultants—specifies the essential functions the capital item must provide. The product specifications may have to be quite detailed and may take considerable effort on the part of the organization to develop. For some items, the institution will have to work with vendors, architects, or designers to prepare realistic specifications. The specifications are critical to the success of the project because they serve as a sort of order form for the vendor or builder. And if the item must be built for the organization, those specifications serve as a blueprint for the vendors to use in generating their bids. The bid price will be honored by the vendor only to the extent that the specifications provided by the customer are complete and accurate blueprints of the desired product. If the organization decides it must add to the specifications after a bid has been accepted and a contract signed, the price may rise significantly beyond what was budgeted. An old rule of thumb in information systems planning is that an entire project should be broken down as follows: 90% planning, 10% implementing. This is usually correct in terms of the amount of time spent in each part of the process. To cut the planning time short is to risk costs spiraling out of control during construction or implementation.

The number of bids required is a variable across institutions, and within a single organization there may be varying rules about how many bids are necessary, depending on the scope of the capital project. For items that can be purchased off-the-shelf and need little or no customization, the manager may be asked to obtain two or three bids. For large-scale building projects, it is not unusual to have an open bidding process in which any interested contractor may be allowed to bid on the project. The number of bids is generally not as important as ensuring that the bidding process is fair to all vendors. If it is suspected by vendors that one vendor is almost certainly going to get the contract, other vendors won't waste time bidding, and the favored vendor will be free to quote almost any price. The purpose of requesting bids is to give vendors an incentive to discount the capital item as deeply as possible while still providing a product that meets specifications. For that goal to be realized, the bidding process must be fair.

Project Evaluation

Health care organizations often use formal mechanics of project evaluation that parallel the capital budgeting methodology used in the vast majority of proprietary industries. These formal methods provide the economic basis for capital budgeting decisions. They are described in the Appendix at the end of this chapter.

This use of formalized, quantitative approaches to capital investment evaluation should not and does not rule out decisions that ultimately defy the economic results. The formal modeling of capital budgeting is mechanical. The methods described in the Appendix to this chapter are sophisticated mathematical approaches capable of providing precise predictions about the economic viability of an investment. Finance officers use these methods by applying them to the capital budget proposals that nurse managers develop and to the data for evaluation that nurse managers generate. However, as with most mathematical models, these methods are totally devoid of judgment and incapable of addressing the human impact of a decision. They look only at dollars and cents.

As the nurse manager, you are responsible for contributing common sense to the decision. Never accept a model's result as a dictate. Consider it only as advice. The formal approaches of capital budgeting can advise you regarding the strict economics of an investment. As a manager, you must take all factors into account when making a final decision regarding an investment. And given the rapid pace of advances in health care science, sometimes capital items must be purchased even though they won't "pay their way" because without them, the facility cannot provide an acceptable standard of care. For example, the new surgical technology that allows for much less invasive surgery is costly, but actually reduces the time in the OR, the need for care in the intensive care unit after the procedure, and may even change an inpatient procedure into an outpatient procedure. This kind of technology may ultimately reduce the hospital's profit from the procedure because of the lower revenue that results from fewer hospitalization days and less time in the OR. Nonetheless, patients must be provided with care that is the local (and often national) standard or the hospital will lose its Medicare certification, and other insurers will not contract with a hospital that is providing care that is more costly, has higher complication rates and recovery time, and causes patient dissatisfaction. Thus, formal models must be tempered with the knowledge of the facility's physicians, nurse leaders, financial managers, and administrators.

What the formal model can accomplish, however, is formal recognition of trade-offs. If the organization decides to make an investment even though the long-run prospect is a loss of money, that decision clarifies two issues. First, there is recognition that a loss will occur and that the organization is willing to bear that loss to gain some qualitative benefit for the organization or its patients. Second, there must be recognition that a profit will have to be earned elsewhere to offset that loss. Without the availability of a profit elsewhere, going ahead with a losing project may be suicidal to the continued existence of the organization.

Even long-term financial suicide may be deemed to be a better outcome than providing inferior care. This is a decision that the management of the organization must make. By combining capital budgeting efforts by clinical managers with modeling by finance, one can determine the likely impacts of making the investment. It is then up to the clinical managers to work together with top management to arrive at decisions that are, in the long run, in the best interests of the organization, its patients, and its employees.

Summary and Implications for Nurse Managers

Capital budgeting refers to planning for the acquisition of resources that are useful beyond the year in which they are purchased. Such capital items require special attention because they usually cannot generate enough revenue in the year in which they are acquired to appear to be financially feasible.

Because they generate revenues over a period of years, their costs should be allocated over a similar period of years. This requires evaluation of the acquisition in a separate plan, called a capital budget. Each year's share of the total cost of a capital asset is allocated to the operating budget for that year in the form of a depreciation charge.

To determine whether the organization can afford the item or project, revenues and expenses must be compared over the lifetime of the asset. Operating budgets focus only on the portion of revenues and expenses that relate to 1 year. It is the role of capital budgeting to examine the long-term financial implications of resources with multiyear lives. Many capital items do not generate any revenue. The costs of these items should also be spread over their useful lifetimes in order to understand the implications of the spending.

Capital budgets evaluate the impact of resources over long periods of time. Because of this, the money spent on the resources cannot be compared directly with the revenues received from using the resource. Dollars earned in the future are not worth as much as dollars spent today because of the time value of money. That is, the money spent on a capital asset could have been earning interest. The revenues received from the project should be great enough to cover that interest cost as well as to return the amount invested. Present value methods allowing the comparison of future amounts to present amounts are available and are discussed in the Appendix to this chapter.

The first step in capital budgeting is to generate proposals for capital acquisitions. The next step is to collect cash-flow information, detailing the amount and timing of cash receipts and cash payments. The final step is to evaluate the cash receipts and payments. Although this should be done using the formalized approaches of analysis discussed in the Appendix, it is also critical to keep in mind that only a clinical manager can have a full perspective on the actual benefits to be received from an investment. Often, these benefits are related to patient care rather than being profit oriented. It is vital that nurse managers consider the financial implications of their proposals, and it is also vital that health care managers consider noneconomic issues such as impact on quality of care.

It may be in the interest of the organization to sacrifice some economic benefits for increased noneconomic benefits. It is important to bear in mind that capital budgeting techniques are merely tools. The economic implications of decisions must be known, but decisions do not have to be made solely on the basis of economics.

In the cases where a proposal is found to fail on the grounds of economic merit, the nurse manager has two potential choices. One choice is to decide that the capital item is not important enough to fight for if it is not economically advantageous for the institution. The other choice is to decide that the purchase is in fact vital and worth fighting for. In that case, the nurse manager should be prepared to offer a clear statement concerning the benefits to be gained from the investment as well as why the cost is outweighed by the non-economic benefits of the item.

References and Suggested Readings

Anderson, J.R., George, H.W., Perrin, R.A. (1991). Capital equipment management planning and control. *Journal of Healthcare Material Management.* 9(4), 24, 26, 28.

Anonymous. (2006). Capital planning: How strategic is your organization? (HCFM Roundtable). *Healthcare Financial Management.* 60(7), 1-4.

Bliss, M. (2005). Average age of nurses increases. *Southeast Missourian,* October 29, 2005. Downloaded on April 7, 2007 from: http://www.semissourian.com/story/1123934.html

Cleverley, W.O., Cameron, A. (2002). *Essentials of Health Care Finance,* ed 5. Sudbury, MA: Jones and Bartlett.

Gapenski, L.C. (1997). *Financial Analysis and Decision Making for Healthcare Organizations: A Guide for the Healthcare Professional.* Chicago: Irwin Professional.

Hardy, P. (2004). Getting a return on investment from spending capital dollars on new beds. *Journal of Healthcare Management.* 49(3), 199-205.

Haugh, R. (2003). Access to capital: Fund-raising's rough turn. *Hospitals & Health Networks.* 77(8), 33.

Healy, W. (2006). Gainsharing: A primer for orthopaedic surgeons. *Journal of Bone and Joint Surgery.* 88(A8), 1880-1887.

Hogan, A.J. (1987). Capital expenditure planning: The value of information to hospitals. *Hospital & Health Services Administration.* 32(1), 21-37.

Krupka, D., Sandberg, W. (2006). Operating room design and its impact on operating room economics. *Current Opinion in Anesthesiology.* 19(2), 185-191.

Lanser, E. (2001). Procuring capital equipment. *Healthcare Executive.* 16(2), 46-48.

Liechter, S. (2004). Capital equipment invest- ments in diabetes care. *Clinical Diabetes.* 22(1), 5-7.

Magiera, F.T., McLean, R.A. (1996). Strategic options in capital budgeting and program selection under fee-for-service and managed care. *Health Care Management Review.* 21(4), 7-17.

Pelfrey, S. (1991). Financial techniques for evaluating equipment acquisitions. *Journal of Nursing Administration.* 21(3), 15-20.

Peterson, P., Fabozzi, F. (2002). *Capital Budgeting.* New York: Wiley.

Pols, A. (1999). Negotiating optimum capital equipment acquisitions. *Healthcare Financial Management.* 53(6), 66-67.

Rosen, L. (2004). Capital purchasing problems. *Hospitals & Health Networks.* 78(8), 14.

Tonges, M., Baloga-Altieri, B., Atzori, M. (2004). Amplifying nursing's voice through a staff–management partnership. *Journal of Nursing Administration.* 34(3), 134-139.

Appendix to Chapter 10
Quantitative Methods for Capital Budgeting

LEARNING OBJECTIVES
The goals of this technical appendix are to:

- Provide specific techniques for evaluating capital budget proposals
- Explain time value of money in detail
- Describe discounted cash flow analysis
- Discuss time value of money calculation mechanics
- Discuss the role of profits in not-for-profit health care organizations

Several different models for capital budgeting are discussed in this Appendix. They are the payback approach, the present cost approach, the net present value approach, and the internal rate of return approach. Capital budgeting often takes the perspective that current expenditures are offset by future cash receipts. The heart of the analysis is whether the future cash receipts are great enough to justify the current outlays financially. This Appendix also recognizes that in health care, many capital acquisitions cannot be matched directly against future revenues. Therefore, a part of the following discussion revolves around outlays for alternative capital items aimed at accomplishing a particular goal. Methods are presented for determining the least costly approach.

■ THE PAYBACK APPROACH

Once all the appropriate cash receipts and cash expenditures have been estimated, the payback approach can be used as a quick-and-dirty estimate of whether the project is financially feasible. The payback approach evaluates how long it will be before the organization receives an amount of cash receipts from the investment that equals the amount of cash put into the investment.

As short a payback period as possible is preferred. For example, if the organization invests $1,000 today and gets cash receipts of $300 in the first year, $700 in the second year, and $500 in the third year, the payback period would be 2 years. On the other hand, if the cash receipts were $200, $400, and $900 for the 3 years, respectively, the payback period would be 3 years. Although the total amount received is $1,500 in both cases, the organization has recovered its $1,000 investment during the second year in the first case but not until the third year in the second case.

There is some intuitive appeal to this approach. The longer the organization has to wait before it recovers the amount it has invested, the more risky the investment. If the organization has to wait many years until it breaks even on an investment, there is the risk that something may happen that was not anticipated. Although some investments are not very risky (e.g., a refrigerator for the nurses' station), technological obsolescence is a common problem in health care that creates significant risk. With any medical equipment, there is the risk that it will have to be replaced before it wears out.

This problem is an especially difficult one because often it is not possible to predict technological change accurately. If the organization knows that a piece of medical equipment could last for 10 years but will be obsolete in 5 years, then it can just anticipate that it will have a 5-year life. But if it anticipates a 5-year life and the equipment becomes obsolete in 3 years, there will be a problem. Therefore, investments that quickly pay back the initial invested amount are relatively safer.

The payback method does have some severe weaknesses, however. The problems with the payback method are that it ignores what happens after the payback period is over, and it ignores the time value of money (TVM). Suppose that one machine would last for 10 years whereas another machine would last for only 5 years. Suppose further that the price for the latter machine is slightly lower. It may well be that the second machine will have a shorter payback period because of its lower price. The first machine, however, will continue to be useful for an extra 5 years. The payback approach is so concerned with risks over time that it pays relatively little attention to the future and ignores events after the payback period.

Further, the timing of payments within the payback period is not of particular concern under this method. Suppose that the organization spends $1,000 to acquire a piece of equipment, and under one alternative it receives $100 in the first year, $100 in the second year, and $800 in the third year. Under another alternative it still spends $1,000 to acquire the equipment, but it receives $800 in the first year, $100 in the second year, and $100 in the third year. According to the payback method, these two alternatives are equal.

In fact, they are not equal. Because it allows for the receiving of $800 in the first year, the second alternative is superior. In the first year, the second alternative returns $700 more than is provided under the first alternative. That $700 can be put in the bank to earn interest in the 2 intervening years.

Suppose further that the first alternative made payments of $100, $100, and $800 for the 3 years, as described. Now suppose that the second alternative made payments of $800, $100, $99, and $1 over a 4-year period. The first alternative would be deemed to be superior because it has a shorter payback period, 3 years as opposed to 4 years. Yet considering the interest earned on the $800 received in the first year under the second alternative, the organization is better off under the second than under the first method, even though the payback is longer.

These problems are serious. As a result, the payback method is often used for a first appraisal—a quick-and-dirty evaluation of the project. If a proposed investment cannot pay back its cost within a reasonable period—certainly not longer than the useful life of the investment—on strictly economic grounds, it should be rejected (although it may be accepted anyway because of qualitative merits). If an investment passes the payback test, more sophisticated evaluation is still needed to determine whether a specific proposal is acceptable or to help select among alternatives.

■ THE TIME VALUE OF MONEY (TVM)

The three remaining approaches for evaluating capital budgeting proposals require formal acknowledgment of the implications of the TVM. Money paid or received at different points in time is not equally valuable. One would always prefer to receive money sooner and pay it later. By receiving money sooner, one can use the money for current needs or can invest it. If the money is used for current needs, less money will have to be borrowed from the bank, and the organization can avoid interest payments. If the organization already has enough money so that it does not have to borrow from banks, it can invest the money in an interest-bearing account. Either way, by paying money later or receiving it sooner, the organization is financially better off. It can either earn interest or avoid having to borrow money and pay interest.

In its simplest form, there does not appear to be much of a problem with the TVM. If the organization receives a $100 payment from a patient today, it is better off than if it does not receive that payment for a year. At the very least, it could put the money in a bank account earning 5% interest. At the end of the year it would have $105 rather than $100.

Therefore, when a nurse manager looks at alternative investment opportunities, there must be consideration not only of how much the organization will put in and how much it will get out but also of when the money will be spent and received. For example, if a nursing unit invests $100 in a new machine and receives $155 over its 5-year lifetime, is it financially better off or worse off than if it had put the money into a 5-year bank account with 10% interest?

That happens to be a complex question, much more so than it may appear to be on the surface. The money invested in the bank earns 10% interest, and 10% of $100 is $10. For 5 years, one may think that the organization would earn five times $10, or a total of $50 in interest. In that case it would have $150 from the bank versus $155 if it bought the machine. But that is not correct. The money in the bank will earn 10% *compound interest*. Most banks compound interest at least once a year and often more frequently than that. Compounding means that the amount of interest that is earned during each compounding period is calculated and added to the initial amount. In the subsequent periods, interest is earned not only on the initial investment but also on any interest previously earned.

In this example, assuming compounding once a year, $10 in interest on the $100 invested in the bank account would be earned by the end of the first year. At that point there will be $110 in the bank—the original investment plus the interest earned. During the second year, the interest earned will be 10% of $110, or $11. During the third year, the interest earned will be 10% of $121 (the $110 from the beginning of the second year plus the $11 interest earned in the second year). By the end of 5 years, the bank account will have $161. In this case, it appears that from a strictly financial view, keeping the money in the bank is better than buying the machine after all.

However, this is not necessarily true. As was noted earlier, this is a complex problem. If the $155 from the use of the machine is received at the end of the fifth year, the bank investment is better, but if that $155 is received during the 5 years, some of it will be available to be invested in another project or in a bank and thus will earn additional receipts. The timing of cash receipts is crucial. As you can imagine, this makes for some complex calculations. The next section discusses these calculations.

■ DISCOUNTED CASH FLOW APPROACHES

The more sophisticated approaches to capital budgeting take into account the TVM. Such methods are referred to as discounted cash flow models. *Discounting* is the reverse of compounding of interest. Today, $100 would be worth $161 in 5 years with 10% compound interest, as noted earlier. In just the reverse process, $161 received 5 years from now would be worth just $100 today if one were to discount the interest earned in the 5 intervening years. Discounted cash flow techniques are designed to take future cash flows and discount the interest to find out what those flows would be worth today. The cash inflows and outflows can then be compared to cash outlays today to determine whether a project is worthwhile financially.

The two most common discounted cash flow models are *net present value* and *internal rate of return*. Before these specific models can be discussed, it is necessary to delve more deeply into the mechanics of calculating the TVM.

Suppose that two investments are being considered. One investment requires an outlay of $10,000 today; the other requires an outlay of only $7,500. Over the life of the investment, the operating costs will be $3,000 per year for 5 years for the first alternative but $3,600 per year for the second alternative over the same 5 years. This might be the situation for the purchase of several air conditioners. Which alternative is less expensive?

Note that there is no revenue in this example. Often in health care, the focus is on cost-efficient ways to accomplish an objective. In this case, different types of air conditioners are being compared. Over the 5-year life of the air conditioners, the organization will have spent $10,000 plus $3,000 per year for 5 years, or a total of $25,000 for the first alternative. The second type of air conditioner is less expensive to buy but is not as fuel efficient. It will cost $7,500 plus $3,600 per year for 5 years, or a total of $25,500. Which alternative is cheaper? The first project requires the organization to spend $500 less over its lifetime. But it does require it to spend $2,500 more at the beginning. That $2,500 could have been earning interest, thus offsetting some of the extra operating costs.

A way is needed to compare dollars spent at different times. Then one would be able to consider not just how much cash is involved but also when it is received or spent. Rather than solve the problem of the air conditioners now, put it aside for the time being. Let us focus attention on the methodology for dealing with cash flows at different times. Then it will be possible to return to the problem of the air conditioner investment later in this Appendix.

Time Value of Money Calculation Mechanics

The key to capital budgeting calculations is to be able to evaluate cash coming and going at different times. The amount of money spent or received today is referred to as the present value (PV). The interest rate is referred to as i%. The number of interest compounding periods is referred to as N. The compounding process is straightforward. Multiply the interest rate (i%) times the initial investment (PV) to find the interest in the first year. Add that interest to the initial investment. Then multiply the interest rate times the initial amount invested plus all interest already accumulated to find the amount of interest for the second year. If the investment were expected to last for 40 years, this simple process would become tedious.

To make matters worse, cash flows (both in and out) often take place monthly. Therefore, for a greater degree of accuracy regarding how much cash is available for use at any time, use i% as a monthly interest rate, N as the number of months, and do compounding on a monthly basis. For a 40-year project, this will require 480 monthly calculations.

However, formulas have been developed that ease the process. The most fundamental of these formulas is:

$$FV = PV \ (1 + i\%)^N$$

This formula allows a one-step determination of the future value (FV) of some amount of money (PV) invested today at an interest rate (i%) for a period of time equal to N. (This formula will not be derived here. Those interested are referred to any of the basic accounting or finance texts listed in this chapter's references.) Many modern handheld business calculators have this and other TVM formulas built in. A nurse manager who wants to know what $100 would grow to in 5 years at 10% interest would input into a calculator that the PV = $100, i% is 10, and N is 5. Then pressing the calculate button would provide the resulting FV.

Calculators are also relatively simple to use if one wishes to compound more frequently than once a year. When compounding occurs more frequently, one is dealing with a greater number of shorter periods. For example, to compound monthly, instead of N being equal to 5 for a 5-year period, it would be equal to 60, the number of months in 5 years. The interest rate cannot be 10%, because that would imply that 10% was earned each month for the 60 months. Therefore, it will be necessary to divide 10% by 12 to get the monthly interest rate for the 60 months. Thus, i% = 10%/12, and N = 60. In order to make these conversions for quarterly, monthly, or even daily compounding, simply multiply the number of years by the number of quarters, months, or days in a year and divide the interest rate by the same number.

So far this discussion has focused on finding out how much an amount of money held today would grow to be in the future. It is also important to be able to take an amount of money to be received in the future and determine what it would be worth today. That requires reversal of the compounding process. This reversal is called discounting, and the interest rate used in the calculation is called the *discount rate*. In the previous example, if 5 years in the future one expected to receive $161, the calculator could be given FV = $161, i% = 10, and N = 5 and could readily solve for the equivalent present value amount, which is $100. That is equivalent to saying that at a 10% compound interest rate; one would have to put $100 aside today in order to receive $161 in 5 years.

What if it is expected that some money will be received or spent every year, rather than all at one time in the future? For instance, what is the value today of receiving $100 every year for the next 3 years? One way to solve this problem would be to take the PV of $100 to be received 1 year from now, plus the PV of $100 to be received 2 years from now, plus the PV of $100 to be received 3 years from now.

Obviously, this has the potential to be a tedious process. Any time payments are to be made or received and the payments are exactly the same in amount and evenly spaced in time, those payments are referred to as an annuity. (Business calculators generally have a key or button marked PMT. This stands for periodic annuity payment.) Although many people are familiar with annuities as being annual payments of round amounts of money, any amount paid over and over at even periods of time forms an annuity.

To calculate the PV of $100 received every year for 3 years, one would calculate that the PMT = $100, N = 3, and i% = 10. The calculator can then determine the PV. Note that FV does not enter into this calculation because there is no single future value but rather a series of payments, all considered by the term PMT.

The Present Cost Approach

To return to the problem raised earlier, recall that there are two potential air conditioners. One will cost $10,000 and will have operating costs of $3,000 per year for 5 years. The other air conditioner will cost $7,500 and will have operating costs of $3,600 per year for 5 years. The problem of choosing one or the other concerns the fact that the total cost of the first alternative is $25,000, whereas the second alternative costs $25,500, but the one with the lower total cost has the higher initial cash outlay.

In today's dollars, the first alternative is $10,000 plus the present value of an annuity of $3,000 per year for 5 years. The second alternative is $7,500 plus the present value of $3,600 per year for 5 years. The appropriate interest rate to use is the subject of some controversy. For now, simply assume an interest rate of 10%. The problems concerning the selection of the interest rate are discussed later in this appendix. At $N = 5$ and $i\% = 10$, the PV when PMT is $3,000 is $11,372. When the PMT is $3,600, the PV is $13,647. Together with the initial outlays, the PV of the first alternative is $21,372 and for the second alternative it is $21,147. Therefore, other things equal, the second alternative would be chosen.

This method is the present cost approach. It considers the PV of the costs of alternative projects accomplishing the same end. Assuming that both projects are just as effective in terms of accomplishing the desired outcome, the alternative with the lower present value cost is superior. This approach is rarely used in most industries because it totally ignores revenues. It starts from the presumption that the project or investment is going to be made and simply determines which alternative will have the lowest effective cost over its lifetime. Most industries are very concerned with the profitability of a project.

Health Care Organizations and Profitability

In order to examine profitability, one must use one of two approaches: the net present value (NPV) or the internal rate of return (IRR). Proprietary organizations in the health care industry are particularly interested in using these methods. They are potentially valuable, however, even for the not-for-profit part of the health care industry. There are many reasons that a not-for-profit organization must actually earn a profit on some of its programs, services, or investments.

Why should a not-for-profit organization want to make a profit? That seems paradoxical. The term "not-for-profit," merely means that the main purpose of the organization is not to make profits. However, it does not mean that the revenues of the organization cannot exceed its expenses. Such profits are needed to offset losses on various services. They are also needed for replacing buildings and equipment and expanding the number and types of services offered.

Inflation and technological change compound this problem. If the organization bought a patient monitor 10 years ago for $50,000, a new one may well cost $100,000. To be able to buy the new one without borrowing money, the organization would have to have made a $50,000 profit during the life of the machine it is replacing. The cash to buy the new, more expensive equipment must come from somewhere.

The bottom line is that the organization must consider whether at least some investments will be profitable to offset losses and for future investment needs.

Furthermore, because resources are limited, it must be able to do more than determine whether a project is profitable; it must have a method of choosing the best project from among a number of profitable alternatives.

Therefore, the NPV and IRR approaches are important for all health care organizations. These methods, like the present cost approach, are discounted cash-flow methods because they analyze cash-flow information by discounting back to the present amounts to be spent or to be received in the future. Both methods aid in choosing the best project from a group of alternatives.

The Net Present Value (NPV) Approach

The NPV method of analysis determines whether a project earns more or less than a stated desired rate of return. That rate of return is the interest rate used in the calculations of the TVM. Recall that the interest rate for finding the PV of money received in the future is referred to as the discount rate. In NPV calculations this rate is often referred to as the hurdle rate or required rate of return. The starting point of the analysis is the determination of this rate.

The Appropriate Discount Rate

The key factor in PV calculations is the interest rate chosen. Yet there is no general consensus about the rate that should be used, especially in the not-for-profit sector. Earlier it was noted that one of the key reasons to consider the TVM is that money could be kept in an interest-earning account. Therefore, one would not want to get involved in a project that did not earn at least that rate.

Most health care organizations do not have the luxury of having large amounts of money in the bank. If the money is not needed for a particular project, there certainly are other pressing needs for which the money will be used. In fact, most health care organizations usually have a certain amount of long-term borrowing. Therefore, it has often been suggested that the appropriate discount rate be the cost of obtaining the funds needed for the project.

This in itself brings up a number of problems. Some funding comes by way of contributions, whereas other funds are borrowed at high rates from banks or through the issuance of bonds. This can lead to inconsistent decisions. Projects that are poor from an economic viewpoint may be accepted in years when contributions are high because the cost of the contributed funds used for the project is zero. On the other hand, fairly good projects might be rejected if contributions are particularly low in a given year.

It is generally agreed that any particular project's inherent merits should not be based on where the funding for that particular project will come from. Therefore, there should be some average rate commonly applied to all projects. The next question concerns whether that common rate should average the cost of borrowing money with the zero cost of contributed funds. This question has no clear-cut answer. On the one hand, one might argue that if all projects can earn a weighted average of the cost of funds, then the organization can survive financially. On the other hand, it means that projects will be accepted that would be rejected if there were no contributions.

For example, suppose that a hospital could borrow $9,000,000 at a 10% rate and that it receives contributions of $1,000,000. The interest cost on the borrowed money is $900,000 per year; on the contributions, the interest cost is zero. The combined cost of the $10,000,000 total would be $900,000, or an average rate of 9%. If this average is used as a hurdle rate, the organization will accept projects with a projected return of 9% or more. It would, for instance, be willing to accept a project with a 9.5% return because it would more than cover its cost. The objection to this is that a for-profit business would have rejected a 9.5% project because it would presumably have no contributions. The 9.5% return is less than the 10% cost of borrowed money. Therefore, from a purely financial standpoint, it is not a good investment.

The contention is that even not-for-profit organizations should make wise resource-allocation choices. This requires them to act as if they were for-profit organizations. The counter to this argument is that a not-for-profit organization by its very nature is willing to undertake unprofitable ventures because of its desire to provide some benefit to society. Furthermore, the contributed funds did not come from individuals hoping the hospital would spend money only when it could make a profit. They were contributed to cover losing operations.

It is advocated here that projects first be evaluated from a strictly economic approach. Can the project bring in enough money to cover the cost if it had had to borrow money to finance it? Such projects can be undertaken, assuming that the organization has the personnel available to implement them, because they will not place a drain on the financial resources of the institution.

Projects that cannot meet this criterion can be evaluated on the basis of what they contribute to the organization and its patients relative to the money it has to spend on them. This results in a more socioeconomic approach. Projects that will yield a return less than that required from an economic viewpoint can be subsidized by projects that earn more than the cost of the borrowed funds needed to support them, plus the money from contributions. Thus, the 9.5% project would not be automatically accepted because it does not surpass the 10% hurdle rate, based on the cost of borrowed funds. It would have to compete with all other projects that earn less than the hurdle rate, based on its qualitative social merit.

The nurse manager does not have to make major decisions regarding appropriate discount rates. The financial officers of the organization have undoubtedly gone over this problem in detail and made some policy decision. If the budget process is extremely efficient in the organization, the discount rate will be included in the set of assumptions that was prepared as part of the budget foundations process. In such cases, the discount rate will be readily available. Many health care organizations are less sophisticated, and it would be necessary to call upon your financial officers to get an appropriate rate.

NPV Calculations
Once the hurdle rate has been determined, the NPV method can be used to assess whether a project is acceptable. The NPV method compares the present value of a project's cash inflows to the present value of its cash outflows, as calculated at a particular hurdle rate. If the present value of the money coming in exceeds the present value of the money going out, the project is earning a rate of return greater than the hurdle rate. In equation form, NPV can be defined as follows:

$$NPV = PV \text{ inflows} - PV \text{ outflows}$$

If the NPV is greater than zero, the inflows are greater than the outflows when evaluated at the hurdle rate. If the NPV is less than zero, the organization is spending more than it is receiving. If the NPV is exactly zero, the inflows are equal to the outflows, and the project is earning exactly the hurdle rate. In most cases, it will be financial managers rather than nurse managers who perform the actual calculations. Nevertheless, nurse managers should understand the evaluation process that capital projects are subjected to prior to approval.

To find the NPV, first sum the PVs of the cash received in each year. Then find the sum of the PVs of the cash spent each year. Then compare the sum of the PVs of the inflows to the sum of the PVs of the outflows.

For example, suppose that the hospital is considering adding a new wing. There is an initial cash outflow of $10,000,000. Assume that the money for the wing could be borrowed at 10%. Suppose that the operating cash expenses (including information about the costs relating to nursing, which you have contributed to the analysis) and the cash revenues for each of the 20 years of the useful life of the wing are as shown in Table 10A-1. Without considering the timing of the cash flows, a total of $16,570,000 is being spent, and $35,435,192 is being received. The project appears to be very profitable. Note, however, that a large amount of money is spent at the beginning of the project, whereas revenues are earned gradually over the 20 years.

TABLE 10A-1 Example of Project Cash Flows and Present Values

| | Cash Flow | | Present Value (PV) | |
	Cash Expenses	Cash Revenues	Cash Expenses	Cash Revenues
Start	$10,000,000		$10,000,000	
Year 1	200,000	$1,000,000	181,818	$ 909,091
2	230,000	1,020,000	190,083	842,975
3	250,000	1,081,200	187,829	812,322
4	270,000	1,146,072	184,414	782,783
5	270,000	1,214,836	167,649	754,318
6	280,000	1,287,726	158,053	726,888
7	290,000	1,364,990	148,816	700,456
8	310,000	1,446,889	144,617	674,985
9	310,000	1,533,703	131,470	650,440
10	320,000	1,625,725	123,374	626,787
11	330,000	1,723,269	115,663	603,995
12	345,000	1,826,665	109,928	582,032
13	355,000	1,936,265	102,831	560,866
14	370,000	2,052,440	97,433	540,472
15	380,000	2,175,587	90,969	520,818
16	390,000	2,306,122	84,875	501,879
17	400,000	2,444,489	79,137	483,628
18	410,000	2,591,159	73,742	466,043
19	420,000	2,746,628	68,673	449,096
20	440,000	2,911,426	65,403	432,765
Totals	$16,570,000	$35,435,192	$12,506,777	$12,662,639

By using PV methodology, the PV of each cash flow can be calculated; then the PVs of the inflows and the outflows can be summed. The result is that the total PV of the inflows is $12,622,639, and the PV of the outflows is $12,506,777. The NPV, equal to the PV of the inflows less the PV of the outflows, is $115,862. This number is greater than zero, so the project is earning more than 10% and is acceptable. However, it is not nearly as profitable as it appeared at first glance.

Even though the net PV is positive, that does not necessarily mean that the organization will go ahead with the project. It may have limited resources and not be able to undertake all projects in a given year, even if they all earn better than the hurdle rate.

Alternatively, projects may exist that conflict. For example, suppose that the organization is considering using a site either for a traditional new wing, a new co-op care wing, or medical office space. Assuming that the land can be used for only one of these three uses, a conflict will exist if all three projects have an NPV greater than zero. Another method of capital budgeting, the IRR, is designed to utilize a ranking system that helps to help make a choice among competing projects. It should be noted, however, that the ranking will be based strictly on economic calculations, and managerial judgment will be needed to make final decisions. There may well be qualitative or political aspects that will affect the ultimate choice. Nevertheless, even if these other aspects are important to the final decision, it is appropriate to make the economic comparison so that the organization's management can fully understand the trade-offs that are being made.

The Internal Rate of Return (IRR) Approach

The principal objection to the NPV approach is that it does not indicate the specific rate of return that a project is earning. It simply indicates whether the proposed investment is earning more or less than a specified rate of return. This creates problems if there are several projects that exceed the hurdle rate. This is especially true when the projects conflict or if there are insufficient funds to undertake all projects with a positive NPV. The IRR method is a mathematical formulation that sets the present value of the inflows equal to the present value of the outflows. This equation holds true only at the exact interest rate that a project is earning. If the equation is solved for the interest rate that makes it hold true, that is the rate of return that the project is earning.

Although the mathematics for calculating the IRR are complex, a calculator or computer can be used to determine the interest rate that any project earns. Unfortunately, IRR mathematics are complex. This is particularly true when the cash flows are not the same from year to year. To solve the problem when the cash flow is different each year requires a trial-and-error approach. There is really no better method for finding the IRR than by trying a variety of rates of return until the one rate that makes the PV of the inflows equal to the PV of the outflows is found. This would be a tedious operation by hand, but there are some business calculators and many computer programs that can perform this process for you.

Project Ranking

One of the advantages of the IRR method is that it allows the organization to list all the projects being considered and rank them in order from the highest return on investment to the lowest. The IRR method reveals the specific interest rate that each project is expected to return. Even if the organization is not-for-profit, it must consider the fact that the projects with the highest return on investment, or rate of return, will provide the largest amount of cash coming into the organization in the future. This cash can in turn be used to allow for additional projects to be undertaken. By listing projects in order from the highest rate of return to the lowest, this ranking makes the project selection process far easier.

Calculators that compute TVM calculations can be purchased for a relatively small sum—in the $30 range or found free online from several websites. The computations can also be performed easily using an electronic spreadsheet program.

■ USING COMPUTER SPREADSHEETS FOR TVM COMPUTATIONS

A number of computer and electronic spreadsheet software programs are available to solve TVM problems. Some of the most popular are Microsoft's Excel, Lotus Development Corporation's Lotus 1-2-3, and Corel's Quattro Pro. They are particularly useful for some of the more complicated calculations. This appendix provides examples of how to solve TVM problems with Excel.[1] The approach of other spreadsheets is similar.

Consider finding the future value of $100 invested for 2 years at 6%. Using Excel, you begin by entering the data that will be used to solve the problem. Note that Excel uses Nper rather than N for the number of compounding periods, and Rate rather than i for the discount rate. In this example, the problem could be set up as shown in Figure 10A-1. This screen shows the data you have and the variable, FV,

[1] The Excel® approach used in this chapter is based on Microsoft Excel 2002 (10.4524.4219) SP-2. Other versions of Excel may differ somewhat in the exact approach, steps, or formulas used, or in the exact appearance of the screen.

Figure 10A-1 Initial data entry. (Excel ® Spreadsheet Software. Microsoft product screen shot(s) reprinted with permission from Microsoft Corporation.)

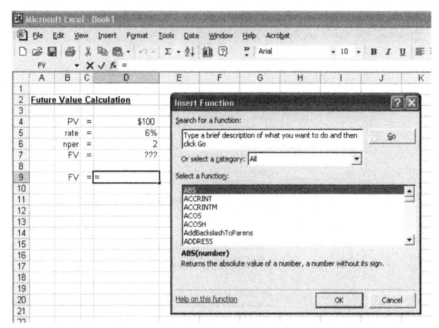

Figure 10A-2 The insert function window. (Excel ® Spreadsheet Software. Microsoft product screen shot(s) reprinted with permission from Microsoft Corporation.)

that you are looking for, and it indicates where the answer will be shown. Once the data have been entered, you move the cursor into the cell where you want the solution to appear. In this case, it is cell D9. Then you press the Function Wizard button, *fx*, which is located on the toolbar at the top of the screen. In Figure 10A-1, the cursor arrow is pointing at the Function Wizard button.

Clicking on the Function Wizard opens a box headed Insert Function (Figure 10A-2). Within the box that has opened, users can search for a function by describing what they are trying to do, such as "find a future value," or they can select a category and a function name. For TVM calculations, the category is always Financial. To solve the above problem, the function is FV (Figure 10A-3.)

Note, in Figure 10A-3, that the Financial category and the FV function have been selected. Next, click the OK button at the bottom of the Insert Function window. A new window called Function Arguments will open (Figure 10A-4). Note that Excel sometimes uses "Pv" to refer to the present value, which is commonly abbreviated as PV, and "Fv" to refer to the future value, which is commonly abbreviated as FV. Excel also sometimes uses "Pmt" to refer to the periodic payment that is more commonly abbreviated at PMT. The Pv, Fv, and Pmt abbreviations will be used in this Appendix when we are specifically referring to an Excel formula. In this window insert the Rate, Nper, and Pv. There is no annuity payment in this problem so you can ignore Pmt. Type refers to whether the payments come at the beginning or end of each period. This pertains primarily to annuities. For now, we can

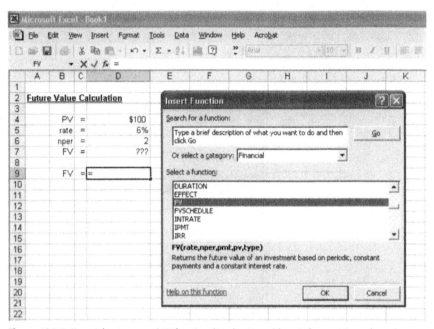

Figure 10A-3 Financial category and FV function. (Excel ® Spreadsheet Software. Microsoft product screen shot(s) reprinted with permission from Microsoft Corporation.)

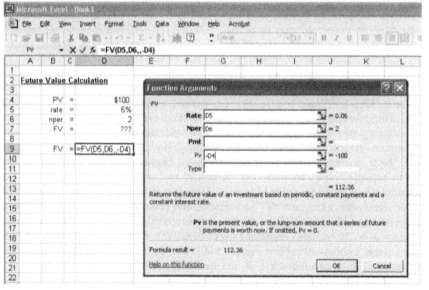

Figure 10A-4 The function arguments screen. (Excel ® Spreadsheet Software. Microsoft product screen shot(s) reprinted with permission from Microsoft Corporation.)

Microsoft Excel - Book1

File   Edit   View   Insert   Format   Tools   Data

D9 fx =FV(D5,D6,,-D4)

	A	B	C	D	E
1					
2	**Future Value Calculation**				
3					
4		PV	=	$100	
5		rate	=	6%	
6		nper	=	2	
7		FV	=	???	
8					
9		FV	=	$112.36	
10					

Figure 10A-5 Solving for future value. (Excel ® Spreadsheet Software. Microsoft product screen shot(s) reprinted with permission from Microsoft Corporation.)

ignore it as well. The variables can be inserted as follows: Rate as 6%, Nper as 2, and Pv as (100).

Note that the Pv in the Function Arguments window is shown as –D4. Excel follows the logic that if you pay out something today, you will get back something in the future. So if the Fv is to be a positive amount, representing a receipt of cash, the Pv must be a negative amount, representing a payment of cash. The same thing could have been accomplished by showing a negative initial present value ($100) in cell D4 instead of showing it as $100. Now the user can click on OK at the bottom of the Function Arguments window. The solution appears in cell D9 in Figure 10A-5. Excel can be used to solve for other TVM variables as well as the FV.

Skipping the Function Wizard

Although it is sometimes helpful to go through the detailed steps just mentioned, a shortcut process may be used. On the screen in Figure 10A-3, near the bottom of the Insert Function window, the Excel formula for finding the FV appears:

FV(rate, nper, pmt, pv, type)

The future value can be solved by simply entering this formula in a cell, beginning with an equal sign. If this shortcut were used to solve the problem above, a blank space must be left for the pmt. The value for the type can be omitted completely. For example, given the cell location of the raw data in the worksheet in Figures 10A-1 to 10A-5, the formula to solve the above problem would be:

= FV(D5, D6, ,–D4)

In fact, looking at the formula bar in Figure 10A-5, one can see that this is the exact formula that the Function Wizard used to calculate the value for cell D9. An advantage of a formula that uses the cell references is that it will automatically recalculate the future value if the numeric value in any of the indicated cells is changed. If one were to change the rate in cell D5 from 6% to 8%, a new future value would immediately appear on the worksheet.

However, another approach is to show the numeric values for the raw data in the Excel formula, such as:

$$= FV(6\%, 2, ,-100)$$

The advantage of this approach is that it not only calculates the answer in the Excel spreadsheet, but also it can be communicated to a colleague who can tell exactly what information you have and what you are trying to calculate. Anyone can drop this into a spreadsheet without needing to know where all the raw data appear in the spreadsheet. For the remainder of this Appendix, TVM Excel problems are discussed in the form of providing the basic Excel formula for a variable, and the numeric value formula, such as:

$$= FV(rate, nper, pmt, pv, type)$$

$$= FV(6\%, 2, ,-100).$$

Note that if you enter = FV(6%, 2, ,–100) into an Excel spreadsheet cell, the solution of 112.36 will automatically be calculated.

Examples

The previous example started with information about the present value, rate, and number of compounding periods and solved for the future value. Using Excel, one can solve for any variable if one has the other information. In fact, Excel can even directly find the NPV or IRR. In each case the basic approach is to click on fx, the Function Wizard, on the formula bar, indicate in the Insert Function window that the category is Financial, and select PV, Rate, Nper, PMT, NPV or IRR, respectively, as the function. As each function is highlighted in the Insert Function window, its Excel formula appears near the bottom of the window. The formulas are:

$$= PV \ (rate, nper, pmt, fv, type)$$

$$= Rate \ (nper, pmt, pv, fv, type, guess)$$

$$= Nper \ (rate, pmt, pv, fv, type)$$

$$= PMT \ (rate, nper, pv, fv, type)$$

$$= NPV \ (rate, value1, value2, ...)$$

$$= IRR \ (values, guess)$$

Present Value
Suppose that you can buy a capital asset that will result in your receiving $15,000, 5 years from now, and that you believe an appropriate discount rate for this specific piece of equipment is 7%. You need to decide the most that you would pay for that asset. What is the PV of that future receipt?

Figure 10A-6 Present value – data. (Excel ® Spreadsheet Software. Microsoft product screen shot(s) reprinted with permission from Microsoft Corporation.)

You can start the solution by recording the raw data in an Excel spreadsheet (Figure 10A-6). Note that the cursor in this screen is pointing at *fx*, the Function Wizard. Click on the wizard, and the Insert Function window appears. Use the dropdown menu to change the category to Financial, and scroll down to PV. The result is seen in Figure 10A-7. Note that you can see in that screen that the formula for the PV is PV (rate, nper, pmt, fv, type). Click OK. Enter the cell references for the Rate, Nper, and Fv. If you want the solution to appear as a positive number, enter a minus sign before the cell reference for the Fv. This will generate Figure 10A-8. Click OK to solve the problem. The resulting screen would appear as Figure 10A-9, and the present value is $10,694.79. If you wish to show the formula with numeric values, it would be = PV (7%, 5, , –15000).

Rate
Suppose that you have $10,000 today, could invest it for 6 years, and need to have $20,000 at the end of that time. What rate would have to be earned? The data setup would be similar to that of the problem just solved, except that you are looking for the rate rather than the present value. You would click on the Function Wizard, and in the Insert Function window, you would select Financial as the category and Rate as the function. The formula appears on the Insert Functions window as Rate (nper, pmt, pv, fv, type, guess). You would then click OK and enter the cell references, as shown in Figure 10A-10. Note that either the PV or the FV must be a negative number. The rate that must be earned for $10,000 to grow to $20,000 in 6 years is shown in Figure 10A-11. The formula for this with numeric values would be = Rate (6%, , –10,000, 20000). Leave a blank between two commas for Pmt because there

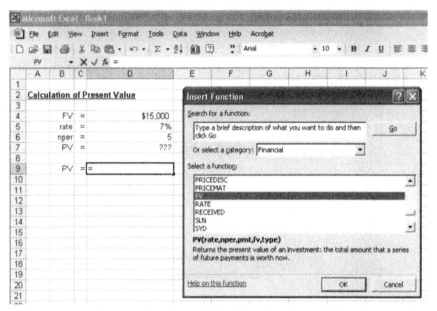

Figure 10A-7 Insert function window. (Excel ® Spreadsheet Software. Microsoft product screen shot(s) reprinted with permission from Microsoft Corporation.)

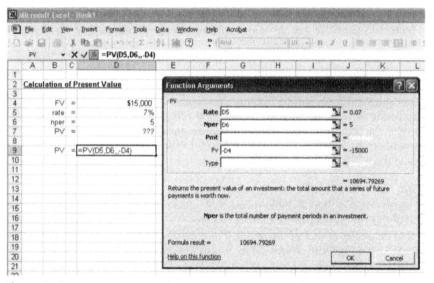

Figure 10A-8 Function arguments window. (Excel ® Spreadsheet Software. Microsoft product screen shot(s) reprinted with permission from Microsoft Corporation.)

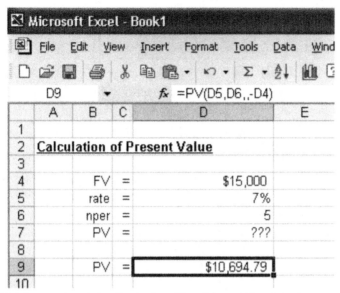

Figure 10A-9 Present value solution. (Excel ® Spreadsheet Software. Microsoft product screen shot(s) reprinted with permission from Microsoft Corporation.)

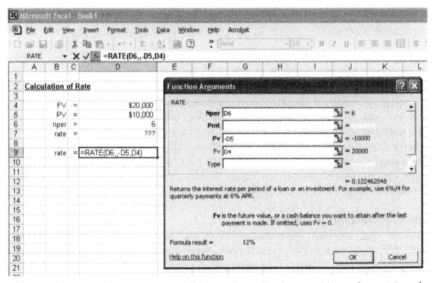

Figure 10A-10 Function arguments window for rate solution. (Excel ® Spreadsheet Software. Microsoft product screen shot(s) reprinted with permission from Microsoft Corporation.)

Figure 10A-11 Rate solution. (Excel ® Spreadsheet Software. Microsoft product screen shot(s) reprinted with permission from Microsoft Corporation.)

is no periodic repeating payment in this problem. You do not need to enter any values for type or guess.

Number of Periods

Suppose that you can earn only 9% per year. How many years would it be before the $10,000 will grow to become $20,000? After setting up the data, you would click on fx, select the Financial category and Nper as the function. The formula that appears is Nper (rate, pmt, pv, fv, type). Then click OK. The Function Arguments window, showing the cell references, is shown on the Excel Screen in Figure 10A-12. After entering the cell references in this window, click OK, and the result is 8.04, or a little bit longer than 8 years. Notice that the result can also be seen at the bottom of the Function Arguments window in Figure 10A-12. The formula with numeric values would be = Nper (9%, , –10000, 20000).

Periodic Payments (in Arrears)

Assume that you can invest money every year for 7 years at 8%. If you need $20,000 at the end of the 7 years, how much would you have to put aside each year? Assume you make the payments at the end of each year. After setting up the data, clicking on the Function Wizard, and selecting the financial category and the PMT function, the formula in the Insert Function window is PMT (rate, nper, pv, fv, type). The Function Arguments window is seen in Figure 10A-13. After clicking OK, you find that you would have to invest $2,241.45 each year. You could also see that result at the bottom of the Function Arguments window in Figure 10A-13. The formula with numeric values would be = PMT (8%, 7, ,–20000)

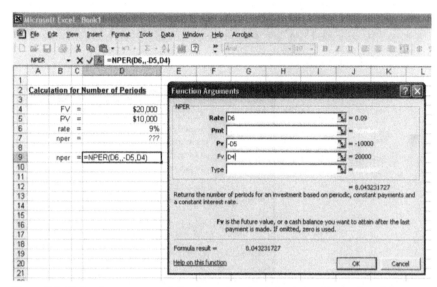

Figure 10A-12 Function arguments window for number of periods solution. (Excel ® Spreadsheet Software. Microsoft product screen shot(s) reprinted with permission from Microsoft Corporation.)

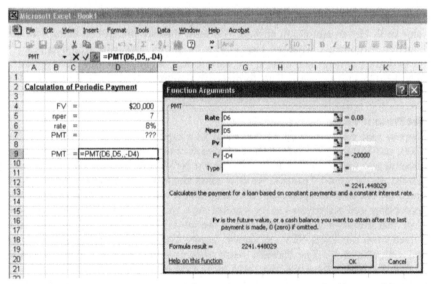

Figure 10A-13 Function arguments window for periodic payments in arrears. (Excel ® Spreadsheet Software. Microsoft product screen shot(s) reprinted with permission from Microsoft Corporation.)

Periodic Payments (in Advance)

However, what if you could put aside money at the beginning of each year rather than the end? That is called an annuity in advance. When payments come at the end of each period, as they do in an ordinary annuity or annuity in arrears, the value for "type" is 0. If you leave it blank, as you have so far, Excel assumes that it has a

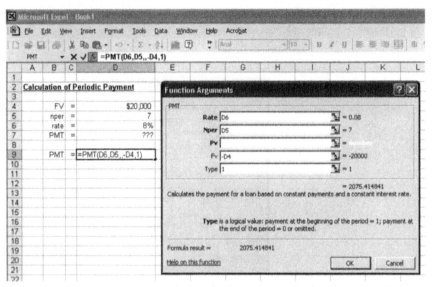

Figure 10A-14 Function arguments window for periodic payments in advance. (Excel ® Spreadsheet Software. Microsoft product screen shot(s) reprinted with permission from Microsoft Corporation.)

value of 0. For an annuity in advance you must indicate the type as being 1 in the Function Arguments window. Figure 10A-14 shows how this would appear. If the periodic payments are made at the start of the year, you would need to put aside only $2,075.41 each year. The formula with numeric values would be = PMT (8%, 7, , –20000, 1).

Net Present Value

Suppose that you can invest $1,000 today in a capital asset and will receive $500, $700, and $800, respectively, at the end of each of the 3 years of the asset's life. Your discount rate for the project is 6%. What is the NPV? After clicking on the Function Wizard, in the Insert Function window select the Financial category and the NPV function. The formula appears as NPV(rate, value1, value2,...). After clicking OK, the appropriate cell references can be entered into the Function Arguments window. Note that the initial outlay **is not** one of the values. The initial outlay must be subtracted from the Excel NPV calculation. Figure 10A-15 shows the problem set-up and cell references. The formula result shown at the bottom of the screen is $1,766.39. After subtracting the outlay of $1,000, the NPV is $766.39.

Internal Rate of Return

What is the IRR of the cash flows described in the NPV section above? After clicking on the Function Wizard, in the Insert Function window select the Financial category and the IRR function. The formula appears as IRR (values, guess). Provide Excel with an initial guess, such as 15%. After you click OK, the appropriate cell references can be entered into the Function Arguments window. Note that the initial outlay is one of the values. In this respect, the IRR function works differently from the NPV function. Figure 10A-16 shows the problem setup and cell references. The formula

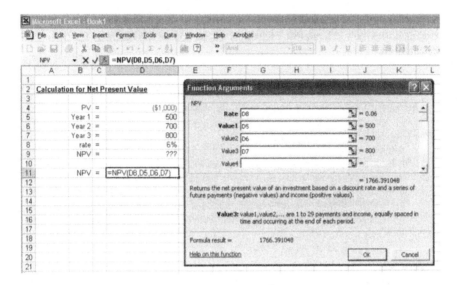

Figure 10A-15 Function arguments window for net present value. (Excel ® Spreadsheet Software. Microsoft product screen shot(s) reprinted with permission from Microsoft Corporation.)

result shown at the bottom of the screen is .404. This means that the IRR for the capital asset would be 40.4%.

Each of the major spreadsheet programs handles the TVM process slightly differently. In fact, within any program, very minor changes in the process tend to occur from one edition to the next. And to some extent the spreadsheet approaches are quirky. For example, not allowing the initial, time zero, outflow to be directly included in the NPV calculation seems odd. Nevertheless, spreadsheets can handle

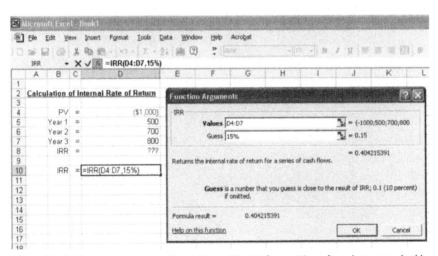

Figure 10A-16 Internal rate of return. (Excel ® Spreadsheet Software. Microsoft product screen shot(s) reprinted with permission from Microsoft Corporation.)

with ease the more complicated numbers found in real-world situations, and most organizations now rely almost exclusively on computer spreadsheets for their TVM calculations.

Summary and Implications for Nurse Managers

Capital budget proposals can be evaluated by several methods. The first of these is the payback approach, which is a rather unsophisticated model that is useful for a first assessment of the capital item but is flawed by the fact that it ignores the TVM.

Discounted cash flow techniques are accurate. These approaches include the present cost, NPV, and IRR methods. All of these discounted cash-flow techniques account for the TVM. The present cost approach is useful for comparing alternative ways to accomplish the same goal. The method does not evaluate revenues. Both the NPV and IRR methods determine whether the cash inflows are adequate to justify the cash outflows from a strictly economic point of view. The IRR method additionally allows for a ranking of projects by rate of return on investment. This method is somewhat more complex to use than NPV.

Reference

http://www.pine-grove.com/financial%20calculators/irr.htm provides a calculator for IRR as well as many other financial formula calculations.

11

Performance Budgeting

LEARNING OBJECTIVES
The goals of this chapter are to:

- Introduce the concept of performance or outcomes budgeting
- Describe the management by objectives (MBO) approach to budgeting
- Identify weaknesses in traditional measures of output and performance
- Create an awareness of the importance of focusing on goals and measuring the accomplishment of goals

- Outline the specific technical steps of performance budgeting
- Provide an example of performance budgeting
- Identify potential output measures for use by nursing in performance budgets

■ INTRODUCTION

The extreme financial pressure faced by health care organizations in recent years has resulted in substantial budget cuts. Managers have had to find ways to make do with less growth in revenues—in most cases, much less. A major concern in this environment is that the quality of patient care is likely to suffer; and this concern has been borne out by the evidence of problems with quality of care. The Institute of Medicine (IOM) published two landmark reports about the serious quality problems they found in American health care: *To Err is Human: Building a Safer Health System* (Corrigan, Kohn, & Donaldson, 2000) and *Crossing the Quality Chasm: A New Health System for the 21st Century* (IOM, 2001). These reports by such a prestigious, federally sponsored agency gained the attention of politicians, policy makers, and the American public. The result has been a strong refocusing of attention from cost control to a dual focus on conserving financial resources while at the same time placing a strong emphasis on quality and outcomes of health care services. Budgeting can help managers by focusing to a greater extent on the results that departments and organizations achieve. This process, called *performance* or *outcomes budgeting*, is the topic of this chapter.

Performance budgeting is a technique that evaluates the activities of a cost center in terms of what the center accomplishes as well as the costs of that accomplishment. It is an approach to budgeting specifically designed to evaluate the multiple outcomes of cost centers rather than a single budgeted output, such as the number of home care visits. Performance budgeting provides a mechanism for gaining a better understanding of the relationships between financial resources and the level and quality of results.

Traditionally, budgets have focused primarily on the resources used by a department or cost center. There is detailed information on the number of nurses working in a unit and their pay rate. Supplies, educational seminars, and publications are all carefully considered. However, these are all inputs. They are the resources the unit needs to achieve its objectives. Unfortunately, there has been little focus on objectives. What are the goals of the unit? What is it trying to achieve? Cost centers often define their goals only in the simplest terms, such as the number of visits, patient days, or procedures. Performance budgeting shifts the focus from the resources the unit plans to use to the various things it is trying to accomplish.

The first step in performance budgeting is to define the objectives or areas of accomplishment for the unit or department. These are called performance areas. Some examples of performance areas are quality of care, nursing satisfaction, patient satisfaction, productivity, and innovation. The second step is to identify the operating budget costs for the cost center being evaluated. In a nursing unit these costs include items such as the salary for the unit nurse manager, salaries for clinical staff, education costs, and supplies. The third step is to determine what percentage of available resources should be used for each performance area. The fourth step is to assign the budgeted costs for the center to the individual performance areas on the basis of those percentages. The fifth and final step is to choose measures of performance for each performance area and to determine the cost per unit of workload based on those measures.

■ MANAGEMENT BY OBJECTIVES

One of the forerunners of performance budgeting was management by objectives (MBO). MBO is a budgeting technique in which a supervising manager and subordinate manager agree on a common set of objectives that will be used as a basis for the measurement of performance. This process requires more than simply developing an operating budget and agreeing to work toward attaining it. MBO programs require that there be a set of specific, measurable goals for each manager. These goals represent the performance of the manager, rather than just the performance of the unit.

A principal reason for introducing MBO was that many organizations were dictating budgets to their department managers. Such an approach gained little support. Managers felt that the budgets were unattainable and reflected little recognition of the realities faced by the department. The MBO approach is one that guarantees more active participation by the manager. There are clear incentive benefits to such an approach. On the other hand, it requires a major commitment of time on the part of the supervisor and the manager to work out a sensible, meaningful set of objectives.

MBO is a potentially useful approach. For those organizations not yet ready for performance budgeting, it provides a middle ground. It allows for better measures of performance without demanding the major time and effort necessary for performance budgeting. Performance budgeting starts where MBO leaves off. It recognizes the need to specify performance in terms of more than simply the typical department cost and general output measure. However, performance budgeting goes beyond MBO in that it allocates a portion of the unit or department operating budget to each of the objectives.

■ WHEN IS PERFORMANCE BUDGETING APPROPRIATE?

In any organization that has multiple goals and objectives, performance budgeting may be useful. Performance budgeting allows the organization to define the various elements of performance that are important. It can then assess managers and departments based on their accomplishments in terms of those elements. Each department can have its own set of performance or outcomes criteria. Most existing budget measures focus on simple criteria, such as the number of patient days. Such measures are incapable of getting at issues such as quality of care per patient day or cost per unit of quality of care.

When nursing budgets are cut or inadequately increased in response to changes in patient acuity, wage rate increases, or other factors, there is often an expectation by top management that at least the same amount of work will be performed. Often this is an unreasonable and unrealistic expectation. Although it is true that the number of patients or patient days may be handled with a smaller budget, the amount of care given almost certainly will not be the same. Performance levels and outcomes are likely to deteriorate. Unfortunately, rarely is there a linkage between the budget or amount spent and the amount of care provided, other than one simplistic measure such as the number of patient days.

If a nursing unit can handle 10,000 patient days in a year with a budget of $2,000,000, what happens if the budget is slashed to $1,750,000? If the unit still provides 10,000 patient days of care, traditional budgeting makes it appear that costs are down and output is unchanged. In reality, only chronically overstaffed units can achieve such a budget cut without reducing some patient care activities. And when patient care activities are reduced, it is highly unlikely that outcomes will remain unchanged. Given the tight budgets of the past 15 to 20 years, very few units today are chronically overstaffed. Indeed, the opposite problem—chronic understaffing—is far more common. Quality of patient care in many health care facilities is known to have declined in a number of dimensions. For example, the incidence of decubitus ulcers in intensive care units is becoming a much greater concern than it was 20 years ago, when that problem was much less prevalent in those units. (Cuddigan, 2001; Romero et al., 2006; Rosen et al., 2006). Today, with the work of the National Pressure Ulcer Advisory Panel, there is some evidence that, at least in some hospitals, the incidence of this nursing-care-sensitive indicator is declining. However, a traditional operating budget focusing on the number of patient days is unlikely to capture any of the changes that have occurred—either in the occurrence of pressure ulcers or in other indicators of the quality of nursing care. A performance budget can help to measure those changes.

■ THE PERFORMANCE BUDGETING TECHNIQUE

Determining Key Performance Areas

Nurse managers attempt to achieve a number of different objectives. Nursing units attempt to provide high-quality care. They attempt to satisfy patient needs and desires. They attempt to control costs. If you do not define clearly the performance that you hope to achieve, you cannot measure your success. The key is to develop a set of performance areas for measurement.

In developing performance areas, one should consider a variety of questions, such as: What important goals should be measured? What elements of a unit's performance are within the control of the nurse manager, and what elements are not? If census and acuity are variable, how should the performance measures be indexed to the variable workload? How should the nurse manager most productively spend working time? How should the nursing staff most productively use their time? How can the performance of a nursing unit be evaluated?

In addressing these questions, it is necessary to categorize the major elements of the manager's and unit's job or function. For example, consider a nurse manager of a 30-bed unit. Some effort should go toward ensuring a high level of patient care. Some effort should go to staffing the unit, some to controlling unit expenses, some to improving productivity, some to increasing patient satisfaction and improving staff morale, and some to innovation and long-range planning. These are some key performance areas for the manager and unit. There may well be other important outcome areas that are not listed here. A performance budget for a nursing home or ambulatory care organization might well have a set of performance areas different from those used by a hospital-based nursing unit. Managers must establish performance areas based on their own unit's or department's specific circumstances.

Technical Steps in Performance Budgeting

Identifying the performance areas of a cost center is the first step in performance budgeting. The second step is to identify the existing line-item budget for the cost center being evaluated. In a nursing unit, this budget includes the cost of items such as the salary of the unit nurse manager, salaries for clinical staff, education costs, and supplies.

The next step is to define how much of the resources represented by each line item are to be devoted to each of the performance areas. This requires that the manager develop a resource allocation model. This process forces the manager to think about what elements of the job are really important and how important they are.

If, for instance, patient satisfaction is very important to the organization, the manager must consider whether an adequate amount of time and effort is being devoted to achieving patient satisfaction. The resource allocation for the performance budget explicitly notes the specific portion of the nurse manager's time, staff time, and other resources that should be spent on ensuring patient satisfaction.

It is up to the nurse manager to decide how to allocate resources among the various processes that are associated with the desired outcomes. How much of the resources should be focused on quality of care? How much on staffing? A percentage of the total effort should be assigned to each of the performance areas. The manager's allocations will probably not be the same for management time, staff time, and other resources. Each resource is allocated on the basis of differing needs. For example, unit nurse managers might allocate 40% of clinical staff time and 90% of supplies to direct patient care. A chart or table should be developed that shows the performance areas and the percentage of each line-item cost being allocated to each performance area.

The allocation of resources to different performance areas should be based on explicit decisions related to organizational priorities. However, when a performance budget is first introduced, it is easier to make allocations based on historical information. This information can be gathered by having all personnel keep a log of their time for several weeks or it can be based on their best guess of how they use their time. Once the performance budget has been developed, more information will be available to the manager, and explicit choices can be made to reallocate resources in a more useful manner.

Once the percentage of each resource to be used to achieve each performance area has been decided, a calculation must be made to determine how much money has been budgeted for each performance area. This can be done by taking the percentage of each line item allocated to each performance area and multiplying it by the total amount of money in the budget for that line item. For instance, if the nurse manager's salary is $90,000 and 10% of the manager's working time is spent on improving quality of care, then $9,000 is calculated ($90,000 × 10%) as being spent on quality. If the staff nurses for the unit earn $1,500,000 in total and they spend 5% of their efforts on improving quality, there is another $75,000 ($1,500,000 × 5%) being allocated to quality improvement. The nurse manager can total all the costs for each performance element. In this case, a total of $84,000 has been budgeted for improving quality of care.

The final step is to choose measures of performance in each performance area, budget a specific numerical objective for each area, and determine the budgeted cost per unit of each objective on the basis of those measures. For instance, suppose that the nurse manager chooses to measure quality of care improvement based on the number of medication variances. Suppose further that the performance budget calls for reducing the number of medication variances in the unit by 60 instances. Because $84,000 has been allocated to improve quality, it can be said that $1,400 has been budgeted per medication variance eliminated. The next year the same amount of money might need to be budgeted just to maintain the level of care.

This approach may be sufficient if eliminating medication variances is a sufficient measure of overall quality improvement. On the other hand, more than one measure of quality may be needed in order to gain the quality improvements that are sought. Just as it is important to select appropriate areas of performance that the manager wants to consider, it is also critical to select good measures of performance to allow the manager to see how well things are being done in each critical performance area.

Note that the performance budget specifies an amount of an outcome to be accomplished. For example, it might budget to reduce medication errors by a specific number. The performance budget also specifies the inputs that will be devoted to achieving that outcome. A certain amount of nurse time is budgeted for accomplishing the reduction in medication errors. Thus, goals are matched with the resources needed for their accomplishment. The process of performance budgeting can be clarified by an example.

■ PERFORMANCE BUDGET EXAMPLE

The first step in developing a performance budget is to determine the performance areas that the nurse manager intends to use. The following is one possible set of performance areas:

- Patient care
- Quality of care improvement
- Staffing
- Cost control
- Increased productivity
- Increased patient satisfaction
- Improved staff morale
- Innovation and long-range planning

The second step is to get the cost information for the unit from the operating budget. Converting operating budget information into a performance budget will give a clearer focus of how the unit spends the budgeted amount of money. The operating budget already gives information such as the number of full-time equivalents by skill level. However, those are inputs rather than outcomes. The performance budget will provide information about results rather than just inputs. Suppose, hypothetically, that the line-item operating budget for a nursing unit is $1,800,000 for the coming year, as follows:

Nurse manager	$ 90,000
Clinical staff salaries	1,500,000
Education	30,000
Supplies	90,000
Overhead	90,000
Total	$1,800,000

The third step is to determine the percentage allocation of operating budget resources to performance areas. The allocation of the nurse manager's time to performance areas might be as follows:

Quality of care improvement	5%
Staffing	15%
Cost control	5%
Increasing productivity	5%
Increasing patient satisfaction	5%
Improving staff morale	10%
Innovation and long-range planning	5%
Personnel and operations management	50%
Total	100%[1]

By developing the allocation to areas of performance, a plan is provided that describes how the nurse manager should spend her or his time and which areas are deemed to be the most important or the most in need of attention.

There is no reason to believe that all resources within a department or unit should necessarily be allocated in the same fashion. The time allocation for clinical staff might be as follows:

Direct patient care	40%
Indirect patient care	30%
Quality of care improvement	5%
Cost control	5%
Increasing productivity	2%
Increasing patient satisfaction	15%
Other	3%
Total	100%

The allocation of time for direct patient care seems low, but this is misleading. A substantial portion of the time spent in quality of care improvement and increased patient satisfaction may in fact be additional direct patient care time, with a specific

---

[1] This simplified example treats the nurse manager's time as if it were all directly under her control. A more realistic calculation might set aside an amount of time such as 20% for administrative mandated activities.

focus on those two goals. Therefore, this allocation might imply that about half of nurses' time on the unit is spent on direct patient care.

To develop a full performance budget for the unit, it also will be necessary to determine how education, supplies, and overhead resources relate to the performance of the unit. Suppose that a reasonable expectation for the role of education in a given year is as follows:

Quality of care improvement	20%
Cost control	20%
Increasing productivity	20%
Increasing patient satisfaction	10%
Improving staff morale	10%
Innovation and long-range planning	20%
Total	100%

Supplies used by a nursing unit are primarily clinical supplies for direct patient care and, to a much lesser extent, administrative forms and other administrative supplies. Suppose that a reasonable expectation for the role of supplies is as follows:

Staffing	2%
Cost control	2%
Direct patient care	90%
Indirect patient care	5%
Other	1%
Total	100%

There is no uniquely correct way to allocate overhead because much of it is assigned to a nursing unit in an arbitrary manner. Ultimately, performance budget measures will be used to assess the cost of devoting resources to a particular activity such as improving quality of care. Overhead is not likely to vary based on how much effort the manager and clinical staff devote to improving quality of care on the unit, so it is reasonable to assign all of the unit's overhead to direct patient care. However, this is an arbitrary allocation, and alternative approaches are possible.

These percentage allocations are summarized in Table 11-1. Every line-item category within the original operating budget has had a percentage assigned to performance areas based on what the manager decides is a reasonable allocation of resources.

The original operating budget can now be assigned to performance areas, as is seen in Table 11-2. This table takes the total cost of each line item in the operating budget and multiplies it by the percentages in Table 11-1 to determine the budgeted cost for each performance area for each line item. For example, staff salary is budgeted at a total of $1,500,000 (see Table 11-2, Total column). Of this amount, 5% is allocated to quality of care improvements (see Table 11-1, Quality column, Staff Salary row). As a result, 5% of $1,500,000, or $75,000, is allocated to quality of care improvements (see Table 11-2, Quality column, Staff Salary row).

The total budgeted cost of each of the performance areas can be assessed. It is expected that the nursing unit will spend $87,300 in total on quality improvement efforts (see Table 11-2, Quality column, Totals row); $15,300 on staffing; $85,500 on cost control; and so on. In Table 11-2, compare the bottom row, which gives the total for each key performance area, with the Total column, which gives the total by line item from the original operating budget. The original operating budget appears to be primarily a fixed budget over which the unit has little control. It shows only the

TABLE 11-1 Summary of Percentage Allocations to Performance Areas

Cost Item	Performance Areas										
	Quality	Staffing	Cost Control	Productivity	Patient Satis.	Staff Morale	Innov.	Direct Care	Indirect Care	Other	Total
Nurse Manager	5%	15%	5%	5%	5%	10%	5%	0%	0%	50%	100%
Staff Salary	5%	0%	5%	2%	15%	0%	0%	40%	30%	3%	100%
Education	20%	0%	20%	20%	10%	10%	20%	0%	0%	0%	100%
Supplies	2%	2%	0%	0%	0%	0%	20%	90%	5%	1%	100%
Overhead	0%	0%	0%	0%	0%	0%	0%	100%	0%	0%	100%

TABLE 11-2 Allocation of Expenditures to Performance Areas

Cost Item	Performance Areas										
	Quality	Staffing	Cost Control	Productivity	Patient Satis.	Staff Morale	Innov.	Direct Care	Indirect Care	Other	Total
Nurse Manager	$ 4,500	$13,500	$ 4,500	$ 4,500	$ 4,500	$ 9,000	$ 4,500	$ 0	$ 0	$45,000	$ 90,000
Staff Salary	75,000	0	75,000	30,000	225,000	0	0	600,000	450,000	45,000	1,500,000
Education	6,000	0	6,000	6,000	3,000	3,000	6,000	0	0	0	30,000
Supplies	1,800	1,800	0	0	0	0	0	81,000	4,500	900	90,000
Overhead	0	0	0	0	0	0	0	90,000	0	0	90,000
Totals	$87,300	$15,300	$85,500	$40,500	$232,500	$12,000	$10,500	$771,000	$454,500	$90,900	$1,800,000

amount to be spent on each input resource consumed. However, the bottom row shows that implicit choices are being made about the allocation of the operating budget resources to different priority areas. Each column in Table 11-2 shows the amount of money budgeted for each performance area. The manager does in fact have at least some ability to modify how these resources are spent. It could be decided that relatively greater efforts should be made in one particular area and less in another. Knowing that $87,300 is budgeted for quality, $232,500 for patient satisfaction, and $771,000 for direct patient care is much more valuable information than knowing that $1,500,000 is budgeted for staff salaries. The focus has shifted from inputs to performance.

Note, however, that a performance budget still has not been fully developed. The allocation of operating budget to performance areas (see Table 11-2) is a valuable plan that provides an indication of whether the unit is planning to proceed in the most appropriate manner. It does not go far enough, however. It is not specific in terms of quantifying the goals for each performance area.

Table 11-3 presents the next step—the actual performance budget. In Table 11-3, the performance areas have been moved from the top row to the left side of the table. The difficult task of choosing a performance measure and quantifying the budgeted level for each performance area must be addressed.

Health care organizations try to produce improved health. This cannot be measured directly in most cases, so proxies such as the number of patient days of care are used. Performance budgets add additional proxies to assess the accomplishment of the organization's goals. In Table 11-3 it is seen that a budget can be developed that gives information about such items as the budgeted cost to attain a reduction in patient care planning errors. In this example, the budgeted cost is $8,730 for each 1% drop in the rate of failure to comply with patient care plan procedures (see Table 11-3, Average Cost column, Quality Improvement row). The next section addresses the issue of developing proxies for performance measurement.

■ DEVELOPING PERFORMANCE AREA MEASURES

To be able to create a performance budget that will be as useful as possible, there must be specific ways to measure accomplishments in each performance area. Some of the measures developed for the various performance areas will appear to be crude metrics at best. However, the measure of patient days is itself a crude proxy for the process of providing health care, which in turn is a proxy for improved health. Yet counting patient days is a useful measure. Over time, performance budgeting will improve as better proxies are suggested and incorporated into the technique. What are some potential output measures for evaluating the results of a nursing unit? Each of the performance areas is likely to have some associated key activities that can be budgeted and measured.[2]

It will take a fair amount of thought to come up with a good set of performance areas and measures of performance. For example, are patients' complaints an appropriate measure of patient satisfaction with the nursing unit? If patients complain about

---

[2] The measures described are a mix of both process and outcome measures. They also overlap to some extent. Eventually, performance budgeting may be refined to a point where such problems can be overcome.

TABLE 11-3 Performance Budget

Performance Catergory	Type of Activity	Description of Output Measure	Amount of Output Budgeted	Total	Average Cost
Quality improvement	Patient care planning	Patient care plan compliance	10% Reduction in failure rate	$ 87,300	$8,730 per 1% Drop in failure rate
Staffing	Daily staff calculations	1) Number of daily calculations	1) 365 Daily calculations	15,300	$41.92 Per Daily calculation
		2) Reduction in paid hours per patient day	2) .2 Paid hours per patient day		$76,500 per 1 Hour reduction/ patient day for the year
Cost control	Reduce cost	Reduction in cost/patient day	$8/Patient day	85,500	$10,687 Reduction for the year
Increase productivity	1) Revise procedures	Reduction in total unit cost per direct care hour	$3 Reduction per direct care hour	40,500	$13,500 Per $1 reduction in cost per direct care hour
	2) Work more efficiently				
Increase patient satisfaction	Respond to needs	Complaints	10% Reduction in complaints	232,500	$23,250/10% Reduction in complaints
Improve staff morale	Respond to needs	Turnover	25% Reduction in turnover	12,000	480 Per 1% reduction in turnover
Innovation & planning	Planning sessions	Number of meetings	12 Meetings	10,500	$875/Meeting
Direct care	Direct patient care	Hours of care	10,000 Hours	771,000	$77.10/Direct care hour
Indirect care	Charting, cleaning, etc.	Number of patient days	7,300 Patient days	454,500	$62.26/Patient day
Other				90,900	
Total				$1,800,000	

nurses, is it because the quality of care or attention to patients is not what it should be or is it simply that the patients are reflecting their general mood related to their illnesses? However, **increases** in the rate of complaints may well be a meaningful performance measurement.

Quality of Care

The quality of care measure will be addressed first because quality always presents a particular measurement challenge. Earlier, the use of medication variances was suggested as one possible measure for the change in quality of care. Another possible approach is to focus on the patient care plan as a quality indicator. If nurses are not skillfully developing patient care plans, ultimately, patient care may suffer. Therefore it is possible to measure the quality of nursing by how well plans are developed. Measurement can be based on the **percentage** of reduction in the number of incomplete care plans, or it can be based on the **number** of incomplete care plans. Many nursing units already measure the quality of their patient care planning. However, with performance budgeting, not only is the quality measured but the measurement is also associated with the expected cost of improving compliance.

In the first row of Table 11-3, it can be seen that one performance area in the budget is Quality Improvement. The measure used for this performance area will be the percentage of reduction in incomplete patient care plans. A 10% reduction is budgeted. As Table 11-2 showed, $87,300 is devoted to this area of the budget. Therefore it is expected that each percentage of reduction in incomplete plans will cost $8,730. This represents the total $87,300 to be spent in this area divided by the volume of output expected; in this case, $87,300 divided by a 10% reduction equals $8,730 per one percent reduction in the failure rate.

This approach recognizes that improvements in performance cost money. It is insufficient simply to dictate that a nursing unit improves its patient care planning without providing additional resources to accomplish this end. Can this unit lower its failure rate even more? Yes, it probably can. However, the performance budget provides explicit information that improved patient care planning requires more attention from the nursing staff. Such additional attention requires real additional resources in terms of increased staffing. If additional staffing is not provided, the only way to improve patient care planning is to devote a greater percentage of the staff's efforts to compliance in this area (unless productivity can be increased). However, this will mean devoting less time to other areas. And if that happens, it will be extremely important for the manager to plan which activities will have reduced time and to project the costs of reducing time in other activities. More typically, administrators have expected that nurses would just absorb the extra duties into their workloads, and no other aspects of their work would suffer quality decrements. This is an unreasonable expectation, and it has as its underlying assumption that nurses are not working hard enough now.

A major threat to quality in any arena, whether it be health care, manufacturing, or other service industries, is variability in performance and outputs. If the manager increases workload in one area for nurses whose time is already constrained, the natural result will be that nurses spend less time in some other aspect of the job. However, not every nurse will select the same job activity to reduce. Thus, the inevitable outcome of failing to manage a change in work expectations is higher variability in how nurses spend their time at work. This will produce higher variability in the quality of nursing services. This reality should impel the nurse manager who has decided to use performance-based budgeting to consider and make decisions carefully about changes in staffing levels to meet the new goals. Or if additional staff are not provided, the nurse manager should ask, "Which work activities are to be prioritized differently when the budget changes in response to new performance goals?" It is important to consider that a change to performance-based budgeting will require the manager to work with the staff to determine how best to meet the performance goals in all areas simultaneously and to avoid the danger of focusing on one goal such that another area of performance suffers.

As an example, consider the case in which a unit is satisfied with its patient care plans. The nurse manager of the unit does not believe that it is worth a substantial effort to improve its patient care planning. However, even maintaining a given level of quality requires staff attention. And if another area of work is deemed to need more attention, it will be important to organize and prioritize the work in such a way that care plan performance does not deteriorate. Thus the performance budget might show a goal of no change in the number of incomplete plans. An explicit portion of the performance budget would still be allocated to the quality area so as to achieve that steady state.

What happens if the overall budget for the nursing unit is cut? The performance budget allows determination of areas in which resources should be cut. If a choice is made to cut resources in an area that affects quality, it would not be surprising to detect later that the number of incomplete patient care plans is increasing. The performance budget would show how the cuts to the unit are expected to affect the various performance areas. Budget cuts must be assigned explicitly to the performance areas to be cut. It is vitally important that managers avoid the expectation that there will be no impact from budget cuts; explicit choices about which performance goals to scale back should be made, and the unit manager should communicate to the administration which outcomes are likely to deteriorate as a result of the budget cut.

Staffing

A nursing unit manager must make many staffing decisions throughout the year as well as manage vacations, holidays, sick leave, and busy and slow periods. In Table 11-3, it is assumed that daily calculations are made for staff adjustments. This requires some managerial time each and every day.

Calculations by the unit manager to adjust unit staffing could conceivably be made weekly or just once a month. If staffing were adjusted only monthly, extra staff might be assigned all month long so that there would be adequate staff for busy days. Less frequent work on staffing would save managerial time but would likely result in higher staffing costs. Monthly calculations would require the unit to devote only about $1,275 of management resources to staffing annually instead of the $15,300 annual cost that results when staffing is adjusted daily. However, the cost of extra nursing staff might offset the savings. The performance budget serves a useful function by making explicit the costs of daily calculations.

The performance budget can also show the benefits of daily calculations. Suppose that it is expected that by adjusting staffing daily, 7 days a week, to the desired staffing level for the actual workload, it is possible to reduce the overall average paid hours per patient day by 0.2 hour (12 minutes). Presumably, by monitoring staffing needs closely, it is possible to avert unneeded overtime, excessive use of agency nurses, and periods of overstaffing. If the 0.2 hour per patient day reduction is achieved by calculating staffing daily, $15,300 of the departmental budget will be devoted to staffing calculations. However, if the nursing unit has an average census of 20 patients, there would be a savings, on average, of four paid nursing hours per day (20 patients × 0.2 hour per patient day), or 1,460 nursing hours per year. The cost of 1,460 nursing hours at approximately $36 per hour is $52,560. That is more than three times the $15,300 investment in daily calculations to adjust staffing. A net savings of $37,260 in unit costs is almost certainly worth the investment of $15,300 to achieve that savings (i.e., $52,560 savings less the $15,300 investment = overall savings of $37,260).

It is possible to calculate the return on investment for this activity. Suppose that in this example, the average nurse wage on the unit is approximately $36 per hour. The total wage savings is $52,560. A return on investment can be calculated by dividing the savings of $52,560 by the cost of $15,300, or 3.43. In other words, $3.43 is saved for every dollar spent by doing staffing adjustments daily.

Cost Control

The purpose of cost control is to reduce or restrain increases in the organization's costs. For health care providers paid under a prospective payment system, such as capitation or diagnosis related groups, reduced costs per patient directly improve the organization's financial health. The performance measure for cost control in Table 11-3 focuses on a reduction in the cost per patient day. The activity, to reduce cost, really represents a goal rather than a description of specifically how the nurses in the unit are to go about accomplishing the goal. However, the budget shows a clear commitment in this area: $85,500 is allocated specifically to accomplishing this end. Referring to Table 11-1, it is possible to see how much of the cost control effort is expected to come from the nurse manager's time, how much from the staff, how much from formal education, and so forth. In this example, each staff nurse is expected to spend 5% of the time, or about 2 hours per week, specifically focusing on cost reduction. This could mean 8 hours at a continuing education program once a month. Or it might mean that small teams of nurses have some scheduled meeting times monthly to brainstorm about the areas they think could be run more efficiently. In this computer age, it might mean that all of the staff participate in an online virtual conference in which the subject of conversation is generating ideas about how to save costs. It does not necessarily mean that each week each nurse will spend 2 hours on cost control.

In Table 11-3, it can be seen that the performance budget calls for a cost reduction per patient day of $8. The cost of the efforts in this area are budgeted to be $85,500. Most of this comes from requiring the staff to make a specific effort to find ways of containing costs. When the $85,500 budgeted cost for cost control is compared with the budgeted cost reduction of $8 per patient day, for each dollar saved in cost per patient day it will cost the unit $10,687.50.[3] That seems rather high. Perhaps the unit is spending more on this activity than it is worth. In some cases the performance budget may make explicit the fact that the unit is spending more to accomplish an end than it is worth.

---

[3] $85,500 ÷ $8 per patient day = $10,687.50 per dollar saved per patient day. Typically we find the cost per unit, such as the cost per percentage reduction in turnover or the cost per percentage reduction in incomplete patient care plans. This is similar to finding the cost per patient day or the cost per discharge.

However, care must be exercised in interpreting the performance budget. If $10,687 is spent to save a dollar per patient day, there must be a consideration of how many patient days there are likely to be. If the unit's average census is 20, there will be 7,300 patient days during the year (20 patients per day × 365 days in a year), and the savings of $1 per patient day would be $7,300, or about $3,400 less than the $10,687 cost. However, if the census is 28, the savings would be $10,220 which is just slightly less than the cost of producing those savings. The census would need to be at least 30 for this investment in resources to produce a small savings of $263 per year.

Cost control is a general goal. Although the cost per patient day is a rough proxy intended to measure success with respect to that goal, it may be that the cost-control efforts are also saving money by allowing patients to be discharged sooner. The shorter length of stay decreases overall costs.

To determine the true payback of cost-control efforts, it would be necessary to combine the savings from the reduced cost per patient day with the savings from the shorter length of stay. The same $85,500 effort to achieve cost control will be working toward both of those ends. For this reason, although it is more complicated, it is often worth using several different measures of performance to assess more completely the unit and its accomplishments. This is discussed subsequently in the Multiple Measures section of this chapter.

Increased Productivity

The desired productivity outcome is for the unit to accomplish more with the same or fewer resources. Procedures may have to be revised to help the staff accomplish this. It is difficult to specify exactly how this can be accomplished, but it is not difficult to establish how to measure success. Assume that the organization is concerned about the cost of direct hours of care per patient day. If the total budgeted cost for the department is divided by the total direct patient care hours, a cost per direct care hour can be determined. It will probably be necessary to do occasional special studies to measure, on average, how many direct patient care hours are being provided.

Performance can then be assessed by the reduction in the overall unit cost per direct patient care hour. Such a reduction would indicate either a reduction in total costs or an increase in direct care hours. This approach has a big advantage over simply looking at the cost per patient day. If the cost per patient day declines, this could mean that patients are getting less care during each day. With this measure, cost of care is directly linked to the number of hours of direct care.

Is it worth it for the unit to allocate $40,500 of resources to attempt to reduce the cost per direct care hour? This comes out to a cost of $13,500 for each $1 reduction in the cost per direct care hour (see Table 11-3). The answer depends on how many direct care hours are provided. Over time, bedside computer terminals are likely to become more sophisticated and more widely used. That will allow direct patient care hours to be easily obtainable information, making this approach practical as well as informative.

Patient Satisfaction and Staff Morale

The key approach to satisfaction is to be responsive to the needs of individuals. Some health care organizations use a formal instrument to collect data concerning patient satisfaction. That would be a good tool to use for performance budgeting. However, even if the organization is not that sophisticated or is unwilling to spend the money on data collection that a formal instrument requires, performance budgeting can still be useful. One simply needs to be a bit more creative in establishing the measurement proxies.

For example, to measure patient satisfaction, the number of complaints could be counted. It may be true that some complaints are unreasonable or are about things that are not controllable. Many dissatisfied patients may not complain to anyone at the hospital. However, dissatisfied patients are likely to spread the story of their dissatisfaction widely (Kurtus, 2006; Wysocki et al., 2001). "It is said that an unhappy customer will tell 13 people about his or her dissatisfaction" (Kurtus, 2006). And those 13 will tell other people. It is not unreasonable to think that 60 people or more might hear of the problem that occurred with your service. For every person who complains, there may be hundreds who are unhappy but do not complain. Therefore, complaints are an important indicator to monitor because they may warn management of serious problems that would otherwise go undiscovered. Despite the relatively small number of people who complain to management, some reduction in the number of complaints may be a means of going about measuring increases in patient satisfaction. As with other areas, it must be determined how much of an increase in patient satisfaction it is hoped can be generated and whether the cost of the increase in satisfaction scores is acceptable relative to the expected level of improvement.

Staff morale might also be measured in terms of complaints. However, turnover rates might be a better indicator. If the hypothetical numbers in the example were correct, taking action to improve staff morale that requires $12,000 of total cost would be worthwhile because it would cost only $480 for each 1% reduction in staff turnover on the unit. This is likely to be a small cost compared with the cost of recruiting and orienting new staff.

Innovation and Planning

Sometimes it is difficult to measure performance. Innovative activity is one example. Proxies for performance in this area tend to be particularly weak. On the other hand, one of the most important things that a manager can do is to be innovative and to foster innovation. By making innovative activity explicitly a part of the performance budget, the necessity of devoting energies to this area can be recognized, even if the proxies available to measure performance are weak.

One measure of innovative activity and accomplishment is the number of procedure changes introduced based on recently published research. Another is the number of meetings related to change—especially if brainstorming and group problem solving are given time on the agenda. The fact that meetings are taking place is probably an indicator that activity is going on in this area. Are the meetings themselves the end goal? No. Do more meetings necessarily mean that more is being accomplished? No. They do, however, provide some sense of the degree of innovative activity.

It is also beneficial to see how expensive meetings are (see Table 11-3). When managers and staff are aware of the cost per meeting, it is likely that more serious work will be done and in less time, with fewer meetings.

Although meetings are used in Table 11-3, it is clearly a measure of process rather than of actual innovation. The number of useful innovative ideas generated might be a better measure. And certainly some formal system of rewards should be developed to give employees an incentive to generate innovative ideas.

Direct Care

The measure suggested for performance evaluation in this area is the direct care cost per direct care hour. Lowering the cost per direct care hour can be achieved either by increasing the number of hours produced for the same cost or by lowering the costs for a given number of direct care hours. This is not the total unit cost per direct care hour. Rather, it considers the total cost for only the hours of direct care provided, divided by the hours of direct care. This will generate information on the cost per hour of the direct care. If this cost can be lowered, it often implies that less overtime was necessary or fewer agency nurses were being used. Another common way to achieve this goal is to substitute less skilled caregivers such as unlicensed assistive personnel for RNs or to substitute less expensive RNs for more experienced, more expensive RNs. However, replacing RNs with unlicensed assistive personnel has been associated with higher mortality rates and higher complication rates, and it may also increase costs in other areas far more than the salary savings to the unit (Aiken et al., 2002; Aiken, Smith, & Lake, 1994; Hinshaw et al., 1981). With the government, the public, and third-party payers focusing more on quality of care since the IOM report, all cost-savings initiatives must be carefully analyzed for their effects on patient outcomes. Some cost-savings initiatives could well result in unintended higher costs in one area than the initiative saves in another area.

Indirect Care

Indirect care is more difficult to measure than direct care because it comprises a wide variety of activities, such as charting and communication with physicians. One approach is to measure the cost per patient day for these indirect activities. Reducing the cost per patient day of indirect activities is likely to indicate improved efficiency, unless the quality of the activities deteriorates. However, if there are a series of quality performance measures, such as patient care planning, adverse patient events, and other checks on quality, such deterioration would probably not go unnoticed.

Other

Some activities do not lend themselves to quantification and analysis. It is preferable to reduce the portion of the budget used for "other" purposes as much as possible. However, although they exist, there is no simple way to measure performance with respect to the use of resources devoted to these activities.

This discussion is not meant to be comprehensive. Rather, it presents some examples of ways in which specific measures can be associated with various performance areas. It is necessary for the nurse manager to manage staff closely so as to ensure that they follow the performance budget as closely as possible. If staff is included in the process of preparing performance budgets, they are more likely to strive to achieve the budgeted targets. One indication of the success of the performance budget approach is the extent to which the unit achieves its performance budget goals.

■ MULTIPLE MEASURES

In most of the cases mentioned, one measurement was used for each of the various performance areas. This is not always an optimal approach. For example, the percentage of patient care plans that are incomplete is not the only measure of quality available to nursing units. Adverse events, such as medication errors or the number of patient falls, could also be measured. As performance budgets become more sophisticated, it would not be unreasonable for the $87,300 allocated for quality to be subdivided. Perhaps half of the quality efforts will be related to patient care plans, one quarter to reducing patient falls, and one quarter to reducing the number of medication variances. In that case, the $87,300 in the performance budget would be subdivided into $43,650 for patient care plans, $21,825 for reducing patient falls, and $21,825 for reducing medication variances. The budgeted cost per fall prevented and the budgeted cost per medication variance avoided could be calculated in the same way as the budgeted cost for reducing failures to comply with patient care plan procedures was calculated earlier.

This multiple-measure approach is clearly superior to using one measure for each performance area. It is likely that the nurse manager will be trying to improve quality in many areas, so assigning all $87,300 to one area is likely to be an overstatement of the cost per unit of performance in that area. It also ignores other important activities. Some quality improvement activities such as providing research-based care may improve several areas of quality, whereas other approaches such as a staff development program about decreasing medication errors may be specific to one area.

Suppose that the quality outcome area is subdivided, and it is determined that 10 medication variances can be eliminated by focusing specific attention on that area. Suppose further that it would cost $14,250 to do this. The cost per medication variance eliminated would be $1,425. Is this too much to spend on this problem? Perhaps it is so low that even more should be spent to try to eliminate additional medication variances. The key is that this approach allows the manager to quantify the financial impact of many activities that are currently being performed without any specific cost-effectiveness measurement. With this method it is possible to assess whether the results in a given area warrant the resource investment in that area.

In some cases, rather than allocating the cost to several different areas, it simply makes sense to aggregate the benefits yielded by the unit's efforts. For example, in the case of cost control, there may be efforts to reduce the cost per direct care hour, reduce supply costs, and also reduce the average length of stay. In real-life situations, it is probably hard to determine how much staff effort goes to reduced length of stay and how much effort to reduced direct hours per day. One solution is to calculate the benefits of both shorter length of stay and reduced direct hours per patient day and combine them. Thus the total benefits can be compared with the total costs.

Summary and Implications for Nurse Managers

There is a wealth of information to be gained from performance budgeting. It is a tool that is likely to improve substantially both the planning and the control processes in hospitals. Performance budgeting represents a proactive approach to management. This approach follows a basic concept of budgeting: managers prepare a plan and attempt to manage according to that plan.

The starting point in performance budgeting is to determine the key performance areas. Next, the operating budget is used to determine the resources available. There is no conflict between the operating budget and the performance budget. They should work together. The operating budget focuses primarily on input resources. How much is going to be spent on RNs, how much on aides, and how much on supplies? The performance budget focuses on both processes and outcomes. How much is being budgeted to improve quality, how much to provide direct patient care, how much to innovate?

Continued

Summary and Implications for Nurse Managers—cont'd

As health care organizations move forward in managerial sophistication, they must move beyond the focus on inputs and begin to focus on performance. Financial pressure to be more efficient can easily lead to deterioration in the quality of care provided. However, cuts in resources do not have to affect performance in a random or arbitrary manner. Performance budgeting can show where resources are being used. Movement toward a measurement focus on the costs of the goals of the nursing unit can allow the manager to make choices and to allocate scarce resources wisely among alternative possible uses.

Performance budgeting is time-consuming and challenging. In some cases, the allocation of money to goal achievement will be inexact or arbitrary. However, it has tremendous potential value in health care organizations. Performance budgets can allow for an indication of the level of quality of care expected in a planned budget. They can explicitly show quality decreases that are likely if budgets are cut without corresponding reduction in patient days. It is likely that as part of the evolution in budgeting, this is an approach that will gain ever wider use.

References and Suggested Readings

Aiken, L., Clarke, S., Sloane, D., Sochalski, J., Silber, J. (2002). Hospital nurse staffing and patient mortality, nurse burnout, and job dissatisfaction. *Journal of the American Medical Association.* 288(16), 1987-1993.

Aiken, L., Smith, H., Lake, E. (1994). Lower Medicare mortality among a set of hospitals known for good nursing care. *Medical Care.* 32(5), 771-787.

Castaneda-Mendez, K. (1997). Value-based cost management: The foundation of a balanced performance measurement system. *Journal of Healthcare Quality.* 18(4), 6-9.

Cuddigan, J., Berlowitz, D., Ayello, E. (eds). (2001). Pressure ulcers in America: Prevalence, incidence, and implications for the future. An Executive Summary of the National Pressure Ulcer Advisory Panel (NPUAP) Monograph. *Advances in Skin and Wound Care.* 14(4, Part 1), 208-215.

Ditmyer, S., Keopsell, B., Branum, V., et al. (1998). Developing a nursing outcomes measurement tool. *Journal of Nursing Administration.* 28(6), 10-16.

Dongsung, K. (2006). Performance-based budgeting: The U.S. experience. *Public Organization Review: A Global Journal.* 5(2), 91-107.

Finkler, S.A., Ward, D.R. (1999). *Cost Accounting for Health Care Organizations: Concepts and Applications,* ed 2. Gaithersburg, MD: Aspen.

Hinshaw, A., Scofield, R., Atwood, J. (1981). Staff, patient, and cost outcomes of all registered nurse staffing. *Journal of Nursing Administration.* 11(6), 30-36.

Kurtus, R. (2006). Dealing with customer complaints. *School for Champions.* Downloaded on September 5, 2006, from: http://www.school-for-champions.com/tqm/complaints.htm.

Leeth, L. (2004). Are you fiscally fit? *Nursing Management.* 35(4), 42-47.

Reed, L., Blegen, M.A., Goode, C.S. (1998). Adverse patient occurrences as a measure of nursing care quality. *Journal of Nursing Administration.* 28(5), 62-69.

Rizzo, J. (1993). Flexible and performance budgeting for the nursing unit. *Hospital Cost Management and Accounting.* 5(4), 1-8.

Roey, K. (1997). *Managing Outcomes, Process, and Cost in a Managed Care Environment.* Gaithersburg, MD: Aspen.

Romero, D., Treston, J., and O'Sullivan, A. (2006). Raising awareness of pressure ulcer prevention and treatment. *Advances in Skin and Wound Care.* 19(7), 398-405.

Rosen, A., Zhao, S., Rivard, P., Loveland, S., Montez-Rath, M., Elixhauser, A., Romano, P. (2006). Tracking rates of patient safety indicators over time: Lessons from the Veterans Administration. *Medical Care.* 44(9), 850-861.

Schmidtlein, F. (1999). Assumptions underlying performance-based budgeting. *Tertiary Education & Management.* 5(2):159-174.

Suthathip, Y., Burgess, J. (2005). Performance-based budgeting in the public sector: An illustration from the VA health care system. *Health Economics.* 15(3), 295-310.

Wysocki, A., Kepner, K., Glasser, M. (2001). *Customer complaints and types of customers.* EDIS document HR 005, Department of Food and Resource Economics, Florida Cooperative Extension Service, Institute of Food and Agricultural Sciences, University of Florida, Gainesville, FL. Downloaded on September 5, 2000, from http://edis.ifas.ufl.edu/HR005.

12

Cash Budgeting

■ WHO'S RESPONSIBLE FOR CASH BUDGETING?

Cash budgeting is not a direct nursing responsibility. The financial officers of the organization must be aware of the timing of the organization's *cash receipts* and *cash payments*. In order to respond to this responsibility, these financial officers prepare cash budgets that predict when excess cash will be available and when the cash balance is likely to become negative if specific actions are not taken. Nevertheless, all managers should understand the relationship between the various budgets in the organization. Cash budgeting is as vital to the survival and well-being of the organization as program, capital, and operating budgets are. The nurse manager should have a reasonable understanding of cash budgets and the cash budgeting process. It is often cash budget problems that force the need for modifications in the budgets that nurse managers have prepared. This increases the importance of a nurse manager's having a basic understanding of the elements of cash budgeting.

■ THE CASH BUDGET

A substantial part of this book has focused on the operating budget and its control. The operating budget is concerned with the revenues and expenses of an organization. Revenues and expenses should not be thought of as being the same as cash receipts and cash payments. For most organizations, revenues and expenses are not recorded in the accounting records at the time cash is received or paid. Revenue, for example, is usually recorded when patients are billed. It may be weeks or months before the patients or a third-party payer such as Medicaid pays the bills. Furthermore, capital expenditures often require substantial cash outlays at the time a capital item is acquired.

The operating budget is defined in terms of revenues and expenses. This allows for an assessment of whether the planned operating budget implies an expected surplus, a break-even situation, or a loss. Determining whether a surplus or loss is expected is critical information for management decision making. To a great extent, this calculation of whether the results of normal operations of the organization are likely to result in a surplus or loss is seen as information more valuable than knowing when the revenues will actually be received in cash or when the expenses will have to be paid in cash. As a result, the operating budget focus is not on when cash comes and goes but instead on the total revenues and expenses for the year.

However, this does not mean that the flow of cash in and out of the organization is unimportant. Administration of the cash flow is a critical function of successful management. In order to pay employees and meet other obligations on a timely basis, the organization's managers must know how much cash is expected to be on hand at any given time. The amount and timing of the cash flowing into and out of the organization can substantially impact the ability of the organization to meet its current cash obligations. Therefore, a distinct and separate cash budgeting process exists. The fact that the process is separate and is conducted primarily by the organization's financial officers should not lead one to believe that the cash budget is not integrally related to the other budgets and decisions of the organization.

The development of the cash budget is based on the necessity of meeting routine cash requirements for salaries and supplies. At times, proper administration of the organization's cash flow will cause the organization to make decisions that seem to make no sense in the way they impact nurse managers. For example, consider a request by nursing to buy new clinic equipment for $200,000. The equipment is expected to have a useful lifetime of 10 years and will generate an extra $40,000 per year in revenues from new patients that the clinic cannot treat without the equipment. The $400,000 of revenues over the 10-year period is enough to make the initial investment of $200,000 profitable. Each year an extra $40,000 of revenue and an extra $20,000 of depreciation expense (one tenth the cost of the equipment would be charged as an expense for each of the 10 years) would be shown. There is a profit of $20,000 per year. (Assume there are no costs for using the equipment.) Yet, the financial officers may say that the organization cannot afford the equipment.

How can this decision make any sense to the staff and managers of the affected departments? Cash flow administration is typically conducted entirely within the department of the chief financial officer, so the reason for the denial may never be communicated to the people in the affected department. This is unfortunate because it can result in morale problems. The department staff—and even the manager—may conclude that the top administrators don't make good decisions or, worse, that they don't care about the welfare of the patients. Because the needs of the cash budget can drive decisions that otherwise may not be comprehensible to department managers and their staff, executives may want to consider communicating financial goals and necessities, including the facts about the cash budget, as part of the overall financial management message they send to the rest of the organization (Hamm, 2006).

It is the job of the chief financial officer to manage the cash budget. Given the long time it typically takes to receive payment from third-party payers in the health care system, health care facilities are often forced to make decisions based more on the cash flow needs of the organization than on the long-term profitability of capital purchases. Even though a profit will be earned each year from new equipment, the organization may not be able to purchase the equipment. The entire price of

$200,000 for the equipment will have to be paid in cash this year, even though the revenues are only $40,000 this year. Where will the cash for the initial $200,000 purchase come from?

The potential for profit does not by itself provide the cash needed to make the investment. Certainly, it might be wise to lease the asset rather than pay all the cash up front. Or maybe the organization can borrow the money from a bank. Or perhaps it can raise the money through contributions. The organization's managers should try to pursue various ways to get the cash for worthwhile investments—whether they are worthwhile because they are profitable or simply because they are good for the patients—but there is a responsibility to the well-being of the organization to avoid committing to major purchases until it has first been determined that there will be sufficient cash available to meet the payments.

Financial officers must carefully consider the cash implications of the operating and capital budgets before those budgets are approved. In effect, various departments submit their operating and capital budget requests. A cash budget is developed based on these requests. One reason departmental budgets may be rejected is that the cash budget may show that the organization would simply run out of cash if it makes all the requested payments. If an organization finds itself without cash to meet its obligations, it may be forced into bankruptcy. Even if the organization is making a profit, without careful management, it may run out of cash and get into financial difficulty.

■ CASH MANAGEMENT

In a well-run organization, cash is actively managed. This means that an initial projection is made regarding the timing of cash receipts from philanthropy, patients, the government, and insurance companies (including HMOs). An initial projection of the dates payments must be made by the organization is also prepared. The cash excess or shortfall is calculated.

If there is a shortfall, it may be possible to go to a bank and arrange for a line of credit to be available at the projected time cash is needed. Before doing that, however, other approaches must be considered. What if the financial managers take actions to process patient billings more quickly and accurately so that payments will be received sooner? Will the extra cost of speedier invoicing be offset by the interest saved by borrowing less money from the bank? What if payments to the organization's suppliers are delayed by 30 days to avoid borrowing money? How angry will this make the organization's suppliers? How much interest will the suppliers charge for that delay? Will late payments cause suppliers to refuse to extend any credit to the facility and demand payment in advance of delivery of supplies? Imagine a situation in which a hospital could not obtain any IV fluid supplies without having to make a decision between paying out the money for the supplies and meeting payroll that week? This is exactly the situation that some hospitals have found themselves in when cash budget difficulties caused them to be chronically late with payments to suppliers. That situation puts any organization in imminent jeopardy of bankruptcy and closure.

Actions taken to speed up the receipt of cash and to slow down the payment of cash are part of the cash management of the organization. Another critical piece of cash management is determining how much cash the organization needs to keep in its bank accounts. Managing cash is much like walking a tightrope. It is important that enough cash be held by the organization to meet its routine needs for payroll and payments to creditors and to provide a cushion of cash to cover any unexpected *contingencies*. On the other hand, when more money is kept in cash, less is available for capital investment and other organizational needs.

The goal is to have enough cash to meet routine needs and contingencies but not any more than that. If there is no immediate use for excess cash, it can be invested to earn interest, used to repay loans, or used to provide more health care services. Thus, financial managers must be careful to ensure that the organization will always have enough cash to meet obligations, but they also must be careful to ensure that the organization is not missing opportunities to provide additional health services because it is keeping too much cash in the bank. Thus, either too little or too much cash leaves the organization in a less than optimal situation.

■ CASH BUDGET PREPARATION

In health care organizations, the cash budget is generally prepared for the entire coming year on a monthly basis. Some businesses such as banks even prepare cash budgets on a daily basis in order to be sure to have cash on hand for particularly busy days of the week or month.

The format of cash budgets is fairly standard. Each month begins with a starting cash balance. The expected cash receipts for the month are added to this. These receipts may be broken down into categories such as inpatient, outpatient, other operating, and nonoperating, or by payer (e.g., Medicare, Medicaid, HMO, other insurers, self-pay patients, donations, and cafeteria sales). The starting cash balance is added to the total receipts to get a subtotal of available cash.

Expected cash payments are subtracted from the available cash. The principal categories of payments include salaries, payments to suppliers, payments for capital acquisitions, and payments on loans. The result of subtracting total payments from the available cash is a tentative cash balance. This balance is considered tentative because the organization will generally have a minimum desired cash balance at the end of each month. This minimum balance is used for cash payments at the beginning of the next month and also serves as a safety net for any required but unexpected cash outlays.

If the tentative balance exceeds the minimum desired balance, the excess can be invested. If the tentative cash balance is less than the minimum desired balance, the organization will borrow funds to meet the minimum level if their credit is good enough. If their credit is poor, the organization may have to liquidate reserves or investment funds to meet cash requirements. The final cash balance is the tentative cash balance less any amounts invested or plus any amounts borrowed. If an organization is in particularly poor financial condition, banks may be unwilling to lend money. Such a situation will lead to a crisis unless all budgeting is done carefully enough throughout the organization that cash *deficits* are not encountered. Generally, this requires severe service cutbacks.

One of the cash management problems health care financial officers have had to cope with in the recent past is commercial third-party payers' deciding to improve their own cash flow by delaying payments. This has been a particular problem for clinical and medical practices. As a result, during the 1990s and the beginning of the new millennium lawsuits have been filed by state attorneys general and health care providers to force the insurers to make payments within 30 days (Barbier & Roberts, 2006; Mercer, 2005; State of Connecticut, 2000).

If a surplus one month is followed by a shortfall the next, it may pay to invest the extra cash in a short-term investment such as a money market fund. In this way, the excess cash from one month can earn some interest, which can be available to meet the shortage the next month. Borrowing can thus be avoided. In general, the interest rate paid on borrowed money will exceed the rate that can be earned on money invested for a short period. The cash balance at the end of any month will be the starting cash balance for the next month. An example of a cash budget for the first quarter of a year is presented in Table 12-1.

In the example, the beginning cash balance for January is $20,000. Combining the beginning cash balance with the $385,000 expected in receipts during January, $405,000 will be available in cash. Subtracting the expected disbursements of $375,000 leaves a month-end tentative cash balance of $30,000. Assuming that $20,000 is desired as a safety cushion, $10,000 is available to invest. In February, cash payments have risen by $25,000, but cash receipts have risen even more. The result is that there is an additional $18,000 available for short-term investment.

The tables turn in March. Cash receipts are down and cash payments are up. What could logically cause this result? Does it indicate a serious problem? Very possibly not. It is reasonable to assume that during December; substantially fewer elective procedures were done because of the holiday season. The March cash receipts from Medicaid patients are likely to be influenced by what happened in December. On the other hand, because January, February, and March may have colder weather, they are quite possibly busy months with high salary payments for overtime and

TABLE 12-1 Cash Budget for One Quarter

	January	February	March
Starting cash balance	$ 20,000	$ 20,000	$ 20,000
Expected receipts			
Medicare	$120,000	$140,000	$115,000
Medicaid	80,000	90,000	75,000
HMOs	90,000	90,000	90,000
Other insurers	42,000	40,000	40,000
Self-pay	40,000	38,000	41,000
Philanthropy	5,000	10,000	8,000
Other	8,000	10,000	9,000
Total receipts	$385,000	$418,000	$378,000
Available cash	$405,000	$438,000	$398,000
Less expected payments			
Labor costs	$170,000	$180,000	$190,000
Suppliers	25,000	30,000	40,000
Capital acquisitions	0	10,000	15,000
Payments on loans	180,000	180,000	180,000
Total payments	$375,000	$400,000	$425,000
Tentative cash balance	$ 30,000	$ 38,000	$ (27,000)
Less amount invested	(10,000)	(18,000)	28,000
Plus amount borrowed			19,000
Final cash balance	$ 20,000	$ 20,000	$ 20,000

agency nurses. But the revenues for the cold months will not be received as cash until 30 to 60 days (or more) after the services were provided. Thus, it is not surprising to see lower cash receipts in a given month and at the same time see cash payments that are rising during that month. Frequently, health care organizations find that in a given month their payments are greatly influenced by the current month's activity but that their receipts are more influenced by workload in earlier months.

The March tentative balance indicates a cash deficit of $27,000. Additionally, there is a desired $20,000 ending balance. This need can be met in several ways. The organization could simply borrow $47,000. A more likely result is that the $10,000 invested in January and the $18,000 invested in February will be used to reduce the amount needed to $19,000. Then the $19,000 will be borrowed.

Planning for necessary borrowing should take place well in advance. The plan developed should include a projection of when it will be possible to repay the loan. Bankers are much more receptive to an organization's needs if it has specific plans and projections than if it simply tries to borrow money when an immediate cash shortage becomes apparent. From the bank's perspective, an organization that can plan reasonably well is more likely to be able to repay a loan than one that does not even know several months in advance that a cash shortage is likely to occur.

Summary and Implications for Nurse Managers

Cash needs are crucial. As much as nurse managers may like to think of health care services as more than a business, if the organization cannot pay its bills, it will be out of business. The role of cash budgeting is therefore vital to the overall budget process.

Although cash budgets are normally prepared by financial managers, nurse managers should be aware of the crucial role that they play in the overall budget process. Cash sufficiency is essential to making the program, capital, and operating budgets feasible. The cash budget will have a direct bearing on the items that will or will not be approved in operating and capital budgets.

Because of the delays in payments by the government, insurers, and self-pay patients and because of the long-term nature of some investments, cash receipts and payments do not neatly match each other within each month. Some months (or even years) produce cash surpluses and others produce cash deficits. Such surpluses and deficits are not necessarily the results of profits or losses. A profitable year may result in a cash deficit because of the need to make loan repayments or because of major capital acquisitions. Nurse managers must budget their resource needs carefully so that in periods of cash surplus, resources can be wisely invested and cash deficits can be covered by the organization without the need for emergency measures.

References and Suggested Readings

Barbier, R., Roberts, M. (2006). Managing managed care: Providers fight back against HMOs. *South Carolina Bar Association.* Downloaded on September 10, 2006 from: http://www.scbar.org/pdf/SCL/Sep01/barbier.pdf.

Berger, S. (2002). *Fundamentals of Health Care Financial Management: A Practical Guide to Fiscal Issues and Activities.* New York: Jossey-Boss.

Briggs, B. (2006). I.T. helps revenue cycle spin faster. *Health Data Management.* 14(6), 54, 56, 58.

Drewniak, S., Nagle, B. (2003). Effective cash management can save time and help boost profits. *Nursing News.* 27(2), 10.

Finkler, S.A., Ward, D.R., Baker, J. (2007). *Essentials of Cost Accounting for Health Care Organizations,* ed 3. Sudbury, MA: Jones & Bartlett.

Hamm, J. (2006). The five messages leaders must manage. *Harvard Business Review.* 84(5), 114-123

Jones, K.R. (1996). Cash management in health care organizations. *Seminars for Nurse Managers.* 4(3), 142-143.

Lofgren, R., Karpf, M., Perman, J., Higdon, C. (2006). The U.S. health care system is in crisis: Implications for academic medical centers and their missions. *Academic Medicine.* 81(8), 713-720.

McLean, R.A. (2002). *Financial Management in Health Care Organizations.* Albany, NY: Thomson-Delmar.

Mercer. (2005). *State high court to consider provider lawsuit against HMOs.* Downloaded on September 12, 2006, from: http://wrg.wmmercer.com/blurb/56366/.

Nowicki, M. (2004). *The Financial Management of Hospitals and Healthcare Organization,* ed 3. Chicago: Health Administration Press.

Pelfrey, S. (1990). Understanding the tools for managing cash. *Journal of Nursing Administration.* 20(10), 23-27.

Rivenson, H., Wheeler, J., Smith, D., Reiter, K. (2000). Cash management in health care systems. *Journal of Health Care Finance.* 24(4), 59-69.

Robertson, B., Raddemann, B. (2006). The monthly reserve valuation process. *Healthcare Financial Management.* 60(5), 113-115.

Robertson, B., Raddemann, B. (2006). Reserve process quality assessment. *Healthcare Financial Management.* 60(6), 111-112.

Runy, R. (2006). Debt financing: an executive's guide. *Hospitals & Health Networks.* 80(6), 41, 43-46.

State of Connecticut. (2000). Attorney General files class action lawsuit against Connecticut HMOs. *Connecticut Attorney General's Office Press Release.* Downloaded on September 12, 2006, from: http://www.ct.gov/ag/cwp/view.asp?a=1775&q=283006.

Zelman, W., McCue, M., Millikan, A., Glick, N. (2003). *Financial Management of Health Care Organizations: An Introduction to Fundamental Tools, Concepts, and Applications,* ed 2. Malden, MA: Blackwell Publishing.

J

13

Variance Analysis

LEARNING OBJECTIVES
The goals of this chapter are to:

- Focus on issues of control, including uses and benefits of control
- Define variance analysis
- Explain the reasons for doing variance analysis
- Distinguish between the concept of an "unfavorable" variance and a bad outcome
- Discuss traditional unit or department line-item variances

- Outline some possible causes of variances
- Explain flexible or variable budgeting
- Introduce a flexible budget notation for variance analysis
- Define volume, quantity, and price variances
- Discuss analysis of revenue variances
- Provide variance analysis tools and examples

■ INTRODUCTION: USING BUDGETS FOR CONTROL

Budgets are plans. So far, this book has focused on budgets, but the title of the book uses the word "budgeting." Budgeting refers not only to making plans; it also refers to using those plans to control operations. If a plan is made and then not used, the organization is worse off than it was without the plan—the time wasted on preparing an unused plan could undoubtedly have been put to better use!

Certainly, making plans forces managers to think ahead and anticipate possible future events. Based on such planning, a manager may have made some useful decisions that would not have been made otherwise. Perhaps changes may have been made in the manner in which the organization is operated. For the most part, however, if budgets are not used to control operations, then budgeting is a fruitless process. Health care organizations prepare sophisticated budgets because they recognize a need to control their expenses. The government has limited the resources available to the health care sector by cutting the reimbursement rates for care provided to Medicare and Medicaid recipients.[1] Further potential cuts in Medicare and Medicaid are an ever-present threat to the finances of health care providers, nursing homes, and hospitals (Darves, 2003; Zwillich, February 2, 2006; Zwillich, February 6, 2006). Control of costs is vital.

---

[1] The total dollars budgeted for Medicare continue to rise, albeit at a slower rate than in the past. However, the rate paid per service for each Medicare patient has been cut.

In most health care organizations, such control is critical to survival. In other organizations, cost control is the only way to ensure continuation of all the things the organization is accustomed to—first class equipment and the ability to provide at least adequate and, hopefully, excellent care.

When resources become extremely limited, an organization has choices. It can reduce the quality of care, it can reduce services, or it can become more efficient. True efficiency means providing the same amount of care and quality of care at a lower cost; it requires avoiding waste of resources. Budgeting allows the manager to plan the resources that are needed to do the job. If the budget is not used during the year to control costs, resources may be wasted and services and quality of care may suffer. Using budgets to control costs will not eliminate all of an institution's financial woes, but without such control, the problems will be far worse.

Using budgets for control can help to locate causes of inefficiency and can help to avoid waste. In addition, in the hands of a skilled person, budgeting can also help to establish a defense for not meeting the budget (if there are valid reasons for the over-budget spending). Budgeting is a very powerful tool. This chapter and those that follow should be of particular interest to nurse managers because they contain important information on methods to defend over-budget spending when that spending is caused by factors outside the control of the nursing unit or department.

■ VARIANCE ANALYSIS

Variance analysis is the aspect of budgeting in which actual results are compared to budgeted expectations. The difference between actual results and planned results represents a *variance*, that is, the amount by which the results **vary** from the budget. Variances are calculated for three principal reasons. One reason is to aid in preparing the budget for the coming year. By understanding why results were not as expected, the budget process can be improved so that it will be more accurate in the future. The second reason is to aid in controlling results throughout the current year. By understanding why variances are occurring, actions can be taken to reduce or eliminate undesirable variances over the coming months. The third reason to calculate variances is to evaluate the performance of units or departments and their managers.

For variance reports to be an effective tool, managers must be able to understand the causes of the variances. This requires investigation, which in turn requires the knowledge, judgment, and experience of nurse managers. Variances can be calculated by financial managers. However, those finance personnel do not have the specific knowledge to explain why the variances are occurring. Without such explanations, the reports are not useful managerial aides.

Variance reports are given by the finance department to nurse managers for *justification*. The word "justification," which is often used, is unduly confrontational. It focuses attention on the evaluation role of variance analysis instead of on the planning and control roles. The goal of the investigation process is to obtain an explanation of why the variances arose. In the majority of cases, the variance report is used to understand what is happening and to control future results to the greatest extent possible. The focus should not be on a defensive justification of what was spent.

If variances arose as a result of inefficiency (e.g., long coffee breaks at the nurses' station), the process of providing cost-effective care is out of control. By discovering this inefficiency, actions can be taken to eliminate it and to bring the process back under control. In this case, future costs will be lower because of the investigation of the variance. The improvement comes, however, not from placing blame on who failed to control past results but on using the information to improve control of future results. It is important to realize that variance analysis provides its greatest benefits when it is used as a tool to improve future outcomes rather than as a way to assign blame for past results.

It would be naive; however, not to realize that in many cases health care organizations do use variances to assign blame for the organization's failures. Therefore, this chapter and the one that follows provide tools that will aid nurse managers and executives not only in explaining variances but also in deflecting blame for any variances that arise because of factors outside their control.

In many cases, variances are in fact caused by factors outside the control of nursing units or the nursing department. For example, increases in the average level of patient acuity may well cause staffing costs to rise. Because most facilities' contracts with payers do not permit the addition of extra charges for higher acuity, the hospital is not typically reimbursed for patients who require much extra care due to certain kinds of comorbidities (e.g., frail elderly patients) or mentation problems such as dementia. Yet these illnesses can sharply raise acuity and, thus, costs. Another example of an outside factor that can cause variances is unanticipated external price increases that cause more spending on clinical supplies than had been budgeted.

Although these factors are out of the control of nurse managers and should be explained as such, their impact on total costs should not be ignored. Competent nurse managers should be aware of the fact that even variances beyond their control may require that responsive actions be taken. Spending in excess of the budget in one area may result in the need to restrict spending in another. Adjustments to the entire budget must be considered and either made or rejected in the overall context of the organization and its financial situation.

On the other hand, if spending increases are the result of an increase in the number of patients, more revenue is likely to be received by the organization. In that case, there should be less pressure to restrict costs. It therefore becomes critical to understand as much as possible about why variances are occurring. Are they controllable or not? If they are controllable, can actions be taken to reduce or eliminate the variances? If they are not controllable, is their nature such that responsive actions are required?

■ TRADITIONAL VARIANCE ANALYSIS

At the end of a given time period, an organization compares its actual results to the budget. Suppose that the organization does this monthly. Several weeks after each month ends, the accountants gather all the cost information and report the actual totals for the month.[2]

The simplest approach is to compare the total costs that the entire organization has incurred with the budgeted costs for the entire organization. For example,

[2] One sign of the quality of a finance department is how quickly it provides department and unit managers with monthly variance reports after each month ends. If finance provides the reports in 2 weeks or less after the end of each month, it is doing an excellent job; 3 weeks after the end of the month is acceptable performance but is not excellent. Longer than 3 weeks indicates the need for improvement. For example, a variance report for the month of Janauary should ideally be received by the manager no later than February 14.

suppose that the Wagner Hospital had a total budget for the month of March of $4,800,000. The actual costs were $5,200,000. Wagner spent $400,000 more than had been budgeted. The difference between the amount budgeted and the amount actually incurred is the total hospital variance. This variance is referred to as an *unfavorable variance* because the organization spent more than had been budgeted. Accountants use the term *favorable variance* to indicate spending that is lower than expected.

Assuming that the Wagner Hospital begins its year on January 1, the variance could appear in a format somewhat like the following:

The Wagner Hospital
March Variance Report

	Actual	Budget	Variance
Current Month	$ 5,200,000	$ 4,800,000	$400,000 U
Year-to-Date	$15,150,000	$14,876,000	$274,000 U

In future examples, the *year-to-date* information will be dispensed with for simplicity. The focus will be on the current month under review. In health organizations, nurse managers are generally provided with information for the year-to-date as well as the current month. The capital U following the variance refers to the fact that the variance is unfavorable. If the variance were favorable, it would be followed by a capital F.

One alternative to using U and F is to use a negative number for an unfavorable variance and a positive number for a favorable variance. Or parentheses may be placed around unfavorable variances and no parentheses around favorable variances (parentheses indicate a negative number). It is important to exercise caution in interpreting variance notation. Any systematic approach can be used to indicate favorable versus unfavorable variances. It would not be wrong to use negative numbers for favorable variances and positive numbers for unfavorable variances, as long as the use is consistent throughout the organization. There is no consistent approach followed by all organizations in the health care industry.

Why has Wagner had a $400,000 unfavorable variance for the month of March? If variance analysis is to be used to evaluate results, it is necessary to be able to determine not simply that the organization was $400,000 over budget but why that occurred. Given this simple total for the entire organization, the chief executive officer has no idea what caused the variance. That officer does not even know which managers to ask about the variance because all that is known is the total amount of the variance for the entire organization.

One solution to this problem would be to have organization-wide *line-item* totals. That is, the total amount budgeted for salaries for the entire organization could be compared to actual total salary costs. The total amount budgeted for surgical supplies could be compared to the actual total amount spent on surgical supplies. The problem with this solution is that there would still be no way to determine what caused the variances. All departments have salaries. A number of departments use surgical supplies. Who should be asked about the variances?

In order to use budgets for control, it must be possible to assign responsibility for variances to individual managers. Those managers can investigate the causes of the variances and attempt to eliminate the variances in the future. The key is that it must be possible to hold individual managers accountable for the variances. This leads to the necessity of determining variances by unit and department. Although the following example uses a hospital, all variance analysis techniques discussed in this book apply equally to clinics, nursing homes, visiting nurse agencies, and all other types of health care organizations.

Unit and Department Variances

The overall Wagner variance of $400,000 is an aggregation of variances in a number of departments. The results for the Nursing Department were:

The Wagner Hospital
Department of Nursing Services
March Variance Report

Actual	Budget	Variance
$2,400,000	$2,200,000	$200,000 U

Apparently, half of the variance at the Wagner Hospital during March occurred in the nursing services area. Now there is more information than there was before. Previously it was known that there was an excess expenditure of $400,000, but it was not known how that excess came about. Now it is known that half of it occurred in the nursing area. The chief nurse executive (CNE) can be asked to explain why the $200,000 variance occurred.

Unfortunately, at this point the CNE has not been given much to go on. The CNE simply knows that there was an expenditure of $200,000 that was not in the budget. Most hospitals would take this total cost for the nursing department and break it down into the various nursing units. Each nursing unit that has a nurse manager who is responsible for running that unit should have both a budget for the unit and a variance report that shows the unit's performance in comparison to the budget.

The variance for one particular nursing unit might appear as follows:

The Wagner Hospital
Department of Nursing Services
Med/Surg 6th Floor West
March Variance Report

Actual	Budget	Variance
$120,000	$110,000	$10,000 U

Line-Item Variances

Once the total nursing department variance has been divided among the various nursing units, more information is still needed as a guide. Is the variance the result of unexpectedly high costs for nursing salaries? Does it relate to usage of supplies? There is no way to know based on a total variance for the unit or department. More detailed information is needed.

In order to have any real chance to control costs, there must be variance information for individual line items within a unit or department. The CNE must know how much of the nursing total went to salaries and how much to supplies. Nurse managers must have similar information for their own units. For example:

The Wagner Hospital
Department of Nursing Services
Med/Surg 6th Floor West
March Variance Report

	Actual	Budget	Variance
Salary	$108,000	$100,000	$ 8,000 U
Supplies	12,000	10,000	2,000 U
Total	$120,000	$110,000	$10,000 U

This is obviously a great simplification. There should be line items for employee-benefit costs. There should be separate line items for each type of employee. LPNs would be separate from RNs. Each major different type of other-than-personnel-services cost could be a separate line item. For example, see Table 13-1. The more detailed the line items are, the more information is available. Variance reports with detailed line-item results for each unit and department are generally available in health care organizations today.

Understanding Variances

The objectives of doing variance analysis are first to determine whether the budget variance is material or immaterial and, second, if the variance is material in amount, why it arose. Nothing can be done with respect to the goal of controlling costs until the nurse manager knows whether the variance is due to expected common-cause variation or whether it is due to a control problem. If the variance is material, the manager must determine where the unit or department is deviating from the plan and why. The more detailed the line-item information, the easier it will be to identify the specific areas where variances are occurring.

Once the variance for each line item in each unit has been calculated, it must be determined whether or not to investigate the variance. Minor variances (considered to be immaterial in amount) can be ignored. Variances that are significant in amount (considered to be material variances) must be investigated. (The issue of how to determine whether a variance is significant enough to warrant investigation is discussed in the next chapter under the heading Investigation and Control of Variances.) By dividing variances into nursing units, each unit manager can be assigned the responsibility of determining the causes of the variances in the unit. The manager of 6th Floor West must explain the causes of the $10,000 unfavorable unit variance.

By dividing the variances into line items, the unit manager can begin the investigation. In the case of this example, $8,000 of the variance is the result from labor costs, and $2,000 is the result from spending more on supplies than the budget allowed. Note that although the $8,000 labor variance is much larger than the supplies variance in absolute dollar terms, the labor variance is 8% over budget, whereas the supply variance is 20% over budget. Both these variances should be investigated and their causes determined. Where possible, corrective action should then be instituted to avoid similar variances in future months.

TABLE 13-1 Sample Variance Report: March 2008

Cost Center: 6th Floor West Med/Surg

This Month			Account No./Description	Year-to-Date		
Actual	Budget	Variance		Actual	Budget	Variance
$ 58,951	$ 53,431	$ 5,520	010 Salaries: RNs	$164,245	$160,296	$3,949
32,110	31,098	1,012	011 Salaries: LPNs	94,930	93,294	1,636
14,124	13,256	868	012 Salaries: Nurses' Aides	41,569	39,768	1,801
4,581	4,088	493	020 FICA	13,742	12,263	1,479
1,081	1,014	67	021 FICA	3,241	3,041	201
351	313	38	022 FICA	1,051	938	113
209	200	9	050 Life insurance	627	600	27
343	350	(7)	060 Other fringes	1,029	1,050	(21)
$111,750	$103,750	$ 8,000	(a) Personnel cost	$320,435	$311,249	$9,185
$ 4,970	$ 3,000	$ 1,970	300 Patient care supplies	$ 8,950	$ 9,000	($ 50)
828	800	28	400 Office supplies/forms	2,484	2,400	84
650	650	0	500 Seminars/meetings	1,950	1,950	0
750	750	0	600 Noncapital equipment	2,250	2,250	0
425	400	25	700 Maintenance/repair	1,275	1,200	75
45	50	(5)	800 Miscellaneous	135	150	(15)
582	600	(18)	900 Interdepartmental	1,746	1,800	(54)
$ 8,250	$ 6,250	$ 2,000	(b) Other than personnel services (OTPS)	$ 18,790	$ 18,750	$ 40
$120,000	$110,000	$ 10,000	(c) Total unit costs (c = a + b)	$339,225	$329,999	$9,225

Note: In this table, unfavorable variances are positive numbers and favorable variances are negative numbers.

Traditional variance analysis requires that the nurse manager proceed to use the unit line-item variance information to attempt to discover the underlying causes of the variances. Consider the $8,000 variance in salaries. Why were salaries $8,000 above the budget? No matter how narrowly defined the line items for salaries are (e.g., separating RNs from LPNs from nurses' aides), the question still arises: Why were salaries $8,000 above the budget?

In the absence of supporting evidence, the 6th Floor West unit manager and nurses may be told that they did not do a good job of controlling the use of staff. This is an unwarranted conclusion. Expenditure for staff in excess of the budgeted amount could have a number of possible causes. Investigation may disclose which potential cause was in fact responsible in a given instance.

One potential cause of the $8,000 salary variance is that the unit manager just did not do a good job in controlling the usage of staff. As a result, more hours of nursing care per patient were paid for than had been expected. Another possibility is that the patients were sicker than anticipated, and the higher average acuity level caused more nursing hours to be used per patient. Another possible cause is that the hourly rate for nurses increased. Nurse managers may have no direct control over base salaries. On the other hand, the higher cost could have been due to increased overtime. Overtime may be necessary because of higher-than-expected use of sick time, forcing the manager to pay overtime to cover the sick leaves. A problem like that may be out of management's control if perhaps there was an influenza epidemic in the community, causing both greater staff utilization and more sick leave.

A possible cause of unnecessary overtime might be something like staff signing or clocking in early (or clocking out late). If the hospital calculates overtime as one tenth of an hour, staff standing at the time clock for 6 minutes waiting to clock out so as to earn one tenth of an hour of overtime can easily become a practice. If the manager does not enforce policies related to clocking in only when the person's shift officially begins and clocking out immediately when the staff member leaves the unit, unnecessary and unauthorized overtime can quickly add up to substantial over-budget dollars. That one tenth of an hour of overtime equals an unnecessary over-time cost for every staff member who does this. Consider that such behavior in a unit with 40 RNs could amount to 40 hours of overtime every pay period (40 staff × 6 minutes per shift × 10 shifts per 2-week pay period = 2,400 minutes of overtime; 2,400 ÷ 60 minutes/hour = 40 hours of overtime). If the average hourly wage for RNs is $25.00 per hour, that wasted overtime, at time-and-a-half, amounts to $1,500 ($25 × 1.5 overtime rate = $37.50 × 40 hours = $1,500) per pay period, or $39,000 per year ($1,500 × 26 pay periods = $39,000).

Another possible cause of the variance is that there were more patients, and the additional patients caused more consumption of nursing hours. This is a case of necessary over-budget salary costs and typically, the extra salary costs are associated with higher patient care revenues. The most serious problem of traditional variance analysis is that it compares the predicted cost of a predicted workload level (e.g., volume of patient days adjusted for acuity) to the actual cost of the actual workload level.[3]

---

[3] The general term "workload" is used here because there is no single, unique measure of workload that is always relevant for budgeting. Sometimes we use the technocratic term "output" interchangeably with workload. If we are dealing with a home health agency, workload is measured by the number of visits. For the radiology department, the workload measure is likely to be the number of radiographs. For a nursing unit, the workload is generally the number of patient days, adjusted for acuity. For an operating room, it might be the number of procedures or hours of surgical procedures.

Unless the actual workload is exactly as predicted, there is little chance that a unit will achieve exactly the budgeted expectations.

Essentially, with traditional variance analysis, an attempt is being made to match actual costs to a budget that is relevant for an expected workload level. But the expected workload level is usually not the same as the actual workload. If a nursing unit has more or fewer patients, the original budget is no longer relevant. If costs fall by 5%, under traditional variance analysis, there is a temptation to praise the manager for coming in under budget. However, if patient volume falls by 20% and costs fall by only 5%, it does not make sense to offer that praise. Such a large patient decline might have warranted a bigger decrease in costs.

Similarly, if patient workload increases by 20% and costs rise by only 5%, it makes little sense to have a variance analysis system that is oriented toward criticizing the unit and manager for having gone over the original budget. The problem with traditional variance analysis is that it is overly focused on the original budget. A *flexible budget* approach allows for more sophisticated analysis.

■ FLEXIBLE OR VARIABLE BUDGETS

Flexible or *variable budgeting* takes into consideration the fact that the actual output level often differs from expectations. Managers must have some way of controlling operations in light of varying levels of activity.

Preparing a budget requires many assumptions and predictions. One of the most prominent of these concerns the workload level. If the volume of services, costs of services, and revenues related to services all rose and fell in equal proportions, this might not create a significant problem. However, that is generally not the case. Revenues may change in a proportion that differs sharply from costs. Managers must be able to anticipate such variations. A flexible budget is a tool to aid managers in this area. Flexible budgets are sometimes referred to as variable budgets.

A flexible budget is an operating budget for varying workload levels. For example, suppose that Best Clinic expects 4,000 visits and had the following operating budget for the coming month:

Best Clinic
Budget for Next Month

Revenues	
Patient Care	$165,000
Expenses	
Salaries	$115,000
Supplies	30,000
Rent	12,000
Other	6,000
Total Expense	$163,000
Surplus	$ 2,000

This budget provides Best Clinic with information that a modest surplus of $2,000 is projected. But what will happen if the number of visits is greater or fewer than expected?

Assume that revenue changes in direct proportion to the number of visits. However, some of the expenses are fixed costs (see Chapter 4 for a discussion of fixed and variable costs). They will not change as the volume of visits changes. For example, rent on the clinic building is a flat monthly amount, regardless of visits. Salary costs may be somewhat variable but often function almost as fixed costs because staff are typically scheduled on the basis of promised full-time or part-time hours rather than on projected patient visits. The risk of losing staff to turnover if they do not receive their promised hours may limit the ability of the organization to require staff to take unpaid days off if the workload is lighter than expected on a particular day. For most organizations, however, some costs are variable. They vary as the volume of visits goes up or down. Best Clinic will have to buy more supplies if it gets very busy. Or it can buy fewer supplies if it has fewer patients. And staff may be offered a paid day off when the workload is light. The advantage of that approach is that the day off is taken when there is no need to replace the off hours with another staff member (who must be paid). Thus, a higher number of paid days off are taken when those vacant hours do not have to be replaced by higher cost overtime or per diem agency salary rates.

A flexible budget takes the basic operating budget and adjusts it for the impact of possible workload changes. Assume that revenues and supplies are the only items that vary with the number of visits. For this simple example, assume that the clinic's staffing is fixed for any likely range of activity. Consider a flexible budget for Best Clinic, assuming that 3,600 or 4,400 visits, a 10% decrease or increase respectively, occur next month:

Best Clinic
Flexible Budget for Next Month
Volume of Clinic Visits

	3,600	4,000	4,400
Revenues			
Patient Revenue	$148,500	$165,000	$181,500
Expenses			
Salaries	$115,000	$115,000	$115,000
Supplies	27,000	30,000	33,000
Rent	12,000	12,000	12,000
Other	6,000	6,000	6,000
Total Expense	$160,000	$163,000	$166,000
Surplus/(Deficit)	($ 11,500)	$ 2,000	$ 15,500

This flexible budget shows that if the number of visits increases by just 10%, a surplus or profit of $15,500 will occur. But a 10% fall in visits will result in a loss of $11,500. This information can serve as a warning to the managers during the planning stage. They must be aware of the potential for losses if volume does not meet expectations as well as of the possible benefits from extra visits.

During the month, if managers see that visits are fewer than expected, they can anticipate the likely financial shortfall without waiting until the end of the month or later to find out. Actions can be taken to increase fund-raising efforts or to find ways to cut costs. Decisions can be made regarding whether the clinic can sustain a financial loss. If it cannot, it may have to find ways to cut costs.

Flexible or variable budgets focus on volume. Nursing units in hospitals have patient days. Home care agencies provide visits. Operating rooms have procedures. In each case, some measure of volume is needed to prepare a flexible budget.

The key to preparing a flexible budget is identification of fixed and variable costs. As volume varies up or down, which numbers in the budget are likely to change and which are likely to remain the same? Will the costs that vary change in direct proportion to volume changes, or will their change be more or less than proportional? Managers must work to understand revenue and cost structures well enough to be able to anticipate the changes caused by volume variations.

Flexible budgets not only are useful for planning but also serve a critical role in variance analysis. By understanding flexible budgets, a manager is able to interpret more accurately why variances occur and to take any required actions as a result of variances.

■ FLEXIBLE BUDGET VARIANCE ANALYSIS

Flexible budgeting is a system that requires a little more work than traditional variance analysis but it can provide nurse managers with substantially more information. The information provided can help managers understand the causes of variances so that they can be controlled. It can also demonstrate that certain unfavorable variances are not the fault of a manager's unit or department but were caused by factors outside of the unit or department's control.

Suppose that the following was the variance report for nursing department salaries:

The Wagner Hospital
Department of Nursing Services
March Variance Report

	Actual	Budget	Variance
Salary	$1,000,000	$1,000,000	$0

It looks like the department came in right on budget. It is probable that the department's managers would be feeling pretty good about this line item for March. Suppose, however, that the budget of $1,000,000 for nursing salaries was based on an assumption of 25,000 patient days, but there were actually only 20,000 patient days. One would expect that the lower patient-day volume should have allowed for a reduction in overtime and the elimination of some temporary agency nurse time. The department should have spent less than $1,000,000. The original budget ignores this fact.

When used for variance analysis, the flexible budget is a restatement of the budget based on the volume actually attained. Basically, the flexible budget shows what a line item should have cost, given the workload level that actually occurred.

In variance analysis the flexible budget is prepared after the fact. The actual volume must be known in order to prepare the flexible budget for that specific volume.[4] Keep in mind that because some costs are fixed and some costs are variable, total costs do not change in direct proportion with volume. One would normally expect that a 10% increase in patient days would be accompanied by **less** than a 10% increase in costs because only some costs are variable and will increase as census does. On the other hand, a 10% reduction in workload would be expected to be accompanied by **less** than a 10% reduction in cost because the fixed costs would not decline.

Using the flexible budget technique allows the variance for any line item to be subdivided to get additional information. Essentially, the variance already calculated

[4] As part of the budget preparation process, some organizations prospectively prepare flexible budgets. This provides the organization with a sense of what costs are likely to be at several different workload levels.

(i.e., the difference between the budgeted amount and the actual result) is going to be divided into three parts: a *volume variance*, a *price variance*, and a *quantity variance*.

The Volume Variance

The volume variance is defined here as the amount of the variance in any line item that is caused simply by the fact that the workload level has changed. For example, if the budget calls for 25,000 patient days when actually there were 30,000 patient days, it would be expected that it would be necessary to spend more. Variable costs would undoubtedly rise. The cost of the resources needed for an extra 5,000 patient days constitutes a volume variance.

A substantial number of unfavorable unit line-item variances may result simply from the fact that workload increased above expectations. Such an increase is generally outside of the control of the nurse manager. For many health care organizations, an increase in workload is a good thing. Higher hospital or nursing home occupancy may mean that there are more patients sharing the fixed overhead of the institution. Similarly, with home health agencies, more visits mean more patients to share the fixed costs of the agency.

Higher volume demands higher cost. The flexible budget approach allows for specific identification of how much of the variance in any line item is attributable to changes in the workload volume as opposed to other causes. If the higher volume was not budgeted for, there will be spending in excess of the budget. Note that revenue will likely be higher than budget as well. Unfortunately, many health care organizations have not linked their expense budgets with their revenue budgets. More often than not, nurse managers are held responsible for controlling costs, but they do not receive any credit for increases in revenues.

The Price (or Rate) Variance

The price (or rate) variance is the portion of the total variance of any line item that is caused by spending more per unit of some resource than had been anticipated. For example, if the average wage rate for nurses is more per hour than had been expected, that would give rise to this type of variance. When the variance is used to measure labor resources, it is generally called a *rate variance* because the average hourly rate has varied from expectations. When considering the price of supplies, such as the cost per package of sutures, it is called a *price variance* because it is the purchase price that has varied. The terms "price" and "rate" are often used interchangeably in practice.

If a unit manager expected to pay $1.00 per roll for bandage tape but actually paid $1.10 per roll, this would give rise to a price variance. Or suppose there is a line item for nurses hired on a temporary basis from an outside agency. If the unit manager expected to pay the agency $45.00 per hour but actually paid an average of $48.00 per hour, this would give rise to a rate variance.

The price, or rate, variance may or may not be under the control of the nurse manager. If the purchasing department predicts all prices used for supplies and then winds up paying a higher price than predicted, it should be possible to measure the price variance so that the responsibility can be placed with the purchasing department. If the nursing department bears the responsibility for price variances on supplies, the purchasing department would have no incentive to find the best prices. On the other hand, if the nurse manager hires temporary nurses directly from the agency, the responsibility for the rate variance may rest with the nurse manager. Were overqualified people hired? Was an attempt made to seek out an agency that would give the best rate? The manager who can exercise some control over the outcome should be the manager held accountable for the outcome.

The Quantity (or Use) Variance

The third general type of variance under the flexible budgeting scheme is the quantity (or use) variance. This is the portion of the overall variance for a particular line item that results from using more of a resource than was expected for a given workload level. For example, if more supplies were used per patient day than expected, this would give rise to a quantity variance because the quantity of supplies used per patient day exceeded expectations.

This variance is also frequently referred to as a *use variance* because it focuses on how much of the resource has been used. For example, if a half roll of bandage tape was used per patient day, and the expected usage was only a quarter roll, there would be a use variance. The terms "quantity" and "use" are often used interchangeably.

■ DETERMINATION OF THE CAUSES OF VARIANCES

Before discussing how these various flexible budget variances can be calculated, there is another critical issue to be considered first. The volume, price, and quantity variances are going to be used to find out more information about why the budget differs from the actual results. Using these variances, it will be possible to find out how much of the variance was caused simply by a change in the workload volume, how much by a change in prices, and how much by changes in the amount of each resource consumed for a given level of workload.

What the nurse manager will not get from this analysis is the ultimate explanation of the causes of the variances. The nurse manager will still have to investigate to find out **why** these variances have occurred. The analysis provides significant new information by pointing a finger in a specific direction instead of waving a hand in a vague direction.

For instance, if twice as many surgical supplies were used per patient day as expected, the nurse manager knows exactly what to investigate. The analysis does not explain why there was a variance, but it does indicate where it occurred. Rather than simply saying that the OR is over budget, it is known that the line item for surgical supplies is over budget. Furthermore, rather than simply noting that too much was spent on surgical supplies, it has been determined that the problem did not occur because there were extra procedures. Nor did it occur because the price of surgical supplies went up. It is specifically known that the problem lay in using more surgical supplies per procedure than had been budgeted for. Managers must take over at this point and investigate why this occurred. Why were more surgical supplies used per procedure than expected? Was it sloppy use? Clear-cut waste? Was it pilferage? Was there a major disaster that did not increase the number of procedures considerably but did bring in patients requiring a great amount of surgical supplies? Is the budget wrong and it is not really possible to get by with the budgeted amount of surgical supplies per procedure?

If answers to these questions were not needed, the variance process could get by with a lot more accountants and computers and a lot fewer nurse managers.

Accountants and computers, however, cannot answer these questions. Ultimately, the nurse manager must find out the actual underlying cause of the variance.

■ THE MECHANICS OF FLEXIBLE BUDGET VARIANCE ANALYSIS

The first step in flexible budgeting is to establish the flexible budget for the actual workload level. Given the actual cost of a particular line item and the original budgeted amount, it must be determined what it should have cost for that line item, given the workload level that actually occurred.

For example, consider the supplies budgeted for and used by the Med/Surg 6th Floor West nursing unit at the Wagner Hospital in March:

The Wagner Hospital
Department of Nursing Services
Med/Surg 6th Floor West
March Variance Report

	Actual	Budget	Variance
Supplies	$12,000	$10,000	$2,000 U

The actual consumption was $12,000. The budgeted consumption was $10,000. Suppose that the budget assumed that there would be 500 patient days for this unit during March, but there actually turned out to be 600 patient days. (For the time being, ignore the acuity level of the patients. Using acuity in the variance model is explicitly addressed in the next chapter.) Assuming that the consumption of supplies would normally be expected to vary in direct proportion to patient days, the planned consumption was $20 per patient day. This is calculated by dividing the $10,000 budget by the 500 expected patient days.

For 600 patient days at $20 per patient day, $12,000 would have been budgeted for supplies. This is the flexible budget. It is the amount the department would have expected to spend had the actual number of patient days been known. Notice that in this case the flexible budget and the actual amount spent are identical:

The Wagner Hospital
Department of Nursing Services
Med/Surg 6th Floor West
March Variance Report

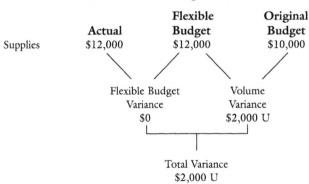

The difference between the original budget and the actual amount spent is the total variance. This is still $2,000 U. The difference between the original budget and the new flexible budget is the volume variance. In this case, the difference is $2,000 U. Note that this volume variance is considered to be unfavorable because the flexible budget requires more spending than was expected. The increased workload may well have been a favorable event for the organization, but the accountant always refers to cost in excess of the original budget as being an unfavorable variance.

The difference between the flexible budget and the actual amount spent can be referred to as a flexible budget variance. Here the flexible budget variance is zero. The entire variance in supplies has been explained by the fact that there was a different volume of patients than had been anticipated.

What about the nursing salaries for the unit? Recall the variance report for nursing salaries:

The Wagner Hospital
Department of Nursing Services
Med/Surg 6th Floor West
March Variance Report

	Actual	**Budget**	**Variance**
Salary	$108,000	$100,000	$8,000 U

To keep the discussion relatively simple at this point, assume that nursing salary costs should vary in direct proportion to the number of patient days. In other words, assume that nursing salary costs are variable. A more realistic example is discussed in the next chapter, once flexible budget mechanics have been fully developed.

Nursing salaries had been budgeted at $100,000, with an expectation of 500 patient days. This is a cost of $200 per patient day. Assuming nursing salary costs are variable, had it been known that there would be 600 patient days, $120,000 would have been budgeted. The variance report can be restated as follows:

The Wagner Hospital
Department of Nursing Services
Med/Surg 6th Floor West
March Variance Report

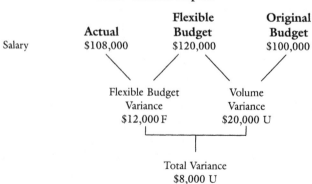

	Actual	**Flexible Budget**	**Original Budget**
Salary	$108,000	$120,000	$100,000

Flexible Budget Variance $12,000 F   Volume Variance $20,000 U

Total Variance
$8,000 U

Subtracting the original budget from the flexible budget, the volume variance is found to be $20,000 U. When the flexible budget is subtracted from the actual cost, it turns out that the flexible budget variance is $12,000 F. Note that the volume variance is unfavorable because the extra patients require more spending. However, the actual amount spent was less than the flexible budget, resulting in a favorable flexible budget variance.

If the volume and flexible budget variances for salaries are combined, there is an unfavorable total variance of $8,000. Note that if both variances were favorable, they could be added together and the result would be $32,000 F. If they were both unfavorable, they could be added and the result would be $32,000 U. Because one of the variances is favorable and one is unfavorable, the smaller one must be subtracted from the larger one to get a combined total variance. The total variance will have the same label (i.e., favorable or unfavorable) as the larger of the two variances. Hence, $20,000 U − $12,000 F = $8,000 U.

At this point in the analysis, there is not yet sufficient information to determine the causes of the flexible budget variance. Suppose that the CNE of the organization had gone to the unit manager in the middle of April and complained about a total lack of cost control on the unit. The unit had a $2,000 unfavorable supplies variance and an $8,000 unfavorable salary variance. Based on traditional variances (without using a flexible budget), there would be no way the unit manager could determine the exact causes of the problem.

Certainly, the unit manager is aware of increased patient volume and would argue that extra patient days were a major factor. But how major? By using a flexible budget, it is possible to find out exactly what dollar impact the extra patient days should have had. In the example, flexible budgeting has shown that the entire variance in supplies is attributable to the extra patient days. The volume variance for supplies was $2,000 U, the same as the amount of the total supply variance. Furthermore, the volume variance was $20,000 U for salaries. The department manager should have expected to spend $20,000 more on nursing salaries than was in the original budget, given the 100 extra patient days. In fact, only $8,000 was spent above the original salary budget. Rather than being blamed for having gone over budget, the unit manager can now show that given the actual number of patient days, the unit actually spent $12,000 less than should have been expected!

Flexible Budget Notation

The next step in the process is to try to determine what caused the flexible budget variance. In order to do this it is necessary to formalize the flexible budgeting process by introducing some notation. The letter A is used to refer to an actual amount. The letter B is used to refer to a budgeted amount. The letter P stands for a price or rate, and the letter Q stands for a quantity. The letter i stands for an input, and the letter o stands for an output or workload.

Inputs are resources used for each line item. If one is considering how much was spent on nursing salaries, the input is nursing time. If one is considering the cost of bandage tape, the input is rolls of bandage tape. *Outputs* are measures of what is being produced. Because improved health cannot be measured readily, proxies are used to measure how much output is produced. Commonly used output measures include patients, patient days, visits, treatments, and procedures.

The notation is combined to form six key variables. Pi stands for the **price** of the **input,** such as $1 per roll of bandage tape or $25 per hour for nursing salary. Qo stands for the total **quantity** of **output**. Qi stands for the **quantity** of **input** needed to produce one unit of output. The letter B in front of other letters indicates a **budgeted** amount. The letter A in front of other letters indicates an **actual** result. The definitions of the notations can be formalized as follows:

- BPi: *b*udgeted *p*rice per unit of *i*nput
- BQi: *b*udgeted *q*uantity of *i*nput for each unit of output produced
- BQo: *b*udgeted *q*uantity of *o*utput
- APi: *a*ctual *p*rice paid per unit of *i*nput
- AQi: *a*ctual *q*uantity of *i*nput for each unit of output produced
- AQo: *a*ctual *q*uantity of *o*utput

The notation can be understood best through an example.

An Example of Volume, Price, and Quantity Variances

Suppose that Wagner Hospital had the following line item in its variance report for a nursing unit for the prior month:

	Actual	Budget	Variance
Nursing Labor	$34,038	$28,800	$5,238 U

The unit manager wants to find out what caused the variance, so the following information is gathered:

- BPi: $24.00 per hour budgeted nursing rate
- BQi: 3.0 hours of budgeted nursing time per patient day
- BQo: 400 budgeted patient days
- APi: $24.40 actual average nursing rate per hour
- AQi: 3.1 hours of actual nursing time per patient day
- AQo: 450 actual patient days

Before proceeding to use these data, consider what is involved in obtaining the information. Information is worthwhile only if it is more valuable than the cost of collecting it. All three of the budgeted items are already known. It would not have been possible to prepare an operating budget without a forecast of patient days, the average rate for nurses, and the budgeted hours per patient day (or at least the total budgeted time, which can be divided by the expected patient days to get the budgeted time per patient day). What about the actual information? The actual number of patient days is readily available. The actual wage rate and the amount of actual paid nursing time is available from the payroll department. Given the nursing time and the actual number of patient days, one can divide to get the nursing time per patient day. Therefore, all the data needed for flexible budget variance analysis is readily available.[5]

---

[5] Note: A nurse manager will save much time and frustration if an electronic, or computerized, spreadsheet such as Excel or Lotus 1-2-3 is used to perform all calculations. Additionally, keeping a budget variance spreadsheet allows the manager to update the data as frequently as necessary. Ideally, the budget reports from the controller's department should be in spreadsheet format so that the nurse manager can avoid reentering numbers into a unit-level spreadsheet. However, few nurse managers receive their budget reports in spreadsheet format, so creating and updating one's own spreadsheet is typically the most efficient way to track the budget performance. See the annotated list of online Excel tutorials at the end of Chapter 8 for assistance with learning to use a spreadsheet.

The first step in utilizing this data is to calculate the original budget in terms of the notation. The original budget is simply the expected cost per patient day multiplied by the expected number of patient days. In this case, the expectation is that nurses will be paid $24.00 per hour; the department will pay for an average of 3.0 hours per patient day. Therefore, the expected cost is $72 per patient day. For the month, 400 patient days are expected, so the budget is $28,800 as follows:

Original Budget

Budgeted Quantity	×	Budgeted Price	×	Budgeted Volume	
3.0	×	$24.00	×	400	= $28,800

In terms of the notation, this can be shown as follows:

Original Budget

$$BQi \times BPi \times BQo$$
$$3.0 \times \$24.00 \times 400$$
$$\$28,800$$

That is, BQi, the budgeted quantity of input per patient day, is 3.0 hours; BPi, the budgeted price per hour of nursing time, is $24.00; and BQo, the budgeted quantity of patient days, is 400. If these three numbers are multiplied together, the result is the originally budgeted amount for nursing labor.

The next step is to find the flexible budget. Keep in mind that the flexible budget is the amount that one would have expected to spend if the actual number of patient days had been known in advance. Therefore, leave the BQi at the budgeted 3.0 hours per patient day, and leave the BPi at the budgeted $24.00 per hour. The only change is from a BQo of 400 patient days to a new AQo of 450 patient days. The flexible budget can then be calculated as follows:

Flexible Budget

Budgeted Quantity	×	Budgeted Price	×	Actual Volume	
3.0	×	$24.00	×	450	= $32,400

In terms of the notation, this can be shown as follows:

Flexible Budget

$$BQi \times BPi \times AQo$$
$$3.0 \times \$24.00 \times 450$$
$$\$32,400$$

Note that the difference between the original budget and the flexible budget is caused by a difference in the number of patient days. Other than that, the calculations are the same. The originally budgeted amount of $28,800 can be compared with the flexible budget amount of $32,400 to determine the volume variance of $3,600 U. Because patient days are higher than expected, costs will be higher than expected. This will give rise to an unfavorable variance. The comparison between the original budget and the flexible budget can be shown as follows:

Original Budget versus Flexible Budget

Budgeted Quantity × Budgeted Price × **Budgeted Volume**
− Budgeted Quantity × Budgeted Price × **Actual Volume**

or

$$3.0 \times \$24.00 \times \mathbf{400} = \$28,800$$
$$-3.0 \times \$24.00 \times \mathbf{450} = \underline{\$32,400}$$
$$\text{Volume Variance} = \overline{\$\ 3,600}\ \text{U}$$

Or, using the notation, this can be shown as:

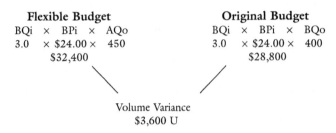

Flexible Budget	**Original Budget**
BQi × BPi × AQo	BQi × BPi × BQo
3.0 × \$24.00 × 450	3.0 × \$24.00 × 400
\$32,400	\$28,800

Volume Variance
\$3,600 U

At this point, the flexible budget can be compared to the actual results in order to find the flexible budget variance. First, consider the actual amount spent:

Actual Cost
Actual Quantity × Actual Price × Actual Volume
3.1 × \$24.40 × 450 = \$34,038

Or, the actual costs in terms of the notation are:

Actual
AQi × APi × AQo
3.1 × \$24.40 × 450
\$34,038

Note that for the actual cost, the actual paid time per patient day, the actual price paid per hour, and the actual number of patient days are used. If desired, the flexible budget can be compared to the actual results to determine a *flexible budget variance.*

Actual Cost versus Flexible Budget
Actual Quantity × **Actual Price** × Actual Volume
− **Budgeted Quantity** × **Budgeted Price** × Actual Volume

or

$$3.1 \times \$24.40 \times 450 = \$34,038$$
$$-3.0 \times \$24.00 \times 450 = \underline{\$32,400}$$
$$\text{Flexible Budget Variance} = \overline{\$\ 1,638}\ \text{U}$$

Or, using the notation, this can be shown as:

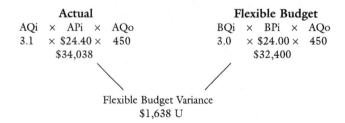

Actual	**Flexible Budget**
AQi × APi × AQo	BQi × BPi × AQo
3.1 × \$24.40 × 450	3.0 × \$24.00 × 450
\$34,038	\$32,400

Flexible Budget Variance
\$1,638 U

The flexible budget variance is $1,638 U. Because the total variance is simply being broken into its component parts, it is possible to combine the volume variance and the flexible budget variance and come out with the total variance. The difference between the original budget and the actual result is $5,238 (i.e., $34,038 − $28,800). Consider all the information available so far in notation form:

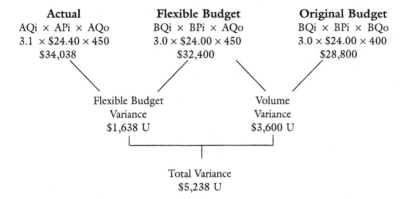

Actual
AQi × APi × AQo
3.1 × $24.40 × 450
$34,038

Flexible Budget
BQi × BPi × AQo
3.0 × $24.00 × 450
$32,400

Original Budget
BQi × BPi × BQo
3.0 × $24.00 × 400
$28,800

Flexible Budget
Variance
$1,638 U

Volume
Variance
$3,600 U

Total Variance
$5,238 U

As can be seen, the total variance still is $5,238, but it has now been separated into a flexible budget variance and a volume variance. If the $1,638 U flexible budget variance is added to the $3,600 U volume variance, the result is the $5,238 total variance. The flexible budget variance is of greater concern to the nurse manager than is the volume variance. The volume variance results from changes in the workload. This is usually outside of the nurse manager's control. The flexible budget variance is caused by the difference between the budgeted and the actual price per hour for nursing services and because of differences in the amount of nursing time per patient day. If possible, more should be found out about what makes up this variance.

In order to find out this extra information, it is necessary to derive something called a *subcategory*. This subcategory is simply a device to allow for separation of the flexible budget variance into two pieces: the price variance and the quantity variance. The subcategory is defined as the actual quantity of input per unit of output, multiplied by the budgeted price of the input, times the actual output level. In terms of the notation, the subcategory can be calculated as follows:

Subcategory

Actual Quantity	×	Budgeted Price	×	Actual Volume	
3.1	×	$24.00	×	450	= $33,480

or in notation:

Subcategory
AQi × BPi × AQo
3.1 × $24.00 × 450
$33,480

If the subcategory calculation is compared to the actual costs, the price variance can be determined. First, consider the following:

Actual
AQi × APi × AQo

Subcategory
AQi × BPi × AQo

What is the difference between the actual and the subcategory calculations? The Q_i, quantity of input per unit of output, is exactly the same for both; it is the actual value. The Q_o, quantity of patient days, is exactly the same for both; it is the actual value. The price or hourly rate is different, however. The actual uses the actual price or rate, whereas the subcategory uses the budgeted price or rate. This is the only difference between the two. Therefore, if the actual amount spent does not equal the subcategory, it must be due to a difference between the price paid for the resource and the price budgeted.

Now insert numbers and see what that variance is:

Actual Cost versus Subcategory

Actual Quantity × **Actual Price** × Actual Volume

−Actual Quantity × **Budgeted Price** × Actual Volume

or

$$3.1 \times \$24.40 \times 450 = \$34,038$$
$$-3.1 \times \$24.00 \times 450 = \$33,480$$
$$\text{Price or Rate Variance} = \underline{\underline{\$\quad 558 \text{ U}}}$$

Or, using the notation, this can be shown as:

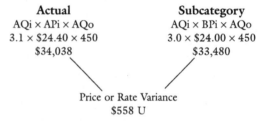

Actual	**Subcategory**
AQi × APi × AQo	AQi × BPi × AQo
3.1 × $24.40 × 450	3.0 × $24.00 × 450
$34,038	$33,480

Price or Rate Variance

$558 U

The price or rate variance of $558 U results from the fact that on average, $24.40 was paid per hour for nursing time instead of the budgeted $24.00. It is possible that this occurred because of poor scheduling, which results in unnecessary overtime. On the other hand, perhaps it resulted from a larger raise for nursing personnel than the nurse manager had been told to put into the budget by the personnel department.[6] Then again, look at the volume variance. Whenever there is a large unfavorable volume variance, it means that the workload was much greater than expected. Such unanticipated increases in workload put a great strain on nursing time, frequently requiring added overtime or the addition of high-priced agency nurses. All these possibilities should be investigated by the nurse manager.

What effect will added patient load have on the quantity of nursing time per patient? It is possible that busy nurses will tire and start to work more slowly. It is also possible that as patient volume increases, the nurses on staff will work harder to cover all of the patients. There may be a favorable variance or an unfavorable variance. Look at the quantity variance, first examining the relationship between the subcategory and the flexible budget:

Subcategory	**Flexible Budget**
AQi × BPi × AQo	BQi × BPi × AQo

---

[6] Typically, the Budget Office makes corrections to the staff salaries in the system when salary raises are granted and then updates all the department budgets with the corrected information. However, if that is not done in the central financial management office, the nurse manager will have to explain that salary variance each month.

What differences are observed between the subcategory and the flexible budget? The P_i, price per hour of nursing time, is the budgeted amount in both cases. The Q_0, quantity of patient days, is the actual amount for both. The only difference between the two is in the Q_i, quantity of nursing time per patient day. The flexible budget uses the budgeted time per patient day; the subcategory uses the actual paid nursing time per patient day. Any difference between the subcategory and the flexible budget must be related to the quantity of nursing time per patient. It is possible to insert values and calculate that variance:

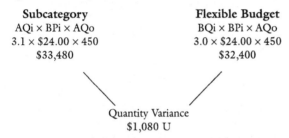

Subcategory versus Flexible Budget

Actual Quantity   ×   Budgeted Price   ×   Actual Volume
–Budgeted Quantity ×   Budgeted Price   ×   Actual Volume

or

$$3.1 \times \$24.00 \times 450 = \$33,480$$
$$-3.0 \times \$24.00 \times 450 = \$32,400$$
$$\text{Quantity or Use Variance} = \underline{\underline{\$\ 1,080\ \text{U}}}$$

Or, using the notation, this can be shown as:

Subcategory	**Flexible Budget**
AQi × BPi × AQo	BQi × BPi × AQo
3.1 × $24.00 × 450	3.0 × $24.00 × 450
$33,480	$32,400

Quantity Variance
$1,080 U

The quantity variance of $1,080 U can be explained in a number of ways. It is possible that because of the substantial increase in patient days above expectations, many part-time nurses were hired. These nurses were unfamiliar with the institution and therefore were not as efficient as the regular nurses. Another possibility is that the population was sicker than anticipated and required more care. Of course, there is also the possibility that supervision was lax and that time was simply being wasted. Again, variance information can only point out the direction; the manager must make the final determination regarding why the variance occurred and how to avoid it in the future.

In order to use flexible budgeting, one should have an idea of how the pieces fit together. Review the price and quantity variances, looking at how, together, they compose the flexible budget variance:

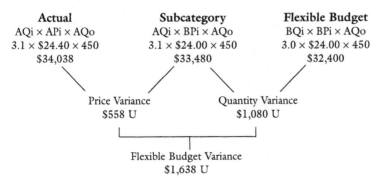

Actual	**Subcategory**	**Flexible Budget**
AQi × APi × AQo	AQi × BPi × AQo	BQi × BPi × AQo
3.1 × $24.40 × 450	3.1 × $24.00 × 450	3.0 × $24.00 × 450
$34,038	$33,480	$32,400

Price Variance
$558 U

Quantity Variance
$1,080 U

Flexible Budget Variance
$1,638 U

Notice that combining the price variance of $558 U and the quantity variance of $1,080 U results in the flexible budget variance. Recall that the flexible budget variance and volume variance add up to the total variance. Figure 13-1 shows that the three individual variances—price, quantity, and volume—add up to the total variance for the line item.

Recall that without flexible budgets, the total variance for the line item would be the only piece of information available for analysis. There was an unfavorable variance of $5,238. Using Figure 13-1, it is possible to determine at the outset that of this total variance, $3,600 was caused by the increase in patient days. It is now also known that $558 of the variance was caused by having paid a higher average rate to the nurses than was anticipated and that $1,080 of the variance was caused by paying for a longer average amount of nursing time per patient day than had been anticipated. Why these specific variances occurred is not known, but there is a much better focus on where the problem areas are.

A generic model for flexible budgeting variances is presented in Figure 13-2. In looking at this model, several things should be kept in mind. First of all, recall that basically all the necessary data are generally readily available. Second, the accounting and information systems departments can calculate all these variances when they do monthly variance reports. If they are not willing to do so, then it is possible to calculate these variances by hand or on a computer.

It sometimes is not obvious whether a variance is favorable or unfavorable. Looking at Figure 13-2, an easy rule of thumb is that as one moves from the right side toward the left, larger numbers on the left indicate unfavorable variance. For example, if the flexible budget amount is larger than the originally budgeted amount, the volume variance is unfavorable. If the subcategory is greater than the flexible budget, the quantity variance is unfavorable. This is true because as one moves from the original budget toward the left, movement is toward the actual result. If the actual result is larger than the original budget, then more was spent than budgeted. The result is an unfavorable variance. Given the way this model is set up, this also holds true for each of the individual variances making up the total variance.

■ MATERIALITY

Virtually all actual budgets will vary somewhat from the projected budget. The question is how large must the variance be to be considered important (i.e., material). For example, consider a department manager whose supplies budget for January was $10,000, but the actual January supplies usage was $10,100. Assuming that the workload was exactly as projected, does that unfavorable budget figure represent a failure to control supplies usage? Or does it represent normal variation in supplies usage for the types of patients served by the department? That $100 figure represents a 1% over-budget situation. There are statistical techniques that can be used to determine not only the amount that should be budgeted, but also the fact that there is not an absolute point prediction or dollar amount that can be made confidently. There is a range around the dollar prediction, and that range is the same thing as a confidence interval around the expected budget figure.

The Quality Management Department can be of great help to department managers here. A dollar figure in a budget projection is actually a mean. It represents the mean cost to provide patient care services for a particular time period. Ideally, it incorporates the flexible budgeting concepts and techniques presented in this chapter.

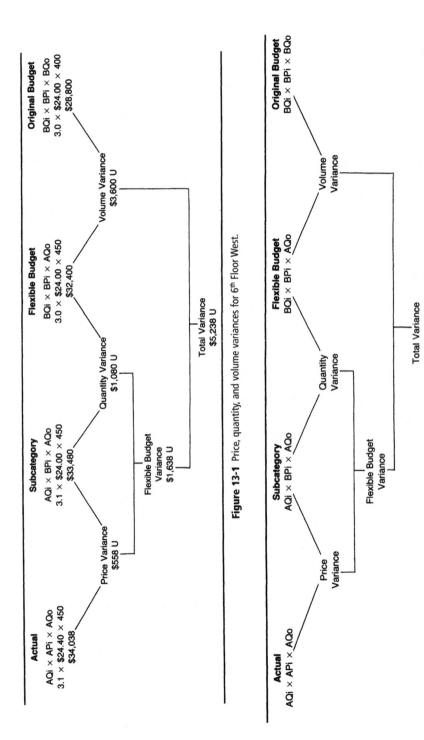

Figure 13-1 Price, quantity, and volume variances for 6th Floor West.

Figure 13-2 Price, quantity, and volume variances for a generic model.

But even with flexible budgeting, there will be variation about the mean cost per visit, cost per patient day, cost per procedure, or any other cost index the institution uses. It should be noted that even when patient mix is considered, patients with the same index rating vary fairly widely within each rating level. Thus, the budgeted staff cost per patient day is a mean, and there is a normal and expected cost range around that mean. It is the range that must be calculated and considered when determining whether a variance is really a variance, or whether the variance is actually within the normal range of variation that should be expected for that particular cost.

The range should not be a guess. It should be calculated from past budgets. Data from the past 2 to 3 years' projected budgets by category (e.g., supplies, staffing costs, overtime costs, medication costs, equipment costs, etc.) along with the actual results should be collected. In this way, the manager can see what the prior budgets were and how much variation the system produced. Then expected variation can be calculated as part of the next year's budget projection. The variation in a current month's budget can be compared to the expected variation to discover whether the dollar amount of the budget variance is outside the range of expected variation. That information provides the manager with information about whether the variation is material (outside expected limits) or immaterial (within expected variation ranges).

In other words, there will always be some random variation. One patient may need a few more supplies than another patient with the same diagnosis. That doesn't necessarily represent inefficiency. It doesn't mean that things are out of control. Due to randomness, there may be a month when a number of patients require a few more supplies than the mean. In another month, there may be patients who need fewer supplies. Over the long run, that random variation will even out. The problem, however, is to determine whether a variance is the result of a random variation or is the result of something that is out of control and should be corrected. This situation is dealt with by calculating expected variations from the budget.

Calculating the Expected Variation in the Budget

Most budget projections are based on past budget experience and are modified by expected changes in volume, program offerings, or other activity changes. There is always some guesswork in budget projections because they are actually statistical estimates based on past performance. In fact, managers often calculate the mean monthly cost of a budget category over the past 2 to 3 years and use the mean plus any price or rate increases as their projection for the next year's budget. However, few managers in nursing today calculate the expected variation around that budget projection. Fortunately, the mathematical calculations are quite simple even if done by hand. And a computer will calculate them automatically if the data and appropriate formulas are entered on a spreadsheet.

Quality management principles state that 95% of all variation will be found within two standard deviations of the mean. What these ranges represent is called normal and expected variation in any system. Variation outside those limits is unexpected (or error) variation. Variation is inevitable because of the myriad factors that individual patients present. Managers ought to expect some month-to-month variation in costs even if patient census and acuity remain constant. However, the over-budget variation in 1 month should be approximately equaled by under-budget variation in some other month. It is only when special circumstances occur that actual expenditures systematically rise or fall. Such things as a prolonged change in census or acuity, patient mix changes, high turnover (leading to higher use of expensive agency staff), and other special and unexpected circumstances that are not part of routine, expected, everyday operations will produce budget figures that deviate seriously from the projected budget. These kinds of changes in the care environment tend to cause much larger budget changes than are seen in the normal monthly random variation. The formula for calculating the expected variation relies heavily on the standard deviation, which is calculated is as follows:

$$\text{Standard Deviation} = \sqrt{\frac{\text{Sum } (X - \overline{X})^2}{n}}$$

Where:

X represents each measure in the dataset (for example, monthly measures would have data from January, February, March, and so on)

$\overline{X}$ represents the mean of the dataset

n represents the count of items in the dataset (for example, if data were collected monthly for 2 years, the count would be 24, given that there are 24 months in 2 years)

If the manager wishes to have a 95% variation range, the upper range of variation is the value of the mean budget cost plus two times the standard deviation. The lower range of variation is the value of the mean budget cost less two times the standard deviation. Table 13-3 represents the projected 2009 budget and the expected range within which the actual budget is expected to fall, assuming a fairly stable workload and other factors. Mathematically, the range is the 95% confidence interval.

The confidence interval is really a function of the standard deviation from the mean of any list of numbers. Typically, we use the 95% confidence interval (two standard deviations above and below the mean) or the 99% confidence interval (3 standard deviations above and below the mean). One way to decide what constitutes a material variance is to calculate the 95% confidence interval; any variance beyond two standard deviations above or below the projected monthly budget must be analyzed and justified. If it is known that patient needs tend to vary widely in that particular unit, the manager may prefer to use three standard deviations, that is, the 99% confidence interval, as the point at which the variance is to be investigated.

When the actual budget expenditures are returned each month during the next year, the manager will be able to use this type of table to determine whether any over- or under-budget expenditures are material because they will be higher than the upper range, or lower than the lower range.

Types of Variance

The rationale for using the 95% confidence interval to determine the materiality of a variance is the understanding that there are basically two types of variation in the environment. The first kind has an identifiable cause. It is called special cause variation, and it is the type of variation that should be the primary target of budget-control efforts. Nurses waiting around the time clock until they clock out late enough to get 6 or more minutes of overtime is an example of a special cause. That practice produces

TABLE 13-2 Calculation of the Standard Deviation of a Supply Budget

Month	Actual Expenditures	Actual Less the Mean	(Actual − Mean)^2
January 2007	$ 10,560	−90	$ 8,100
February	9,987	−663	439,569
March	11,002	352	123,904
April	10,122	−528	278,784
May	10,035	−615	378,225
June	11,022	372	138,384
July	10,840	190	36,100
August	9,988	−662	438,244
September	9,992	−658	432,964
October	11,023	373	139,129
November	11,100	450	202,500
December	10,845	195	38,025
January 2008	8,999	−1,651	2,725,801
February	9,658	−992	984,064
March	9,978	−672	451,584
April	10,559	−91	8,281
May	10,698	48	2,304
June	10,911	261	68,121
July	11,465	815	664,225
August	11,895	1,245	1,550,025
September	10,585	−65	4,225
October	11,405	755	570,025
November	12,001	1,351	1,825,201
December	10,924	274	75,076
Sum	$ 255,594	0	$ 482,619
Average (Mean)	$ 10,650		
Mean ÷ by n = Variance			$ 20,109*

*The standard deviation is the square root of the variance. Therefore, one standard deviation for this supply budget is the square root of $20,109. That equals 141.8067 which we will round to $142. Two standard deviations are required for the 95% range, and thus our 95% interval will be ± $284

overtime costs that lead to an unnecessary over-budget staffing situation. Other sources of special cause variation include things like changes in the patient mix or in the types of procedures performed by the surgeons in the operating room, or perhaps even a dispute between the facility and an HMO that results in loss of that HMO's subscribers.

The second kind of variation is called common cause variation. Common cause variation recognizes that just about everything in the world that can be measured varies from month to month. The causes of random variation are many, and they depend upon the phenomenon being measured. Scientists expect some random variation in every dataset. Budget measurements are no different. The question is: "How much variation is attributable to the many known and unknown vagaries in the universe (i.e., common cause variation), and how much variation is due to special causes?"

TABLE 13-3 2009 Projected Budget and Expected Range

Month	Projected Expenditures	Upper Range for Month (Upper 95%)	Lower Range for Month (Lower 95%)
January 2009	$10,560	$10,844	$10,276
Febuary	9,987	10,271	9,703
March	11,002	11,286	10,718
April	10,122	10,406	9,838
May	10,035	10,319	9,751
June	11,022	11,306	10,738
July	10,840	11,124	10,556
August	9,988	10,272	9,704
September	9,992	10,276	9,708
October	11,023	11,307	10,739
November	11,100	11,384	10,816
December	10,845	11,129	10,561
Annual Budget	**$126,516**	**$129,924**	**$123,108**

Both kinds of variation may be the result of uncontrollable factors, but common cause variation is more often due to factors beyond nursing's control. For example, high staffing costs one month may be caused by an unexpectedly lengthy search for a replacement nurse, forcing the manager to use more agency staff hours than planned. Fortunately, variations due to common cause variation tend to be relatively small if the system being measured is well in control. "In control" means that the manager controls operations such that supplies are not regularly diverted to personal use, wasted, or otherwise not controlled. Only if the manager allows the budget to go out of control will there be large month-to-month variations in the budget, assuming workload, patient mix, and staffing are all stable.

Budget variances that are material in amount are more typically due to special cause variation. Special cause variation should always be investigated. It means that part of the system of care provision in the unit is no longer in good management control, or perhaps it means that conditions have changed such that the original budget is no longer valid. Common cause variation is likely to have many small causes. Often these causes are related to unavoidable requirements presented by individual patients. Common cause variation in the budget is much more difficult to control and is likely to produce variation that stays within the upper and lower ranges of expected budget variation. This does not mean, however, that common cause variation should be ignored. Examination of common cause variation may assist the manager in finding ways to economize by further reducing wastage, eliminating excessive use of supplies, reducing salary costs by more effective scheduling of personal and vacation days, or other means to reduce the variation and perhaps the average cost of providing care in the department.

Long experience has demonstrated that common cause variation accounts for about 95% to 98% of all variation resulting from the vagaries of the universe. When variation exceeds the amount represented by the 95% confidence interval for more than two or three months in a row, there is a very high probability that special cause variation is occurring. The good news is that the source of special cause variation can often be discovered and addressed through the variance analysis process. Often, the causes of material variances are readily recognized by the staff who lived through the period represented by the material variance, and if asked, they can pinpoint the cause. Then, if the variance is unfavorable (over budget), corrective actions can be planned. If the variance is favorable (under budget), it may be important to find out what was done so well so that the improved performance can be structured into the system and perpetuated. The key to successful variance analysis and justification is to first differentiate between material and immaterial variances. It is an utter waste of time and often highly damaging to morale to spend a lot of time trying to correct immaterial variances that are nothing more than normal, random variation in the data.

Many hospital administrators, including nurse executives, make five serious mistakes when analyzing budget variances with their department managers:

1. They fail to discriminate between unimportant and important variances.
2. They do not require units that experience important budget variances to establish working groups to investigate the root causes of those variances.
3. They attend only to over-budget conditions, even though it is equally important to explain under-budget conditions.
4. They fail to provide volume/workload-adjusted budget variance reports to departments whose costs are highly dependent upon volume and workload.
5. They do not assist nurse managers in understanding variances by providing information on the relationship of staffing cost variances (which tend to cause the greatest budget variances in a hospital unit) to workload, turnover, vacancies, and the use of high-cost agency staff.

We have just discussed the first of these five points. Our confidence intervals can allow us to discriminate between important and unimportant variances. We now turn our attention to the remaining four of these five areas.

Team Ownership of the Variance

The second key to successful variance analysis is to find the source of material variation. Sometimes, the nurse manager knows even prior to receipt of the budget report that there will be an important variance due to some special cause issue in the department the preceding month. In other cases, some investigation will be necessary to discover the source of the special cause variation. When it is not obvious why the budget was materially over or under the amount that was expected, the manager may have a much better chance of quickly discovering the source of the variance through team brainstorming with the department's staff. The staff are closest to the operations of the department and may well be the people who will be in the position to carry out any control efforts needed to bring the budget back into control. Team meetings focused on problem identification and resolution can be scheduled so that the thinking and problem solving capabilities of the entire staff can be mobilized.

Managers are responsible for controlling the budget. However, many managers are somewhat removed from the actual day-to-day operations of the unit. Even if intimately involved in unit operations, a manager is only one person with a single brain and perspective. Most systemic problems are more easily recognized by the staff, and quality management studies have repeatedly demonstrated the advantages of submitting work unit problems to the unit's work team. Involving the staff in the resolution of problems that affect their work is also often associated with improved morale and higher levels of cooperation in getting the process back into control.

Analysis of Favorable Budget Variances

All too often managers are asked to justify only over-budget conditions. This is a great mistake. A material under-budget condition is sometimes even more important than an over-budget condition. It may be caused by saving money at the expense of an important quality factor. For example, if a department manager in a retirement facility drastically dimmed the hall lights at night to save on electricity, the facility might end up with a lower electric bill but suddenly incur much higher staffing, radiology, and physician costs because of injuries due to falls. A common condition in people of advanced age is vision impairment resulting from macular degeneration and other eye problems. The visual impairment caused by these conditions is typically exacerbated by dim lighting. Noting the under-budget condition in the electric bill might alert administrators to an unsafe condition that could be corrected before the environmental quality problem led to a large number of injuries.

Another example of the importance of justification of an under-budget condition is cost savings produced by a new program. Consider the following scenario. Suppose a unit experienced an unusually low number of infections during the months of February and March but then rebounded to normal during April. Having a team meeting to consider all possible differences produced the observation that a group of nursing students rotated through the unit during February and March. An interview with the instructor revealed the existence of a new dressing-change technique the instructor had taught the students after learning about it from an article in *Nursing Research*. Based on that discovery, the unit asked the instructor to provide an in-service to train the entire staff in the new dressing-change technique. During the following months, the lowered infection rate was achieved and became the new baseline nosocomial infection rate for the unit. The lower cost of care achieved through lower infection rates might never have been realized if the manager had not recognized the importance of analyzing the under-budget situation just as carefully as she analyzed over-budget situations.

Volume-Adjusted Budget Reporting and Budget Ranges

Although the situation is improving, the standard budget reporting methodology in hospitals may ignore the effects of volume variation in clinical units. Thus, sometimes there is the absurd spectacle of a nurse manager's being called to account for being over-budget in nursing wage costs when an increase in patient days not only accounted for the variance but also produced higher revenues that more than paid for the higher wage costs. It is an unfortunate reality that nurse managers may be given incentive by the organization to pursue actions that have a negative effect on profitability so as to avoid being over budget when volume and workload are not adjusted in the budget report.

If actual volume is significantly above projected volume, variable expenses, such as nursing hours, overtime, and clinical supplies, **should** exceed budget projections within the range calculated as the 95% confidence interval. If these elements do not rise when volume increases, one must ask why. Refusing to provide additional nursing hours when there is a significant increase in occupancy or acuity most often results in insufficient nursing care to maintain clinical quality. A decrement in quality is inevitable if the department is staffed for a particular quality level, and then staffing is reduced relative to the actual patient load that is encountered.

It ought to be obvious that a unit staffed to provide a particular level of nursing care cannot maintain that level if there is a reduction in the number of nursing hours per patient. Some care will have to be omitted. Nurses, like everybody else, have 24 hours in a day and no more. So if the number of nursing hours is held constant while the number or acuity of patients increases, some or all of the patients will have fewer nursing hours available to them. It seems strange that so many managers in health care institutions act as if they did not understand this simple equation. Managerial directives and punitive measures cannot change the facts of time-related physics.

Assisting the Manager to Understand Budget Variances

Managers need data if they are to understand material variances. Although many managers observe changes in their departments that they know will produce budget variances, they need data on those changes to make accurate, reliable decisions about how to better control their operations so that future variances do not occur. Staffing variances tend to produce the largest dollar differences between a planned and an actual budget. If the manager is to invest in remedies to solve a staffing budget variance problem, it is vital to have data on such factors as:

- Turnover rates and trends in turnover rates
- Actual hours per patient day delivered (and budgeted)
- Increase in patient census, visits, or procedures
- Number of sick calls by staff member
- Number of overstaffed shifts
- Number and duration of staff vacancies
- Number of overtime hours paid to cover vacancies
- Number of agency nurse hours paid to cover vacancies
- Reasons for staff terminations
- Numbers of orientees not counted in the budget and total hours of non-budget orientees

These data allow the manager and facility administration to understand why there is a staffing variance problem. Efforts to rectify over-budget problems are more likely to succeed if the manager understands exactly why the over-budget condition arose. If there were an unexpectedly high number of voluntary separations, the manager may well need the assistance of the human resources department to review and analyze exit interviews so as to discover whether there is a morale problem that can be addressed. Or perhaps a competitor started offering significantly higher salaries, and that led to resignations. These two different root causes require very different solutions. Analysis of budget variances is a process that is best achieved collaboratively among managers, administration, human resources, and other departments that can provide information necessary to a successful analysis and problem resolution process.

■ REVENUE VARIANCES

The nurse manager's primary variance analysis effort focuses on expenses. This is predominantly because managers of health care organizations have a greater degree of control over expenses than they do over revenues. However, the information that revenue variance analysis can yield is also important. For example, changes in revenue that result from changes in patient volume may be outside the control of the organization and its managers. Such changes, however, may require management actions or reactions to protect the organization's financial position.

Revenue variance methodology follows the same pattern as expense methodology. There is a traditional variance that tends to focus on the total revenue expected and actually achieved for a unit or department. There is also a flexible budget methodology that helps to identify the various underlying causes of variances. The total revenue variance for a unit, department, or organization can be broken down into a volume variance, a mix variance, and a price variance. The *patient mix variance* refers to changes in the types of patients for which services are provided. For example, if a particular clinic has served primarily retired persons with chronic conditions typical of the elderly, and a new housing development attracting primarily young families with children opens in the clinic's service area, it is likely that the mix of patients served by the clinic will change. The clinic will almost certainly have to expand hours to serve an employed customer base, and it may need to open (or expand) a pediatric service. Those kinds of changes in the patient mix will have implications for revenues and, of course, for expenses.

Consider an outpatient surgery department that has budgeted revenues of $1 million for the month just ended. Actual revenues were $850,000. Traditional variance analysis identifies a $150,000 unfavorable revenue variance. What caused the $150,000 shortfall?

The first step in flexible budget revenue variance analysis is to identify the revenue per patient. Unlike costs, which may be fixed or variable, in most health care organizations, all revenues are variable. Therefore the total $1 million budget could be divided by the number of patients budgeted to arrive at an average revenue per patient. This allows calculation of a volume variance. Suppose that 800 patients were expected for the month. In that case the average revenue per patient was expected to be $1,250 (i.e., the $1 million total revenue divided by 800 patients = $1,250 of revenue per patient; Figure 13-3).

If there were actually only 750 patients, a flexible budget for revenue of $937,500 (i.e., 750 patients × $1,250 price) would be calculated. The revenue flexible budget indicates the amount of revenue that would have been budgeted if the number of patients had been forecast exactly. The difference between the original budget for 800 patients and the flexible budget for 750 actual patients is an unfavorable volume variance of $62,500. Less revenue than expected is considered unfavorable.

The next calculation concerns the mix of patients. Not all patients would be expected to be charged $1,250. That figure represents an average. Assume that half the patients were expected to be type A patients charged $1,000 and half were expected to be type B patients charged $1,500. Any number of different types of patients with different prices is possible, but for this discussion we will limit it to just types A and B.

Suppose that of the 750 actual patients, 450 were type A and 300 were type B. Not only are there fewer patients than expected, but the mix of patients has changed as well. Less than half the patients are the more highly priced type B patients. Based on the actual number of patients and the actual mix, revenues would be expected to be $900,000 (i.e., 450 patients × $1,000 + 300 patients × $1,500). If one compares the flexible budget of $937,500 (the revenue that would have been expected for 750 patients) to this new "subcategory" value based on the actual mix, the difference is $37,500. This is the mix variance, which is unfavorable. The variance is unfavorable because there is a greater proportion of low-revenue patients.

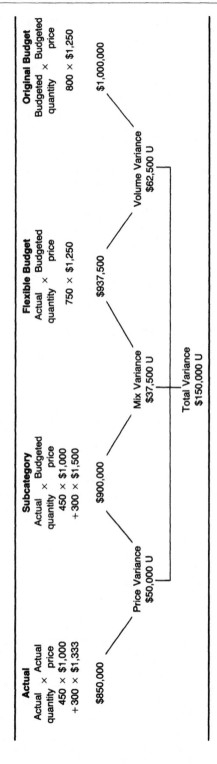

Figure 13-3 Revenue variances.

This still leaves an unexplained variance of $50,000. This is a price variance. It is a result of charging a different price than expected. Although the outpatient surgery intended to charge $1,500 for type B patients, it is possible that because of government regulation or negotiated rates with insurance companies, the average price for type B patients was only $1,333.33. In that case, actual revenue would be $850,000 (i.e., 450 patients × $1,000 + 300 patients × $1,333.33). The $50,000 difference between the $900,000 from the mix calculation is an unfavorable price variance. It is unfavorable because the price was less than budgeted.

The calculations for these variances can be seen in Figure 13-3. Note that in each case the number of patients is multiplied by the price per patient. For the budget and flexible budget, the total number of patients and the budgeted average price per patient are used. For the subcategory, the mix of patients is used, splitting the total into the number of actual patients of each type. For the subcategory, the budgeted price for each type of patient is used. For the actual costs, the actual number of each type of patient and the actual prices for each type of patient are used.

In the past, the patient mix has not been a factor nurse managers dealt with much except to ensure that proper staffing, equipment, and supplies were used for the patients served. The mix can change for a variety of reasons. Some of those reasons result in rapid changes in mix, whereas others are much slower. For example, if a particularly bad flu unexpectedly affects many members of the community, there may be a month or two when there are many flu patients, dramatically altering the patient mix for those months. Or perhaps a hospital is successful in attracting three cardiologists from the competitor across town. The mix of cases such as cardiac catheterizations is likely to rise dramatically as compared to those foreseen by a budget prepared before the cardiologists started using that hospital. In suburban areas, new housing developments can change the mix within a few short months.

Often revenue variances are calculated based on the contribution margin (price minus variable cost) rather than on the revenue. Revenue places too great a focus on the total charge for different types of patients rather than on the profit implications of each type of patient. A patient producing high revenue could have even greater expenses and cause losses. Another patient who produces only modest revenues could be quite profitable. Managers do not need information solely about changes in revenues. They also need to know whether the revenue changes are in profitable areas or unprofitable ones.

It is possible therefore to use the budgeted contribution margin rather than the revenue in all the calculations just discussed. There still would be a volume variance. Fewer patients would imply a lower overall contribution margin. There still would be a mix variance. However, whether the mix variance is favorable or unfavorable would depend on whether there is a greater or lesser proportion of the types of patients with higher contribution margins. The price variance would still depend on the actual price charged for each type of patient.

Knowing whether variances are caused by changes in prices, the mix of patients, or the volume of patients is important information that managers can use in taking actions to respond to increases or decreases in revenues. If the number of patients is falling, steps should be taken to find out why and to make sure that there are corresponding reductions in organizational expenses. If the mix of patients is changing, it may be necessary to shift resources within the organization. If prices differ from budget, an effort must be made to understand why it has occurred and its overall implications for the organization's finances.

Summary and Implications for Nurse Managers

Budgeting is a process of planning and controlling. If a budget is prepared but is not used to control results, a substantial part of the potential benefit of budgeting is lost. The key issue to remember, however, is that organizations do not control costs; people do. Organizations must take steps to ensure that their employees are motivated to accomplish the organization's objectives.

The difference between the budget and what actually occurs is called a variance. Comparing actual results to budgeted expectations and analyzing the resulting variances should be done monthly. This can allow for midstream corrections that will improve the year-end results. It also provides information for preparing the coming year's budget and for evaluating the performance of units, departments, and managers.

Many health care organizations prepare variance reports by comparing the information in the original budget to the actual results. There are several problems with that type of comparison. First, it does not tell as much about the cause of the variance as one would like to know; for instance, traditional variance analysis does not indicate whether a variance is caused by more resource use per patient or by higher prices for resources used. Second, traditional variance analysis ignores the fact that resource consumption would be expected to vary with workload volume. One can compare the budgeted cost for an expected patient volume to the actual cost for the actual patient volume. Part of the variance, therefore, will just be the result of changes in workload levels, rather than being related to efficiency.

This has caused many health care organizations to start using a method called flexible budgeting. Flexible budgeting establishes an after-the-fact budget; that is, what it would have been expected to cost had the actual workload been known in advance. Using flexible budgets, it is possible to break down a unit's or a department's line-item expense variances into components caused by (1) changes in prices or salary rates from those expected; (2) changes in the amount of input used per unit of workload or output, such as the amount of nursing time per patient day; and (3) changes in the workload volume itself. It is also possible to divide revenue variances into the portion caused by volume, mix, or price changes.

Managerial expertise and judgment are still needed to investigate and evaluate the variances that are determined by using flexible budgeting. Ultimately, this technique can make the manager's job easier by segregating the variance into its component parts. This allows the manager to spend more time understanding and explaining why the variance occurred.

References and Suggested Readings

Carey, R., Lloyd, R. (2000). *Measuring Quality Improvement in Health Care.* Milwaukee, WI: American Society for Quality.

Cavouras, C.A., McKinley, J. (1997). Variable budgeting for staffing analysis and evaluation. *Nursing Management.* 28(5), 34-36, 39.

Cohen, J. (2006). Take the fear out of the figures. *Nursing Management.* 37(4), 12.

Darves, B. (2003). Medicare cuts forcing some hard choices. *American College of Physicians-American Society for Internal Medicine Observer.* Downloaded on September 26, 2006, from http://www.acponline.org/journals/news/jan03/medicare_cuts.htm.

Dayhoff, N., Moore, P. (2005). It's all about cash flow. *Clinical Nurse Specialist.* 19(3), 127-128.

Dunham-Taylor, J, Pinczuk, J.Z. (2006). *Health Care Financial Management for Nurse Managers.* Sudbury, MA: Jones & Bartlett.

Felteau, A. (1992). Budget variance analysis and justification. *Nursing Management.* 23(2), 40-41.

Finkler, S.A., Ward, D.R., Baker, J. (2007). *Essentials of Cost Accounting for Health Care Organizations,* ed 3. Sudbury, MA: Jones & Bartlett.

Foley, R. (2005). Use key strategies for successful budgets. *Nursing Management.* 36(8), 28-34.

Henderson, E. (2003). Budgeting, Part II. *Nursing Management.* 10(2), 32-36.

Horngren, C.T., Datar, S.M., Foster, G. (2005). *Cost Accounting: A Managerial Emphasis,* ed 12. Englewood Cliffs, NJ: Prentice-Hall.

Maitland, D. (1993). Flexible budgeting and variance analysis: Why leave staff nurses in the dark? *Hospital Cost Management Accounting.* 5(9), 1-8.

Swansburg, R.C. (1997). *Budgeting and Financial Management for Nurse Managers.* Boston: Jones & Bartlett.

Wilburn, D. (1992). Budget response to volume variability. *Nursing Management*. 23(2), 42-45.

Zwillich, T. (February 2, 2006). House OKs Medicare, Medicaid cuts. *WebMD Medical News*. Downloaded on September 26, 2006: http://www.webmd.com/content/article/118/112913.htm

Zwillich, T. (February 6, 2006). Medicare faces cuts in Bush budget. *WebMD Medical News*. Downloaded on September 26, 2006: http://www.webmd.com/content/article/118/112982?src=RSS_PUBLIC.

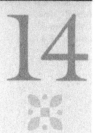

14 Variance Analysis: Examples, Extensions, and Caveats

LEARNING OBJECTIVES
The goals of this chapter are to:

- Provide additional variance analysis examples
- Provide insight into the problems encountered when variance information is aggregated
- Introduce the concept of exception reports and explain their benefits
- Explore further the interpretation of variances
- Explain how flexible budgeting can be used even if staffing patterns are rigid
- Provide a tool for determining the variance due to changes in patient acuity
- Reiterate the dependence of flexible budget variance analysis on variable costs
- Discuss causes of variances
- Discuss when a variance is large enough to warrant managerial attention and investigation
- Discuss variance analysis as related to performance budgeting

■ INTRODUCTION

Chapter 13 presented the basic mechanics of flexible budgeting. This chapter provides several exercises to help the reader become more familiar with the notation and process of flexible budget variance analysis. Flexible budgets differ from original budgets because some costs are variable. Those costs should be expected to change as workload levels change. Therefore, one may have questions regarding how to integrate flexible budgets with fairly rigid staffing patterns. Integration of acuity measures into flexible budgeting will be of interest to many as well. These extensions are discussed in this chapter. Finally, issues concerning fixed versus variable costs, the causes of variances, variance investigation and control, and variance analysis of performance budgets are addressed in the last part of this chapter.

■ AGGREGATION PROBLEMS

Nearby Hospital had the following results for labor costs for the last month:

Salary	Actual	Original Budget	Variance
All departments	$499,700	$500,000	$300F

Should the hospital administrator investigate this variance? Is more information about the variance required? Your immediate reaction is probably to leave well enough alone. The total amount of the variance is small—and favorable at that. Why worry about a $300 variance?

The problem with these results is that when variances are combined, there is a tendency to lose information. Some of the favorable and unfavorable variances may offset each other. The net result is small, and the two variances cannot be observed. For example, assume that the departmental breakdown of the $300 variance is as follows:

Salary	Actual	Original Budget	Variance
Operating Room	$150,000	$125,000	$25,000 U
Dietary	100,000	125,000	25,000 F
Nursing	124,900	125,000	100 F
Lab	124,800	125,000	200 F
Totals	$499,700	$500,000	$ 300 F

Given this extra information, it becomes apparent that it would be a mistake not to investigate further. In this case, which departments need to be investigated? It is fairly obvious that one should be especially concerned with the operating room. And, even though the dietary variance is favorable, it would be wise to find out what is happening in that department as well.

However, focus attention on the nursing department. Suppose that the following information for the nursing department is available[1]:

BPi:	Budgeted nursing rate is $20.00 per hour
BQi:	2.5 hours of budgeted nursing time per patient day
BQo:	2,500 budgeted patient days
AQo:	2,000 actual patient days
Budgeted Total Cost:	$125,000
Actual Total Cost:	$124,900

Although the variance for the nursing department is only $100 and is favorable, the number of patient days is down substantially from expectations.

What variances can be calculated? Is all the desired information available? What is meant by a favorable variance in this context? The original budgeted cost was $125,000, and the actual cost was $124,900. Looking only at the total budgeted and actual **dollars** spent, it would appear that everything is fine because there is a $100 favorable variance. However, even though the total dollars were close to the amount budgeted, it is useful to calculate the price, quantity, and volume variances to see if everything is in fact okay.

To calculate a volume variance, it is first necessary to determine the flexible budget (i.e., the amount that would have been budgeted if the actual workload level had been predicted accurately). The flexible budget is the budgeted quantity of input, multiplied by the budgeted price of inputs, multiplied by the actual quantity of output.

---

[1] Recall that the notation from Chapter 13 was as follows:
BPi: budgeted price per unit of input
BQi: budgeted quantity of input for each unit of output
BQo: budgeted quantity of output
APi: actual price paid per unit of input
AQi: actual quantity of input for each unit of output produced
AQo: actual quantity of output

Information about all those variables is available, and the volume variance can be calculated as follows:

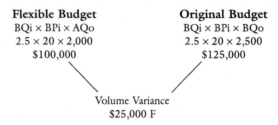

Flexible Budget
BQi × BPi × AQo
2.5 × 20 × 2,000
$100,000

Original Budget
BQi × BPi × BQo
2.5 × 20 × 2,500
$125,000

Volume Variance
$25,000 F

The volume variance is a favorable $25,000. This means that the workload was down substantially. If it is assumed that nursing staff costs are variable (this assumption will be relaxed later in the chapter), a volume variance should be accompanied by reduced spending. For most hospitals, a reduction in patient days from the expected level would often be an *unfavorable* event. It probably means that admissions and revenues are down substantially. It is called a *favorable* variance because treating fewer patients implies that less would be spent. However, that does not mean that something good has happened. It is important for managers to be aware of favorable volume variances as quickly as possible, so that adjustments can be made to staffing if necessary.

In order to calculate price and quantity variances, it is necessary to be able to calculate the subcategory value. This requires multiplying the actual quantity of input by the budgeted price by the actual quantity of output. Information on the actual quantity of input was not given, so it is not possible to calculate the subcategory value. However, the actual spending can be compared to the flexible budget to determine a flexible budget variance.

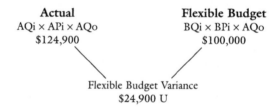

Actual
AQi × APi × AQo
$124,900

Flexible Budget
BQi × BPi × AQo
$100,000

Flexible Budget Variance
$24,900 U

This variance is unfavorable. It is not known why it has occurred, and there is not enough information here to break this variance into its price and quantity components. It is possible, however, that the reduced patient load was not accompanied by reduced staffing. If staffing was kept virtually the same, the amount of nursing time available per patient day would rise, and an unfavorable quantity variance would occur. This means that workload and possibly revenue are falling but that costs are not decreasing. This will result in financial losses.

The point of this example is not to be able to determine what really happened at Nearby Hospital but to get a good understanding of the problems that get buried when variances are aggregated and evaluated in total. When the overall variance for the hospital was examined, the offsetting variances in the operating room and dietary departments were not apparent. Variance information for each department separately is needed. One would certainly want to investigate the large unfavorable variance in the operating room. Even though the variance in the dietary department is favorable, it is important to determine what caused that variance as well. Certainly the favorable variance might be due at least in part to the lower patient days. However, other factors may be at play in this situation. As noted, favorable variances are not always good variances. Other sources of the variance such as replacing a higher cost food supplier with a lower cost food supplier may be the reason for the variance, or replacing higher quality food with lower quality food might be the source of the price decrease.

However, looking at department variances did not point out the problem within the nursing department. It is possible that different units in the nursing department might have variances that would offset each other. So it is really necessary to look at variances for each unit. Within a nursing unit, it is possible that an unfavorable salary variance could be offset by a favorable supply variance. Managers must look at each line item of each unit. Traditional variance analysis would allow that.

In this example, however, falling patient volume was offset by a flexible budget variance. A manager who simply examined the line-item variance for nursing salaries in a particular nursing unit would not be aware of that problem. Only by using flexible budget variance analysis can the manager get more information about what is going on within a line item. Once managers have such information, they can investigate the variances. In this example, the flexible budget variance might have been the result of a failure to reduce staffing as workload decreased. It might have been the result of a salary rate increase. It might have been the result of a change in patient mix or a deliberate decision to invest in training the operating room (OR) nursing staff to care for a new population of surgery patients. For example, the hospital might plan to expand the orthopedic surgery service by offering joint replacement services. The expertise of the manager is needed to make the final determination. However, the ability of managers to use their knowledge and expertise is substantially enhanced if price, quantity, and volume variances are calculated for each line item for each unit.

■ EXCEPTION REPORTING

Aggregation problems create substantial difficulty. The only way to be sure that one variance is not being offset by another variance is by examining every single price, quantity, and volume variance of every single line item of every single unit of every single department of the organization. This creates a potentially unmanageable burden. Should the chief executive officer (CEO) examine every individual variance for the entire organization? Should the chief nurse executive (CNE) have to examine every individual variance in all units of the nursing department? The time required would be enormous. A solution to this problem is the use of *exception reports*.

Assuming a computer prepares all the variances for each cost element, it is a simple process to have the computer prepare a list for the CEO of only those individual variances that exceed a certain limit. This is called an exception report. It lists only the variances that are large. How large depends on the desires of the individual CEO. When tight, centralized control is desired, smaller variances are of interest. For example, whereas some CEOs might be interested only in monthly or year-to-date variances that are greater than 20% of the budget or $50,000, a CEO running a more centralized operation might be interested in variances greater than 10%, or $10,000.

This does not mean that variances less than $10,000 must go unnoticed. Each department head, such as the CNE, would get a report for the department at a more detailed level, perhaps 5%, or $1,000. Continuing the process, nurse managers would receive detailed exception reports for the variances in units under their supervision. Ultimately, the nurse manager who has direct control over a unit would want to review all variances for that unit. In all cases, if a nurse manager feels that a particular variance indicates a problem that is likely to grow worse in future months, the higher levels of nursing administration should be alerted to the problem rather than waiting until the variance is great enough to appear on the CNE's exception report.

■ INTERPRETATION OF VARIANCES

Assume that you are the nursing administrator for a medical group. This may be either a fee-for-service organization or a prepaid-group practice. Suppose that the organization is expecting a severe outbreak of the Hoboken flu this winter, so it has hired extra agency nurses to treat the patients and administer shots. The budgeted expectation was that 1,000 hours of part-time services would be needed at $40.00 per hour, for a total cost of $40,000. It was also expected that the part-time nurses would average a half hour for each of 2,000 patients. The results at the end of the flu season are as follows:

Salary	Actual	Original Budget	Variance
Part-time nurses	$50,000	$40,000	$10,000

Would this be considered to be a favorable or an unfavorable variance? On the surface, more was spent than was expected; therefore, it would be recorded as an unfavorable variance from an accounting viewpoint. The physician director of the medical group may well be complaining about the total lack of budget control exhibited by the unexpected $10,000 excess cost. At this stage, however, there is more to the variance than simply what was expected to be spent and what was actually spent. Consider how much work was done for the $50,000 actually spent.

Suppose that 2,600 patients were actually treated by the part-time nurses, who worked a total of 1,200 hours. What are the variances that can be computed from this information? The original budget is $40,000 and the actual cost was $50,000. The number of patients actually treated was 2,600, the budgeted time per patient was one-half hour, and the budgeted hourly rate was $40.00. Therefore, the flexible budget would be $52,000 (½ × $40 × 2,600). The subcategory would compare the actual quantity of hours required to treat the actual number of patients at the budgeted hourly rate of $40.00. The actual time taken to treat the actual number of patients has been given as 1,200 hours. For 2,600 patients to be treated in 1,200 hours, an average of 0.461 hours must have been used per patient (1,200 hours divided by 2,600 patients = 0.461 hours per patient). Therefore, the subcategory is $48,000 (0.461 hours per patient × $40 per hour × 2,600 patients).

The resulting variances are shown in Figure 14-1. Although the actual wage rate is not known, it is known that the actual costs were $50,000. The rate variance is $2,000 U, the quantity variance is $4,000 F, and the volume variance is $12,000 U. Let's discuss the volume variance first because it is the largest. That variance is attributable to the fact that there were 2,600 patients instead of the expected 2,000 patients.

Is this result good or bad for the organization? What is the likely effect of these extra patients on revenues? If the medical group is a *prepaid group plan*, such as an HMO, the volume variance is bad news. It means that the number of patients treated has gone up substantially without any increase in revenue. On the other hand, if it is

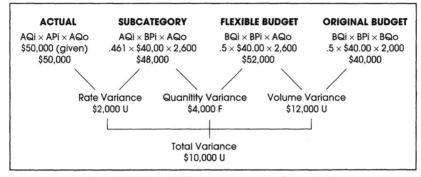

ACTUAL	SUBCATEGORY	FLEXIBLE BUDGET	ORIGINAL BUDGET
AQi × APi × AQo	AQi × BPi × AQo	BQi × BPi × AQo	BQi × BPi × BQo
$50,000 (given)	.461 × $40,00 × 2,600	.5 × $40.00 × 2,600	.5 × $40.00 × 2,000
$50,000	$48,000	$52,000	$40,000

Rate Variance $2,000 U   Quanitity Variance $4,000 F   Volume Variance $12,000 U

Total Variance $10,000 U

Figure 14-1 The medical group agency nurse salary variances.

a *fee-for-service* organization, the extra cost will be associated with increased billings. The number of patients treated is 30% greater than expected. Therefore, even if the actual costs were $12,000 more than the budgeted $40,000 (i.e., the budgeted $40,000 × 30% = $12,000), the organization still would be better off if it makes a profit on each patient.

In any case, a clear argument can be made that the portion of the unfavorable variance caused by increased patient flow is beyond the control and therefore beyond the responsibility of the nursing administrator.

What about the two remaining variances—the $2,000 unfavorable rate variance and the $4,000 favorable quantity variance? Certainly, one can come up with several possible scenarios. For instance, because more part-time hours were needed than had been expected, some experienced RNs were hired rather than just new graduates (i.e., there were not enough new graduates available to fill the need). The experienced RNs, however, were so skillful that their higher wage rate (resulting in the unfavorable rate variance) was more than offset by the speedy efficiency with which they worked (resulting in the favorable quantity variance). If this was in fact the case, the organization should learn for the future that it may be more cost-effective to use experienced RNs.

An alternative scenario would be that the rate variance was simply the result of overtime wages. Once the patients started coming, there was not enough time to hire anyone else, so the organization just worked the agency nurses it had for longer hours, resulting in an overtime premium. However, the rate variance resulting from the overtime premium was more than offset by the fact that there were so many patients that the nurses never had idle time. Because some idle time had been built into the budget, the favorable quantity variance resulted.

This can also indicate something about the future. Perhaps the nurses were thrilled that they did not have to sit around bored. In this case, fewer nurses should be hired in the future and they should be kept relatively busy. On the other hand, one possible implication of a favorable quantity variance is a reduced level of quality of care, with each patient receiving less time and attention. Reduced quality of care normally shows up as a favorable quantity variance. If quality of care suffered, one would want to avoid that situation in the future. Another possibility is that the nurses worked hard and fast (the patients were lined up right out into the hall, so it was continuous work), but they are so angry at being overworked that they will never work for the organization again. A "favorable" quantity variance does not always mean favorable things for the organization.

Nothing can be concluded for certain about the rate and quantity variances in the medical group because the reader was not actually there and knows little about the organization. A truly useful variance report can be developed only by someone with knowledge of the specific situation. The value of flexible budgeting, however, should be reasonably clear.

The methodology does help to separate out the elements that are totally beyond the unit's or the manager's control such as the number of patients. It is then possible to see clearly the magnitude of the rate and quantity variances. If they are substantial, the manager can turn attention to finding out why they occurred. This information is needed for two reasons: first, so that the organization can be managed more efficiently in the future; and second, so that the manager can reasonably defend the way the department or unit was run.

■ RIGID STAFFING PATTERNS

The medical group example presents an extreme because nurses were hired by the hour. Flexible budgeting makes the assumption that if one more patient is treated; it is possible to consume just one more tongue depressor, a quarter roll more of bandage tape, or a half hour more of nursing time. This may be true in the case of tongue depressors and bandage tape, but it implies a lot more flexibility of nurse staffing than most organizations have.

Health care organizations often have some flexibility to transfer nurses from one shift to another or from a unit with a temporarily low occupancy to one with a higher occupancy. In some cases, however, such flexibility may be limited. This is particularly the case at unionized organizations with strong work rules. The key to flexible budgeting is that if the workload (such as patient days) increases or decreases, costs should increase or decrease as well. But nursing costs cannot be reduced if patient days are just one or two fewer than expected. Nurse staffing tends to be variable only if there are more substantial workload changes. One heuristic is that because nurses can work up to 30% faster during a short-term understaffing situation, the use of floating or per diem nurses is not considered until the unit has a nursing hours excess or shortage of at least 4 hours of direct nursing care (McHugh, 1988; McHugh, 1997; McHugh & Dwyer, 1992). In fact, the need to bring in per diem nurses or request overtime from the current staff will be judged on both the number of nurses available to pick up the extra work and the type of work needed.

For example, in a large hospital medical unit where there are 10 RNs on duty, a shortage of 4 hours of nursing care would not require replacement. If only 7 of the nurses worked 10% faster, the shortage would be more than covered. On the other hand, in the OR, if those 4 hours meant that a room would not have a circulator, the hours would have to be replaced even if there were 10 other RNs working in the OR that day. In that instance, the ability of nurses to work faster is not relevant. Room coverage is what must be accomplished.

Suppose that a department has rigid work rules. No nurses can be shifted into or out of the department. Either new nurses are hired or nurses are let go if the patient volume changes significantly. Obviously, for small changes in workload, a manager will not change staffing levels. However, flexible budget variance analysis can still be used.

For simplicity's sake, this example examines variances for an entire year, using annual full-time equivalents (FTEs) and annual salaries. (In practice, one would want to find the variances on a monthly basis.) Suppose that the staffing pattern is as follows:

Staffing Guide

FTEs (RNs)	Patient Days
4	0– 6,000
5	6,001– 7,000
6	7,001– 8,000
7	8,001– 9,000
8	9,001–10,000

Further assume that for the year just past:

	Actual	Original Budget	Variance
Nurses salaries	$286,000	$320,000	$34,000 F

Also assume for that year, that:

$$
\begin{aligned}
\text{Expected patient days} &= 10{,}000 \\
\text{Expected salary per FTE} &= \$40{,}000 \\
\text{Actual patient days} &= 7{,}750 \\
\text{Actual salary} &= \$44{,}000 \\
\text{Actual FTEs} &= 6.5
\end{aligned}
$$

Although the variance is listed as $34,000 F, one can readily see from the staffing guide that for the actual workload of 7,750 patient days, staffing should have been 6 FTEs. The so-called favorable variance may stem largely from a volume variance, and there may be underlying price and quantity variances that would warrant investigation.

With a rigid staffing guide, there is no need to find both the quantity of input per unit of output (Q_i) and the quantity of output (Q_o) and then multiply them to find the total quantity of input. The staffing guide can be used to simplify this process.

The original budget is concerned solely with budgeted amounts. At the BQ_o of 10,000 patient days, the staffing guide calls for 8 FTEs. This can be referred to as the TBQ (total budgeted quantity of input). If the TBQ is multiplied by the budgeted price per FTE, the result is the original budget (Figure 14-2).

Both the actual results and the subcategory are based on the actual quantity amounts. In this example, the actual total quantity consumed is 6.5 FTEs. Refer to that as the TAQ (total actual quantity of input). If the TAQ is multiplied times the

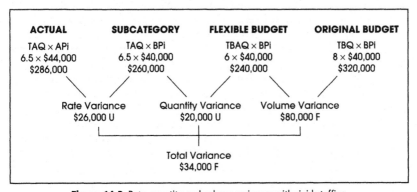

Figure 14-2 Rate, quantity, and volume variances with rigid staffing.

actual price per FTE, the result is the actual value; if TAQ is multiplied by the budgeted price per FTE, the result is the subcategory value.

The flexible budget is what would have been budgeted had the actual workload level been known. In this case, patient days were actually 7,750. According to the staffing guide, 6 FTEs should have been used for that number of patient days. Refer to that as the TBAQ (total budgeted quantity of input for the actual quantity of output). If TBAQ is multiplied by the budgeted price per FTE, the result is the flexible budget.

Looking at Figure 14-2, one can now find the variances. Notice that the Pi shown in each case is the cost per FTE, not per hour of nursing time. This is necessary because of the rigid nature of the staffing patterns, where quantity measures are given as the number of FTEs rather than in hours.

Figure 14-2 indicates that the actual cost of $286,000 came about because 6.5 FTEs were used at an actual rate of $44,000 each. The same quantity of nursing labor (6.5 FTEs) at the budgeted salary of $40,000 per FTE would have cost $260,000. There is a $26,000 rate variance because the average salary paid exceeded expectations by $4,000 per FTE. The flexible budget next compares the actual amount of labor used with the amount of labor that would have been budgeted had the actual number of patient days been known in advance. Thus it is seen that there was a $20,000 unfavorable variance as a result of having used 0.5 FTE more than would have been budgeted for 7,750 patient days.

The largest variance is the volume variance. This is a favorable variance only in the sense that the unit expected to need 8 FTEs for 10,000 patient days. In fact, the unit should have needed only 6 FTEs for 7,750 patient days. If the manager had reacted immediately, $80,000 less would have been spent. Spending less implies a favorable variance even if the workload decline is bad for the organization.

Now the results can be evaluated in the same way as they would be if nurses could be moved around by the hour, but one must be cognizant of the implications of the staffing pattern. The volume variance is not of much interest, assuming that it is outside the manager's control. This may not always be the case. There are situations in which poor management can keep beds empty when there are patients waiting to fill them. In such cases, the volume variance may be at least partly a nursing responsibility.

The quantity variance is of some concern. Did the nurse manager of this unit do a good or bad job of controlling staffing costs? Despite the large unfavorable variance, there is strong reason to believe that the manager did a reasonably good job. In order to come down to 6 FTEs, a full 25% of the unit's staffing had to be either laid off or permanently reassigned elsewhere. Given the high costs associated with attracting, training, and retaining qualified nurses, a manager must be most reluctant to let a nurse go unless there is evidence that a downturn in patient days is not merely a passing aberration but rather a permanent trend. Finishing the year with additional consumption of only 0.5 FTE would appear to indicate that the manager sized up the situation and acted reasonably quickly.

What about the rate variance? Certainly, if it is the result of overtime or unexpected shift-differential increases, that might indicate poor scheduling control in light of the decrease in patient days. A much more plausible explanation is that the two nurses who were released had the least seniority and the lowest pay rate. The six nurses who were retained are likely to have been earning a higher rate. This would raise the average rate and therefore cause the price variance.

Thus, even in a case where staffing patterns are relatively rigid, managers can still benefit from flexible budget variance analysis.

■ FLEXIBLE BUDGETING AND ACUITY

Acuity measures can lead to substantial improvements in budgeting and reimbursement. The budgeting improvements stem from the recognition that different patients require different amounts of nursing care. If patient acuity can be measured and predicted, the amount of staffing budgeted can be adjusted on the basis of both the number of patients or patient days and the degree of illness of the patients and their likely requirement for nursing inputs.

If acuity is used in preparing the operating budget, acuity should be included when that budget is used as a tool for control. If average acuity is different from the expected level, it is logical that resource consumption in terms of nursing requirements will also differ from the budgeted amount.

Acuity can be built into variance analysis through the flexible budget model (Figure 14-3). Begin on the right-hand side of the figure, with the original budget. The budgeted quantity of input per unit of output, BQi, has been replaced by BQiBA, which is the budgeted quantity of input per unit of output at the **budgeted acuity level.** In other words, BQiBA is the amount of nursing time budgeted per patient day, assuming a particular expected acuity level. The BPi and BQo are the same as in the earlier model.

Moving to the left, you find the flexible budget. The only change between the original budget and the flexible budget is that the budgeted quantity of output has been replaced with the actual quantity of output. Thus, the flexible budget indicates what the cost would have been expected to be had the actual output level (e.g., number of patient days) been known when the budget was being prepared. This assumes that the model is using the actual output level but the expected acuity level. The difference between the original and flexible budgets is the volume variance.

The next category is a new one: the acuity subcategory. The price of inputs and the quantity of outputs are the same for the flexible budget and the acuity subcategory. However, the flexible budget uses the budgeted quantity of input per unit of output for the budgeted acuity level, BQiBA. The acuity subcategory uses the

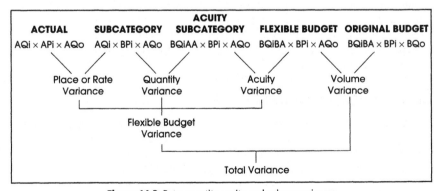

Figure 14-3 Rate, quantity, acuity, and volume variances.

budgeted quantity of input per unit of output for the actual acuity level, BQiAA. The difference between the flexible budget and the acuity subcategory is called the acuity variance.

The acuity subcategory represents what would have been budgeted for the actual output and acuity. The flexible budget represents what would have been budgeted for the actual output level, using a budgeted acuity level. Because the quantity of output in both cases is the actual and the price of inputs in both cases is the budgeted, the difference between these two categories must be attributable to the fact that the actual and budgeted acuity levels do not agree. If the acuity subcategory is larger than the flexible budget, the actual acuity was greater than expected. The logical outcome of greater acuity is that there would be the need to consume more resources. The result is an unfavorable acuity variance.

Moving to the left, you find the subcategory, which is the same as the subcategory that has been used up until now. The AQi (actual quantity of input per unit of output) inherently represents the actual quantity of input per unit of output for the actual acuity level. The resulting quantity variance indicates whether more or less input per unit of output was used than expected, given the actual acuity level. The price variance is unchanged.

It is important to note that if the price, quantity, acuity, and volume variances are totaled, the total variance is the same as it would have been if acuity had not been used in the model. Additional amounts of variance have not been added. Rather, the variance has been subdivided so that the causes of the overall variance can be more easily determined. Where did the acuity variance come from? Until this discussion, the acuity variance was buried in the quantity variance. What has been done here is to separate the quantity variance into the part caused by a change in acuity and the remainder, which resulted from other causes, such as number of patient days or clinic visits or the number of procedures.

This is a significant separation if in fact nursing resources are supposed to be added as acuity increases. Suppose that the department has an unfavorable overall variance. How did that variance arise? The part of it caused simply by increased patient days (the volume variance) or by a larger than anticipated hourly raise (the rate variance) can be identified. But what if most of the unfavorable variance resides in the quantity variance? Was that unfavorable variance the result of factors beyond the control of the nurse manager?

In Figure 14-3, it is possible to separate the portion caused by an unexpected change in the acuity level. Thus, it is a little easier to determine whether the remaining quantity variance is the result of controllable or uncontrollable events. The reader should keep in mind that the quantity and acuity variances combined in Figure 14-3 would equal the quantity variance if the acuity component were not being segregated.

■ FIXED VERSUS VARIABLE COSTS

The basic approach surrounding flexible budgeting is that the original budget assumes a specific level of workload, such as a fixed number of patient days. If the actual level differs from that expected, the amount of resources consumed should change. The starting point for a flexible budget analysis, therefore, is that we assume that resources will be consumed in some direct relationship to output. However, with respect to fixed costs, this is not the case.

By definition, a fixed cost is one that does not vary with the level of output. Examples include the depreciation on a hospital building or the salary paid to a nurse manager. These costs do not change in proportion to the number of patients or patient days. This does not mean that they will not have any variances. They may well have variances. For example, if heating costs are allocated to the unit, and it is an especially cold winter, the heating costs may well vary unfavorably from the budget. However, no part of the variance can be related specifically to any workload volume measure. As a result, there cannot be a volume variance.

Furthermore, in the case of fixed costs, it may be difficult to determine what portion of the variance represents a price variance and what portion a quantity variance. In some cases, price and quantity variances can be calculated for fixed costs. The cost of heating a clinic can be evaluated in terms of the price of fuel and the quantity of fuel. In many cases, however, there will be only one variance for fixed-cost items. Although flexible budgeting can be very helpful in the case of costs that vary with output levels, the reader should be aware of this limitation with respect to fixed costs.

■ CAUSES OF VARIANCES

Throughout the past several chapters, there have been numerous examples of variances and suppositions as to what might have caused them. It is important to be aware that variance analysis is only a tool that points in the right direction. The nurse manager must make the investigation and the final determination of what caused a variance to arise.

Common internal causes of variances include shifts in the quality of care provided, changes in the technology used, changes in the efficiency of the nurses, changes in the organization's policies, or simply incorrect standards. Variance analysis can highlight a quantity variance, but it cannot indicate whether quality of care is improving or whether coffee breaks are getting longer. Both might show up as unfavorable quantity variances. Poor staff scheduling may have produced excessive overtime, or pay raises may have increased labor costs. Both would show up as unfavorable rate variances.

External causes of variances commonly include price changes for supplies, volume changes in workload, and unexpected shifts in the availability of staff. Flexible budgeting is somewhat more helpful in these cases than in internally caused variances. Shifts in workload can be isolated in the volume variance. Going over budget on supplies can be isolated in the price variance if the problem is in the purchasing department as opposed to lax nursing control over the quantity of supplies used.

In any event, flexible budget variance analysis can greatly ease the problem of determining the cause of a department's overall variance. It can even simplify the problem of determining the cause of the variance in any one specific line item. However, the final responsibility for determining the cause of the variance ultimately rests on the shoulders of the nurse manager.

■ INVESTIGATION AND CONTROL OF VARIANCES

Probably the most difficult aspect of variance analysis is determining when a variance is large enough to warrant investigation. As has been shown in this chapter, even a small variance can hide significant problems when variances are aggregated. But suppose that variances have not been aggregated and information is available on each individual price, quantity, and volume variance for each cost element. Should a manager investigate $5, $50, $100, or $1,000 variances? How big a variance is too big to tolerate without investigation?

It must be kept in mind that budgets are "guesstimates" of the future. They cannot be expected to come out exactly on target. Small variances can generally be ignored. It is to be hoped that over the course of a year, the small unfavorable variances will be balanced out by small favorable variances.

This still does not indicate when to investigate a variance. Unfortunately, there is no set answer. A good heuristic is to investigate any variance that lies outside the 95% variability probability (see Chapter 13). However, some variances smaller than the 95% variability level might need investigation. Other, larger variances may be planned and understood and so need no investigation (for example, consider the case described earlier in which the OR staff needed extra training to handle new orthopedic procedures). The solution we favor is as follows: when a manager looks at a variance, it should be assumed that it will occur in the same amount month after month until the end of the year. For instance, suppose that a $500 unfavorable variance was found for January for nurses' aides' salaries. If that variance occurred every month, it would total $6,000 for the year. If $6,000 is an unreasonably high variance, investigate the $500 January variance as soon as possible.

Suppose that the January variance was only $100 and that $1,200 is a variance that would be acceptable for the year. No immediate investigation would take place. In February, the variance might be $200, but perhaps the unit can live with a $2,400 variance as well. If the variance is $300 in March, the manager must be concerned, even if $3,600 would be an acceptable level. The monthly increase in the variance indicates a growing problem. There is a **trend** for the budget to exhibit unfavorable variances. At this point, the manager would probably investigate the variance to make sure that it does not continue to grow even further out of control.

The key to controlling variances is to be timely, to correct behavior if necessary, and to use the information from variances to correct rates promptly.

If variances are not investigated promptly after each month's variance report is received, the budget will serve only as a planning tool, not a tool to help the organization control its operations. Information about last month's performance should be used to improve the performance for the remaining months of the year.

Such improvement is likely to depend on taking actions to correct behavior when necessary. This may mean meeting to discuss areas of waste, tightening rules on coffee breaks or on personal use of supplies, and so forth. For the most part, the key to improvement is simply a heightened awareness of the budget throughout the year. Everyone is enthusiastic about meeting the budget for the first month or two, but then they gradually slip back into old, sometimes wasteful habits. By bringing budget variances to the attention of relevant employees whenever the variances start to get out of line, the manager can reinforce the beneficial motivating aspects of the budget that were prominent right after the budget was adopted. If necessary, more forceful means should be used to modify behavior when budget variances are the result of employees' not doing their jobs properly.

Finally, in some cases, it will be found that the variances are simply out of the control of the unit or the manager. A shortage of a key raw material may drive the price of supplies up. If there appears to be a protracted change that is outside the control of the manager and that will result in continuing unfavorable variances, it is important to bring this change to the attention of the organization's rate-setting personnel. The sooner the change is recognized and the rates are corrected upward, the better it is for the financial stability of the organization.

■ PERFORMANCE BUDGETS AND VARIANCE ANALYSIS

Performance budgeting was the topic of Chapter 11 of this book. In a sense, most of this chapter on variance analysis revolves around performance budgeting. Flexible budgets are attempts to match actual costs incurred with the costs that should have been incurred based on the actual workload. By looking at the actual workload rather than the original budgeted expectations, variances are being calculated with at least some measure of performance being taken into account. However, in developing the performance budget, Chapter 11 went beyond the flexible budget. Performance budgets were established based on a variety of key performance areas.

In the example in Chapter 11, it was suggested that a percentage of the cost of each line item could be allocated to each key performance area. For example, 15% of the nurse manager's time might be devoted to quality improvement (see Table 11-1). Based on these percentage allocations, a cost could be budgeted for each key performance area. For example, $87,300 might be budgeted for quality improvement (see Table 11-2). A budgeted cost could then be determined for each unit of output in each key performance area. For example, the budgeted cost might be $8,730 per 1% drop in the rate of failure to comply with patient care plans (see Table 11-3). How can these performance budget calculations be compared to actual results? And how can variances between the budget and the actual expenses be determined?

The first step is to assess how much output was actually accomplished in each key performance area. In establishing the performance budget, one chooses output measures that are quantifiable. For example, at the end of the month or year, the percentage of reduction in failures to comply with patient care plan procedures can be determined and compared with the budgeted reduction. Similar measures are used for the other key performance areas. For example, the number of patient complaints can be compared with the budgeted number of complaints; the nurse turnover rate can be compared with the budgeted turnover rate. Thus, finding a variance in terms of volume of output achieved is readily possible.

The next step is to compare the actual cost per unit of work accomplished to the budgeted cost. For instance, suppose $87,300 was budgeted for reducing patient care plan errors, with a budgeted goal of a 10% reduction in the rate of failures to comply (a budgeted cost of $8,730 per 1% drop in the failure rate). Suppose that the actual results were that the failure rate fell by 12%. If the total actual cost for this quality improvement is divided by 12, the actual cost per 1% drop can be determined and compared to the budgeted cost of $8,730.

Unfortunately, it is difficult to calculate the actual amount that was spent on quality improvement. This amount consists of a percentage of the cost of each line item. The actual costs for each line item will be known. This cost information is used in the traditional and flexible budget variance analyses discussed earlier. However, there is no ready mechanism for determining the exact percentage of each line item that actually was devoted to each key performance area.

Consider the following information abstracted from the tables in Chapter 11. It includes the budgeted percent effort (just for the quality improvement key performance area) for each line item (see Table 11-1), the budgeted cost for each line item, and the budgeted cost for quality improvement (see Table 11-2). A total of $87,300 was included in the performance budget for quality improvement.

Line Item	Line Item Total Cost		Percent Effort Devoted to Quality Improvement		Cost Budgeted for Quality Improvement
Nurse manager	$90,000	×	5%	=	$ 4,500
Staff	1,500,000	×	5	=	75,000
Education	30,000	×	20	=	6,000
Supplies	90,000	×	2	=	1,800
Overhead	90,000	×	0	=	0
Total					$87,300
Divided by budgeted outcome (% reduction in failure to comply with patient care plan)					÷10
Budgeted cost per percent reduction in failures					$ 8,730

In the example, the nurse manager was budgeted to devote 5% of her total effort to quality improvement. Did she or he, in fact, devote 10%? Or perhaps only 2%? In most organizations (if not all), the data collection systems are not nearly sophisticated enough to capture such information. Therefore, it is generally necessary to estimate the actual percentage allocations.

Suppose that the nurse manager was budgeted to cost $90,000 but that, because of a change in fringe benefit rates, the actual manager cost was $91,000. Also suppose that the manager makes an ex post allocation of her total time and estimates that 10% of her effort was devoted to quality improvement. In that case, instead of the budgeted $4,500 of manager cost for quality improvement, the actual manager cost for quality improvement was $9,100 (total nurse manager cost of $91,000 multiplied by 10% effort on the quality area).

Assume that the actual results for each line item in the quality improvement area were as follows:

Line Item	Line Item Total Cost		Percent Effort Devoted to Quality Improvement		Actual Cost for Quality Improvement
Nurse manager	$91,000	×	10%	=	$ 9,100
Staff	1,545,000	×	5	=	77,250
Education	30,000	×	15	=	4,500
Supplies	98,000	×	1	=	980
Overhead	94,000	×	0	=	0
Total					$91,830
Divided by actual outcome (% reduction in failure to comply with patient care plan)					÷12
Actual cost per percent reduction in failures					$ 7,652

The actual cost information would come from the unit's regular variance reports. The percentages of actual effort would be based on estimates by the unit manager and the unit's staff. The budgeted cost for quality improvement was $87,300, whereas the actual cost was $91,830. The difference between these two numbers represents an $4,530 unfavorable variance. However, this variance does not consider actual work accomplished.

Just as with the flexible variance analysis discussed earlier, it is necessary to consider more than simply the absolute amount of money spent. In terms of accomplishing the goal of reducing the rate of failures to comply with patient care plans, the budgeted cost was $8,730 per 1% reduction in the failure rate. The actual result was a cost of $7,652 per percent reduction in the failure rate. The cost per percent dropped because even though costs were over budget, the failure rate dropped by 12% rather than 10%.

Had one anticipated the 12% reduction, the budgeted cost would have been $104,760 ($8,730 multiplied by 12). Although there is a total variance of $4,530 unfavorable, the volume variance was $17,460 unfavorable ($87,300 budgeted minus $104,760 flexible budget for a 12% reduction). The cost for the actual volume was less than would have been expected for that volume.

In analyzing performance budget results, it is also interesting to look at each line item. In this case, staff salaries of $77,250 were devoted to quality improvement. In the original budget, the amount was $75,000. This greater effort has apparently led to a greater reduction in the failure rate. Even though the cost per percent reduction was less than budgeted, this result would require careful scrutiny by the nurse manager. If greater efforts were being made in this area, where were efforts less than budgeted? Perhaps this represents more attention to charting and less direct patient care. In that case, this may not be considered to be a favorable use of time. A unit could have perfect, failure-free patient care plans but poor-quality care because of insufficient direct care time. On the other hand, if the reduction in effort elsewhere was in the area of other indirect time, this may represent a favorable outcome.

As with all areas of variance analysis, the calculations provide raw information about what has occurred. The judgment and experience of competent managers is needed to interpret the variances and determine both their underlying causes and whether they represent favorable or unfavorable events for the unit and organization.

Summary and Implications for Nurse Managers

Flexible budget variance analysis is a useful but complex tool. Care must be taken to make sure the analysis helps the manager. For example, the aggregation of variances can hide serious problems. Offsetting variances are quite common. If variances are aggregated, offsetting variances may go undetected. Exception reports are particularly useful to keep large variances from going unnoticed.

Flexible budgeting assumes that costs are variable. With fixed costs, there will be no volume variance because fixed costs by definition do not vary with volume. However, nursing labor costs, even with rigid staffing patterns, can be evaluated in a flexible budget analysis. Varying levels of acuity can also be readily built into the model.

Variances are generally caused by internal changes in efficiency, technology, or quality of care or by externally caused changes in workload volume or prices. Whatever the causes, efficient management requires investigation and evaluation of variances on a timely basis, followed by actions to correct variances whenever possible.

References and Suggested Readings

Dunham-Taylor, J., Pinczuk, J.Z. (2006). *Health Care Financial Management for Nurse Managers.* Sudbury, MA: Jones and Bartlett.

Felteau, A. (1992). Budget variance analysis and justification. *Nursing Management.* 23(2), 40-41.

Finkler, S.A., Ward, D.R., Baker, J. (2007). *Essentials of Cost Accounting for Health Care Organizations,* ed 3. Sudbury, MA: Jones and Bartlett.

Horngren, C.T., Datar, S.M., Foster, G. (2005). *Cost Accounting: A Managerial Emphasis,* ed 12. Englewood Cliffs, NJ: Prentice-Hall.

McHugh, M. (1997). Cost-effectiveness of clustered versus unclustered unit transfers of nursing staff. *Nursing Economic$.* 15 (6), 294-300.

McHugh, M. (1988). Comparison of four nurse staffing patterns using computer simulation. *Proceedings of the Third International Symposium on Computer Use in Nursing.* Dublin, Ireland.

McHugh, M., Dwyer, V. (1992). Measurement issues in patient acuity classification for prediction of hours in nursing care. *Journal of Nursing Administration Quarterly.* 16(4), 20-31.

Voss, G.B., Van Ooij, A., Brans-Brabant, L.J., Limpens, P.G. (1997). Cost-variance analysis by DRGs: Technique for clinical budget analysis. *Health Policy.* 39(2), 153-166.

Budgeting for Information Systems

■ INTRODUCTION

Hospitals have used computers for a long time. Originally, they were used primarily for business applications, such as payroll, billing, and tracking patients. In the 1960s and 1970s, computers were used primarily to process large amounts of data such as hours worked and to print reports such as patient bills. Throughout the 1980s and 1990s, rapid development allowed computers to do much more complex tasks. A significant development was the advent of *database management systems (DBMS)* that allowed vast amounts of data to be stored quickly and retrieved almost instantly. Along with improved database systems, computer hardware (the machinery) and software (the programs that tell the computer what to do) advanced at an amazing rate—the personal computers that sit on so many people's desks at home and work and cost about $2,000 or less can now do more work than large mainframe computers costing several million dollars could do in the 1970s. Computer hardware and software—and machines like heart monitors and EKG machines that have computer chips—are often referred to as information technology (IT).

By the middle of the 1970s, computer hardware was much less expensive, and software technology had developed to the extent that in some businesses, people at the point of service could enter data into a computer as they completed transactions. In some hospitals, nurses entered data about bed availability into those early systems. The computer was able to record the data directly into the databases so that a clerical person was no longer needed to transfer the handwritten data into the computer database. These complex systems that can gather, store, and retrieve large amounts of data, support human work processes, and produce reports are called information systems (IS). Although the costs of computer equipment steadily decrease every year, the costs of the complex computer programs—the software—needed to support clinical computing remain high, and health care facilities must budget for these systems as capital acquisitions.

In this chapter we focus on the various costs involved in a large system project. Examples of large systems include an electronic medical record (EMR), a pharmacy system, a laboratory system, or a system that combines several of these systems, which is sometimes called a total hospital information system (HIS). Acquisition and implementation of any of these systems constitutes a large and expensive IS project for which careful budgeting will be necessary.

■ IMPORTANCE OF NURSE'S INVOLVEMENT IN THE SELECTION AND IMPLEMENTATION OF HEALTH CARE INFORMATION SYSTEMS

Health care facilities have been slow to implement computer systems designed to support the patient care work of nurses. Budgets have been strictly constrained, and large information systems are expensive. However, since the 1990s, a steadily increasing number of hospitals have purchased *clinical information systems (CIS)*. These are computer systems with programming that allows care providers to enter patient data—often at the bedside or using a hand-held computer—and to retrieve that information either on the computer screen or by printing it out as part of the paper chart. Systems designed to support patient care will increasingly become a much more important part of the hospital environment over the next 10 years for a variety of reasons, including new and emerging federal regulations and the demands of the third-party payers that provide health insurance (Wall Street Journal, 2006). Some hospitals and other health care facilities have fully computerized part or all of their clinical information, but others are just now investigating the possibility of moving from a paper-based patient record to a computerized record.

Because IS usage will become more widespread in the health care environment, health care facilities and their managers, including nurse managers, will have to become more involved in selecting and budgeting for these products. Nurse managers must know about budgeting for IS because many aspects of the acquisition and maintenance of the systems involve the nursing department. Certainly the chief nursing executive (CNE), as part of top management, will be involved in strategic decisions, including the financing of such systems, which involve the purchase of health care IS. Nursing department managers, from the CNE to the unit managers, will be represented on the committees that plan for these systems, evaluate the products available, and select the systems to be installed in their nursing units. To function as effective nursing leaders, nurses must understand the basics of the systems' selection and implementation processes and must understand the costs of the various phases of the selection and implementation process. Nursing's voice is a critical component of these committees. Nurses form the largest user group of patient care systems, and to participate as credible, effective members of the selection committee, nurse managers must understand the processes and the costs involved. The danger to nursing, if nurses are not directly involved in the system selection process, is that the new systems will interfere with nursing practice rather than support clinical nursing.

Budgeting for a new IS product is a complex and multistep process. New systems are far more likely to be successful if the organization's top management, including the CNE and IS department managers, understand the budgetary needs of new system projects. A good model for IS project budgeting is the systems' life-cycle model. The components of the systems' life cycle for which management must prepare budgets include the following:

1. Planning and project management
2. Systems analysis
3. Systems design and testing or systems selection and purchase (this phase must also address security issues for the new systems)
4. Systems implementation
5. Systems evaluation
6. Systems maintenance and upgrades

Each of these phases requires specific budget line items, and there are budget items that span the entire project. The total project budget consists of the overall project items and the budgets for each of the phases. It should be recognized that the activities, and thus the budget implications, of each phase of the systems' life cycle are quite separate and distinct. This chapter focuses on the work processes, supplies, equipment, and people for which budget line items will be necessary during each phase of the systems' life cycle and how to plan and budget for each of those factors.

Planners must understand that purchasing and implementing new systems are only two components of a multistep process. Systems implementation tends to be the shortest part of the whole systems' life cycle. It should occur only after time has been spent evaluating needs and after a careful design and product selection process. Yet it is not uncommon for managers to expect to be able to purchase and implement systems in a short period of time after deciding that a new system is necessary. That view of the timeline necessary for the planning, acquisition, and implementation of a major new IS product is seriously flawed and typically it leads at best to a difficult transition to the new IS and at worst to a complete failure that forces the removal of the new system. Experienced systems experts recommend that the planning, design, and purchase of new IS (phases 1 through 3) should consume between 70% and 80% of the project's timeline. The implementation and stabilization of new IS should take no more than 10% to 20% of the total project timeline. When the first three phases are cut short, the results are usually not optimal. In fact, many case studies in the management literature have reported that the single most common cause of failure of an IS project is failure to invest sufficient time and effort into the first three phases of the project. Therefore, this chapter delineates the work that should be done in each phase so that the reader can budget for the project in a way that enhances the probability of success when implementing new systems.

IS are already an important presence in the health care industry and are likely to grow significantly in importance and as a percentage of the total budget over the next 20 to 30 years. Most other major industries and government operations in the United States are fundamentally dependent on their computerized IS (Ward & Peppard, 2002). In fact, most business sources report that they invest between 10% and 12% of their budgets on IS. However, most health care facilities currently invest only between 2% and 4% of their budgets on IS products and support. Consequently, the health care industry is far behind other areas of the economy in computerizing its data and operations. It is somewhat ironic that an industry that always seeks out the newest and best technology when producing its services (e.g., the newest MRI scanner, etc.) lags behind in using technology for managing the organization itself.

This lack of investment in IT may be a double-edged sword. Health care facilities have far less ability to access and use their data strategically, but they also have fewer legacy systems to contend with as they move toward increasing computerization of their work processes and information processing. Legacy systems are the old computerized systems still in use in some organizations. They are the systems that were developed when programming languages, computer hardware, and software development techniques were very different from today's technology and processes.

The negative effect of so little investment in the IT area is that few health care facilities can retrieve and analyze their operations data (which means patient care data) in such a way as to support management decision making. Much of the patient care data in health care facilities are stored on hand-written paper charts. It is an enormously expensive endeavor to retrieve the charts, read the information, and convert that narrative information into coded information suitable for computer storage. It is also costly and time consuming to write the programs that can then prepare reports based on data that have been extracted from the database and analyzed so that the raw data have been converted into usable information. The data are physically available, but they are so expensive to retrieve and analyze from paper charts that the data are not economically available. Essentially, the clinical information stored in those paper records might as well be stored on Jupiter for all the help it can provide to decision makers. As a result, decision makers in health care facilities frequently have to base their decisions on unsupported opinions of what is happening in their operations. Worse, those clinical data constitute an economically unavailable gold mine of information that could be used to make decisions about clinical practice and quality improvement as well as about management decisions—decisions that today have to be made with, at best, just a few days of prospective data collection instead of months or years of retrospective data derived from the patient charts. It is well known that decisions that have to be made in the dark, so to speak, are far less likely to be successful than decisions based on evidence.

Another problem with the lack of computerized patient records is that transferring information from one facility to another is costly. It is expensive for a hospital or clinic to pay an employee to physically retrieve a paper record and to copy the relevant portions (or the entire record) when the patient must have it sent to another doctor or hospital. Anecdotally, we have heard of instances where patients have been unable to have their records transferred at all because some health care organizations ignore patient requests until faced with a subpoena to produce the documents. This problem will be greatly eased when hospitals and clinics institute all-electronic patient records. The records can be downloaded on media such as the patient's own memory stick or onto a CD-ROM or smart card so that patients have their own copies of their medical records and can give them to their specialists or new doctors whenever necessary. One advantage of digital media is that images, such as MRIs or radiographs, can easily be stored on electronic storage media. In addition, having personal health records (PHRs) carried in a wallet or purse—just like a credit card—might prove very important in an emergency room situation. In fact, several insurance companies and large employers are working on building a multimillion-dollar data warehouse that links hospitals, doctors, and pharmacies and allows patients to access and download their own information so that patients can be in greater control of their own health information (Wall Street Journal, 2006). It is important to understand that hospitals and clinics will have to make a considerable investment of money and human resources in a variety of IS projects to obtain these benefits of computerization of the patient record.

It is also important to recognize that some of the people working on the IS project will need release time from their other duties in order to accomplish the work of the project. Others will be able to absorb their project work into their regular workload. In order to fully understand the costs of the new system, the time invested by all members of the project team should be included in the project budget. But even if the time of people who absorb their project work into their regular workloads is not listed as part of the project budget, some of the members of the project team will have to devote so much time to the project that temporary replacements will have to be retained.

A success factor in any large IS project is an adequate budget, including the costs of people who must be temporarily relieved of their regular duties and replaced with someone else. It absolutely must be recognized that if some people are not relieved from their regular duties to participate in the project, the likelihood of success declines significantly. Department heads will be more inclined to cooperate in reassigning their staff members' duties if they are given the resources to replace those members temporarily. If they are expected to absorb the extra cost into their budgets, resistance can be expected. That may lead to failure to release employees from their regular duties so they can devote time to the project. The employee torn between the project and regular duties is most likely to stop attending meetings and quit the project. Personnel budgets are a touchy subject in most health care organizations, and early planning to acquire the necessary human resources is absolutely essential to the success of a new IS project.

■ THE LEGACY PROBLEM

Although many health care organizations have the advantage of relatively few legacy systems, such systems are not rare in health care facilities. Virtually all hospitals and clinics have one or more legacy systems upon which they are dependent for operations such as payroll, billing, accounting, and personnel. Some of these systems date back as far as the 1970s, when operations were first being computerized in the organization. Legacy systems are still in use and are performing vital functions for the organization. However, old systems may be difficult to maintain and difficult or impossible to upgrade. It is usually difficult or impossible to interface legacy applications with new systems because the technology of new systems is so different from that of legacy systems. Sometimes the strategy for implementing a new system includes a plan to transfer (or migrate) data and processes from a legacy system to the new system. System migration is usually an expensive, frustrating, and time-consuming effort.

Legacy systems were never developed with the idea of migrating to newer products. They were programmed in older, third-generation[1] languages such as COBOL, which are not typically used for newer business programs. Every year, there are fewer programmers who know how to write or maintain the legacy program languages (although COBOL is still taught in many engineering and computer science schools). More problematic is the fact that the source code necessary to support the program may not be available. Sometimes the legacy systems were developed in-house, and the

---

[1] The first-generation language is *machine language* and consists entirely of number codes; the second-generation language is *assembly language*, which is very like machine language except that some words are used. Third generation languages are less numerically based but are still obscure to the lay person. As the generation number increases, the language tends to become more English-like.

developers are long gone from the organization. For other legacy programs, the company that originally developed them has gone out of business or merged with another company, and the product hasn't been externally supported for years. These factors make linkage of old systems with new systems difficult or impossible.

For maximum efficiency, it is typically necessary for the new systems to use data that are contained in the legacy systems. If the two systems cannot be interfaced or integrated, it may be impossible to electronically transfer data between the old and new systems. The alternative is to have an employee type the data contained in the old system into the new system. There are two problems with that approach. First, it is expensive. Transcription work is detailed and tedious and it is necessary to have certain technical skills to type the data into the new system. Thus, the person employed to do the work tends to be a relatively expensive clerical person. The process takes a considerable amount of time, and if the old system is continuously generating or collecting data, the transcription process is ongoing. Second, no human being can perform transcription work without error. Old studies from the 1970s found that keypunch operators made an average of one error for every thousand keystrokes. Thus, the transcription process inevitably introduces error into the new system's data. Electronic transmission may create an error, but typically the systems are programmed with checks to discover and correct most errors so that electronic transmission typically produces error-free data in the new system.

Given the problems of moving data from older systems to new ones, the reader should always consider that implementation of a new product may force the organization to get into a bigger project than had originally been considered. Not only will the new systems have to be budgeted, but also the organization may have to add on a project that integrates the data from the old systems with those of the new systems. The organization may even find that it must replace one or more legacy systems if it is to obtain the desired benefit from the new systems. That, of course, will require the planning team and management to consider the expense of implementing both the originally desired new systems and any old systems that must be replaced as part of the transition.

■ PLANNING AND PROJECT MANAGEMENT

The size of the budget for the planning phase is dependent on the size of the system being considered. For a very small system that does one constrained but repetitive task, the planning committee may consist only of the department director, a member of the IS department, and one or two of the people who will be using the system. In the case of a very small localized product, the personnel on the planning committee may be able to incorporate the work into their existing schedules. These projects tend to create small applications that nurse managers use for things like supporting their budget calculations, tracking requested capital equipment bids and the like. These probably don't need a budget or a selection process. In fact, many managers just use Excel for those types of applications. If the manager needs the assistance of a staff person from the IS department, that person's time is usually budgeted out of the IS department, and the costs may or may not be charged to the department. Those smaller projects may be reviewed by the IS department committee that prioritizes requests, but they do not cross multiple departments and are not a major cost. Therefore, there is no need for an organizational planning committee. It is only when the new systems will be very costly (perhaps $100,000 or more) or when they will affect multiple departments that a special project planning committee will have to be created.

For a large system that will have effects on several departments, the planning process will be time consuming and will demand very significant amounts of time from members of the project committee. The examples in this chapter focus primarily on large systems that affect multiple departments and have far-ranging effects on the organization's processing support for operations. The following list of large systems that nurses may help to evaluate includes (but is not limited to): *nurse staffing* and *nurse scheduling systems; provider* (or *physician) order entry systems (POES), electronic medical records systems (EMR), electronic health records (EHR), personal health record (PHR), hospital information systems (HIS), clinical information systems (CIS),* perioperative support systems, obstetric documentation systems, and *object-oriented clinical data repositories.* A large systems project will be far more likely to succeed if the project budget includes release time for key project personnel, including staff nurses who represent the nurse end-users who will use the system to document patient care. In addition to personnel, other items such as project management software, clerical assistance, copying expenses, and other resources should be budgeted.

The activities that the planning committee will pursue include (but may not be limited to) the following:

- Analyzing the organization's strategic goals and priorities and how the new system will facilitate meeting those goals and priorities.
- Precisely defining the problem that the new system will solve. For example, is a new system needed because the federal government has mandated that medical information be computerized, or perhaps because the current system is outdated and will no longer be supported by the vendor? Perhaps a new system is needed because technological advancements have greatly increased the productivity (efficiency, scope, quality) of new products over the product in place or because the old system does not support billing and third-party payer information requirements. Whatever the problems are, they should be specified precisely so that prospective products can be evaluated on the basis of their ability to resolve the problems identified in the current system. The product of this activity will be a document that specifies the requirements of an acceptable solution.
- Performing a feasibility study. A feasibility study is a preliminary analysis of the likelihood of success of the project. It identifies and evaluates possible alternatives to solving the problem and selects the best alternative—whether that be to remain manual, to build a system in-house, or to purchase a system from a vendor. The feasibility study must answer at least the following five questions.

    1. Is there a solution that is technically feasible? This means that the planners must ascertain whether technology is sufficiently advanced to provide any solution at all.
    2. Is a large system economically feasible for the organization at this time?
    3. What scheduling issues will arise, and is there a schedule for acquiring and implementing a new system that is feasible for the organization? For example, it would not make much sense to schedule a large new systems project if the administration anticipated the organization might merge with another organization during the systems project.
    4. Is such a project feasible within the organization as it currently stands? This addresses the question of whether the organization has or can acquire personnel with the requisite skills to handle the project and

whether the organization's administration will support the project adequately.

5. Is the project feasible from the point of view of an organization's culture? That is, will the people in the organization be able to absorb this change along with any other changes it is handling at the same time? Too much change too fast can cause exhaustion among the people of the organization, and the feasibility study should examine the proposed change within the context of everything else that is happening in the organization and, of course, the amount of resistance to change likely to be encountered by the management and the end-users.

There may be other questions to be addressed by the feasibility study, but it is absolutely essential to answer these five questions in the process of planning for the implementation of a large system.

Other activities that must be completed during the planning phase if the feasibility study indicates that the project should go forward include the following:

- Preparing the project schedule.
- Preparing a project budget and obtaining administrative approval of the budget.
- Identifying the people to be involved for each of the phases of the project.
- Determining architecture requirements for a new system. This activity will focus on comparing the organization's current systems architecture (e.g., the type of hardware used to support the organization's computer systems) to the requirements of systems available for purchase. If the organization has older models of servers, mainframes, and network software, upgrades or new hardware may be necessary if any new systems are to be supported.
- Acquiring suitable project management software to assist with managing the project.
- Determining the physical office and work spaces that will be needed for the project, and requisitioning furniture, equipment, and supplies for the project. In addition, the planning committee must specify the clerical support that will be needed for the project and negotiate with administration for all these needs.
- Conducting a search of the products available in the market that might meet the needs and obtaining contact information for the vendors of these products.

Budgeting for Planning Committee Personnel

The first budget item for the planning phase addresses planning phase personnel requirements. The following are the minimum positions that must be filled on the planning committee: Project Director, Systems Expert, Department Managers' Representative, Informatics Nurse Specialist, Administration Liaison (from the financial management department), and End-User Department Representatives (one from each department that will be using the system). The first budget item for the planning phase addresses planning-phase personnel requirements.

Project Director
The Project Director (PD) will manage the entire project from start to finish. Therefore, this appointment is critical; the PD will have to be able to devote a significant amount of time to the project and will usually continue in the role of director

for the entire length of the project. The PD is the person responsible for organizing meetings; defining and scheduling tasks; and serving as the liaison among members of the project team, the administration, the IS department, and external consultants and vendors. The person in this role must have sufficient authority to summon team members to meetings, to set and enforce deadlines, to negotiate a project budget, and to negotiate with the organization's administration for the resources needed for the project. As the size of the project increases, the PD's time commitment on the project must increase. At times, the PD will have to work on the project full time, but for much of the project, the time allocation will be less than 100%. In general terms, one should begin by planning to assign the PD to the project at least 50% of the time.

Although it is possible that the organization could contract with an outside consulting organization for a PD, in most cases, the PD will be a member of the organization's top level administration or IS department staff. The project will have to budget the PD's direct and indirect costs. Typically, this expense is paid out of the IS department budget. However, other models exist. Sometimes the project will have a special budget that is a component of the administrative budget under the heading Special-Project Budgets. Regardless of the budgeting strategy used, the time of the PD must be released to the project. This may mean that the IS department hires another person on a temporary basis to pick up the duties the PD would otherwise be doing in his or her regular job. What will not work is to assume that the PD can simply absorb these duties into an already full schedule. Something will fail if release time isn't provided, and all too often, it is the new system that is shorted in such a way that the project ends up with a solution that is far less than optimal.

If the PD's only role in the acquisition of the new system is to manage the process, that person should be budgeted to spend about 25% to 50% of the time during phases 1 through 4, depending on how the work is divided, and 20% of the time during the evaluation phase. If he or she is also the system analyst, it makes sense to budget a great deal more time for the PD. One possible means of allocation might be as shown in Table 15-1.

Systems Expert

The systems expert (SE) may be the director of the organization's IS department or a member within the department who has systems life-cycle skills and who is familiar

TABLE 15-1 Example of Planning Phase Time Allocation for Project Personnel

Project Phase (assuming that a product will be purchased and not developed in-house)	Percent of Director's Time Allocated to the Project
Planning Phase—6 months	50%
Systems Analysis Phase—6 months	50%
System Selection and Staff Preparation Phase—6 months	100%
Implementation and Testing Phase (During the go-live period, this will be a 100% time commitment)—4 months	50%
Evaluation Phase—1 to 3 months	25%
System Maintenance—assuming the Director works in the IS Department and maintains oversight over the system.	10%

Note: During upgrades, if the Project Director works for the IS Department, the time commitment may increase temporarily to 100% if the Project Director manages the upgrades.

with the organization's key computer systems, including hardware, software, and the network. The SE must also have experience with vendor relations, with bid and contract preparation, and with new systems projects. The SE will bring to the project a macro view of the organization's computer systems and its data warehouse. This is important because new systems almost always have to be integrated into an existing network of computer systems and must be able to share data with other systems already in use in the organization. A reasonable allocation of the SE's project time includes 40% during planning, 100% during the analysis phase, 50% during the system selection phase, and 100% during the implementation phase. However, each project and each facility is different and each will have to determine the time allocation for each committee member on the basis of its own situation.

Department Managers' Representative

Managers of the departments most affected by the proposed system should be on the planning team themselves. However, because most department managers do not have the time to serve as regular members of the project team, a knowledgeable member of the nursing team may be named to represent their interests. Because most department managers do not have the time to serve as regular members of the project team, a representative on the team must be named to represent their interests. Commonly, this is a department manager with an interest in the project or whose department is a key user of the proposed system. The Department Manager Representative position on the team may not have to extend for the full life of the project. However, because their departments will be most affected by the new system, and because they will have to assign some of their departments' personnel to various tasks during the new system process, department managers must be sure that their interests are represented on the planning team. The representation may be accomplished through direct participation by department managers affected by the change, or by a representative of the group that will serve on the planning team and communicate regularly with the department managers about the project Department managers' time on the project is usually not budgeted separately because they absorb this activity into their regular workloads. However, the time of the Department Managers' Representative may be budgeted to the project.

Informatics Nurse Specialist

If the nursing department is significantly affected by the new system, there should be a nurse on the planning committee who will represent the interests of the nursing department in the planning process. A nursing department representative who has an overview of the entire nursing department must serve on the project committee throughout the life of the project. Typically, this person is an Informatics Nurse Specialist (INS). That is, the person is a registered nurse who has training and expertise in computers and IS. Ideally, the INS has a master's degree in health care informatics and is certified in informatics by the American Nurses Credentialing Center. However, there are a number of nurses working as informatics nurses in health care facilities who have on-the-job training and experience in nursing information systems. The INS may report through the IS department or through the nursing department. In either reporting situation, the INS is the primary liaison between nursing and the IS technical people and can translate nursing needs to the computer specialists and the computer specialists' needs to nurses. In addition, with a clinical background, the INS may also be responsible for communicating with the organization's physicians about the new system project. The amount of time the INS spends on the project will depend on how great an impact the system will have on the nursing department. For example, if the proposed system is an electronic medical record, the INS may be assigned full-time throughout the life of the project. During the planning phase, the INS will be deeply involved in the feasibility study. The INS will have to be involved during the evaluation of technical feasibility and may take the lead during the organizational and cultural feasibility portions of the study because those topics relate to the clinical departments. For smaller systems that affect only a single nursing unit, the INS may spend 20% to 50% time on the project.

Administrative Liaison

The position of Administrative Liaison may or may not be a position separate from that of the PD. The role, however, is somewhat different. Typically, the Administrative Liaison is a member of the finance department. Major computer systems are expensive, and the Administrative Liaison must lead activities related to financing the system. The Administrative Liaison advocates for the project within the organization's administrative structure and keeps the other administrators up-to-date on the progress of the project. Because the Administrative Liaison is often the chief financial officer (CFO) or an assistant to the CFO, this person is typically involved in the regular meetings of administrative personnel and will regularly report to senior management on the progress of the project. This person will absorb the project in his or her regular workload and will not be budgeted for separately in the project budget.

End-User Department Representatives

A key to the success of any new IS project is involvement in the project by the people who will be the primary users of the system once it is up and running. These people are called end-users. There should be a minimum of one end-user representative for each department or group that will constitute the users of the new system as part of their jobs. End-user representation throughout the new systems project is essential to the success of the project. Managers and project leaders must understand that end-users are experts in the work processes of the organization and have an essential view of how work proceeds on a daily basis in the patient care units.

There should be some end-user involvement in the planning phase. However, it may be that some of the end users are involved in the meetings of the project team primarily for informational purposes. Thus, they will probably be able to absorb the meetings into their regular workloads. Nurses cover for each other during lunch periods and can cover for another nurse during a 2-hour meeting every other week or once a month. Depending on nursing work schedules, it may also be possible to schedule late-afternoon meetings if the nurse members get off work at 3:30 pm. This obviously will not work if the organization's nurses work 12-hour shifts. In that case, some other arrangement will be needed so that patient care personnel can attend the meetings.

The main reason that these end-users must be involved is that the probability of a successful acquisition and implementation drops dramatically if the end users are not heavily involved in the process. Another benefit of involving staff nurses is that they can help keep the rest of the nursing staff up-to-date on the progress of the project so the nurses feel included in the process. More important, they can share ideas from the meetings with other staff and get input from the rest of the nurses about what is needed and what will work in that particular organization. Nursing buy-in will be critical to the success of any system that nurses have to use, and the nursing department end-user representatives will be key opinion leaders with regard to the new system.

The end-user members of the committee may not need much release time during the planning phase, but they will need considerably more time for the project during the systems analysis and system selection phases. At that point, they will have to be released from their patient care duties 1 or 2 days a week to participate in the systems analysis. Replacement nurses will have to be paid to take over patient care duties, and this is a cost the organization should have in its project budget. It is unwise to ask the department manager to add the extra nursing hours into the department budget because that may engender resistance on the part of the manager to paying for a replacement nurse. That in turn, may lead to loss of the end-user input into the project—and ultimate problems with the implementation of the new system.

The end-user representatives may be drafted as super-users for the new system. In this context, the phrase *super-user* means a user who is a trained expert in the use of the system, and usually a super-user has some administrative privileges in the system that regular users do not have. However, the super-users in this context do not have full administrative access to the system. If the end-user representatives are the designated super-users of their departments, they will also have to spend extra time during the systems selection process to learn more about how the systems will be used. Once the product has been chosen, they will need special training—often off-site—to learn to be expert users of the new system. They will then become trainers for those in their departments. During the go-live phase, the super-users may have to be assigned to training and support full-time until all the staff members become comfortable using the new system. That may take from a week to a month to accomplish. The project budget must reflect this kind of time commitment to the project on the part of end-user representatives.

Budgeting for Other Planning Committee Needs

In addition to personnel, the planning committee will need space. The committee will meet regularly, perhaps on a weekly basis for the first month or two and every other week or monthly thereafter. Most facilities have adequate meeting space, and rooms can be scheduled as needed. But for employees who work full-time on the project during the design, analysis, implementation, and evaluation phases, a separate space might be beneficial. The office space should have its own dedicated file cabinets and perhaps a dedicated computer or two. Furniture, phones, and computer connections will be necessary for that dedicated space. Office supplies such as paper, file folders, pencils, pens, notepads and the like will be needed as well. Clerical support should be explicitly budgeted. Usually the work is assigned to an administrative support person who takes on the project as an extra workload. If some of that person's duties have to be reassigned so that the project work receives adequate attention, plans for that work redistribution should take place early in the planning process.

It is likely that members of the planning committee will have to travel to other facilities that have in place systems that are similar to the prospective system. Different members of the team will have to travel during the planning stage, but at least the PD, SE, INS, and one to three members of the end-user representative group should be included in visits to other installations. A good rule of thumb is to plan for airfare, ground transportation, and meals and tips. At least two trips should be expected, and perhaps a total of five to eight members will travel. Approximately $500 per person or more will be necessary per trip (depending on how far the group has to travel and on prevailing airfare and hotel rates in the city to which the group travels). In the budget example in Table 15-2, the assumption is that eight people travel twice

TABLE 15-2 Electronic Medical Record Project Budget

PLANNING PHASE BUDGET

Personnel	Base Monthly Salary	Fringe Benefits	Monthly Total	Time on Project (%)	Planning Phase (Months)	Planning Phase (Costs)	Replacement Costs[1]	Total Costs
Project Director	$9,167	$2,567	$11,733	50	6	$35,200	$10,000	$45,200
Systems Expert	8,417	2,357	10,773	40	6	25,856	0	25,856
Chief Financial Officer	20,833	5,833	26,667	20	6	32,000	0	32,000
Informatics Nurse Specialist	5,833	1,633	7,467	50	6	22,400	0	22,400
Clerical Support	2,500	700	3,200	10	6	1,920	0	1,920
Department Managers								
Med-Surg Nursing	8,667	2,427	11,093	5	6	3,328	0	3,328
Peds and OB Nursing	8,167	2,287	10,453	5	6	3,136	0	3,136
Peri-Ooperative Nursing	8,833	2,473	11,307	5	6	3,392	0	3,392
ICU Nursing	9,000	2,520	11,520	5	6	3,456	0	3,456
Psychiatric Nursing	8,083	2,263	10,347	5	6	3,104	0	3,104
Emergency Nursing	8,250	2,310	10,560	5	6	3,168	0	3,168
Medical Staff Chief	25,000	7,000	32,000	5	6	9,600	0	9,600
Chief of Surgery	33,333	9,333	42,667	5	6	12,800	0	12,800
End-User Representatives								
Med-Surg Nursing	5,167	1,447	6,613	5	6	1,984	0	1,984
Peds and OB Nursing	5,000	1,400	6,400	5	6	1,920	0	1,920
Peri-Operative Nursing	5,417	1,517	6,933	5	6	2,080	0	2,080
ICU Nursing	5,458	1,528	6,987	5	6	2,096	0	2,096
Psychiatric Nursing	4,833	1,353	6,187	5	6	1,856	0	1,856
Emergency Nursing	5,250	1,470	6,720	5	6	2,016	0	2,016
Total Salary Costs								**$181,312**
Other Costs								
Travel								$18,400
Office furniture								1,035
Office supplies, postage, misc.								200
Two dedicated computers								4,630
Total Other Costs								**$24,265**
Planning Phase Costs								**$205,577**

[1] This category is for costs over and above the person's salary and benefits if the replacement person is paid a higher rate for temporary work.

and that they travel a relatively short distance to a city where hotels and meals are not in the high-cost bracket.

■ SYSTEM ANALYSIS PHASE

A detailed analysis of the system to be replaced will allow the planners to understand what kinds of processes must be accomplished by the new system. No new system will completely replicate (on a computer) the processes in place, nor should it. Ideally, the new system will improve the existing processes. However, until the nature of the work being done with the existing system is thoroughly understood, it will not be possible to evaluate prospective products for their suitability for the organization.

The system analysis phase is time-consuming for the Systems Expert, the INS, and the end-users involved in the project. Current work processes are examined through observations of the work and interviews with end-users. In this phase, the work that must be done is specified precisely. The "what" of the work the new system must perform is identified in this phase. The scope of the work is defined, the domains in which the work proceeds are specified, examples of scenarios that the system must support are prepared, and both usual and extreme workloads are detailed.

In order to participate effectively in this process, the end-users will require some training in the procedures of structured systems analysis. The INS will be important in this process because as a person who knows both computing systems and nursing care processes, the INS will be responsible for ensuring that the computer people understand the importance of the processes of nursing care. Additionally, the INS will have to translate computer-specialist language to the end-user representatives and to the nurses working in the units. Nurses may resent or feel threatened by the engineering personnel who perform the observations of their work. Therefore, the INS will have to prepare the nursing personnel for the observational studies and explain that the engineers are not there to judge them or report on their work to their superiors. Observations will be made on specific nurses, but their anonymity will be maintained because no nurse will be identified by name in the work-process study reports. It will be explained that the purpose of the observations is to understand what work has to be done relative to the new system so that the product brought in will actually support rather than interfere with their work.

The management engineers will conduct interviews with the staff, or the organization may choose to train the End-User Representatives to conduct the interviews. In either case, the purpose of the interviews is to discover parts of the process that may not be visible to the observers. Members of the staff will be asked what they want and need in a system, and they will also be asked about any experiences they or their friends have had with similar systems. It will be important to discover attitudes toward the new system and to incorporate end-user ideas into the system's specifications. The product of the system analysis will be a report on the functional requirements of the system.

This phase of the project is likely to be expensive. Several members of the project team will have to work full-time on the project, and management engineers with expertise in work-flow observation and documentation should be brought in for the observational studies. The number of observers will depend on the number of units and the speed with which the organization wants to have the study completed. One approach is to use the same observers for all units and to have the units observed sequentially. In that case, two to four observers should be sufficient. They will observe one unit and then prepare their report of the functional requirements for that unit. They will then go to another unit and observe it. They will then prepare a report of any differences in functional requirements between the two units. They will continue that process until all units have been observed and documented. Typically, the INS will explain work processes to the observers (who have no clinical background). The engineers may also observe physician operations and any other type of operations relevant to the proposed system.

In addition to conducting an analysis of the work system in place, the engineers bring their expertise to bear on helping the project committee visualize possibilities for improvements of which they may not have been aware. Once the systems analysis is complete, the PD and SE work with the other engineers to prepare a list of functional specifications for the new system. At this time, the committee finalizes its list of vendors who will be asked to submit proposals. Therefore, the work of identifying potential vendors must be completed during this phase. Another task of the committee is to learn more about the products available on the market so that their requests to the vendors for proposals are realistic in terms of what the existing products can do. It is possible that the team will discover that it is unlikely that any system available will perform all the desired functions. Should that be the case, the team will have to decide whether a partial solution is better than the existing system. If not, the committee will submit a report to management recommending that no change be made at the present time. Otherwise, the committee will prepare requests for proposals (RFPs) and send them to the vendors who have been chosen as potential project partners. The RFP lists all the functions the system must support and may also include a wish list, that is, a list of desirable functions that are not mandatory. Then the RFPs are sent to the prospective vendors.

The budget for the systems analysis phase will have to include 1 full-time week per End-User Representative (including a replacement per diem nurse at whatever cost the replacement person will incur).[2] In the subsequent example, each end-user continues to attend the now monthly project meetings (this adds up to 12 meeting hours during the 6 months). In addition, the end-users will receive 6 hours of training in systems analysis and interviewing. They will then spend 40 hours conducting interviews during a 1-week period and an additional 40 hours with the engineers during the week the engineers survey units in their departments. This adds up to a total of 96 hours during that 6-month period, which is a 10% time commitment for the 6 months.

The end product of the systems analysis phase is a set of functional specifications for the new system. The functional specifications consist of the following documents:

1. The list of goals that the new system must achieve.
2. A prioritized list of user requirements of the new system, and a wish list of non-essential but useful functions for the new system.
3. An environment specification that identifies the architecture in which the new system must function and any other specifics, such as number of buildings to be connected and so forth.
4. A request for proposal that defines these functional and environmental specifications to the vendors who will be asked to submit a proposal for their product.

[2] Note that the budget for per diem nurses includes only the extra cost incurred over and above what the department would normally pay the End-User Representatives. For the purposes of this example, $30 per hour is budgeted for each per diem nurse as the cost over and above the hourly cost of the regular staff nurse.

TABLE 15-3 Electronic Medical Record Project Budget

SYSTEM ANALYSIS PHASE

Personnel	Base Monthly Salary	Fringe Benefits	Monthly Total	Time on Project (%)	Analysis Phase (Months)	Analysis Phase (Costs)	Replacement Costs[1]	Total Costs
Project Director	$9,167	$2,567	$11,733	50	6	$35,200	$10,000	$45,200
Systems Expert	8,417	2,357	10,773	100	6	64,640	0	64,640
Chief Financial Officer	20,833	5,833	26,667	5	6	8,000	0	8,000
Informatics Nurse Specialist	5,833	1,633	7,467	100	6	44,800	0	44,800
Clerical Support	2,500	700	3,200	10	6	1,920	0	1,920
Department Managers								
Med-Surg Nursing	8,667	2,427	11,093	5	6	3,328	0	3,328
Peds and OB Nursing	8,167	2,287	10,453	5	6	3,136	0	3,136
Peri-Operative Nursing	8,833	2,473	11,307	5	6	3,392	0	3,392
ICU Nursing	9,000	2,520	11,520	5	6	3,456	0	3,456
Psychiatric Nursing	8,083	2,263	10,347	5	6	3,104	0	3,104
Emergency Nursing	8,250	2,310	10,560	5	6	3,168	0	3,168
Medical Staff Chief	25,000	7,000	32,000	5	6	9,600	0	9,600
Chief of Surgery	33,333	9,333	42,667	5	6	12,800	0	12,800
End-User Representatives								
Med-Surg Nursing	5,167	1,447	6,613	10	6	3,968	0	3,968
Peds and OB Nursing	5,000	1,400	6,400	10	6	3,840	0	3,840
Perioperative Nursing	5,417	1,517	6,933	10	6	4,160	0	4,160
ICU Nursing	5,458	1,528	6,987	10	6	4,192	0	4,192
Psychiatric Nursing	4,833	1,353	6,187	10	6	3,712	0	3,712
Emergency Nursing	5,250	1,470	6,720	10	6	4,032	0	4,032

Replacement (Per Diem) Nurses[2]

Med-Surg Nurse	2,400
Peds and OB Nurse	2,400
Peri-Operative Nurse	2,400
ICU Nurse	2,400
Psychiatric Nurse	2,400
Emergency Nurse	2,400

Observation study personnel

Four engineering graduate students (assuming they will work full time for 8 weeks conducting the observational study)	38,400
Total Salary Costs	**$283,248**

Other Costs

Office supplies, postage, misc.	$200
Total Other Costs	**$200**
System Analysis Phase Costs:	**$283,448**

[1]This category is for costs over and above the person's salary and benefits if the replacement person is paid a higher rate for temporary work.

[2]Replacement nurses are budgeted at 1 week per end-user department while the end user is conducting interviews.

An example of the systems analysis budget is presented in Table 15-3. Notice that the hospital will use per diem nurses to replace the end-users during the 2 weeks they will need to work full-time on the work process study. Other members of the project team are budgeted as presented in Table 15-3.

■ SYSTEM SELECTION PHASE (OR SYSTEM DESIGN PHASE)

The work to be accomplished in the system selection phase is a bit more complex than is implied by the title. Not only does a product have to be chosen, but also there is usually a need for customization of the product, and super-users must be trained so well on the new system that they can teach and support the other members of the staff who will use the system. Also, after the product is customized, it must be tested to be sure the modifications work. Documentation must be prepared for the IS department and for the end-user groups. Only after all those processes are complete is the system ready for implementation.

First, the project committee must receive the formal proposals from the vendors. During the design phase or early in the selection phase, an evaluation tool is developed. The tool will list all the requirements of the system, and possibly options that are desirable but not mandatory for the system to be usable in the facility. This evaluation typically has several parts. There will always be a set of end-user functions to be evaluated (Table 15-4). There will usually be a set of computer architecture (hardware and software) specifications to be evaluated, and there will probably be a cost-evaluation tool for the financial officer. The vendor's proposals are evaluated according to the specifications listed on the evaluation tools. Those proposals that meet minimum specifications are retained, and those that fail will cause a rejection letter to be sent to the vendors whose products did not make the cut.

Usually, two or three proposals are retained as possibilities and the rest rejected. Once the project team decides which vendors have products that could possibly meet the requirements, those vendors will be asked to come and demonstrate their products. The project team members who must attend the product demonstrations include the

TABLE 15-4 Example of a Small Portion of a Product Evaluation Tool

Requirements for Nurse Charting	Met Fully = 5 pts	Met Partially = 3 pts	Not Met = 0 pts	NA
1. Uses an ANA-approved vocabulary				
2. Uses a flow-chart format for entry of nursing data				
3. Permits employee access via name-badge bar code				
4. Allows clinical record access to be restricted to patients in units defined by name-badge department				
5. Automatically signs user off after 5 minutes of non-use				
6. Incorporates error traps for data that can be magnitude limited (e.g., maximum systolic BP = 300)				
7. Incorporates error traps for data that are either numerical or alphabetical (e.g., no letters or symbols can be entered where numerical data should be entered)				
8. Allows text comments to be recorded with coded data				
9. Provides a graphic representation of vital signs				

PD, SE, INS, CFO, medical staff team members, and End-User Representatives. In addition, it may be useful to schedule the demonstrations in a room large enough that other interested members of the organization can attend to get some idea of the products the project team is considering. Department managers and members of the IS department, in particular, may want to attend the product demonstrations.

This phase will be especially time-intensive for the PD and the SE. It may also be time-intensive for the INS, depending on the nurse specialist's role in product selection. It is not unreasonable to expect the PD and the SE to spend virtually 100% of their time on this project during the system selection phase. The organization will have to budget additional travel moneys for this phase. The purpose of travel during this phase is to inspect other installations of the products in which they are most interested. On the other hand, the time investment of the end-users will not be as great as during the analysis phase. There may not need to be monthly project team meetings during this phase because the members of the team will be able to talk about the products they have just seen after the demonstrations. However, there will be ad hoc meetings of each user group that has attended a presentation so they can evaluate the product (using the evaluation tool).

During this phase, users may discover that products have functions of which they were not aware but which they realize will greatly enhance the quality and usability of the product. They may decide to add those functions to the evaluation tool and to revisit earlier product evaluations to consider them in terms of the added function. This may require contacting other vendors to determine whether those vendors also offer the newly recognized function. The PD or SE will handle all vendor contacts for continuity and fairness in the product selection process. It is likely that end-user representatives will spend as much as 10% of their time on product evaluation activities. However, that time will not often occur in blocks of a full day unless they travel to visit product installation sites. Therefore, there may or may not have to be replacement staff during this phase. It should be noted that all visits to product installations should include at least some end-users who will be able to see things that nonusers are unlikely to understand.

Once a product is selected, the PD will work with the CFO to negotiate a contract with the vendor. It should be noted that the purchase price is not included in the project budget. Systems vary widely in cost, and the price negotiations will include not only the hardware and software necessary to run the system but also vendor support for the product. Part of that support will include training. The people scheduled to serve as super-users will probably be sent to the vendor's home office for training. This training must be timed with care. It must not be so long before the system is scheduled to "go live" that the trainees forget what they have learned, but there must be enough time for them to become skilled in the use of the new system prior to the actual installation of the system in the patient care units. The go-live time is the moment after the system has been installed when it is turned on and the staff start using the system to do their work. Given the training time needed, this phase is also expensive, even without considering the cost of purchasing the product. A sample budget for the systems selection phase is presented in Table 15-5.

■ SYSTEM IMPLEMENTATION AND TESTING PHASE

System implementation includes not only installing the hardware and software but also the work involved in customizing the system for the organization. Once a system has been customized, it must be tested to ensure that the custom programming

TABLE 15-5 Electronic Medical Record Project Budget

SYSTEM SELECTION PHASE

Personnel	Base Monthly Salary	Fringe Benefits	Monthly Total	Time on Project (%)	Selection Phase (Months)	Selection Phase (Costs)	Replacement Costs[1]	Total Costs
Project Director	$9,167	$2,567	$11,733	100	6	$70,400	$10,000	$80,400
Systems Expert	8,417	2,357	10,773	100	6	64,640	0	64,640
Chief Financial Officer	20,833	5,833	26,667	10	6	16,000	0	16,000
Informatics Nurse Specialist	5,833	1,633	7,467	50	6	22,400	0	22,400
Clerical Support	2,500	700	3,200	10	6	1,920	0	1,920
Department Managers								
Med-Surg Nursing	8,667	2,427	11,093	5	6	3,328	0	3,328
Peds and OB Nursing	8,167	2,287	10,453	5	6	3,136	0	3,136
Peri-Operative Nursing	8,833	2,473	11,307	5	6	3,392	0	3,392
ICU Nursing	9,000	2,520	11,520	5	6	3,456	0	3,456
Psychiatric Nursing	8,083	2,263	10,347	5	6	3,104	0	3,104
Emergency Nursing	8,250	2,310	10,560	5	6	3,168	0	3,168
Medical Staff Chief	25,000	7,000	32,000	5	6	9,600	0	9,600
Chief of Surgery	33,333	9,333	42,667	5	6	12,800	0	12,800
End-User Representatives								
Med-Surg Nursing	5,167	1,447	6,613	10	6	3,968	0	3,968
Peds and OB Nursing	5,000	1,400	6,400	10	6	3,840	0	3,840
Peri-Operative Nursing	5,417	1,517	6,933	10	6	4,160	0	4,160
ICU Nursing	5,458	1,528	6,987	10	6	4,192	0	4,192
Psychiatric Nursing	4,833	1,353	6,187	10	6	3,712	0	3,712
Emergency Nursing	5,250	1,470	6,720	10	6	4,032	0	4,032
Total Salary Costs								**$251,248**
Other Costs								
Travel								$18,400
Office supplies, postage, misc.								200
Total Other Costs								**$18,600**
System Selection Phase Costs								**$269,848**

[1] This category is for costs over and above the person's salary and benefits if the replacement person is paid a higher rate for temporary work.

works and does not interfere with the overall operation of the system. This phase includes training all the end-users in the use of the new system and supporting them during the go-live phase.

Two kinds of changes are made to most new large systems: system customization and user-interface customization. The system customization concerns programming that permits the system to be integrated with the rest of the organization's systems. Interface programs that link the new system to existing systems, such as the financial management system and other clinical systems, such as lab and pharmacy systems, may have to be written. Some work may be needed to fit the new system to some existing hardware and to link it with the organization's internal network (intranet). Adjustments may be needed for the security programs that protect the organization from malicious intrusions, computer viruses, spyware, accidental or deliberate data destruction, and other aspects of system security.

After these types of changes have been made, the new system will have to be tested extensively to make sure that the new programming does not interfere with the system's functioning and performance. The IS people must work with the vendor to make sure that the new programming doesn't cause a *system crash*.

The term "user interface customization" relates to customizing data input screens, report screens, and paper reports generated by the system. Most major systems work right away, but few organizations would be happy with a system that didn't permit them to do any customization of the user interfaces, especially data entry screens and reports. In fact, some products require the purchaser to design the screens and reports to be used in the new site. The informatics nurse typically leads the nursing committee charged with designing the nursing screens and reports and may work with physicians and members of the other clinical services to assist in the design of the screens and reports. The INS and perhaps the super-users will have administrative permission to change the screens so that they can perform the customization work as they make design decisions.

During this phase, the super-users will train all the staff that will use the system. This is an expensive undertaking for most organizations, and there is a strong temptation to cut training short, hoping users will learn as they go. Given the training time required, this approach is extremely unlikely to be successful. It is a serious mistake to cut training time short, but given that the staff will probably have to be paid overtime for the training time, it is an expense that seems to unduly upset many managers. The reality is that failure to train adequately can actually sabotage the success of the entire project. And compared to the total expense of the project, training costs are one of the smaller costs. But those costs are wise investments in the success of the new system. An example of an implementation phase budget is presented in Table 15-6.

■ SYSTEM EVALUATION PHASE

Once the system is running well and the users are adequately skilled in its use, the system can be said to have reached steady-state functioning. This means it is functioning the way it is expected to continue functioning for the foreseeable future. Once this state has been achieved, it is time to evaluate the system. The primary questions in the evaluation concern the extent to which the system is meeting the original goals of the project.

The most important aspect of the evaluation is measuring the extent to which the new system meets the needs of the end-users. Are they able to complete their

TABLE 15-6 System Implementation Phase Budget

SYSTEM IMPLEMENTATION PHASE BUDGET

Personnel	Base Monthly Salary	Fringe Benefits	Monthly Total	Time on Project (%)	Implementation Phase (Months)	Implementation Phase (Cost)	Replacement Costs[1]	Total Cost
Project Director	$9,167	$2,567	$11,733	100	4	$46,933	$10,000	$56,933
Systems Expert	8,417	2,357	10,773	100	4	43,093	0	43,093
Chief Financial Officer	20,833	5,833	26,667	5	4	5,333	0	5,333
Informatics Nurse Specialist	5,833	1,633	7,467	100	4	29,867	0	29,867
Clerical Support	2,500	700	3,200	10	4	1,280	0	1,280
Department Managers								
Med-Surg Nursing	8,667	2,427	11,093	5	4	2,219	0	2,219
Peds and OB Nursing	8,167	2,287	10,453	5	4	2,091	0	2,091
Peri-Operative Nursing	8,833	2,473	11,307	5	4	2,261	0	2,261
ICU Nursing	9,000	2,520	11,520	5	4	2,304	0	2,304
Psychiatric Nursing	8,083	2,263	10,347	5	4	2,069	0	2,069
Emergency Nursing	8,250	2,310	10,560	5	4	2,112	0	2,112
Medical Staff Chief	25,000	7,000	32,000	5	4	6,400	0	6,400
Chief of Surgery	33,333	9,333	42,667	5	4	8,533	0	8,533
Super-Users								
Med-Surg Nursing	5,167	1,447	6,613	10	4	2,645	0	2,645
Peds and OB Nursing	5,000	1,400	6,400	10	4	2,560	0	2,560
Peri-Operative Nursing	5,417	1,517	6,933	10	4	2,773	0	2,773
ICU Nursing	5,458	1,528	6,987	10	4	2,795	0	2,795
Psychiatric Nursing	4,833	1,353	6,187	10	4	2,475	0	2,475
Emergency Nursing	5,250	1,470	6,720	10	4	2,688	0	2,688

Replacement (Per Diem) Nurses[2]

Med-Surg Nurse	2,400
Peds and OB Nurse	2,400
Peri-Operative Nurse	2,400
ICU Nurse	2,400
Psychiatric Nurse	2,400
Emergency Nurse	2,400
End-user training costs (assuming there are 100 users, each of whom will need 8 hours of training on overtime; also assuming an average salary cost of $25.00 per hour plus benefit costs of 28%)	30,000
Total Salary Costs	**$224,832**

Other Costs

Travel costs	$15,000
Office supplies, postage, misc.	200
Total Other Costs	**$15,200**
System Implementation Phase Costs	**$240,032**

[1]This category is for costs over and above the person's salary and benefits if the replacement person is paid a higher rate for temporary work.

[2]Replacement nurses are budgeted at 2 weeks per super-user.

work with the new system as well as or better than they could with the old system? Are they able to enter and retrieve data as needed. Are there functions the system should have provided but that are being performed manually or through some other system? If the project concerned a clinical system, the evaluators will want to measure the extent to which high-quality patient care is supported by the system.

A key component of the evaluation will be the financial results of the project. The CFO will direct this component of the evaluation. Areas examined will concern whether the project stayed within budget and whether the new system reduces costs, increases costs, or maintains costs. Not every new system is expected to reduce costs. Many new systems in hospitals will have to produce clinical data electronically because of new federal regulations. The cost may be higher, but the new federal regulations could not be met with the old system. In other words, the new system was a necessary cost of doing business. In some cases, the new system may save the organization money. In that case, the evaluation will address how much money is saved and whether or not there is a break-even point for the new system.

Finally, there will be an evaluation of the process of the project. Questions to be addressed may include such elements as: Was training adequate and well suited to the learners? Was the planned time frame for the project appropriate for the scope of the project? How smoothly was the transition from the old system to the new system made at the time the new system went live? Were people helped to make the transition in an efficient way with as few hurt feelings and bruised interdepartmental relations as possible? How could the process have been better managed? What were the strengths of the process? These kinds of questions will not only help to complete the evaluation of the total project, they may also serve as learning opportunities for the organization. In that way, it is hoped that the next large project will benefit from what was learned from this project. A sample budget for the evaluation phase is presented in Table 15-7.

■ SYSTEM MAINTENANCE AND UPGRADES

Once the system has been successfully implemented and evaluated, the project team is disbanded. The system has become part of "the new way we do our work here."

TABLE 15-7 Sample Evaluation Phase Personnel Budget Electronic Medical Record Project Budget

SYSTEM EVALUATION PHASE PERSONNEL BUDGET

Personnel	Base Monthly Salary	Fringe Benefits	Monthly Total	Time on Project (%)	Evaluation Phase (Months)	Evaluation Phase (Cost)
Project Director	$9,167	$2,567	$11,733	20	2	$ 4,693
Systems Expert	8,417	2,357	10,773	50	2	10,773
Chief Financial Officer	20,833	5,833	26,667	5	2	2,667
Informatics Nurse	5,833	1,633	7,467	20	2	2,987
Clerical Support	2,500	700	3,200	10	2	640
Total Salary Costs						21,760
System Evaluation Phase Personnel Costs						$21,760

System maintenance costs include replacing printers, monitors, and printer paper and training new staff. These items are usually incorporated into each department's operating budget. But as anyone who has owned a personal computer for more than 5 years knows, software is upgraded on a regular basis. Who has not dealt with the need to learn a new operating system for a personal computer? Upgrades are a fact of life for business and clinical systems too.

If the organization does not regularly purchase and install the upgrades from the vendor, it may find itself, in a very few years, in the undesirable position of having a system the vendor no longer supports. Therefore, part of the contract for a new information system almost certainly addresses the costs of upgrades and vendor support for installing the upgrades and training the super-users in changes that affect the staff. Additionally, most contracts contain clauses (and costs) that provide for vendor support and training for periods of up to 5 years. Those contractual agreements often include a fixed price for any upgrades released during the first year or two after purchase, and they may include fixing the price for upgrades for as long as the contract lasts. Other costs that may be included in the contract are items such as membership in a national user group, regular retraining for super-users and system support people in the IS department, remote and on-site service contracts, and perhaps even some hardware-replacement costs. These kinds of maintenance costs are often allocated to the IS department budget, but the salaries and benefit costs of the super-users may remain within those users' departments after the end of the implementation phase. It is important for managers, administration, and the IS department to agree on how those costs will be allocated during the system planning phase so that there are no problems later in including system maintenance and support costs in the organization's budget.

Summary and Implications for Nurse Managers

The process of introducing a new system into an organization is called the system life cycle. It consists of the following five phases: planning, analysis, design/selection, implementation, and evaluation. The project budget is a compilation of the budgets of each of the five phases. It is critical that adequate budget consideration be given to each of the phases, because underfunding any part of the process reduces the probability that the new system will be successfully implemented.

The PD and the Administrative Liaison are responsible primarily for preparing the project's budget and for obtaining adequate funds for each phase of the project. Some sensitivity will be needed in negotiations with managers of departments affected by the new system. Some of their personnel will have to devote time to the project, and it will be important to gain the support of the managers so that those employees have adequate time to perform their project duties. Because the use of staff time has budget implications, it is wise to budget overtly for the staff time needed. In a large system acquisition and implementation project, it is unreasonable to expect people to add project work to their already heavy workloads. That will produce a situation in which the project becomes a low priority, and the work may not be done in such a way as to enhance the probabilities of success. Such an approach is penny wise and pound foolish. Large systems may cost $1 million or more to purchase from the vendor. Failure to budget for and acquire the necessary staff resources to plan for and implement the system adequately may lead to the loss of that investment.

Total failure of a new system, such that the entire product has to be scrapped, is not common. Nevertheless, it is an unpleasant possibility that has been reported in the business literature. So it is a possibility that should be kept in mind as plans and budgets are prepared for the project. The PD and Administration Liaison should explain to management the possible consequences of project underfunding.

Continued

Summary and Implications for Nurse Managers—cont'd

It is better to scrap the whole idea of a new system than to handle the acquisition in such a way that it leads to disastrous results for the organization—and underfunding any of the phases of the new system development process decreases the probability of successful implementation. Fortunately, there are a variety of books and journal publications that address strategies for successful implementation (most of the references at the end of this chapter address this topic). Additionally, most large hospitals and clinics have IS professionals on staff, and smaller facilities either have them or can hire them from consulting firms. The skills necessary for a successful information systems project are readily available, and the people with these skills understand the importance of adequate budgeting for each phase of the project. The wise organization recognizes that an investment in planning, analysis, and careful system selection sets the stage for successful implementation, and the first requisite for a successful system project is an adequate budget.

References and Suggested Readings

Brumleve, R. (2006). The benefits of a preimplementation phase in an electronic medical record implementation project. *Computers in Nursing.* 25(5), 253-255.

Dennis, A., Wixom, B., Roth, R. (2005). *System Analysis and Design*, ed 3. New York: John Wiley & Sons.

Faron, M., Hale, T., Jesberg, L. (2006). The pitfalls of introducing electronic medical records. *Annals of Internal Medicine.* 144(3), 220.

Grady, J. (2006). *System Requirements Analysis.* New York: Academic Press.

Hay, D. (2002). *Requirements Analysis: From Business Views to Architecture.* Upper Saddle River, NJ: Prentice Hall.

Kendall, K., Kendall, J. (2005). *Systems Analysis and Design*, ed 6. Upper Saddle River, NJ: Prentice Hall.

McHugh, M. (2004). Computer software and systems. In: Saba, V., McCormick, K., eds. *Essentials of Computers for Nurses*, ed 4. New York: McGraw Hill.

McLane, S. (2005). Designing an EMR planning process based on staff attitudes toward and opinions about computers in health care. *Computers in Nursing.* 23(2), 85-92.

Personal communication. (2006). Report of a patient who was unable to acquire her cardiology records from one hospital when transferring to another hospital because the first hospital's policy was not to transfer records without a subpoena—due to copying costs. January 23, 2006.

Wall Street Journal. (2006). Big employers plan electronic health records. *Wall Street Journal*, November 29, 2006.

Ward, J., Peppard, J. (2002). *Strategic Planning for Information Systems*, ed 3. New York: John Wiley & Sons.

Wasson, C. (2005). *System Analysis, Design, and Development: Concepts, Principles, and Practices.* New York: Wiley-Interscience.

Wikipedia. (Updated November 8, 2006). COBOL. Downloaded on November 12, 2006 from http://en.wikipedia.org/wiki/COBOL.

Yamamoto, L., Khan, A. (2006). Challenges of electronic medical record implementation in the emergency department. *Pediatric Emergency Care.* 22(3), 184-191.

Budgeting for the Operating Room

Marilyn Bowman-Hayes and Mary L. McHugh

LEARNING OBJECTIVES
The goals of this chapter are to:

- Identify the key stakeholders in the operating room (OR) budget planning process
- Determine the special budget needs of the OR
- Forecast future technological developments and their cost impacts on the OR budget
- Explore the factors involved in capital equipment decisions
- Explain the special factors related to budgeting for staffing needs in the OR
- Plan for marketing the OR's services

■ INTRODUCTION

This chapter takes a close look at budgeting in a specific department, the operating room (OR). There are many characteristics of the OR that make it particularly complex and interesting from a budgeting perspective, and therefore worthy of some individual attention. However, this chapter contains many elements that are germane to most departments. Readers who are interested primarily in areas other than the OR will also learn a great deal of useful information from reading this chapter.

There are two primary characteristics of the budgeting process in ORs that tend to be different from budgeting processes in other clinical areas. First, budgeting is constantly on the mind of the department director because even an approved budget is never really finished in the OR. Second, budgeting is much more collaborative in the perioperative area than in other units. In order to expedite the budgeting process at budget time, it is imperative that the OR management team actively plan for both the current and the next year's budget every day of the year. Even while working on the next year's budget, the manager is dealing with the interface between the current year's budget and the following year's budget. Specifically, the OR manager must identify those items on the current budget that can be delayed until the next year's budget period—and perhaps on moving items planned for the next year to a higher priority for this year's budget.

This happens in the OR budget because every year some equipment breaks or wears out unexpectedly early and must be replaced by using this year's money. In addition, in the OR more often than in other clinical units, new equipment comes onto the market and must be purchased immediately. The standard of care in surgery is changing rapidly as newer, less invasive surgical techniques and procedures are developed. But to offer the new surgical services, the surgeons usually require specialized equipment and perhaps differently trained staff—or even more staff. It may happen that new (i.e., unplanned-for) equipment ends up having a higher acquisition priority than some of the items on this year's budget. Therefore, some of the items scheduled for purchase this year get pushed back into the next year's budget. There is seldom sufficient money to purchase all the equipment that the OR would like to have, and priorities have to be determined. In the perioperative area, far more than in other clinical units, the staff, the director, and the surgeons must continually think about staffing, instrument, and equipment needs and how to prioritize those needs for both the current year and for the next fiscal year's budget.

The OR budget typically includes significant personnel and equipment costs, and it must be developed as a collaborative effort among a variety of stakeholders. The people who provide information necessary to the budgeting process include the OR Director, the surgeons who use the OR, the OR staff, staff from other hospital units, the hospital's administration—including members of the board of directors or trustees—the local business community, local politicians, sales representatives, and perhaps other stakeholders such as the fire department (if there is a burn unit in the hospital). The reasons for including the hospital-based people are obvious. But sometimes nurses forget that local businesses have an interest in the quality of care provided to their employees. Local businesses often have input into the kinds of services offered because they cannot attract or retain key employees if those key employees do not believe that they and their families can get adequate medical care services from the local hospital. Therefore, local business people can provide important input into the kinds of services their employees need and expect. Additionally, local business leaders often assist with fundraising for the hospital. Therefore, they expect to be consulted on important changes in services and in special equipment needs that they might be able to help with.

Local politicians (and sometimes state politicians) may take a strong interest in the local hospitals and the services they can offer. Politicians know that good health and hospital services are important to their constituencies. Politicians also can be a source of fundraising support, and they expect to be kept informed about changes that may affect voters in their districts. They also may want to have input into the kinds of health services (and necessary equipment) offered to the voters. A relationship with local leaders is especially important in a small rural community. The wise OR Director in a rural community where there is only one hospital will have at least some relationship with members of the local Chamber of Commerce and perhaps with a member of the City Council who has an interest in health care issues. There may be other leaders in the community who are interested in health care issues and who would be interested in working with the OR Director to improve surgical services.

Once the key players in the budget planning process are identified, it is important to consider the various categories of budget that typically fall within the OR budget. Like all departments, the OR budget will have an operating budget with the same components that other clinical units have: a personnel budget; a supplies budget that includes things like sutures, dressings, and OR supplies; and it may also include building costs, such as utilities and square footage charges for space. The OR will have a large capital equipment budget. However, the OR budget will also have to include items such as sterilization and instrument cleaning and a significant equipment maintenance budget, and it may also have to include the cost of implants, organ transplant costs, and perhaps special costs for surgeon recruiting.

▇ COLLABORATION IN THE BUDGET DEVELOPMENT PROCESS: KEY STAKEHOLDERS

Budget planning is a collaborative process in the OR. The director of the perioperative department cannot simply project the next year's budget from the previous year's budget. The OR budget must be responsive to rapidly changing surgical techniques, which impose changing equipment and instrument requirements. It must also be sensitive to the expectations of the OR staff and the surgeons. It must be responsive to the cost-control concerns of the hospital's administration and board of directors. The OR Director also has to be aware of the expectations, ideas, and opinions of members of the local community and its political and business leaders.

The Accounting Department

When planning the OR budget, the OR Director should schedule time with the member of the accounting staff who is responsible for assisting with the OR budget. This person is usually responsible for compiling the current budget and several years of past budgets for the OR Director. These documents should be reviewed with the accounting person to plan for the following year. This time should be scheduled prior to the formal planning sessions that are held with the facility's administration during the budget-preparation process. The accounting team member will be able to review the current budget and information that the manager brings to the table in regard to projections for the following year. After this meeting, the manager will have a better idea of the target numbers the hospital expects for the following year. The accounting person will be able to prepare preliminary budget projections that the OR Director can use to prepare a proposed budget for the next year.

Throughout the entire budgeting process, the OR Director will benefit from the advice and support of the accounting team's OR support person. Through this collaboration, the OR Director may be able to obtain advance projections of expected surgery group expansions, planned surgeon retirements, the hospital's plans for new surgeon recruitment, and other aspects of the administration's plans that may affect OR services. It may help to have a standing monthly meeting with the accounting person. It is not unusual for the OR support member of the accounting team to be able to advocate for the OR Director's requests once the need for new personnel, equipment, and supplies is made clear. This person will certainly know a great deal about budget justification and may be able to assist the OR Director to write persuasive justifications for the OR budgets. This should be viewed as a key relationship in the budget-planning process.

Operating Room Staff

The OR staff are often the first source of information about the budget needs of the department. The circulators, surgical technicians, and other people who staff the OR rooms are the first to know if equipment gets broken, if they are running into too many situations where two cases need the same equipment at the same time, or some staff are borrowing items from other rooms to set up their own cases because their packs contain insufficient numbers of some instruments. They will know if the flash sterilizer is being overused rather than having equipment properly cleaned and autoclaved in the instrument processing department. They know if the OR is frequently borrowing from other hospitals and if cases are being delayed or rescheduled due to insufficient equipment.

The OR staff knows if they are spending more time planning with teams from other rooms about when one case will be finished so that special equipment can be flash-sterilized and reused immediately in another case. They can tell the OR Director if the controls on a particular OR table are being repaired often (and that perhaps that table needs to be replaced) and if OR teams are opening extra instrument packs to retrieve just one or two instruments for a case.[1] All of these situations call for changes in the instrument pack setups and perhaps requests for additional equipment. Learning about this type of information from the OR staff assists the OR Director in preparing a budget that will allow cases to proceed on schedule and with the correct equipment and instruments needed for patient safety.

Clinical Specialists and Charge Nurses

A special category of staff that should be involved in the budgeting process is the clinical specialists and first-level managers in the OR (these staff may be called charge nurses, service specialists, or service coordinators). In ORs that have specialty teams, the team leaders fall into this category. The team leaders have particular knowledge of both current problems and future trends. They are especially helpful to the OR Director in setting priorities for the instruments and equipment to request in the budget. They are more likely to be aware of new procedures and techniques that are being discussed—and the nursing implications of those new procedures and techniques. So they can advise the director about possible personnel changes as well as about new instruments and equipment that the surgeons might need to provide the best patient care. These types of nursing specialty staff also know what instrument sets are being flashed, what drills need replacing, and the frustrations that are being expressed in the ORs or halls. They know which problems the staff and surgeons face when preparing for a case, during the procedure, and after the procedure is concluded. They learn first-hand about the frustrations surgeons, staff, and anesthetists experience with equipment and supplies, and they can communicate these types of problems to the OR Director. This information may not always be disseminated back to the manager because once emotions have settled; the staff and surgeons may forget to bring the problem to the attention to the OR Director.

---

[1] Instrument packs are sets of several (or many) instruments packaged together because that grouping of instruments is used for particular cases. When certain instruments are not available, sometimes the sterile-processing personnel have to make up a pack with insufficient instruments. Then another whole pack must be opened to retrieve a few needed instruments. That is a very costly solution to obtaining instruments, because once opened, the whole pack of instruments has to be resterilized. In other cases, changes in surgical techniques may mean that certain procedures are using more of some instruments than are contained in the pack and are perhaps not using as many of other instruments. In that case, the instruments that are almost never used are an excess cost while the OR runs up higher processing costs because extra packs are opened to obtain just a few instruments. The solution is obviously to reevaluate instrument needs by procedure and realign the items in the packs. But somebody has to inform management that the existing pack guides (that tell the people in the sterile processing department what items to put in each pack) need to be updated. The scrub techs and circulators are the staff members who know this information.

The Physicians: Surgeons and Anesthesiologists

The next group that can provide important information to the OR Director is the physicians—the surgeons who perform the surgical procedures and the anesthesia staff who keep patients comfortable or "asleep" during the procedures. The surgeon and anesthesia staff will talk about equipment and instruments needs and preferences during the procedures. These are critical members of the budgeting planning team. Surgeons and anesthetists notice when there are problems with the instruments they use during procedures. In addition, surgeons are especially likely to keep up with new surgical techniques. It is not unusual for a surgeon to go to a surgery conference, hear about improved equipment, and ask the OR Director to obtain that improved equipment. Surgeons may also travel to another hospital to acquire training in a new surgical technique or procedure and, in the process of that training, learn about new instruments and equipment. And it is common for the surgeon to need different instruments and equipment in order to be able to perform the new procedures or techniques. Anesthesiologists also attend conferences and learn about new techniques and equipment. Therefore, both the surgeons and the anesthesiologists are important sources of information about equipment and instrument that should be included in the budget.

The OR Director might have a special problem in gaining and evaluating information from the physicians in the OR. Surgeons may not always express their needs and wants to the OR Director but may instead take their requests directly to the hospital's administration or even to members of the board of directors. This creates a problem when selecting appropriate items to include in the budget and when prioritizing equipment and instruments in the budget. In the OR, as in many other settings, there is a danger that "the squeaky wheel will get the grease." This is an issue the OR Director and hospital administrators must deal with directly because some very poor purchase decisions can be made when the loudest or most aggressive person is the one whose wishes are granted. First, if equipment of lower priority is purchased, it may not be possible to purchase other more critical equipment because the budget has been depleted by the purchase of the lower priority items. Poor choices about purchasing instruments and equipment for the OR can lead to poor-quality care for some patients. Worse, they may lead to a situation in which the quieter physicians who prefer to follow a more logical and orderly process leave and take their patients elsewhere. It is not unusual for surgeons who make their needs known in a calm, professional manner to find that their requests go unfilled because other surgeons who threaten and raise their voices succeed in having their items purchased. Then there is nothing left in the budget for the quiet surgeon's items.

Developing the Budget Prioritization Process

It is simply poor financial management to base the OR budget on personalities rather than on sound analysis and planning. The OR Director must set the stage for a good budget process by establishing lines of communication for all of the stakeholders in that budget. Then the director must gain the buy-in of the administration and the board of directors of the OR budget process. The process should consist of the following steps:

1. Gather information about instrument and equipment needs. Ask OR staff, surgeons, anesthetists, and other key stakeholders to submit equipment and instrument requests and to include justifications for their requests.

Provide early feedback on their requests and, if necessary, on the adequacy of their justifications.

2. Prioritize the requests according to some system of prioritization that is agreed upon in advance by the surgery committee and the hospital's administration (and the board of directors, if relevant). An example of one possible system for prioritizing requests is as follows:

   a. The first priority is replacement of new equipment and instruments without which the surgeons cannot continue to operate or cannot perform new procedures or techniques that are important for quality patient care or for maintaining the required standards of care.

   b. The second priority applies to instruments and equipment that are needed to improve the quality of care, improve patient comfort or satisfaction, or improve the efficiency of the OR. These may include extra supplies of instruments and equipment so that there is less demand for the flash sterilizers or so that cases aren't being delayed or cancelled because someone else is using the required items. These items are not essential for staying in business but are important to keep the OR competitive.

   c. The third priority includes items that the surgeons could function without but that they want for a variety of possible reasons. For example, the item may make procedures go more quickly or be in some other way better but not absolutely essential for patient safety or to maintain standards of care. These are the "wants" that are requested and that may well provide some advantage to patients, surgeons, other members of the OR team, and the OR as a unit. But the third-priority items are not essential for staying in business or for maintaining care standards.

3. Publish the draft budget and provide the key players with opportunities for final input into the portions of the budget that are of concern and over which some discretion can be exerted (i.e., second- and third-priority items). At this point, somebody may provide information that moves a second or third item to a higher priority level. However, it is safer to make all prioritization decisions in the context of a surgery committee so that one individual cannot easily distort the process.

4. Finalize the budget and submit it for administrative approval.

Other Hospital Staff and Managers

Other people who can provide important information about the budget to the OR Director are the nurses and nurse managers of other clinical units in the hospital. These units care for patients prior to and after surgery, and they have a vision of the kinds of laboratory tests, imaging studies, and other noninvasive and invasive procedures that the physicians are ordering for patients who need surgical procedures. They may have information that, combined with information in the hands of the OR Director, may be used to reduce costs and improve the quality of patient care.

For example, there was a situation in which one hospital was transporting its pacemaker patients to an affiliated hospital for pacemaker insertion because the cardiologist was used to the cardiac catheterization laboratory there and had never inquired about whether the procedure could be done at the first hospital. The staff of the cardiac step-down unit from which the patients were being transferred discussed the situation with both the director of the catheterization lab and the surgical services director. After a discussion about the requirements of the patients, it was discovered that the first hospital was fully capable of handling the pacemaker insertion procedure. An analysis of the hospital's costs for ambulance transportation to and from the affiliated hospital was performed and shared with the physician. In negotiations with the physician, it was discovered that some additional supplies and a particular pacemaker type would be needed if he were to perform the procedure at the first hospital. The necessary equipment and supplies and staff training were taken care of so that the procedure could be performed at the first hospital. This saved not only the cost of transport, it also saved the family and patient the inconvenience of having to be transported to a different hospital for the pacemaker insertion procedure.

Hospital Administrators and the Board of Directors

The hospital's administrators and board of directors have the final authority to approve budgets in hospitals. It is their shoulders upon which lies the ultimate responsibility for the survival of the organization. Additionally, administrators are responsible for developing the organization's mission and goals and for strategic planning designed to fulfill the mission and goals. They can assist the OR to understand the hospital's objectives for its future and to recognize where the OR department and its services fit into those plans.

Equipment and instruments for the OR tend to be high-cost items. Therefore, it is the OR Director's duty to work with administrators and sometimes the members of the board to negotiate for items in the OR budget. Ideally, the relationship is one of mutual respect and willingness to learn from each other. The OR Director must be able to teach administrators and members of the board about clinical standards and the people and items necessary to maintain acceptable standards of care. Administrators and members of the board must be willing to learn about the realities of managing and equipping a surgical department. On the other hand, the administrators and board members tend to know the realities of running an entire hospital. They must be willing to explain the hospital's financial situation to the OR Director respectfully, and that director must be equally willing to learn from them. The OR Director ought to share appropriate information about the budget process with the OR teams so that reasons for decisions do not seem capricious or unfair, or worse, uncaring of patient care.

Some items within the OR budget are not subject to negotiation. If the director cannot provide essential instruments, equipment, and personnel, the surgeon cannot operate. But other items and personnel are subject to negotiation. For this reason, the OR Director must develop skill in evaluating resources in terms of whether they are essential to the OR's functioning or whether a particular item can be delayed until resources permit its acquisition. Part of evaluating resources is calculating their potential benefits in light of their costs. Surgery is a business, and the most important part of justifying a resource to an administrator is displaying a careful analysis of the likely benefits—especially financial benefits—of acquiring the resource and the financial costs of the resource. Other benefits may include improved quality of care, increased surgeon satisfaction, improved staff morale, improved patient and community satisfaction, and other such intangible benefits.

The intangible benefits are important and should be presented to the administrators. But they must accompany an analysis of the financial results of acquiring the resource too. This does not mean that every resource must produce a direct financial return on investment, but most intangible benefits can be translated ultimately into cost savings or higher return on investments. For example, if the key benefit of a new piece of equipment is improved staff morale, that piece of equipment will probably not produce a direct financial gain. If, however, the OR Director can estimate a reduction in turnover or absenteeism as a benefit of the acquisition of the equipment, a dollar figure can be estimated for the reduction in costs of turnover or absenteeism. That is the kind of information expected by administrators, and the wise OR Director learns to provide those kinds of data during budget negotiations.

The OR Director must be realistic in relationships with administrators. Administration will not always support the OR manager's ideas for volume growth. That lack of support does not necessarily mean that the OR Director's ideas are not good. There may be other factors influencing administrators' decisions, factors that have nothing to do with the OR or the OR Director's presentation. Regardless of the excellence of the OR Director's budget justifications, administration may ask that costs be lowered. Administrators have to balance requests from the OR with requests from the rest of the hospital. It is simply a fact that no hospital has all the money it wants.

Finally, administrators and members of the board can be important allies of the OR Director, for acquiring resources and for managing disappointed surgeons when they learn that their desired resource is not in the budget for the coming year. Administrators and board members may have influence with charitable foundations or community business leaders that can help get resources the hospital could not otherwise acquire. Sometimes surgeons ask for equipment more because they have been "sold" than because it is important for patient care or surgical technique. The OR Director is typically not in a position to negotiate with a surgeon who is threatening to take his patients elsewhere if he or she doesn't get some item of equipment requested. Furthermore, administrators may carry more credibility with a surgeon if they explain that the hospital simply does not have the money to acquire the resource requested. The chief executive officer or chief operating officer typically has the authority to negotiate with a surgeon about what can be done to resolve a situation in which the surgeon cannot have exactly what is wanted. Perhaps other arrangements can be made that will satisfy the surgeon, but typically, the OR Director is not in a position to do what essentially amounts to negotiating a contract with a surgeon.

Vendor Representatives

Representatives of the companies that manufacture implants and other specialized equipment used in the OR are an important part of the patient care team. The relationship between vendor representatives and the OR Director is challenging. The OR Director must always be aware that the vendors' primary goal is selling their wares and that this motivation can conflict with the director's two most basic goals of excellent patient care and cost control. Nonetheless, the vendor representatives generally are very knowledgeable about the best ways to use their products. They know whether improvements or upgrades of a product are in manufacturing (so waiting to purchase a replacement is the wisest choice). They are often called upon to train the OR staff and surgeons in the proper use and maintenance of their products. And of course, they know about new products of which the OR Director may not be aware.

Vendor representatives often know what is going on in other hospitals in the community. They might be aware of which hospital is going to start a new surgical program, such as a new open-heart surgery program. They may well know what technology is in use or is being purchased by competing hospitals. For example, perhaps the hospital across town has purchased new three-dimensional imaging technologies to make their craniotomy surgeries more successful. Vendor representatives might know which hospitals' surgeons have recently trained to perform new, minimally invasive total joint procedures. They may also know which surgeons are looking to jump ship from one hospital and take their business to another. The sales representatives also know about the research and development their companies (and perhaps other companies) are performing and where their product changes are headed—and what their competition is doing. All of this information can be very useful to the OR manager for budgeting as well as for other types of strategic planning. Therefore, maintaining a good relationship with vendor representatives can be a useful management strategy.

It is, of course, critically important that nurse managers assess for validity all information received from a vendor representative. If the information is valid, it will assist a nurse manager in planning, in budgeting, and in discussing possible strategic changes in the OR with the hospital's administrators and with the surgeons. To get the vendor representatives to share this kind of information, the OR Director must cultivate a good relationship with them. On the other hand, the OR Director must maintain a professional disinterest in their sales presentations because it is the OR Director's job to be a discriminating consumer. OR managers walk a tightrope in their relationships with vendors. They must remain impartial so that they can professionally evaluate all products presented to them for possible purchase. At the same time, managers must ensure that the vendor representatives feel comfortable sharing this kind of information with the OR Director—and that is most likely to happen when the representatives feel that they are welcome and valued elements of the OR team.

Community Leaders

Business leaders in the community and local politicians can be important boosters for the hospital in general and the surgery program in particular. For example, in one hospital with a particularly tight budget, the director of the burn unit was able to acquire equipment the hospital did not have the budget for by working directly with the local fire chief. The fire department organized a fundraiser for the burn unit and within a very short time raised the money needed to buy the equipment. This ended up providing much good publicity for both the fire department and the hospital. Business and local political leaders have stakes in their communities and want to find ways to improve conditions for the people who live there. Surgery seems a bit dramatic to most people, with its high-tech equipment, scrub attire, and the mystery of being able to cut deeply into a body and have the patient not only survive but live a much better life afterwards. The OR Director, in collaboration with the hospital's public relations department, is in a position to create important relationships with local leaders so as to improve the situation of the hospital and its OR department.

An OR Director may wish to consider joining local business groups as a way to meet and develop friendships with local business leaders. Most people are interested in health care in general and hospitals in particular. People want to believe that the care they will receive at the local hospital is up-to-date and that the surgery department is well equipped to provide the best possible care. And business leaders are typically willing to use their knowledge of the community and their organizational skills to help with fundraising when necessary equipment cannot be acquired through the regular budget process. Additionally, the OR Director can personally learn a lot about good business practices through those relationships.

Political leaders are another group of people who are in a position to support the local hospital. They are usually well connected with the business community and with other key constituencies such as local churches and social organizations. They know how to seek consensus in the community about what issues are important to support. If they believe that the local hospital needs and deserves community support or additional funding, they may be able to mobilize the necessary support. In addition, political leaders may have the authority to pass legislation that can assist the local hospital. They can seek community support to issue bonds and to increase taxes in order to ensure that the local hospital has the ability to provide the kind of care that the community wants and expects. Although the OR Director may not personally have a relationship with local politicians, members of the hospital's public relations team and administration cultivate these relationships. The OR Director will want to communicate with those in the hospital who have relationships with key politicians so that the director can make the OR's needs known and learn about any community initiatives and expectations that will affect the OR services and budget.

Maintaining a Wide Community Network

There are any number of people who can provide the OR Director with information that has importance for the budget. One never knows who might share information about a new surgical service. Hospital employees, volunteers, patients, and their visitors are members of the community the hospital serves, as are the local political and business leaders. Information from any one of these individuals might bring to the attention of the OR Director new technology or procedures that are of interest. In addition, some of these individuals will identify needs for their health care that are not yet available locally. Many potential customers have developed computer skills and search the Internet diligently for information about treatments for their own or another person's health care. They may become aware of options in regard to surgical procedures even before the surgeons and OR Director have heard about them. It is important that the OR Director, the hospital's surgeons, and the hospital's administrators keep abreast of the health-related interests and concerns of people in their communities in order to budget appropriately for OR services.

■ SPECIALIZED ASPECTS OF THE OPERATING ROOM BUDGET

Special Budget Planning Considerations

There are important differences between the budget planning in a non-OR department and the budget planning processes in an OR department. Trend evaluation in particular is a much more critical part of the OR budget planning process than it is in just about any other area in health care. When planning the OR budget for the next fiscal year, it is useful to have both the current year's and the prior year's budgets available. Those two budgets will assist the OR Director to identify trends in the various areas of the OR budget. It may be useful to have available the budgets for the 3 years prior to the previous year's budget, so that 5-year trends can be examined. More than any other department, the OR budget must be sensitive to changes in practice because those changes always have budgetary implications. In some clinical units it **may** work to simply take the current year's budget and add an inflation factor as a way to prepare for the next year's budget,[2] but this is a recipe for financial disaster in the OR budget. Recognizing cost and usage trends in the OR is an essential part of the OR budgeting process.

Planning Processes

The first step is to work with the person in the accounting department who supports the OR budget to examine changes between last year's budget and the current budget and to evaluate how those changes affected the current year's budget. It is especially important to note the ways in which the projected revenue and expense budgets differed from the actual budgets. Identify the items in the prior year's budget that were transferred onto the current year's budget, and identify items in the current year's budget that have been transferred onto the coming year's budget. Is there a pattern in the types of items that are being delayed? If so, it may be useful to seek the assistance of the person in the financial planning office with which the OR Director works on budget planning to determine whether a different budgeting strategy can be used to prepare a more accurate budget for the next year.

As part of the trend analysis process, the OR Director should identify possible changes in the OR environment or in other areas of the hospital that might produce changes in supply costs or staffing requirements. Such changes include plans to introduce new procedures, plans for providing entirely new types of services, and plans to recruit new surgeons (either to offer new services or to expand existing services). The OR Director will want to talk with the finance department to find out if there are any expected changes in contracts the facility has with third-party payers (medical insurance providers) that may have effects on the volume of surgical procedures. The financial planners may be in contract negotiations with insurers, and the results could greatly increase the number of people who can use the hospital for their surgical services. Perhaps the hospital is negotiating with the city about ambulance services that will change the number of trauma patients treated at the facility. Activity in the emergency department (ED) can have enormous implications for the OR budget.

Consider the implications for the OR budget if the hospital is planning to change the ED from a level III trauma center to a level II or even a level I trauma center.[3] A surgeon with research credentials may have to be recruited. All of those

---

[2] Based on earlier chapters, the reader will know that the authors of this book do not support that as a way of budgeting. As was made clear previously, budgeting is an important planning tool, and the authors believe that simply adding an inflationary factor is too simplistic an approach to yield a reasonable budget in most cases.

[3] Trauma center levels range from highest to lowest. Level I offers the highest level of trauma service and has a research program; level II offers the highest level of trauma service but has no research program; level III "does not have the full availability of specialists, but does have resources for the emergency resuscitation, surgery and intensive care of most trauma patients. A level III center has transfer agreements with level I and/or level II trauma centers that provide back-up resources for the care of exceptionally severe injuries" (Wikipedia, 2007). A level IV trauma center provides only emergency stabilization and treatment of trauma patients in preparation for transfer to a higher level trauma center.

kinds of changes will affect the number and types of surgeries as well as the time of day surgeries take place. And that, in turn, will have implications not only for supplies and equipment, but also for staffing.[4] Trauma often occurs in the late evening hours and on weekends. A facility that increases its ED service level to handle a higher level of trauma will need a different level of OR staff availability. The director may have to budget for permanent evening and night shift staff in the OR and to consider the needs of surgeons who have to be in the hospital all night. Conversely, if the hospital decides to reduce its trauma services, there will probably be less demand for emergency surgery, and the OR Director may be able to reduce evening and night staff or on-call requirements.

Standards of Care in the OR

Standards of care in the OR have a significant impact on the budget because they are likely to require, at the least, additional staff training and may require additional staffing, different instruments or equipment, and changes in practices in the perioperative area. These changes typically increase the costs of some budget items. Perioperative care standards change fairly often as new procedures and technology are introduced. They also change as the priorities of regulatory bodies and professional organizations change. An OR Director must keep up with the literature from the various bodies that set standards for the perioperative area. A substantial number of patients who are served by the ORs in America use Medicare and or Medicaid as their payment source. The primary organizations that set standards, policies, and guidelines for the perioperative area are the Centers for Medicare and Medicaid Services, The Joint Commission (TJC),[5] and the Association of periOperative Registered Nurses (AORN).

The Centers for Medicare and Medicaid Services (CMS) administer the standards for Medicare and Medicaid patients. Although the Office of Civil Rights administers the Health Insurance Portability and Accountability Act (HIPAA), the CMS does have a role in ensuring that the health information privacy articles of that act are carried out for Medicare and Medicaid patients. The OR Director must be aware of and comply with the CMS standards and guidelines as they apply to surgical patients. The CMS Website at http://www.cms.hhs.gov/ offers a great deal of information relevant to payment standards, clinical standards, and standards for various types of facilities.

The Joint Commission regularly updates standards in a variety of ways that affect the perioperative areas, including the preoperative care area, the OR, and the postoperative recovery area. A search of the Joint Commission's Website in January of 2007 revealed that at least 10 standards that directly affect the perioperative area were under review or recently updated; a few of them were standards for the timing of histories and physical examinations in hospitals, revisions of the 2008 national safety

---

[4] A high proportion of traumas occur in the late evening and at night. Therefore, changes in the ED's trauma level rating will have implications for evening and night scheduling of OR personnel. EDs with trauma level ratings of III or IV may be able to provide only on-call availability because the ED will try to stabilize seriously injured patients and transfer them to a higher level trauma center. But a level I or level II trauma center is required to provide 24-hour availability of all essential services, supplies, and equipment. That means that the OR must be able to handle major trauma surgery 24/7, and that means the OR Director must staff the OR to meet that requirement.

[5] Formerly known as the Joint Commission on Accreditation of Healthcare Organizations.

goals, standards for the management of conflict, standards for handling disruptive behavior, standards for organ transplant centers, and the emergency management standards (Joint Commission, 2007). In addition to the Joint Commission, AORN works with OR nurses throughout the world to set nursing standards for the OR. These standards are published in *Standards, Recommended Practices, and Guidelines* (AORN, 2006). In the 2006 edition, it can be seen that 26 of the 80 standards—approximately one third—of the recommended practices and guidelines have been updated since 2005. Many of the changes mentioned have implications for the OR budget.

It should be noted that the American College of Surgeons and the official organizations of the various surgery specialties also set a variety of types of standards. For example, the American College of Surgeons provides a booklet on its standards for cancer treatment. The American Academy of Orthopaedic Surgeons provides standards for implantable devices, orthopedic devices, and medical devices. Changes in these standards may bring the Chief of Orthopedic Surgery into the OR Director's office with the need for new devices or supplies that may cost more than those the hospital currently supplies. The OR Director must obtain information that will allow differentiation between equipment and supplies that a surgeon **wants** versus equipment and supplies that the surgeon **needs** in order to meet professional standards. The OR Director, who may not have independent access to the standards of each surgical specialty, will have to collaborate with the surgeons to determine the standards they have to meet.

Special Items in the Operational Budget

The OR budget has all the same categories that other clinical units' budgets have, and those are discussed in prior chapters. As a brief review, those items include the personnel budget, the supplies budget, and perhaps a budget for building and utility costs. But in addition, an OR must have at least the following categories:

- Instruments (new and replacements for worn-out or broken surgery instruments)
- Sterile processing (but only if that service area is within the OR Director's budget)
- Procedure set-up processing
- Implants (items such as tissue implants, joint replacement implants, etc.)
- Maintenance and repair contracts for OR instruments and equipment
- System support and upgrade contracts for specialized OR computer equipment and software

Not only does the OR Director budget for these additional categories, it should be recognized that the supplies budget itself is a substantially higher cost item in the OR than in other units. Supplies in the OR budget will have to include all drapes, dressings, tapes, suture materials, many of the smaller instruments (unless purchased in large lots or sets such that they become capital items), scrub clothing, and many other items not used in other units at all or used only in relatively small quantities.

Instruments

The word **instruments** in surgery generally refers to steel implements such as retractors, forceps, scalpels, and other nonelectric items that are used by the scrub tech and surgeon and that can be cleaned, sterilized, and reused over and over. This word is distinguished from **equipment,** which in surgery tends to be used to mean larger items that may be electrical in nature and, although cleaned and reused, are too large or too delicate to go through the autoclave for sterile processing. The word **supplies** generally refers to smaller items that are disposable and generally not reused. Although the cost of each individual instrument may be fairly low, given the number of instruments needed for a busy surgery department, the investment in instruments overall is quite large.

Not only do instruments have to be purchased, they also have to be sterilized after each use, and some instruments need regular maintenance, such as sharpening or adjusting. Sterilization and maintenance are very expensive components of providing surgical care. Many instruments are quite durable and may last several years, but because the cost of an individual item is low, instruments in general are listed on the operational budget under supplies rather than on the capital budget. However, sometimes instruments are purchased as large sets, in which case the cost may put the purchase into the capital budget.

Instruments may not be listed in the OR budget at all. In some hospitals, surgical services and sterile processing are two separate departments, each with its own budget. If instruments are placed in the budget of a separate sterile-processing department, the OR Director has to collaborate with the manager of sterile processing to ensure an adequate instrument budget. In many facilities, however, the instrument costs are included in the OR budget. In either case, the costs of instruments are conceptually divided into three different types of purchases. (Note that these three categories are not budget categories but categories of instrument acquisition.) These categories are a) purchase of new instruments for new surgical services or procedures or because new instruments are required by changes in practice standards; b) purchase of replacement instruments for those that break or wear out, and maintenance of instruments that need regular attention such as sharpening or adjusting; and c) repair of instruments that have broken but can be repaired.

To develop the instrument budget, the OR Director (or manager of sterile processing) should have already investigated the possibility that entirely new surgery programs or services will be instituted or that some existing services will be expanded. Ideally, the manager will have already worked with the surgeon and the materials manager to obtain cost information for the new instruments that will be required for any additional services or program expansions. If necessary, bids should have been obtained from the instrument suppliers for those items. The timing of the expected expansions or new services should be considered. It is a waste of money and space to purchase instruments in January if the new surgeon who will need those instruments will not arrive at the hospital until June. On the other hand, it will be a serious black mark against the manager if those instruments are not on hand when needed. Therefore, quotes and bids from suppliers should include not only the cost of the items but also the expected time span between submission of the order and delivery of the instruments to the OR.

To complete the instrument budget, the manager should look especially closely at the prior year's history of replacement and repair costs by month. Preparing graphs of the number of service calls or of the amount of time instruments and equipment items are out of service due to breakage or performance problems can provide excellent support for the OR Director's justifications for budgeting new instruments and equipment and for changes in service contracts related to keeping those items in service. The following questions should be answered in preparation for developing the next year's budget: Are replacement and repair costs fairly even across the last 12 months? If not, are there certain months when costs were unexpectedly high or low? Or did costs rise steadily or fall steadily during the past 12 months?

If replacement and repair costs are fairly even across the year, the manager can simply add an inflation factor to the total and then divide the new cost figure by 12, thus budgeting for an equivalent level of repair services for each of the next 12 months. However, if the costs were not evenly distributed throughout the year, then some investigation may be necessary. If one or more months had especially high or low instrument costs, it is important to know why. Was that the result of a special situation that is unlikely to be repeated? In that case, those low (or high) costs may not have to be replicated in the next year's budget. However, if those variations represent real differences in monthly activity, the projected budget should reflect that reality.

If costs rose steadily, it is important to find out whether that increased expense was balanced by an increase in the number of surgeries performed, so that the cost is related to increasing profits. On the other hand, if instrument costs are rising while department activity is remaining stable, there may be a problem. The OR Director and sterile-processing manager will have to try to find out whether instruments are being diverted by someone, or if there is excessive breakage. These two problems require managerial intervention with the staff. Another possibility for increasing instrument costs may be that the instrument pack contents do not match current instrument usage. When that happens, staff members may have to open an entire pack to obtain just one or two instruments. In that case, the pack contents may have to be updated so that a surgery pack contains all the instruments that will typically be needed for each surgeon and each type of surgery. It is extremely expensive to open a whole pack for just one or two instruments and if this is a problem, the OR manager may need to ask the clinical educator to present a program on pack costs at the next OR team meeting. If the nurses identify a problem with pack contents, an ad hoc committee will probably be set up to review existing pack lists and update them as needed.

Finally, the budget reports for the prior year should be examined to identify how much time elapsed between purchase of new (or replacement) instruments and the first time those instruments needed repairs. Ideally, either the OR Director or the sterile-processing manager will have kept records on the various types of instruments and how often those instruments needed replacement or repair. Those data should be used to project the instrument costs for the next year. They should also be compared with the OR instrument repair and replacement costs of similar hospitals. Only by comparing one's own department's usage with that of a benchmark[6] facility or with averages of other hospitals will the OR Director be able to assess whether the current usage is typical or unusually high or low. If replacement and repair costs are excessive, it will be important to conduct some studies to determine the cause of the excess usage and to address that cause through staff education or whatever means are necessary.

Facilities have various methods of developing line-item categories. Generally, it is better to have greater detail in the budget because cost overruns are more easily identified and investigated. Note the different types of information to be gained from Tables 16-1 and 16-2. In both tables, there is a $16,500 unfavorable variance, and it

---

[6] Please refer to Chapter 17 for additional discussion of benchmarking and how it is used in health care budgeting.

TABLE 16-1 Grouped Instrument Budget

Account Number	Account Description	January, 2008		
	Item Type	Actual ($)	Budjet ($)	Variance ($)
1000	Instruments	101,000	103,000	2,000
9000	Instrument repairs	46,500	28,000	(18,500)
9090	Instrument maintenance contract with Dupuy Co.	10,000	10,000	0
TOTAL		156,500	141,000	(16,500)

is clear most of the variance is due to an unexpectedly high instrument repair cost. However, there was a $2,000 favorable variance in instrument purchase costs. That is a relatively small amount of variance, and thus it might seem that everything except instrument repairs is right on target. In Table 16-2 it can be seen that the repair line item was not the only line with an unfavorable variance. There was actually a sizable unfavorable variance in spinal instruments, which was offset by the favorable variance in orthopedic instruments. With this additional information, the manager can identify the reasons for all the favorable and unfavorable variances and use that information to plan the next year's budget while working to reduce the causes of the cost overruns.

If the budget currently groups all instruments and repair costs into single categories, the OR Director may wish to ask the accountant who works on the OR

TABLE 16-2 Detailed Instrument Budget

Account Number	Account Description	January, 2008		
	Item Type	Actual ($)	Budget ($)	Variance ($)
1000	Instruments			
1001	ENT instruments	5,000	7,000	2,000
1003	Endoscopy instruments	15,000	15,000	0
1021	Spinal instruments	20,000	16,000	(4,000)
1032	Ortho instruments	15,000	20,000	5,000
1035	Neuro instruments	6,000	5,000	(1,000)
1090	General surgery instruments	40,000	40,000	0
1000–Subtotals	Instruments	101,000	103,000	2,000
9000	Instrument Repairs & Maintenance			
9001	ENT instrument repairs	3,000	3,000	0
9003	Endoscopy instrument repairs	18,500	2,000	(16,500)
9021	Spinal instrument repairs	4,000	3,000	(1,000)
9032	Ortho instrument repairs	6,000	6,000	0
9035	Neuro instrument repairs	4,000	4,000	0
9040	General surgery instrument repair	11,000	10,000	(1,000)
9090	Instrument maintenance contract with Dupuy County	10,000	10,000	0
9000–Subtotals	Instrument repairs/maintenance	56,500	38,000	(18,500)
TOTAL		157,500	141,000	(16,500)

budget if it is possible, in future years, to report instrument costs according to the subcategories that define the surgical service areas. This reporting change will allow the OR Director to immediately target instrument expenses each month and to investigate unexpected high costs in one area.

For example, consider the unfavorable repair costs. In Table 16-2, it can be seen that most of the overruns in repair costs were caused by repair of endoscopy instruments. Suppose the OR Director discovers that in one month, the flexible bronchoscope had to be repaired three times at a cost of $5,500 per repair. Further, it is discovered that those repairs were occasioned by somebody's mishandling of the equipment. The OR Director points out to the staff that the cost of those repairs could have purchased an automobile or an extra quarter full-time equivalent of nursing time. The nursing staff, in turn, explains that one surgeon has been particularly rough in his usage of the endoscopes. This leads to the OR Director to bring in the endoscope sales representative for a training session that includes all staff and endoscopy surgeons. The surgeon who has been rough with the equipment learns about the delicacy of the instruments and the proper way to handle them. Following the training session, that surgeon handles the equipment properly and after that, repair costs stay in line with expectations. Without the detailed information provided by separate lines in the budget for both instruments and repair costs, it is doubtful that the OR Director could have pinpointed the problem and provided the necessary training, and the problem probably would have continued for much longer.

Implants

Implants include a variety of prosthetics, tissues, and devices. Overall, the implants portion of the budget is likely to encompass high dollar figures. Different organizations handle the budgeting of implants differently. As with instruments, some organizations place all implants together in a single budget code. Others separate them into surgery product lines, each with its own unique budget code and category name. For instance the budget may look like Tables 16-3 and 16-4.

As with all other parts of the OR budget, the director has available prior years' budgets so that trends can be evaluated. This process is made more productive if the budget is prepared and reported by service line rather than having a single figure for each item category in the entire perioperative department. In fact, a service such as orthopedics, which uses a wide variety of implants, from tissue implants to joint prostheses, may require several different line listings for each type of implant, as is shown in Table 16-4.

When budgeting for implants, certain questions must be asked:

- Which implants are on contract?
- Of the implants that are on contract, what is the compliance rate?[7]
- If contracted implants are not being used regularly by all surgeons, why not?

---

[7] This asks the question, "Of all implants used, what percentage was purchased through the contract and what percentage was purchased off contract because of special requests by the surgeons?"

TABLE 16-3 Grouped Implants Budget

Account Number	Account Description	January, 2008		
Implants	Item Type	Actual ($)	Budget ($)	Variance ($)
4000	Implants	5,985,000	5,947,000	(38,000)

TABLE 16-4 Detailed Implants Budget

Account Number	Account Description	January, 2008		
	Item Type	Actual ($)	Budget ($)	Variance ($)
4000	Implants			
4001	ENT implants	20,000	25,000	5,000
4021	Spinal implants	225,000	227,000	2,000
4032	Orthopedic implants—general	65,000	70,000	5,000
4032.2	Total hip implants	2,150,000	2,140,000	(10,000)
4032.3	Total knee implants	3,300,000	3,250,000	(50,000)
4032.4	Shoulder joint implants	50,000	52,000	2,000
4032.5	Finger joint implants	71,000	76,000	5,000
4032.6	Achilles tendons	19,000	22,000	3,000
4035	Neurosurgery implants	45,000	50,000	5,000
4040	General surgery implants	40,000	35,000	(5,000)
TOTAL		5,985,000	5,947,000	(38,000)

- Is there a materials management committee that has surgeon input in regard to implant selection? The end users of implants need to be involved in this committee if a problem with implant contract noncompliance is to be avoided.
- If the OR Director is working within the constraints of a multihospital corporation, what is the methodology for contract implant selection (i.e., corporate- or hospital-based)? The OR Director in a multihospital system should know the corporate person in charge of implant contracts so that surgeons' opinions and concerns can be transmitted to the person or committee that makes the decisions about implant contracts. In this situation, it is important to work with the surgeons to acquire reliable data and facts about the effects of non-contract implants on the quality of patient care and patient care outcomes.
- Does the OR own its implants or are the implants on consignment?[8] It is important to keep in mind that the design of implants changes frequently. If the facility owns its implants, it may end up with outdated inventory that must be wasted.
- What inventory management system has been established for maintaining par levels of implants and extra parts such as plates and screws? Is it effective in providing the implants and equipment when needed? Does it produce a situation in which implants are kept on the shelves until they are outdated? Keeping adequate inventory without keeping so much that some is wasted is a difficult problem, and it is best handled through communication between the OR Director and the Director of Materials Management.
- In regard to refrigerated items like tissue and grafts, what are the par levels and rates of outdates? Are there a certain number of items that are consistently wasted because of the expiration dates of the tissue and grafts? Can

[8] When the OR acquires an implant on consignment, it means that the hospital doesn't actually purchase the implant. The vendor allows the hospital to keep inventory of the implant in the hospital, and the vendor is paid only when the implant is used.

a method be found to reduce or eliminate the wastage without forcing delay of surgeries due to insufficient inventory?

- Is there a nearby hospital with which a partnership could be arranged such that more efficient par levels can be achieved by sharing implants (other than tissue or refrigerated items)?

- How many different types of essentially the same item (for example, hernia meshes) are on the shelves? Is there a way to work with the surgeons to decrease the variety of brands in the selection so as to reduce wastage of excess inventory?

- Are there plans for new procedures that will affect the implant budget?

- Are all of the implants FDA-approved? If not, how did the unapproved implants end up in inventory, and what steps need to be taken to avoid acquisition of nonapproved implants in the future?

- Are all the implants in inventory approved for reimbursement?

- Are all the implants approved by the CMS? If some are not, is there a method of ensuring that only approved implants are used on Medicare and Medicaid patients, or that the requisite paperwork is filed with the CMS on the patient's behalf if a nonapproved implant is more appropriate for quality patient care?

Accounting is usually very helpful in performing analyses of the relationship between the cost of each implant and its reimbursement rate. If the OR has a computerized charging and inventory control system, reporting on the cost and reimbursement rates, usage rates, and other issues with each type of implant can be done on a monthly basis. This reporting frequency can help to alert the manager of changes and can perhaps provide trended data and graphics for the OR Director to use in controlling the implant budget. Cost analysis should be performed regularly in cases that involve implants, and this analysis should include both the cost of the implant and other patient care costs as well. In fact, the implants service line should be closely monitored on a month-to-month basis, and the analysis should include all costs, from admission to discharge. The analysis should include data on the number and percentage of implant patients who are acutely ill inpatients and those who are essentially healthy outpatients. This type of information is important for the accounting department to have available for insurance contract negotiations and to appeal to the CMS when higher costs are incurred for specialized implants and for care of acutely ill patients.

Because implants are so costly, and reimbursement can be very complex, it is imperative that the OR Director stay current with new techniques and procedures. All have budget implications. For example, as of the year 2007, spinal implants are becoming more widely used in patients with back problems, and more orthopedic surgeons and neurosurgeons are obtaining training in how to provide spinal implant services. The cost of those implants will become a more important line item in many OR budgets. It is important for OR Directors to identify these kinds of innovations, understand which are likely to be in high demand, and be prepared to analyze the potential cost of the implants, the reimbursement rates, and any alternatives in the situation so that the new implants do not produce financial losses and become a drain on the OR's budget.

Maintenance and Repair Contracts

Today's OR is an extremely high-technology environment. It is in the nature of high-tech devices that many need regular service for optimal performance, and the rather delicate nature of high-tech equipment means that repairs are needed on a regular basis. Adding to the need for high-tech service support is the growing number of computers in the perioperative department. Most ORs are increasing their use of computers to support activities such as inventory control, surgery scheduling, staff scheduling, quality and outcomes monitoring, Internet access, communication, vendor identification and certification for OR access, cost analysis, financial and other support for OR management, instrument and equipment tracking, and a whole host of other applications. Computer systems have to be supported; the hardware sometimes needs maintenance and repair, and software support is essential. Some of these service requirements may be handled by the hospital's biomedical engineering department, but the number and complexity of the instruments and machinery in the OR is such that no hospital can support all the needs of the OR. As a result, every OR must have some after-sale service contracts with the vendors, and in addition to the support provided by the hospital's service personnel, there are usually additional contracts with external biomedical companies that can maintain and repair the OR's specialized and very expensive devices.

A major consideration of any service contract is hours of service. Many hospitals' ORs provide services 24 hours a day, 7 days a week (this is called 24/7 coverage). If service for equipment is available only Monday through Friday from 8:00 am to 5:00 pm, the OR Director must be sure that the inability to obtain service for several hours or days will not create a major disruption in surgical services. This can be a very serious consideration if the equipment is absolutely required for emergency surgery—which frequently occurs during the night and weekend hours.

Equipment Maintenance and Repair Contracts

There are a large number of surgical instruments, high tech equipment, fluoroscopy machines, endoscopes, microscopes, and other expensive items in the OR. All these items must be maintained and sometimes repaired. Not only will the sales representatives of the vendors work with the hospital to sell the devices, they will also offer service contracts and work with the OR Director to obtain timely maintenance and repair services. Some equipment may be supported by an in-hospital biomedical engineering department. But there will still have to be contracts with external service companies for some of the maintenance and repairs. Just keeping track of the number of contracts and which service company supports what equipment can be a challenge. Therefore, the OR Director must account for those contracts during budget planning.

The cost of service contracts is not trivial, but without that support, many of the machines used in OR would soon be nonfunctional. Prior to the time the budget is due, the OR Director must confirm the status of maintenance agreements and contracts in regard to OR equipment and computer software. During budget planning, the biomedical engineering department also evaluates whether it is more economical for the facility to continue to perform some types of maintenance and repair services. This decision depends partly on whether that department's personnel have the necessary skills and certifications required to maintain the OR's high-tech equipment. If not, it may be decided that it is necessary or more economical to outsource maintenance and repairs on selected equipment. In fact, because of the increasing complexity of the OR's equipment, that decision may be made for them. It may not be possible to recruit technicians or to obtain all the training necessary to keep them fully certified to work on OR equipment. If the biomedical engineering department decides to outsource maintenance, it must to be determined whether the cost of those contracts will be budgeted in the surgery department's budget or in the biomedical engineering department's budget.

Regardless of where those contracts are budgeted, the OR Director should have an established working relationship with whatever department negotiates the contracts for the maintenance and repair of OR equipment. Budget preparation time is a good occasion to ask whether any major contracts are up for renewal and whether changes in those contracts will affect the OR's services. Unfortunately, it is not unusual for contracts held in other departments to be changed in a way that causes problems in the OR. Managers of other departments may not understand the special requirements of the OR and may not realize that an apparently trivial change to a contract will cause problems in the OR. For that reason, the OR Director must participate in the negotiation of any equipment maintenance and repair contracts that include changes that affect surgical services.

Service Contracts for Computer Systems

Computer software and hardware service contracts are typically needed to support the OR's special computer systems. Some of these contracts provide either on-site or in-store repair services for the hardware. Other contracts from the software vendors are designed for full support of the computer programs. These support services typically include some training of the OR's Informatics Nurse, who will be responsible for upgrading the skills of the rest of the staff. In addition, the software vendor's service contract provides product support if there is a problem with the software's performance (i.e., the software crashes, loses data, or otherwise fails to perform as expected). An important add-on to these contracts addresses software upgrades. Typically, they include pricing for upgrades to the software whenever there is a product repair patch (for one of the problems described above), and many include an agreement to supply upgrades at a lower price when a new version of the software is released.

Computerization is becoming a major source of operational support to the OR; the OR Director should check with the software vendors about any new programs they plan to offer and find out whether any improvements of or changes in current software are expected. It is important to ascertain whether those changes are covered by the current service contract. Some of the questions the OR Director might ask within the department or of software vendors include: Is the surgical services department fully utilizing the computerized charting capabilities of the existing software, or are the programs used only used for surgery scheduling and to maintain surgeon preference cards?[9] Is it time to have the anesthesia department move to computerized charting? What integration exists between anesthesia documentation and nursing documentation, in both the OR and the recovery area and in the other nursing units in the hospital? Are computer kiosks available for patients to enter their health self-assessments or demographics? If the OR is already using computerized charting, are additional interfaces needed such as the ability to retrieve lab results electronically? What new programs or modules are available from the vendors of the

---

[9] Preference cards are lists that identify what instruments and supplies are to be put in the procedure carts. There are different lists for each type of procedure performed in the OR, and the cards are often individualized for every surgeon as well as procedure.

OR's current systems? For example, does the current OR scheduling system offer a new inventory-control module, and if so, is this a good time to budget for purchasing and implementing additional modules? Is there new software on the market that might save time and money in the perioperative department by automating some of the manual processes?

As with any capital purchase, new software has to be justified. The most typical justifications for a software investment include cost savings, improvements in quality of patient care, and improved patient safety. Cost savings are most often realized through a reduction in the personnel hours required to perform work manually (because the new software will perform some of the work). In some instances, new software may be used to support new services or procedures that would otherwise require the hiring of new personnel (this is called cost avoidance because the cost of hiring new people is avoided). A financial analysis will be needed to determine the break-even point for the software purchase and to determine how much money will be saved by the new software (and its service contract) and in what time period the cost savings will be realized.

Sometimes, new software costs more than can be directly recovered through salary savings. In that case, it may have to be justified on the basis of improvements in patient safety or quality of care. It is important to try to put a dollar figure on the value of quality and safety improvements. Safety improvements are often easy to justify because safety problems typically carry consequences, such as additional treatment for the injuries, increased length of stay, malpractice suits, and the costs of dealing with regulatory bodies that may investigate the safety problem. Consider, for example, a problem with patients' being exposed to substances they are known to be allergic to (i.e., latex or penicillin). Sometimes information about patient allergies (and other special needs) is lost as the patient passes from one unit to another and from one care provider to another. OR systems are often not integrated into a total hospital information system, and thus information is transferred by written documents. A computer system that integrates information across units and providers may result in less lost information than occurs through human communicators. For example, consider the cost of having to admit a patient to the intensive care unit after a routine outpatient procedure because somebody failed to notice that the patient was allergic to latex; the OR team used latex gloves, and the patient suffered a serious allergic reaction to the latex. The justification for new software should always contain information about exactly how the software will be used to save money and how much cost savings are expected.

There is limited time for developing new interfaces and training staff in how to use complex new software. Therefore, the OR Director will want to know if the new software is "plug and play," which means that other than purchasing the product and having the information technology staff install and test it, there will be essentially no other costs. On the other hand, costs must be calculated and added to the purchase price if the software will require an implementation team, extensive training, or additional hardware. Then the maintenance costs, including service contracts, will have to be considered.

Those are the key the issues to be considered in regard to computer service contracts. The information technology department must be involved in the selection and purchase of the software and in the negotiation of contracts for after-sale service and support. That department has the experts who can evaluate software products and vendors and who know what the industry standards are for computer-related service contracts (refer to Chapter 15 for a review of contracts for computer services). And equally important, they are familiar with the other software owned by the facility and are able to determine whether any new interfaces will be necessary to allow the new software or software upgrades to work satisfactorily with other hospital systems and achieve optimal performance.

Capital Budget Items

The information presented in Chapter 10 on budgeting for capital equipment is relevant to the OR's capital budget. However, given the type of equipment required by the OR, there are a few additional considerations that the OR Director must address for the capital budget. Not only must the manager justify capital items in terms of return on investment, quality of care, patient safety, and necessity for conducting business, but the OR Director may also have to ask for items on the basis of new standards of care, regulatory agency requirements, community demand, and surgeons' requests. Most facilities have their own form for submitting and justifying capital budget requests. The form displayed in Figure 16-1 can be used to support the justification process for specialized OR capital equipment.

■ SPECIAL STAFFING ISSUES IN THE OR

Staffing analyses in surgical services are somewhat different from staffing algorithms in other clinical areas. Most facilities tie OR staffing to the specific procedures performed and to the amount of time it takes to turn over a room.[10] The average time it takes for each type of procedure offered is calculated on a regular basis, and this figure is used to help determine how many people are needed to staff the OR. In addition, nonprocedural time is required to run an OR, but sometimes it is difficult to explain room turnover and nonprocedural time requirements to nonclinical administrators. Administrators often obtain benchmark data from another OR and expect the OR Manager to meet those standards. If the benchmark's OR staffing is approximately the same, the OR Director should have little trouble meeting the administration's expectations. However, this is seldom the case. More typically, the OR Director is presented with staffing expectations that are significantly below the current staffing in the OR.

When the OR Director is presented with the information that another OR is operating more efficiently in terms of full-time-equivalent staff per procedure or per operating room minutes, it is vital to obtain the name and location of that facility. The OR Director will want to consult with the OR Director of the benchmark facility and perhaps even visit that facility to find out what processes are different in the benchmark facility. This is one way an OR Director can discover better ways of operating the department.

However, it is important to compare "apples to apples" in terms of how the two different ORs function. For example, one common finding when an OR is found to be "inefficient" is that staffing allocations to departments are not the same for the two facilities. A typical scenario is that in the benchmark facility, the people who clean and prepare the operating suites between procedures are budgeted through environmental services, whereas in the OR Director's facility, they are included in the

[10] "Turnover" refers to the time it takes to clean a room after a procedure is finished and get the room ready for the next surgery patient.

CAPITAL EQUIPMENT INSTRUMENTATION JUSTIFICATION QUESTIONS

1. Describe the equipment/instrumentation and how it will be used.

2. What is the purchase cost quoted by the sales representative?
    (Attach copy of the quote)

3. Who will be performing the maintenance on the equipment/instrumentation?
    Is a service contract included or required?

4. Is this piece of equipment/instrumentation available through a contracted vendor?

    4.1 If not, who is the vendor?

    4.2 If yes, who is the vendor and is the vendor a contracted vendor?

        4.2.1 If not, why was a non-contracted vendor selected?

5. Who is the requestor of this piece of equipment/instrumentation?

6. What is the projected volume of additional cases this piece of equipment/
    instrumentation will add?

7. What is the projected additional cost per case in supplies for this procedure
    attributable to this item?

8. What is the projected operating room time of the procedure related to this item?

9. If this piece of equipment/instrumentation will not bring additional cases to the
    operating room, what is the benefit of its purchase?

10. What is the projected timeline of purchase, installation and utilization of this
    equipment/instrumentation?

11. What are the effects of not purchasing this piece of equipment/instrumentation?

12. What education and training is required for this equipment/instrumentation?

    12.1 Who will conduct this training?
    12.2 Are there additional costs involved in the education and training?

13. Will the Marketing Department be involved in making the community aware that the
    hospital owns this equipment/instrumentation?

14. Is there a regulatory issue, patient safety or standard of care issue that is involved in
    the justification of this item?

Submitted by:_____ Submit Date: _____

Figure 16-1 An OR capital budget request guide.

OR's budget. Thus, costs appear to be much higher in one facility than in another. But when those environmental services personnel costs are added to the OR budget for the benchmark hospital, the cost differences between the two facilities disappear.

Another common scenario is that the people who transport patients to the OR are in the OR budget in one facility but under a separate transportation department in another facility. Yet a third possible difference may be that housekeeping may be a contracted service in one facility so that those full-time equivalents are not counted in the OR budget, but in another facility they are allocated (or charged directly) to the OR budget. These examples demonstrate how important it is to compare the two budgets line by line to discover where the cost differences lie. The OR Director must be open to the possibility that there is a more efficient way to run the OR but must also ensure that the benchmark facility's OR budget is directly comparable to his or her own budget. To negotiate for adequate staff, the OR Director needs data and credible evidence to show exactly how the OR's current staffing compares with the benchmark facility's staffing.

Following are some items of additional information that may be helpful to the OR Director in planning and budgeting staffing. These bulleted items include links to Websites and some questions to think about as the OR Director works to establish the staffing plan and justify it.

Resources for OR staffing information:

- AORN has a *Position Statement on Nurse-to-Patient Ratios* that is published on its Website: http://www.aorn.org/about/positions/ratios.htm. This and future AORN guidelines on perioperative staffing are evidence of national OR staffing standards and can be used to assist in the staffing justification process.

- The American Society of PostAnesthesia Nurses (ASPAN) provides staffing recommendations for departments that include adult and pediatric patients; its publication, *Standards of Perianesthesia Nursing Practice: Resource 3*, can be ordered from the Website: http://www.aspan.org/Resource3.htm. ASPAN also publishes a set of clinical guidelines that addresses standards of care (which affect staffing): *Standards of Perianesthesia Nursing Practice*; it too can be ordered through the Website: http://www.aspan.org/.

- If the facility is certified as a Level I or Level II trauma center, the OR director should obtain from the ED (or from the department that certifies trauma centers in your state) a copy of the requirements that must be met by the OR to maintain that certification. There are requirements for staffing that should be included in the staffing justification report. If the ED is not a Level I or Level II trauma center but your facility accepts trauma patients, the state guidelines for the type of trauma you treat should be obtained to ensure that staffing meets state guidelines.

- Networking with sister hospitals and other OR facilities in your area and nationwide is valuable (this may be facilitated if your facility is part of a national system). Often, area facilities that are not sister hospitals are reluctant to share business operations information because the hospitals are in competition with each other. Therefore, it is useful to build a regional and national network of colleagues with whom you can share advice and information. The Internet and e-mail greatly ease this part of the OR Director's job.

Questions to answer in order to obtain information relevant to determining and justifying staffing levels:

- What is the case mix of your patients? How does that compare to the case mix of your benchmark OR?
- What are the hours of operation of the OR?
- Is there in-house staffing on weekends?
- What level of downtime versus active time does the room utilization report indicate?
- How do the surgeons and anesthetists perceive the turnover time? The physicians often work at more than one facility and may be able to provide information about whether room turnover times are different at other institutions. They may even know how better room turnover times are achieved if they believe your room turnover time is excessive.
- What is the average room turnover time for the procedures done most frequently? Room turnover varies based on the acuity of the procedure, so it is important to benchmark the turnover times with information found in the literature and through benchmark and peer institutions—and that information is most helpful if it reflects the type of patients your OR serves.
- What do the patient satisfaction surveys for your department indicate about the performance of the OR team from the patient's viewpoint?
- If there is an educator or business manager position in the department, which department's budget are those positions under?
- What is the utilization level of per diem and traveler staff?
- What is the staff turnover rate, and how does it compare with that of other regional facilities and national benchmark statistics?
- What are the orientation and continuing education costs?
- What are the time and costs associated with keeping up with surgeon preference cards, service specialist duties, staff time in meetings, and performance improvement activities?
- What are the technologies utilized in the procedure mix?
- Are additional personnel required for some surgical procedures? What percentage of cases require a third person? These data must be determined in order to calculate core staffing.
- Is the OR staffed with an all-RN staff or is there a combination of RNs and surgery technologists?
- Who makes up the indirect staff and what are their roles? Specifically, which department's budget contains the room turnover staff and the environmental services/cleaning staff?
- OR staff, like all other department staff are entitled to lunch breaks, meeting breaks, morning and afternoon breaks, and the like. In most hospital units, staff are not replaced while on breaks; another member of the staff simply covers their patients until they return. The situation in the OR is quite different. Surgeries do not stop while staff members take breaks, so relief time must be budgeted. Computing the allocation of relief time must account for the fact that when circulating or scrub staff relief is

given, time must be allowed for the relief staff to scrub, gown, and glove and to receive a report prior to providing relief. In addition, the individual relieved must scrub, gown, glove, and receive a report upon return. Relief staff must be included in the core daily staffing levels.

Many facilities that have an ER but are not certified trauma centers rely on on-call staff to handle emergency surgeries that must be performed after the OR's regular hours. The costs of on-call staffing should be budgeted separately from regular staffing costs so that they can be tracked and evaluated during the budget planning process. The OR Director should regularly review the utilization of call-back[11] hours to determine whether on-call staffing is insufficient, adequate, or excessive. If the situation frequently arises that more staff are needed for emergency surgeries even after all on-call staff have been called back, then more staff should be placed on call, or it may be time to consider night and weekend OR staffing. ORs in facilities with Level I and II trauma centers must be staffed 24 hours a day, 7 days a week. But many other hospitals do not perform enough emergency procedures to justify employing permanent night and weekend staff. However, if members of the OR staff are already assigned all the on-call time that is reasonable to expect and are regularly (and consistently) getting called back to work, a reevaluation of staff usage is in order. On-call is not popular with many staff, who expect to be allowed to have private lives outside the hospital; excessive use of on-call staff can be a major source of staff turnover, and it is prudent to monitor carefully the frequency with which on-call staff actually get called back to staff emergency procedures. Whenever that situation arises, the wise OR Director will evaluate the situation and decide whether there is a need for night and weekend staffing.

The staffing budget is created by using national guidelines and evidence of OR activity levels to establish the necessary levels of staffing. The staffing needs of a hospital that has 24/7 coverage will be different from those in an OR that is not staffed after 5:00 p.m. or 11.00 p.m. hours. The decision will have to be made whether there are to be one, two, or more staff placed on-call or whether there is a need to place specialty team members on call.

One concern not yet addressed is whether on-call staff members who were called back are expected to work their regular shifts the next day. This can be a very serious patient safety issue because it may easily result in a nurse's being required to work 36 consecutive hours. This happens whenever nurses who have been scheduled for two or three 12-hour day shifts (with 12 hours off at night) get called back during their 12 hours off. Conceivably, a nurse could work a regular 12-hour day shift and be called back (or have to remain) for the next 12 hours to take care of one or more trauma patients (for example, after a multiple-car accident), and then be required to remain and work the following 12-hour day shift. By the end of the third shift, the nurse will have worked 36 hours straight. There is ample research that documents the fact that people become extremely forgetful and error prone after working far fewer consecutive hours than 36. Forcing a nurse to work such hours is a poor management practice, not only because the nurse is certainly unsafe to practice due to exhaustion, but also because such a practice may greatly increase staff turnover costs. If such a situation happened several times to the same nurse, it is likely that the OR would lose that nurse to some other facility that has more humane staffing practices.

---

[11] Callback is a term that means the on-call staff member had to come back to the hospital to staff an emergency surgery during the time he or she was otherwise scheduled to be off. Usually there is an on-call hourly payment that is considerably less than the nurse's normal hourly rate, but is paid to the on-call nurse even if not called in for a surgery. If called in for surgery, a higher rate applies.

A nurse working 36 straight hours is probably not even cost-effective, aside from the consequences for quality of care and turnover. Having another nurse work a shift at time-and-a-half overtime wages instead of allowing the first nurse to exceed 24 straight hours may seem costly, but the productivity of a nurse after 24 straight hours of work may be so low that it will cause costly delays in turnaround and other areas that may actually result in increased salary costs for many other workers. This would be true, for example, if the start of a case is delayed and a number of staff members are waiting for that case to start.

If the nurse is to be released from the regular day shift after working an on-call case during the night, how will that slot be filled for the next shift? Will such a policy force the OR scheduler to cancel some surgeries because of insufficient staffing? Will the OR Director have to budget for agency (per diem) staff to cover that slot?[12] If addition personnel are needed to cover release time for on-call people so that they are not working for prolonged periods of time, that extra staffing must be calculated into the staffing budget. For budgeting purposes it is necessary to know the on-call rate of pay, hours of on-call status throughout the year, and the call-back pay rate, and this information must be computed for the RN salary and the surgical technologist salary. Once the hours of call coverage have been decided and the number of personnel assigned to on-call status per week has been determined, computation of the on-call cost factor is not difficult.

■ OTHER ISSUES IN BUDGETING FOR SURGICAL SERVICES

The following two sections present suggestions and tips for the OR Director that are relevant to the OR budget planning and implementation process. The first section addresses informal strategies that will support budget planning, and the second section addresses marketing the OR. Without marketing, many hospitals' ORs would lose case volume because competing hospitals have acquired higher visibility in the community through their advertising.

Nonstatistical Methods for Future OR Budget Projections

Financial forecasting has been addressed in Chapter 6. However, there are a variety of sources that the OR Director may want to tap to obtain information about trends and procedures that are available primarily through journal articles and the personal network the director has developed. The OR Director is the person most responsible for guiding the OR to a successful future. Case volume is the force that drives OR profitability. Case volume also has a profound effect on some of the other areas of the hospital, such as the postsurgery nursing care units, radiology, the laboratory, and the dietary department. Therefore, anything that affects case volume is of critical importance for the OR Director to consider in managing and planning for the future of the surgical services department. But to consider information about factors that lead to changes in case volume, the OR Director must be aware of the information.

When the OR volume is down for several weeks, such as can happen during the summer when many surgeons and their patients take summer vacations, it is not unusual for the OR Director to be asked by someone from administration, "What is going on? Census is down all over the hospital." Consider the effect on the organization's profitability if the OR becomes a place where surgeons do not wish to operate and patients do not want to come because at this hospital they cannot get the

---

[12] In fact, it may not always be possible to fill that slot with temporary or part-time personnel. Given the nursing shortage, such staff are not always available, especially in rural hospitals.

up-to-date services they want and demand. It is a key responsibility of OR Directors to find out about trends and changes that will affect their departments' case volumes. There are a variety of strategies the OR Director can employ to gain this knowledge.

Every OR Director should regularly read journals, newspapers, and other published materials to find out about trends that might affect perioperative operations. Other media sources such as television, with its many medical programs and news reports, are a good source of information. Many patients learn about issues in surgery through the mass media and ask questions about what they have learned. For example, when public television presented a program about patients under general anesthesia being able to hear and store memories of what transpired during their procedures, OR nurses were presented with questions about awareness under anesthesia by their patients the very next day. This concern by patients could have been quickly allayed if the OR Director had worked with the anesthesia department to ensure that bispectral index monitors (BIS monitors)[13] were used for every patient. When BIS monitors were first introduced in 1996, the forward-thinking OR Director would have asked, "Are these going to become the standard of care for all patients who receive general anesthesia?" and would have planned future budgets accordingly. Anesthesiologists and surgeons are usually eager to share information about innovations and to collaborate with the OR Director in the effort to acquire equipment that will improve the OR's performance. To be able to discuss new technology and procedures intelligently with the anesthesia and surgeon groups, the OR Director must be well informed about the costs, benefits, and potential drawbacks of innovations.

Members of the facility's administration team attend a variety of conferences, and they can bring back an array of materials, such as booklets, advertising materials, handouts, and brochures for new products. At presentations and meetings, they may hear about innovations that will affect the OR. Most administrators are willing to share this information and collaborate with the OR Director to use the information to make sure that the facility retains (or improves) its competitive position in the perceptions of its customers. The Director of the Ambulatory Surgery Center (ASC) is another person with whom the OR Director should interact. The ASC Manager may know of procedures that are likely to be moved to the ASC in the near future, and that change will have implications for OR case volume and for the budget. The ASC Manager will need information from the OR Director about how the transfer of procedures to ASC will affect their supplies, implants, and staffing, and whether the ASC will need to plan for more overnight stays.

Trending OR activity is a part of volume forecasting. Nurses who have worked in the OR for more than 3 years can usually predict when OR volume will be slow and when the busy times will occur during the year. Case volume trends depend partly on the region of the country. For example, in ski country, the small hospitals experience higher volumes during the winter months and decreases in volume during the summer, and their budgets should reflect those trends. Other volume changes are likely to occur during the times when the general public tend to take vacations and during national conferences that surgeons attend. One good tip is for the OR

---

[13] A BIS monitor is a machine that monitors a patient's level of consciousness through continuous computer analysis of the patient's electroencephalograms during surgery. The depth of anesthesia is associated with the patient's awareness of sounds or sensations during surgery and the ability to form memories while under anesthesia. It can also provide information that assists the anesthetist to protect the patient from excessively deep anesthesia levels, which lead to difficulty in waking the patient after surgery. The BIS index ranges from 0 (no brain activity) to 99 (fully awake and aware). A BIS index of 40 to 60 generally indicates adequate levels of general anesthesia.

Director to make notes on a calendar about what was occurring during the times when volume was unusually high or low. This helps in analyzing monthly or seasonal volume changes during budget planning. This information also assists the OR Director in recognizing temporary changes due to vacations and conferences versus permanent changes such as the opening of a new ASC. The specific trends differ among facilities, but most ORs experience some seasonal volume changes. OR budgets should be based on the OR Director's best predictions of what monthly changes in volume and costs to expect during the next budget year. With the variations due to seasons, regions, lifestyles of the consumers, and elective versus emergency surgeries, the volume in the OR is likely to vary; therefore, the budget must reflex the changes in volume over time.

Marketing the OR

Rare is the OR that has all its rooms full, short turnover times, and excellent payment contracts with health insurance companies and is the only OR provider in town. If your OR is in that enviable situation, marketing may not be important for you. For everybody else, marketing is an important part of maintaining and increasing case volume. Good marketing strategy begins with meetings with the facility's marketing department. An overall marketing strategy should be developed, along with specific plans for marketing in the next budget year. Most facilities centralize marketing efforts and the marketing budget in the marketing department. Therefore, OR marketing may be embedded in marketing activities that promote the entire hospital. If the OR director wants to obtain funding for targeted ads that highlight the OR services, the project must be negotiated through the marketing department. One type of marketing that is low cost involves staff volunteer activities at local public events such as community health fairs. Generally, the OR will be allowed to have a poster or banner and may be able to hand out flyers with information about the services offered.

Within the hospital, events such as National Nurse Week in May and Perioperative Week in November, as well as PeriAnesthesia, CRNA, Surgical Technologist and Sterile Processing Weeks can provide opportunities for marketing. Marketing efforts can be as simple as setting up table tents in the cafeteria and displaying posters the hospital's lobby and in public areas of the surgery department. Table tents and posters can be customized with information on OR statistics, photos of the staff, and announcements of special projects. Take pictures. With printers and digital cameras, a professional look can be obtained. Marketing personnel can assist with these efforts. Work with the marketing department to send letters to local high schools offering to provide a speaker on careers in the OR on career day or to health careers class. This is an inexpensive marketing tool and may also count as community service. When seeking opportunities to make presentations about the OR, consider volunteering to make a presentation to students at the local elementary schools. The key is to make sure that the activity or topic is appropriate for the age group to which you are presenting and that it meets with the approval of the instructor. Remember, topics that hospital personnel may discuss on a regular basis may be inappropriate or not approved by parents for the classroom setting, so take care to edit your topic. One easy tool that keeps children and adults interested are the laparoscopic trainers. The company that supplies your trocars and laparoscopic instrumentation will have one that you can borrow. Have small pieces of wrapped candy or mini candy bars available so the participants can pretend to be surgeons and practice using the monitors and laparoscopic instruments to pick up the candy.

Visit the surgeons' offices. Get to know their schedulers and office managers. Patients may be limited by their insurance companies in terms of which hospital they may use for services, but if they have choices, make your hospital their hospital of choice. The schedulers and office managers hear the frustrations of the surgeons, experience difficulties in getting cases on the schedule, and hear the frustration of the patients. These are opportunities for improvement that may eventually lead the surgeons to prefer using your facility when there is a choice.

Word of mouth can be a powerful marketing tool. The wise OR Director will want to ensure that patients and their family members are satisfied with their surgery services. They will talk about their experiences to their friends and acquaintances, and it is important that the message they communicate about the facility be positive. Managers should take the time to visit the waiting room and the preop area on a regular basis and get to know the volunteers who assist the families. Once they know you, they will be more comfortable sharing information about patients' and families' concerns. Provide families and guests of patients with the business card of a member of the OR team who can respond quickly to their concerns and any problems that arise. This card should bear a phone number that allows them to reach immediately a person with the authority to address problems. Family members and guests must know that if they are worried about what is going on, the volunteer will help them to seek assistance.

The OR staff must be reminded regularly of the importance of professional courtesy and good public relations. For example, family members in the waiting room appreciate occasional updates on the progress of their loved one's surgery, especially in longer procedures. These are inexpensive ways to broadcast the message to the rest of the hospital and to the public on a regular basis that the surgical services are excellent in your facility.

A more expensive marketing strategy is to develop an RN liaison role that involves making the rounds to all the service areas (including preop, OR, postanesthesia care, and the waiting room) and to be available to answer questions, solve problems, and update families. The RN liaison should be available to intervene immediately when there are issues or problems in any area of the perioperative department. For example, an RN liaison could explain to patients why cases are running late and could do so without risking a violation of HIPPA regulations by revealing information about another patient that should remain confidential. If a patient complains of unrelieved pain in the recovery room (RR), the RN liaison is free to call the anesthesiologist to obtain orders for more pain medications or for different treatment modalities. In fact, policy might stipulate that the liaison nurse must be summoned if a patient is asking for pain relief and the RR nurse has given all the pain medication ordered. The RR nurse cannot leave the unit to find an anesthesiologist, but the liaison nurse has no such restriction. The liaison nurse can summon a chaplain to comfort the families of trauma patients in the waiting room, or if a patient is not doing well in surgery. The objective of the RN liaison is to help keep patients, family members, and guests calm and satisfied with perioperative services.

Summary and Implications for Nurse Managers

Planning for the OR budget is a collaborative process between the OR director and the various constituencies of the OR. Key stakeholders, such as the surgeons, anesthesiologists, OR and other hospital staff, vendors, administrators, and members of the community all provide information that is

Continued

Summary and Implications for Nurse Managers—cont'd

vital to the development of a workable OR budget. It is especially important for the OR budget to include some method of prioritizing requests for staff, equipment and instruments, and capital budget items. It is rare that any OR has enough money to buy all the resources the OR Director would like to have. Therefore, some budget requests will have to be denied and others delayed to a future budget.

OR budgets contain some categories that are unique to the perioperative department. Such things as medical implants, sterile processing, many maintenance and repair service contracts, and extensive on-call expenses are typically not found in other hospital departments. Although most hospital departments have computer systems, many do not have such specialized systems that are separate from the main hospital information system as does the OR. Many ORs are now finding that they must have one staff member trained in informatics in order to properly support the clinical computer systems in the perioperative department.

Many aspects of the OR personnel budget are similar to the personnel budgets in other departments. However, staffing requirements are calculated differently in the OR than in other nursing units. In addition, most ORs require on-call service from most of their staff, and that must be budgeted. Given that an on-call nurse may be called back to work for long periods of time, the staffing plan must address how to provide relief for those staff who are called back. In addition, OR staff may include not only the nurses and scrub technicians for the OR, but also the personnel who clean up the OR rooms between patients and set up for the next patient. The OR department budget may also include the costs of the sterile-processing department, and they can add considerable complexity to the OR personnel budget.

Finally, it is important to plan marketing for the surgical services department. The OR Director should ensure that there is some budget for advertising and for activities that keep the OR's reputation positive and high in the community's awareness. Most people are interested in the types of surgical services available in local hospitals, and a variety of low-cost initiatives can help to keep the community informed and positive about their local hospital or ACS's services.

Budgeting for the OR is a specialized and work-intensive process. The need for trend evaluation and analysis is important for projecting and budgeting new or expanded services. There is so much change in the numbers and types of surgical procedures offered today that the OR budget is a highly changeable plan. Items planned for purchase this year may have to be delayed in order to offer a cutting-edge service this year. The costs of the equipment and instruments needed for operating a modern OR are significant. Therefore, the work involved in developing the OR budget is extensive.

References and Suggested Readings

American Society of PostAnesthesia Nurses. (2004). *Standards of Perianesthesia Nursing Practice 2006-2008.* Cherry Hill, New Jersey: ASPAN.

Association of periOperative Registered Nurses. (2006). *Standards, Recommended Practices, and Guidelines.* Denver, CO: AORN, Inc.

Association of periOperative Registered Nurses (2006). *Finance: Budgeting.* Denver, CO: AORN, Inc.

Beglinger, J. (2006). Quantifying patient care intensity: An evidence-based approach to determining staffing requirements. *Nursing Administration Quarterly.* 30(3), 193-202.

The Joint Commission. (2007). *Field reviews and draft standards.* Downloaded on January 6, 2007: http://www.jointcommission.org/Standards/FieldReviews/.

Taylor, K., Jackson, S. (2005). A medical equipment replacement score system. *Journal of Clinical Engineering.* 30(1), 37-41.

Thorgrimson, D., Robinson, N. (2005). Building and sustaining an adequate RN workforce. *Journal of Nursing Administration.* 35(11), 474-477.

Wagner, C., Budreau, G., Everett, L. (2005). Analyzing fluctuating unit census for timely staffing intervention. *Nursing Economic$.* 23(2), 85-90.

Wikipedia. (2007). Trauma center. *Wikipedia: The Free Encyclopedia.* Downloaded on January 6, 2007: http://en.wikipedia.org/wiki/Trauma_center.

Benchmarking, Productivity, and Cost-Benefit and Cost-Effectiveness Analysis

LEARNING OBJECTIVES
The goals of this chapter are to:

- Define benchmarking
- Explain the benchmarking technique and the critical steps in the benchmarking process
- Define productivity and productivity measurement
- Provide tools for productivity analysis
- Discuss productivity standards
- Introduce the concept of unit costing

- Explain the relationship between productivity standards and unit-costing
- Explore the notion of productivity improvement
- Define the concepts of cost-benefit analysis and cost-effectiveness analysis
- Explain the principles of cost-benefit analysis and cost-effectiveness analysis

■ INTRODUCTION

Budgeting is not simply about preparing a plan for the organization to do what it has always done in the way it has always done it. Rather, budgeting should help the organization constantly get better—be more effective and efficient in providing its services. Benchmarking, productivity measurement, and cost-benefit/cost-effectiveness analysis are approaches that organizations use to become better at what they do.

Benchmarking is a technique aimed at finding the best practices of other organizations and incorporating them into an organization. Benchmarking is the first major topic covered in this chapter.

Many health care organizations today are also concerned with *productivity*. As financial resources become more constrained, improvements in productivity represent one way of cutting fat rather than lean. The area of productivity measurement, however, remains something of a mystery in many industries, not just health care. In health care, the difficulties are compounded by problems related to quality and outcomes measurement.

As an organization works to improve productivity in health care, one must always guard against the motivation to sacrifice mission so as to achieve productivity increases. It is possible to reduce the number of hours of care per patient day. Some health care administrators consider such a reduction to be evidence of increased productivity. However, if the reduction decreases the quality of patient care or patient outcomes, then productivity has not really improved. It may, in fact, have declined. Productivity is defined as the number of units of output produced per unit of input. Input units are usually expressed as dollars. Output has two factors. It involves both the number of outputs and the quality of those outputs. If quality is decreased, productivity is reduced (McHugh, 1989). Therefore, true productivity improvements are those that enable the organization to use fewer input resources for each unit of service of a particular level of quality provided. In recent years there has been a trend to reorient the focus of nursing productivity measurement from hours per patient day or full-time equivalents per adjusted occupied bed[1] toward the cost per unit of service provided. The essence of this *unit-costing* is that if it is possible to lower the dollar cost of providing a unit of a specific service, it is not necessary to worry about things such as the number of care hours used to provide the service. Unit-costing is discussed in the productivity section of the chapter.

The chapter concludes with a discussion of *cost-benefit analysis* and *cost-effectiveness analysis*. These are two techniques that are frequently used by managers as they attempt to improve the productivity of their departments. The techniques are defined and their basic principles are discussed.

■ BENCHMARKING

One of the roles of budgeting is to help the organization continuously improve over time. The budget should incorporate changes that will allow it to provide services more efficiently. Ultimately, such constant improvement helps the organization to accomplish its mission better, while at the same time providing it with an edge over its competitors. Benchmarking is a technique that many organizations employ to help set the direction for change. Simply stated, benchmarking is a technique that organizations use to find the best practices and to incorporate those practices within the organization.

Benchmarking is linked closely with a variety of process-improvement techniques, such as Total Quality Management (TQM) and Continuous Quality Improvement (CQI). However, those techniques may be employed using a totally internal focus on an organization's processes. The essence of benchmarking is the examination of what others are doing. When the organization forces itself to look beyond itself, many useful approaches developed elsewhere can be used to benefit the organization. This means that an organization may benefit from rare insights or avoid the costly trials and errors of others. It allows the organization to avoid spending substantial resources to reinvent the wheel every time it needs to improve in some area.

Benefits of Benchmarking

There are a number of different ways that benchmarking leads to improved organizational results. Some of the most prominent focuses of benchmarking studies are in the areas of meeting customer requirements, developing accurate measures of productivity, and improving competitiveness.

As health care becomes increasingly competitive, it becomes more important than ever to concentrate on the customer. Knowledge of the services that other organizations are providing to customers is incredibly valuable. To remain competitive, organizations must be aware of what the competition is doing. If it can be determined

---

[1] Adjusted occupied beds is a measure that combines both inpatient days and outpatient care by using a formula for the number of outpatient visits considered to be the equivalent of one inpatient day.

that elsewhere in the country a service is provided that is not offered by any local competitors, the organization can gain insights into how to provide its customers with even more than they expect. The most successful organizations are those that are proactive rather than reactive. The organization that introduces new services first has an edge over those that follow. Because the health care industry is largely localized, one does not have to invent every new service it offers. Rather, organizations should strive to keep abreast of innovations around the country and to have the flexibility to be "the first ones on the block" to offer those services.

One of the greatest difficulties in assessing productivity is trying to determine the right level of productivity. How long should it take to do a certain procedure? It is possible to measure productivity in terms of improvement over time. However, some would argue that an organization cannot be productive unless it has some optimum standard for comparison. Benchmarking evaluates the level of productivity of other organizations. This allows the organization to compare itself to the best organizations, creating productivity targets that are challenging, yet attainable. Productivity is discussed later in this chapter.

Rates of change within organizations are highly variable. Some organizations change rapidly. Others tend to maintain what they believe is a good way of providing care. It is surprising that, despite the rapid change in clinical techniques, health care management techniques often tend to be stagnant. It is difficult to spend a great deal of time being innovative while at the same time trying to complete the day's work that has to be done. Benchmarking helps by allowing organizations to change without having to invent all the changes. This not only reduces the amount of effort required to find changes that truly result in improvements but also allows the organization to leapfrog over competing organizations.

Benchmarking Approaches

There are three primary approaches to benchmarking. These three approaches are competitive benchmarking, cooperative benchmarking, and collaborative benchmarking.[2] Competitive benchmarking involves finding specific information about individual organizations that provide the same services your organization provides. Cooperative benchmarking involves seeking information from organizations in other industries. Collaborative benchmarking involves finding information within your industry but based on industry-wide statistics.

When people think of benchmarking, they often focus their thoughts on competitive benchmarking. Hospital managers may want to determine how a specific function is done at the hospital that does that function best. A visiting nurse agency may want to know the best practices related to supplies inventory used at other home care agencies. This is the hardest type of benchmarking data to obtain. Naturally, organizations are reluctant to share their secrets with the direct competition. For this reason, it is often easier to fly across the country and observe several organizations that are not in direct competition with the organization than to observe practices of direct competitors in the same area as the organization. It is not unusual for

[2] American Society for Training and Development. (1992). *Understanding Benchmarking: The Search for Best Practice.* 92(7), 5-6 (Info-Line).

exchanges to be worked out in which organizations that are similar but in different markets allow visitors to examine their procedures.

Multihospital organizations often use their outcomes data to identify which facilities in their organization have the best success rates in each of a wide variety of performance indicators. For example, one facility in New York may have the best performance outcomes for open-heart surgery, whereas a different facility in Ohio has the best performance outcomes for treatment of sepsis. Once the New York facility has been identified as the organization's benchmark for open-heart surgery, the individuals who monitor quality for the organization determine the protocols the New York facility uses to achieve their success. Then those protocols are shared with other facilities as best practices for open-heart surgery. Managers and clinicians from other facilities within the organization might visit the benchmark to learn how to implement the best-practice protocols, and thus quality increases throughout the organization.

Many healthcare organizations that do not belong to a multifacility corporation have banded together to form consortia that share best practices for both financial and clinical performance indicators. One example of this type of consortium is the University HealthSystem Consortium (UHC) located in Oak Brook, Illinois. Begun as a group purchasing plan to reduce the costs of equipment and supplies for member hospitals, it is now known also for its work in patient care quality and safety (UCH, 2006, 1). It publishes an annual report on the top performers of their 95 academic medical centers and 139 affiliated hospitals—the benchmark facilities—for various clinical variables (UCH, 2006, 2). These types of corporate health care system and health care consortia benchmarks are designed to improve quality throughout their systems by facilitating access to data and information that make competitive benchmarking easier for all of their facilities.

Sometimes competitive benchmarking is done without direct permission. This can occur through informal observation or by using a variety of publicly available information. Health care providers generally issue many reports to the public and government that can be useful in assessing their approaches. Consultants have access to many organizations and are often willing to share the best practices that they have observed. As Pavlock notes, "The goal is to find out what the competitors are doing, how, and how well in order to compare their practices with the benchmarker's operations."[3] Agency nurses often work for many different providers. They can be an invaluable source of information about how other organizations do things.

Cooperative benchmarking takes a substantially different approach. Rather than focusing on specific competitors, it looks at organizations in dissimilar industries. Although this might seem odd at first, it actually has great merit. Suppose that a health care provider finds that it consistently ranks low in customer satisfaction. A cooperative benchmarking approach would be to select an organization that is known for its great customer service. For example, the department store, Nordstrom, has long had a reputation for excellent customer service. Spending some time visiting Nordstrom, learning their philosophy and how they operationalize that philosophy and maintain high customer satisfaction might be enlightening. Why should Nordstrom agree to let you do this? For several reasons. First, everyone loves flattery.

[3] Ernest J. Pavlock. (2002). *Financial Management for Medical Groups.* Englewood, CO: Center for Research in Ambulatory Health Care Administration, p. 588.

And seeking to learn from any organization certainly flatters that organization. Second, many organizations view helping health care providers as an act of public service. Third, health care organizations do not compete with Nordstrom. And fourth, the time may come when you will have some information that might benefit Nordstrom.

It is important to bear in mind that as long as benchmarking is limited to the benchmarker's industry, you never really become a leader. You are always following someone in your industry. By going outside of the industry, you gain the possibility of becoming the industry leader yourself.

Some organizations actually make a business of allowing themselves to be used for benchmarking purposes. Disney now offers a formal program called The Disney Approach to Quality Service for Healthcare Professionals. In a 3½-day program costing about $4,000 per participant, Disney offers "A Unique Benchmarking Opportunity." In the program, Disney provides not only information about how Disney does things but also linkages to how their approaches can be employed in the health care industry (Disney Institute, 2006).

Collaborative benchmarking is a process whereby a number of organizations in the same industry pool data so that all members of the pool can determine where they stand relative to the best members of the pool. Generally there is confidentiality, with members of the pool being anonymous. Each organization sees its own data and where it stands relative to everyone else but does not know who has better or worse ratings.

This collaborative approach is more of a **how much** approach rather than a **how** approach. With competitive or cooperative benchmarking, the benchmarker tries to learn as much about the best practice process so as to make it easy to adopt that practice. Collaborative benchmarking doesn't allow for an understanding of process. On the other hand, if collaborative benchmarking is used, it can help highlight weaknesses. The organization can then move aggressively into one of the other approaches of benchmarking to find ways of converting that weakness into an area of competitive strength.

The Benchmarking Process

The process for benchmarking has been summarized by Camp as having ten steps[4]:

1. Decide what to benchmark.
2. Identify organizations with best practices.
3. Collect data for comparison.
4. Assess the gap between best practice and your performance.
5. Project likely improvement in best practices over the next 3 to 5 years.
6. Communicate findings.
7. Establish goals.
8. Create specific plans for improvement.
9. Implement plans.
10. Reestablish benchmarks as they change over time.

[4] Robert C. Camp. (1989). *Benchmarking: The Search for Industry Best Practices That Lead to Superior Performance.* Milwaukee, WI: American Society for Quality Control, pp. 9-12.

Every organization does too many things to be able to benchmark all processes. Benchmarking usually focuses on problem areas. The organization must first decide where it is most in need of outside comparison (step 1). The focus should start with areas for which a difference in performance will lead to a difference in achievement of mission. That is, one must select areas where change might result in a meaningful impact.

For example, consider two opportunities for change. In the first, the organization can achieve a 50% improvement in performance. In the second, it can produce only a 10% improvement in performance. The initial impulse is to attack the 50% area. However, that may not be the best approach. The manager must also consider the organizational impact of the improvement. Assume that the area where the organization can achieve a 50% performance improvement is in reduced incidence of pneumococcal infections among do-not-resuscitate cases transferred from a local nursing home. The area where the organization can achieve a 10% performance improvement is in reducing the transmission of impetigo in the pediatric ward. But consider that there are only 2 cases of pneumococcal infections per year, whereas there are 60 cases of nosocomial impetigo in the pediatric unit. That 50% reduction of pneumococcal infections means only one patient is affected. But in the impetigo situation, 6 patients are affected by the 10% reduction in impetigo. Assuming the effort and cost are the same for addressing each problem, the improvement efforts in the pediatric unit produce a larger change than the improvement efforts for the elderly patients who have pneumoccal infections. The organization gets "more bang for its buck" from the 10% improvement than for the 50% improvement.

How does the organization discover its areas of weakness? This is a difficult chicken-and-egg problem. How do you know where you fall short until you benchmark? How do you know what to benchmark until you know where you fall short? Collaborative benchmarking can highlight areas where problems are likely to exist. However, ultimately, managers must thoroughly understand their own processes. It can be especially beneficial to focus efforts on those areas that are costly (because they have the most potential for cost savings) and those areas that are creating morale problems.

Second, the benchmarker must select organizations with best practices (step 2). This requires a fair amount of investigation. Reading publications, asking around, talking to consultants, and general networking are essential to this step. Pavlock suggests that you "talk with industry experts, the firm's employees, customers, suppliers and others knowledgeable about the areas or business practices being targeted. Ask whose products, services or business practices are similar in some way to the benchmarking firm. A benchmarking consultant may be helpful."[5] The more you have to offer in return to a benchmarking partner, the more likely they are to allow you to review their organization. So part of the selection process must include consideration of what you have to offer in exchange and who would be likely to want it.

Step 3 concerns data collection. The data collection process involves not only data but also people. In collecting data about your own organization and the comparison organization it is critical to involve the right people. That includes the managers most familiar with the existing processes at both organizations as well as the person responsible for implementing any changes. To the extent possible, the staff

[5] Pavlock, ibid., p. 589

members who will ultimately have to make any changes succeed should be involved in the process. If they do not view the changes as their changes, they will not have a vested interest in having them succeed. The data to be collected must be usable. So before collecting the data, one should question what types of changes might be needed. Although this cannot be answered fully before the data are collected, it will help to formulate the measurement instruments so that the data are collected in a usable form.

Change is difficult and costly. If the gap between best practice and your performance is not great, it may not be worthwhile trying to implement change. So it is important to assess the gap between current and best practices (step 4). If the measurement tools are well designed and a sizable gap is evident, the benchmarker will be able to see where change is needed.

Knowledge of the gap allows the organization to set targets for improvement. However, the targets should not necessarily be set at the level that exists in the best practices organization now. That organization is likely to make improvements during the period when the benchmarker is implementing changes. Therefore, the benchmark established should be set at the level that will be likely to exist at the best practices organization several years in the future (step 5).

It is critical that the findings of the benchmarking process be widely communicated (step 6). There will undoubtedly be ripple effects resulting from any change. The more support developed for changes; the more likely they are to succeed. But support is not possible without clear communication of what was found and why the findings dictate that changes would be beneficial.

Step 7 is the establishment of goals. These goals should be those that the study team believes are appropriate in order to maximize the benefit gained from adopting the best practices. These goals should be developed with a careful eye toward both the existing gap and the estimation of where the best practices organization will be in several years, as discussed earlier.

The goals must be translated into objectives that form the basis for specific plans for improvement (step 8). To the extent possible, all persons who will be involved in the implementation of the changes should be involved in designing the plan for the changes.

Next comes the actual implementation of the plans (step 9). Assuming that the new benchmarks are well communicated and the action plans well designed, the organization should start to make progress fairly quickly. If progress is not visible in a short time, staff may become discouraged and fall into old patterns of behavior. Although the process of gathering the benchmarking data can be challenging and time-consuming, one cannot relax once the data have been collected. Unless the actual implementation is supervised carefully, all the preceding efforts may turn out to have been wasted.

The final step is to reestablish benchmarks as they change over time (step 10). One of the fundamental principles on which benchmarking is based is that change is essential. There is no one correct way to do things. It is not as simple as getting all aspects of the organization to reach that correct plateau. Rather, processes need to be improved continuously. Even if the organization achieves the status of an industry leader that everyone wants to evaluate for its benchmarking efforts, continued improvement is essential.

Requirements for Successful Benchmarking

One thing that should be clear from the previous discussion is that benchmarking is a big deal. It is not a brief activity undertaken at little cost. It involves the time of many managers over substantial periods of time. Benchmarking is unlikely to work unless there is a strong management commitment to the process. Managers in the organization must study their current processes. It is difficult to change to something unless you first know where you are now. And there must be a willingness to change. Such willingness is much harder to obtain than we may expect. Someone once described change as being similar to heaven: everyone is ready to extol its virtues, but no one is actually in much of a rush to get there.

■ PRODUCTIVITY

Contrary to rumor, productivity is not focused primarily on getting people to work harder. The concern, rather, is to have employees' efforts be more productive. What is meant by productivity? The most common productivity measure is the amount of output produced by each unit of input. This can be calculated as follows:

$$\text{Productivity} = \frac{\text{Total Outputs}}{\text{Total Inputs}}$$

For example, suppose that a nurse practitioner can see 250 patients during a month when 100 hours are devoted to seeing patients. The productivity measure would be:

$$= \frac{250 \text{ Patients}}{100 \text{ Hours}} = 2.5 \text{ Patients per Hour}$$

If the practice can be reorganized to allow the nurse to see more patients per hour, productivity would improve, assuming that the care provided remains at the same level. For example, suppose that the nurse practitioner currently records everything manually in the patient chart after the visit. However, a computer program is available with a touch-screen function that allows for faster data entry and chart updating. When less time is spent charting, more patients can be scheduled. Suppose that after the implementation of the computer system, the nurse can now see 270 patients in the same 100 hours. Productivity has improved to:

$$= \frac{270 \text{ Patients}}{100 \text{ Hours}} = 2.7 \text{ Patients per Hour}$$

If the cost of each hour is the same and visits per hour rise from 2.5 to 2.7, the practice is more productive. Note that this model assumes that the quality of patient care remains stable after the change. This means that the lower number of patients per hour was achieved through reduced time spent charting and not because the practitioner spent less time and care evaluating the patients. Assuming that the extra visits per hour generate more revenue, it is more profitable as well. (Note that we have not yet considered the cost of the computer. That will be addressed later in this chapter.)

Productivity Standards

In the above example it was hypothesized that a nurse practitioner used computers to improve productivity from 2.5 patients per hour to 2.7 patients per hour.

One problem with such a measure of productivity is that the only comparison is related to time. Managers often prefer to have a benchmark or standard for comparison as well. Standards can be based on broad industry-average experience, on best industry practice, or simply on the organization's budget.

For example, suppose that the nurse practitioner believes that an ideally functioning practice would see 3 patients per hour. The nurse practitioner has determined this on the basis of reading many articles about similar practices and also by talking to peers around the country. Productivity can be measured by comparing the actual results of this practice to that standard. For example, originally the practice productivity was 2.5 patients an hour. Compared to the standard, this represents an 83% productivity rate calculated as follows:

$$\frac{\text{Actual Productivity}}{\text{Standard Productivity}} \times 100 = \text{Productivity Percent}$$

$$\frac{2.5 \text{ Patients per Hour}}{3.0 \text{ Patients per Hour}} \times 100 = 83\%$$

After the innovation of computer charting, the practice productivity rose to 90%.

$$\frac{2.7 \text{ Patients per Hour}}{3.0 \text{ Patients per Hour}} \times 100 = 90\%$$

If an industry standard cannot be found, the productivity percentage can be calculated as a percentage of the budget or of some perceived ideal. It should be noted, however, that the resulting percentage must be interpreted according to the type of standard used. If the budget is used as the denominator of the fraction, the goal should be to attain 100% productivity or better. That would imply that the organization is achieving or exceeding its budget. In contrast, what if the denominator of the fraction is based on a perceived ideal? It is highly unlikely that an ideal result can ever be attained. Therefore, the manager must bear in mind that productivity can always be expected to be less than 100%, and performance should be assessed based on how close one comes to 100%.

Unit-Costing

In the previous example, productivity rose from 83% to 90% after computer charting was introduced. However, one must still question whether that productivity change is an improvement. In recent years there has been a movement to stop looking at productivity simply in terms of inputs and outputs and to make sure that the cost per unit of service is considered in the calculation. This approach is called unit-costing.

For example, hospitals have long used hours per patient day (HPPD) as a productivity measure. This is actually an inversion of the typical productivity measure. Consider a nursing department that consumed 10,000 hours of nurses' time in a month when it provided 2,500 patient days of care. The standard productivity measure would be outputs divided by inputs to find the amount of output per unit of input. For the nursing department the calculation would be:

$$= \frac{2,500 \text{ Patient Days}}{10,000 \text{ Hours}} = 0.25 \text{ Patient Days per Hour}$$

The result here is cumbersome because each unit of output (i.e., a patient day) requires more than one unit of input (an hour of care). One quarter of a patient day of care is generated by each hour of nursing care. By inverting the fraction, one can measure the HPPD:

$$= \frac{10,000 \text{ Hours}}{2,500 \text{ Patient Days}} = 4 \text{ HPPD}$$

This is a common hospital productivity measure. However, in today's environment of tight financial resources, this measure fails to indicate the cost of care, which is critical. If all LPNs were replaced by RNs, it is possible that the HPPD could be reduced. But would that make the organization more productive? That is a complicated question. An RN can do activities that an LPN cannot do. But the cost per hour for an RN is also higher than it is for an LPN. Consider the following example. Suppose that an RN earns $35 per hour, including benefits, and an LPN earns $25 per hour, including benefits. Suppose further that an LPN requires 20% more time to accomplish activities than an RN would require for the same activities. (Some activities can be performed only by an RN.) Assume that currently one has 100 hours of RN time and 120 hours of LPN time, and there is an output of 50 patient days. The HPPD under the current staffing would be:

$$\frac{100 \text{ RN Hours} + 120 \text{ LPN Hours}}{50 \text{ Patient Days}} = 4.4 \text{ HPPD}$$

and the cost per unit of service would be:

100 RN Hours × $35	= $3,500	
120 LPN Hours × $25	= 3,000	
Total Cost	= $6,500	
	÷50 Patient Days	
Cost per Patient Day	$ 130	

If one shifted to an all-RN staff, one could replace the 120 LPN hours with 100 RN hours. The HPPD would then be:

$$\frac{100 \text{ RN Hours} + 100 \text{ RN Hours}}{50 \text{ Patient Days}} = 4.0 \text{ HPPD}$$

The HPPD have fallen from 4.4 to 4.0. But is the unit more productive? What has happened to the cost of care provided?

200 RN Hours × $35 = $7,000
÷50 Patient Days
Cost per Patient Day $ 140

Productivity is difficult to assess in absolute terms. Shifting from a staff with RNs and LPNs to an all-RN staff resulted in fewer required hours of care for each patient day in the previous example. But the cost per patient day rose from $130 to $140. Clearly, measuring productivity based simply on HPPD does not make sense. HPPD can fall while cost per patient rises. One cannot say this makes a unit more productive. On the other hand, productivity measures should take quality of care into consideration. The previous calculations used only direct salary costs per patient day in the formula. Shifting to the all-RN staff did raise the cost per unit of service, but it may also have raised the level of quality of care. When the value of the increased quality is evaluated, it is possible that the nurse manager may discover that ultimately, the costs per patient day will have decreased. For example, if nosocomial infections decreased such that patients suffered fewer unreimbursed complications, the change may have materially reduced the cost of care per patient. So one cannot say clearly that the increased cost per patient day reduced productivity.

On the other hand, one could identify an acceptable level of quality of care. As long as that level of quality is maintained, reductions in the cost per unit of service would be considered to be productivity increases. In the previous example, if the care being provided by 100 RN hours and 120 LPN hours was of acceptable quality, the shift to an all-RN staff would reduce productivity because it increases the cost per patient day. One cannot let traditional productivity measures such as the reduction in HPPD from 4.4 to 4.0 lead to the belief that productivity is improving when the cost per patient day is increasing. Financial resources are too limited to allow for focus solely on measures such as HPPD. The productivity measure provided by cost per unit of service is much more meaningful to managers who are trying to make the best use of their limited financial resources.

Therefore, at least one author has called on health care organizations to shift their measures of productivity toward the cost per unit of service, or unit-costing. This calls for replacing measures of input with measures of cost.[6] Rather than thinking about the HPPD, one could consider the cost per patient day. Similarly, in various situations, it is possible to measure productivity in terms of the cost per patient, cost per procedure, or cost per visit.

For example, consider the case of the nurse practitioner and the rise in productivity percentage from 83% to 90% after the purchase of a computer. Did productivity really rise or fall? Maybe the cost of the computer was greater than the benefit. Suppose that the total costs of the practice for the month (including the salary of the nurse practitioner) without the computer system were $8,000. The computer system was leased for $300 per month (for all hardware and software). The cost of the practice rose from $8,000 to $8,300. What happened to the cost per unit of service? Originally it was

$$\frac{\$8,000 \ Cost}{250 \ Patients} = \$32.00$$

After the computer implementation, the cost per unit of service was

$$\frac{\$8,300 \ Cost}{270 \ Patients} = \$30.74$$

[6] Barron, J. Productivity and cost per unit of service. In Spitzer-Lehmann, R, ed. (1994). *Nursing Management Desk Reference*. Philadelphia: W.B. Saunders, pp. 260-277.

It turns out that productivity has indeed improved as a result of the computer because the cost per visit, even including the cost of the computer, fell from $32.00 to $30.74.

Notice also that the approach of using cost per unit of service does not require the measurement of the number of different resources used. In the example as initially stated, it was assumed that the nurse practitioner worked 100 hours in both situations. Most likely, the number of hours spent seeing patients would vary from month to month. However, it is possible to calculate the productivity of the practice from month to month without having to track the number of hours worked or the amount of other resources used. All that is needed is the total cost for the services provided each month and the number of units of service provided.

On the other hand, the measurement of costs can be complicated. The last chapter in this book looks in some detail at costing-out nursing services. If it is desirable, the methodologies of that chapter can be used to measure costs in a fairly sophisticated manner. However, in many instances, simple measures of cost can be used. For example, an operating room department or outpatient surgery unit can simply divide its total costs by the number of hours of surgery to get a cost per hour or cost per minute. If the cost per hour of surgery falls from month to month, productivity is improving, assuming that case mix is constant. Similarly, a home care agency could calculate the cost per home care visit by dividing total costs by the total number of visits. Such measures can be tracked over time or compared to some budget or standard, as discussed earlier.

The problem with this approach is that one must be willing to accept some averaging. For instance, if a home care agency provides visits by aides, LPNs, and RNs, the average cost per visit may be misleading. What if the number of visits by RNs is falling and the number of visits by aides is rising? It is likely that the cost per visit will fall. But that may not be indicative of true productivity improvement. This is especially so if the profit on RN visits is greater than the profit on visits by aides.

One way to handle such a situation is to divide the costs of the health care unit or organization into separate categories and measure productivity for each category. One could measure the costs of RN visits, costs of LPN visits, and costs of aide visits, and then divide those costs by the number of visits of each type to assess productivity. For example, suppose that the costs for the agency for the month were $100,000 and there were 4,000 visits. One productivity measure would be

$$\frac{\$100,000 \text{ Cost}}{4,000 \text{ Visits}} = \$25 \text{ Cost per Visit}$$

but a more sophisticated approach would be to determine the volume and cost by type of visit and calculate productivity as

$$\frac{\$50,000 \text{ Cost of RN Visits}}{1,000 \text{ RN Visits}} = \$50 \text{ Cost per RN Visit}$$

$$\frac{\$30,000 \text{ Cost of LPN Visits}}{1,000 \text{ LPN Visits}} = \$30 \text{ Cost per LPN Visit}$$

$$\frac{\$20,000 \text{ Cost of Aide Visits}}{2,000 \text{ Aide Visits}} = \$10 \text{ Cost per Aide Visit}$$

Over time one could track changing productivity for each type of visit.

The difficulty in such productivity measurement is in assigning costs to each group. Clearly, the cost of RN visits would include the cost of RNs, the supplies they use, and their travel and charting costs. The problem is determining what share of rent, supervision, billing, and other costs to assign to one group versus the other groups. There is no simple rule for such allocations. Overhead costs can be allocated based on the number of visits (if half the visits are by aides, assign half the overhead to aides) or based on the revenue from visits (if half the revenue comes from RN visits, assign half the overhead to them) or based on a number of other approaches. No one approach is more valid or correct than any other.

Although many organizations use arbitrary ways to allocate overhead or indirect costs, an alternative approach is to ignore overhead costs. Productivity could be measured based on just the direct costs per unit of service. This approach helps to assess productivity improvement or declines related to direct costs. Unfortunately, it does not provide information about changes in productivity in overhead areas of the organization such as the billing department. This is especially important if changes in RN productivity are associated with changes in overhead departments. However, it is possible to measure productivity for overhead separately by measuring things such as the cost per bill issued.

As you can see, productivity measurement is complex. Managers cannot simply apply productivity formulas blindly. Thought must go into deciding how to measure productivity and also how to interpret productivity measures. Nevertheless, unit-costing is feasible. One must define the unit (such as patient day, RN visit, or nurse practitioner treatment) and divide the number of units of service into the cost of providing that service. One can have broad average costs or more specifically measured costs based on approaches discussed in Chapter 18.

Barron nicely summarizes the issue related to productivity measurement as follows: Managers cannot be held to both dollar and hour limits. Either they manage the hours and watch what happens to the dollars, as is the common practice, or they manage the dollars and watch what happens to the hours. Past practice has led to tightly controlled hours and escalating dollars. A dollars per unit of service system tightly controls dollars while allowing flexible hours.[7] Barron's point is important because it focuses on the fact that productivity is unlikely to improve in health care organizations until management changes its thinking. If the goal is to control costs, finance should not persist in holding managers accountable for measures such as HPPD. That thinking stifles innovation instead of encouraging it. Executives who say that they support innovation and creativity but then evaluate employees based on adherence to a measure such as HPPD clearly are not putting their money where their mouths are. They are forgetting that people respond well to the incentives that an organization provides. If the goal is to control spending per visit, per treatment, or per patient, the productivity measurement and evaluation must be based on those units of service as well.

Unit-Costing and Productivity Standards

If unit-costing is used to assess productivity, it is still possible to employ productivity benchmarks or standards. For instance, in the home care agency example referred to

[7] Barron, op. cit., p. 271.

earlier, one could assess the cost of each visit versus a benchmark. If it is believed that the ideal cost per RN visit is $44, one could divide the actual $50 cost (see previous calculation) into the ideal $44 cost as follows:

$$\frac{\$44 \text{ Ideal Cost}}{\$50 \text{ Actual Cost}} \times 100 = 88\% \text{ Productivity}$$

As the actual cost per visit declines, one gets closer to 100% productivity. Such measures require careful thought about what should go in the numerator and denominator to get a meaningful indicator.

Productivity Improvement

For most health care organizations, the focus on productivity does not exist simply for the purpose of measuring the level of productivity. Rather, the concern is with improving productivity. Such improvements can be accomplished by forcing staff to work harder. Generally, however, such efforts are self-defeating. They result in declining morale. Research into human performance has found that people have a work pace with which they are comfortable. The pace varies a bit with each person, but an individual's work pace is thought to be more a function of the individual's biology than either learned or purposeful behavior. Additionally, people can work up to one third faster when necessary. However, it is not possible to sustain those faster work rates for very long. After a short period of time—perhaps a week or so—the individual tires and work rate returns to the normal work pace (McHugh, 1989). True and sustained productivity improvements are a function of reengineering work processes or work technology. Technology may improve productivity directly through labor saving, by changing the type of work to be done, or through the elimination of some work processes. It also improves productivity by improving the quality of work outcomes (Harrison, 2006). What often happens, unfortunately, is that managers insist that employees work harder to improve productivity. Although short-term improvements may be possible as a result of such strategies, in the longer term, declines in productivity may occur as a result of the pressures placed on employees. Further, the quality of care provided is very likely to decline as a result of physical tiredness and the emotional pressure on employees.

Working smarter, not harder, is the key to improving productivity. Productivity measurement should be used to generate information and to follow the progress of serious process-improvement efforts and the introduction of new, productivity-enhancement technology. New technology and process reengineering approaches are likely to result in permanent productivity gains and should not require increased and often unsustainable individual efforts by employees.

The key to working smarter, not harder, lies in changing technology and changing the work processes. Benchmarking, discussed earlier in this chapter, is one approach to improving productivity. Adopting the best practices of others is likely to change care processes in a way that increases productivity by improving quality outcomes. Reengineering, TQM, CQI, rapid-cycle CQI, and value-added approaches similarly are aimed at improving underlying processes. The essence, however, does not lie in the use of one specific technique such as TQM or CQI but rather in a review of the way the organization provides its services.

Managers must be given the time and support necessary to promote change. Productivity improvement will not happen without some kind of change in the way work is accomplished. The organization must foster an environment that encourages change. Managers must know that innovation is expected from them. If the message given to managers is that they are overseers of an existing operation, then they will simply oversee that static provision of care. Improvement is likely to occur only when innovation is actively supported, encouraged, financed, and rewarded.

Productivity improvements also require an understanding of why resources are consumed. It is necessary first to know why an organizational unit exists. What is the mission of the unit or department? Next, the unit must be examined to determine whether all the resources it consumes are really necessary to accomplish that mission. This is not to say that some resources are simply wasted. Rather, one must take a cost/benefit perspective. Are the benefits of each of the unit's activities great enough to justify the costs of those activities? Some long-standing practices may have to be eliminated because their costs have risen so high over the years that they can no longer be justified.

For example, for each activity of the organizational unit, one might ask:

- When is it performed?
- How often is it performed?
- Where is it performed?
- Who is performing it?
- Is it necessary to perform it at all?[8]
- And finally, is there technology that can reduce the cost of this activity?

The answers to these questions may provide the information needed to make changes that will result in productivity increases without substantial reduction in the services provided. One might find that a function always handled by one department has been superceded by an activity now performed with new technology for a lower cost in another department. The old activity not only may be duplicative but also may be providing information inferior to that already available in the other department.

The old saying "It takes money to make money" is as true in health care productivity as it is in high finance. Managers must be given time to work on improving the efficiency and effectiveness of work processes. They must be provided with time and money for travel occasionally if they are to investigate benchmark organizations that have used new technology and reengineered work processes to improve productivity. They must have some money available to pay members of their staff to participate in quality- and productivity-improvement efforts. All too often, non-nurse managers are reluctant to pay for staff release time for these kinds of efforts. Instead, senior management brings in productivity consultants rather than using the intelligence and intimate knowledge of the organization's work processes held by their own staff. Using external consultants may not be a good strategy. The history of quality circles in Japan has shown that few outsiders can produce the productivity improvements that internal staff can bring about, given time and encouragement to work on the problem (Kelly, 2006; Propenko, 2000).

Over time, space needs change as well. Productivity relates to all resources consumed, not just to labor. If the organization is not using space wisely, then it is possible that money is being wasted. Organizations often grow haphazardly. Space is allocated based on immediate necessity rather than on careful planning. It may be

---

[8] Pavlock, op. cit., p. 595.

worth an organization's time to have a space planner examine operations and reallocate space. It is possible that space savings will occur, and that might allow the organization to rent less outside space, thus saving money.

For example, the past decade has seen substantial movement in hospitals from inpatient care to outpatient care. While new outpatient facilities have been built, what has happened to the excess space formerly needed for inpatients? It is possible that much of that space is being used in suboptimal fashion. Spending some money for redesign and even remodeling could result in substantial reductions in the cost of space and could even make provision of care more efficient, resulting in reduced labor costs as well.

At this point we have questioned the need for the organization to exist and have evaluated its activities to see if they could be eliminated or performed differently. The facilities used by the organization have also been considered. Finally, productivity improvement requires careful evaluation of the staff and supplies used. It is often difficult to assess whether staffing patterns are appropriate. Collaborative benchmarking, as discussed earlier, can be helpful. By considering issues such as the number of visits per home care worker at other home care agencies, one can get a sense of the organization's productivity in the use of staff. This information can be a starting point in getting at least a sense of where an organization is on the continuum of resource consumption.

However, it is critical to keep in mind that collaborative benchmarking results in "how much" information rather than "how" information. Many consulting firms tell health care providers that they can provide their services with fewer staff because others do so, but they don't provide the "how" piece of information. It may be that there are unique factors relating to the organization's physical structure, patient mix, or even culture that make direct application of another facility's staffing structure an extremely poor decision.

For example, suppose that abortions are relatively inexpensive compared to other obstetrical procedures. Hospitals that perform more abortions in their labor and delivery departments need fewer RNs per 1,000 patients than hospitals that perform fewer abortions. Suppose that a hospital that performs many abortions has a ratio of 2 RNs per 1,000 obstetrical procedures. Suppose further that the average hospital that does some abortions uses 2.5 RNs per 1,000. A consultant tells a Catholic hospital that does no abortions that best practice for obstetrics calls for the use of 2 RNs per 1,000 procedures. The Catholic hospital currently has a ratio of 2.7 RNs per 1,000. How useful is that information? Not very. And it may be destructive if top management blindly calls for departments to use benchmarked data without an understanding of how the numbers were achieved. Productivity improvement requires careful analysis rather than simplistic pursuit of targets that are not well understood.

Finally, supplies and equipment should also be considered when an organization is trying to assess productivity improvement. For example, a thorough review of the process related to supplies may find that the hospital does not get the best buy on supplies. Or it may show that it does get good prices but purchases too much and then has to dispose of some supplies that have reached their expiration dates. Or it may show that the hospital buys the correct amount but has trouble distributing the supplies to the places where they are needed, when they are needed, creating bottlenecks that delay patient treatment. Often, productivity improvement requires nothing more than a careful examination of how the organization does things, a determination of where problems are occurring, and development and implementation of solutions to avoid the problems in the future.

Where is room for productivity improvement found? Pavlock notes that "scheduling modifications for patients, staff and physicians are probably the most important way to improve the overall productivity."[9] This requires a delicate balance. Patients do not like to wait for care. However, if caregivers have to wait for patients to arrive, they are being paid for time when they are not productive. This problem is exacerbated by the fact that it takes different amounts of time to treat different patients, and the time needed for any one specific patient cannot be anticipated accurately in advance.

All productivity improvement efforts should include a component to ensure that quality is not negatively impacted. Productivity measures implicitly assume that quality is held constant. If a car maker shifts from producing luxury sedans to economy models, the cost per car made will decline. However, that doesn't represent a productivity gain. The company is simply making a different, less expensive product. In health care, it is incorrect to consider a reduction in hours or cost per treatment to be a productivity gain if it was accomplished by reducing quality.

■ COST-BENEFIT AND COST-EFFECTIVENESS ANALYSIS

Cost-benefit analysis (CBA) and cost-effectiveness analysis (CEA) are methods that are used to consider the advantages and disadvantages of decisions. These techniques are often used in assessing the implementation of best practices based on a benchmarking study or other changes designed to improve productivity. They are employed in a variety of other situations as well.

CBA is a method that compares the benefits related to a decision to the costs of that decision. The method holds that the decision makes sense if the benefits related to the decision will exceed the costs. In terms of numbers, if

$$\frac{\text{Benefits}}{\text{Costs}} > 1$$

the project has a positive benefit/cost ratio and adds value. In order to determine the ratio, it is necessary to assign values to both the costs and the benefits in monetary terms. In practice, it is difficult to assign monetary values to health care outcomes. We have trouble measuring the value of a life and even more difficulty measuring the difference in health outcomes that do not involve life or death.

CEA is not as ambitious as CBA in that it does not require a measurement of the value of the benefits. Rather, it relies on using comparisons. One considers whether a project is cost-effective in comparison with some alternative approach. An approach that achieves a specific desired outcome for the least possible cost is considered to be cost-effective.

Cost-Benefit Analysis

Cost-benefit analysis, as its name implies, compares the costs and benefits of an action or program. The method is used primarily by the government because it can take into

[9] Ibid., p. 597.

account not only private costs and benefits but public ones as well. However, many health care organizations use the method. Cost-benefit analysis has been defined as being an

> analytical technique that compares the social costs and benefits of proposed programs or policy actions. All losses and gains experienced by society are included and measured in dollar terms. The net benefits created by an action are calculated by subtracting the losses incurred by some sectors of society from the gains that accrue to others. Alternative actions are compared, so as to choose one or more that yield the greatest net benefits, or ratio of benefits to costs. The inclusion of all gains and losses to society in cost-benefit analysis distinguishes it from cost-effectiveness analysis, which is a more limited view of costs and benefits.[10]

In the minds of many people, cost-benefit analysis is associated with large-scale public projects such as the building of a dam. However, the technique can be extremely useful even for evaluating small purchases such as a personal computer. Health care **policy makers** will be likely to include the impact on society in their cost-benefit analyses. Health care **managers** are more likely to focus specifically on the impact of a decision on their organization.

All organizations attempt to determine if the benefits from spending money will exceed the costs. If the benefits do outweigh the costs, it makes sense to spend the money; otherwise it does not. Careful measurement of costs and benefits provides the information needed to support a spending decision.

There are several key elements in performing a cost-benefit analysis:

- Determine project goals.
- Estimate project benefits.
- Estimate project costs.
- Discount cost and benefit flows at an appropriate rate.
- Complete the decision analysis.

Determine Project Goals
In order to determine the benefits, it is first necessary to understand what the organization hopes the project will accomplish. So identification of goals and objectives is essential. Suppose that a home care agency is trying to decide whether it should acquire a van that would drop off nurses and aides at patients' homes. The first question is: why does it believe that it would be better off with a van? The goals may be few or numerous, depending on the specific situation. Perhaps staff currently have difficulty parking. They spend a lot of time searching for parking and often incur parking tickets for illegal parking because there are no legal spaces available. The agency may wish to reduce the cost of parking lots and parking tickets and to save the time staff spend searching for parking.

Estimate Project Benefits
Once the goals have been identified, the specific amount of the benefits must be estimated. The benefits should include only the incremental benefits that result from

[10] J.L. Mikesell. (1995). *Fiscal Administration—Analysis and Application for the Public Sector*, ed 4. Fort Worth, TX: Harcourt Brace College Publishers, pp. 559-560.

the project. For instance, the manager would not include the benefit of providing existing services to existing customers because the services are already provided. However, if freeing up staff time allows for more patients to be cared for, the revenue from that extra service should be included in the analysis. Benefits may also arise from cost reductions. All additional benefits should be considered, estimated, and included in the cost-benefit calculation.

In the home care agency example, it is likely that the manager will be able to calculate the benefits fairly directly. For example, the agency may have logs showing travel time separately from visit time. It can use that information to calculate the labor cost of time spent by staff searching for parking. It certainly knows the amount it currently pays for parking lots and parking tickets. Measurement of other benefits is more complicated. If the agency is able to see more patients, the benefit would really be the profit from those additional patients, rather than the entire revenue.

Estimate Project Costs

Projects have costs as well as benefits, and those costs must also be estimated as part of the cost-benefit analysis. In the case of the van, the primary costs relate to the acquisition of the van and the labor cost of the driver. However, care should be exercised to include all costs, such as the cost of gasoline and maintaining the vehicle. Some consideration is also needed for coverage when the driver is sick or on vacation. In cost-benefit analysis it is also critical to consider opportunity costs—the fact that when a decision is made to do something, other alternatives are sacrificed. In the case of buying a van, the agency buys the van with cash that might have been used to pay rent on a new office location in an adjoining community. Perhaps the money in that alternative use would generate many more patients and great amounts of additional revenues and profits.

Discount Cost and Benefit Flows

Often project benefits and costs occur over a period of years. This creates a calculation problem because money has a different value at different times. Money is more valuable today than the same amount of money in the future. If one pays $40,000 for a van today and receives $15,000 of net benefits per year over the 4-year life of the van, one cannot compare the $40,000 to the sum of $15,000 for 4 years. At a minimum, the agency could have invested the $40,000 and earned interest each year.

This creates a problem in comparing benefits and costs. They cannot simply be totaled for the life of the project and then compared to see if the benefits exceed the costs. The timing is critical. This is especially true because projects often have higher costs in early years and higher benefits in later years. Simple addition of total benefits and total costs could lead to improper decisions. The approach to dealing with the problem is referred to as "discounting cash flows." This approach uses an interest rate, referred to as the discount rate, to convert all costs and benefits into their value at the present time. See Time Value of Money in the Appendix to Chapter 10 for additional discussion related to the discounting of future cash flows.

Complete the Decision Analysis

Once all the relevant costs and benefits of a project have been estimated and adjusted in a discounting process, they can be compared to each other in the form of a ratio. Generally, benefits are divided by costs. If the result is greater than 1, it means that the benefits exceed the costs and the project is desirable. The greater the benefit-to-cost ratio, the more desirable the project.

Cost-Effectiveness Analysis

As noted earlier, an approach that achieves a specific desired outcome for the least possible cost is considered to be cost-effective. If one does not have a basis for comparison, difficulties occur. Consider, for example, a project that will save lives. If one knows that it is possible to save lives at a cost of $50 per life, would it be considered cost-effective? Certainly. However, in drawing such a conclusion, one is implicitly placing at least a minimum value on a human life by implying it is worth more than $50. This creates difficulty in trying to establish a cutoff point. Is a project that saves lives at a cost of $10,000 per life cost-effective? How about $1 million per life? How about a cost of $1 billion per life saved?

Some might argue that there are many alternative options that could save lives for less than $1 billion per life saved. Therefore, the project that costs $1 billion per life is not cost-effective. In comparison with alternatives, the billion-dollar-per-life project costs more to accomplish the outcome of saving lives than alternatives cost. The problem with assuming that $50 per life saved is cost-effective is that it puts a value on the benefit rather than simply holding the benefit constant. A more CEA-oriented approach would consider different methods of saving a life and find out which one costs least. That would be the cost-effective alternative.

Therefore, to operationalize CEA, one must compare alternatives that generate similar outcomes. For example, suppose that a hospital has been treating a certain type of patient using a particular approach. Now an alternative approach is suggested. Is the new approach cost-effective? One must first establish that the clinical outcomes are equal. Then one must show that the new approach costs less money than the old approach. If a new approach generates the exact same outcome for less money, then it is cost-effective.

Note how this avoids the problem of measuring the value of the benefits. Because the benefits are held constant, any approach that costs less must inherently be superior to other approaches. In reality, however, it is difficult to find different techniques that yield the exact same health care outcomes.

As a result, researchers have developed a variety of techniques to enable the comparison of outcomes across interventions, conditions, and diseases. Researchers have been able to model the long-term effects of clinical treatments on patients. With this ability, CEA can now go beyond simple comparisons of the cost per life saved to more precise comparisons of cost per life-years saved, cost per quality-adjusted life-years, and cost per disability-adjusted life-years. The latter two outcome measures assume that a life-year in a fully functional state is different from (more valuable than) a life-year in an impaired state.

Will this approach work in all cases? No. It is possible for an alternative to yield an improved health benefit but to cost more. Will that approach be deemed cost-effective? No, even though the improved health may be worth the extra cost, it is not considered cost-effective because it costs more. CEA is limited to evaluating less costly alternatives with at least the same outcome. It cannot comment on the advisability of more costly alternatives that provide better outcomes.

Finally, many managed care programs are looking at CEA as a guide for deciding what treatments will be covered. CEA provides information to assist in decision making. It does not provide the answer. Although strictly allocating resources based on the results of CEAs may be problematic politically or ethically, CEA at least brings information to the table to inform the decision-making process. If an alternative is shown to be cost-effective, then we know that it is a superior alternative because we get at least as good a result for a lower cost.

Summary and Implications for Nurse Managers

Budgeting in the 21st century requires a lot more than simply "minding the store." Nurse managers must find ways to improve the performance of their units proactively. To do this, managers can benefit by understanding productivity and productivity measurement and by using the techniques of benchmarking and cost-benefit and cost-effectiveness analysis.

How does an organization get to be outstanding? It must foster and facilitate innovation and improvement. Unless there is an environment that is supportive and even encouraging of change, progress is likely to be hampered severely. Many organizations like to say that they believe in innovation, but the culture they create stifles change rather than rewarding it. Suggestions for change are viewed as criticism of the way top management is doing its job. Often, such criticism is not welcomed. Staff quickly learn that it is wiser to be quiet and allow the waste and inefficiency they observe to continue. It should not be surprising that the most significant changes in organizations occur only after the top management has been replaced. At those times the new top management can admit openly to problems and the need for change. After all, the existing problems can be attributed to those who have just left.

For change to occur, it is critically important for managers to assess their current situations. The better existing processes are understood, the easier it is to be willing to take the risk of replacing some of them. Benchmarking is an invaluable aid, especially for organizations that are looking to make quick, significant improvement. The task of undertaking a benchmarking study is involved and can be costly. Most organizations are well advised to use benchmarking (at least competitive and cooperative benchmarking) only when they feel there is potentially room for significant improvement.

The true benefit of benchmarking does not come from knowing **how much** the benchmarking organization differs from the best practices organization that it studies. The benefit comes from an understanding of **how** it differs. Knowing that another organization has a lower cost does not really motivate managers to match that cost. It frustrates them because they have no idea how to match that cost. Clear efforts must be made to ensure that benchmarking is not just a tool for leverage to try to make staff work harder. Benchmarking should be used to show the way to true improvements in productivity.

Productivity assesses the amount of inputs needed to produce an organization's outputs. Health care organizations must work constantly on reducing the resources needed to provide high-quality patient care. Such improvements may come about through implementation of technological change or through low-tech changes in procedures. Nurse managers must develop an approach to measuring productivity so that changes in productivity can be monitored. And the measure should be meaningful. As discussed in the chapter, measures such as hours per patient day may be inadequate. If the real goal of improved productivity is to decrease the cost per patient, that goal must be incorporated into the measurement. One approach is to focus on unit-costing. Ultimately, however, it is not measurement but improvement in productivity that is essential for healthy organizations.

Two techniques that are sometimes used by managers to help assess whether changes are likely to improve productivity are cost-benefit and cost-effectiveness analysis. Cost-benefit analysis is a technique that compares the benefits of a change to its costs. If the benefits are greater than the costs, the change is worthwhile. Often, however, managers will not be able to measure benefits. Benefits are particularly hard to value when human life is involved. What is a life really worth?

Cost-effectiveness analysis has an appeal because it requires only that the manager estimate costs. In the cost-effectiveness approach, an alternative is evaluated to see whether it produces at least as good a benefit as another alternative but for a lower cost. Nurse managers may frequently find themselves faced with whether or not to make a change in the way a unit or organization does something. CEA is helpful because if the change will keep results at least as good as they currently are, the analysis needs to focus only on whether the change will cost less.

References and Suggested Readings

Allred, C.A., Arford, P.H., Mauldin, P.D., Goodwin, L.K. (1998). Cost-effectiveness analysis in the nursing literature, 1992–1996. *Image— the Journal of Nursing Scholarship.* 30(3), 235-242.

Amalberti, R., Auroy, Y., Berwick, D., Barach, P. (2005). Five system barriers to achieving ultrasafe health care. *Annals of Internal Medicine.* 142(9), 756-764.

American Society for Quality (ASQ). (2006). Benchmarking. Excerpted from Camp, R.C. (1989). *Benchmarking: The Search for Industry Best Practices That Lead to Superior Performance.* Milwaukee: American Society for Quality Control.

Buerhaus, P.I. (1998). Milton Weinstein's insights on the development, use, and methodologic problems in cost-effectiveness analysis. *Image—the Journal of Nursing Scholarship.* 30(3), 223-227.

Disney Institute. (2006). *The Disney Approach to Quality Service for Healthcare Professionals.* Downloaded on November 22, 2006 from: http://www.mlgma.org/scholarship/Disney%20 quality%20service.pdf

Ellis, J. (2006). All-inclusive benchmarking. *Journal of Nursing Management.* 14(5), 377-383.

Finkler, S.A. (1986). Productivity measurement. *Hospital Cost Accounting Advisor.* 1(8), 1-4.

Hampton, T. (2006). Performance measurements stressed as benchmarks for improving US health care. *Journal of the American Medical Association.* 295(3), 264.

Harrison, J. (2006). The role of clinical information systems in health care quality improvement. *The Health Care Manager.* 25(3), 206-212.

Horngren, C.T., Datar, S.M., Foster, G. (2005). *Cost Accounting: A Managerial Emphasis,* ed 12. Englewood Cliffs, NJ: Prentice-Hall.

Infoline. (1992). Understanding benchmarking: The search for best practice. *American Society for Training and Development,* 92(7), 5-6.

John, L., Eeckhout, L. (2005). *Performance Evaluation and Benchmarking.* Boca Raton, FL: CRC Press.

Kelly, M. *Electronic Manufacturing and Packaging in Japan.* Report of National Science Foundation Cooperative Agreement ENG-9217849, Loyola University, Maryland. Downloaded on December 5, 2006 from: http://www.wtec.org/loyola/pdf/ep.pdf.

McHugh, M. (1989). Measuring productivity in nursing. *Journal of Applied Nursing Research.* 2(2), 99-102.

Mikesell, J.L. (2002). *Fiscal Administration— Analysis and Applications for the Public Sector,* ed 6. Fort Worth, TX: Harcourt Brace College Publishers.

Mittelman, M., Haley, W., Clay, O., Roth, D. (2006). Improving care-giver well-being delays nursing home placement of patients with Alzheimer disease. *Neurology,* 67(9), 1592-1599.

Mylotte, J., Keagle, J. (2005). Benchmarks for antibiotic use and cost in long-term care. *Journal of the American Geriatrics Society.* 53(7), 1117-1122.

Patterson, P. (1986). Mastering the fundamentals of OR productivity monitoring. *OR-Manager.* 2(2), 1, 6-7.

Pavlock, E.J. (2002). *Financial Management for Medical Groups,* ed 2. Englewood, CO: Center for Research in Ambulatory Health Care Administration.

Platt, R. (2005). Toward better benchmarking. *Infection Control and Hospital Epidemiology,* 26(5), 433-434.

Pierre, J. (2006). Staff nurses' use of report card data for quality improvement: First steps. *Journal of Nursing Care Quality,* 21(1), 8-14.

Propenko, J. (2000). *Productivity Promotion Organizations: Evolution and Experience.* Productivity and Management Development Programme of the International Labour Organization. Downloaded on December 1, 2006 from: http://www.ilo.org/public/english/employment/ent/papers/npo.htm.

Talmor, D., Shapiro, N., Greenberg, D., Stone, P., Neumann, P. (2006). When is critical care medicine cost-effective? A systematic review of the cost-effectiveness literature. *Critical Care Medicine,* 34(11), 2738-2747.

University HealthSystem Consortium. (2006). *Five Members Receive Top-Performer Awards at 2006 Quality and Safety Fall Forum.* Oak Brook, IL: University HealthSystem Consortium. Downloaded on December 1, 2006 from: http:// public. uhc.edu/pmail/fulla.asp?folder=publicweb/ uhcnews/2006/nov06&file=003709915.asp.

University HealthSystem Consortium. (2006). *Recognized as Top Performers in the 2006 UHC Quality and Accountability Ranking.* Oak Brook, IL: University HealthSystem Consortium. Downloaded on December 1, 2006 from: http://public.uhc.edu/publicweb/About/Resources/All5PressRelease.pdf.

Wilson, C.K. (1998). Implementing best practices. *Aspen's Advisor for Nurse Executives.* 13(5), 2.

Costing Out Nursing Services

LEARNING OBJECTIVES
The goals of this chapter are to:

- Discuss the various reasons for costing out nursing
- Explain why costing nursing was not always done
- Consider the potential role of computers in costing out nursing
- Identify patient classification systems as one basis for costing out nursing

- Discuss the use of DRGs in costing nursing
- Provide a specific RVU approach and example for costing out nursing services
- Discuss the limitations of an RVU approach
- Introduce product-line costing and budgeting

■ INTRODUCTION

As financial pressures faced by health care organizations continue to grow, the focus on costing out nursing services has increased. Ideally, by costing out nursing, one would like to find the dollar value of the resources consumed to provide nursing care. However, this is a complex problem—one in which even the goals are unclear.

The goal is not to find out what it costs a facility to employ a nurse. The purpose is to find out the cost of providing nursing services to patients. However, it is well known that the cost of providing nursing care varies by patient acuity, type of surgical procedure, primary diagnosis, and by diagnosis plus comorbidities. The facility may need to know the cost of providing nursing care per patient day or per acuity-adjusted patient day. It may need to know the cost per hour or even the cost per minute in a unit such as the operating room. It may need to know the cost per diagnosis-related group (DRG), and clinics and other ambulatory care facilities may need to know the cost per visit.

The cost per patient (or visit or treatment) is the simplest approach. It merely requires dividing total nursing costs by the number of patients (or visits or treatments). However, this method provides little information to aid management in decision making. Knowing the cost per patient tells the manager little about which types of patients require particularly costly nursing care services—nor does it provide information about why those patients incurred higher costs.

Acuity-adjusted measures attempt to separate patients into homogeneous groups for staffing and costing purposes. This information is more sophisticated. For example, the cost for a day at patient classification level 1 can be distinguished from a day at level 2 or 3. However, one must consider whether the organization makes decisions about groups of patients in a particular patient classification level.

Hospitals, for example, are more likely to make decisions on the basis of DRGs for two reasons. First, DRGs are groupings used for setting prices or charges. Second, decisions can be made about whether to provide care for patients with particular DRGs. A hospital could decide it is losing a lot of money on open-heart surgery and stop offering the associated DRGs. A DRG is, in effect, a form of a service line, and hospitals can and do make decisions about what services to offer. It would not be feasible for a hospital to decide that it loses money on patients when they are at patient classification level 3 and to decide to treat patients only when they are classified as 1, 2, and 4.

The problem of costing nursing services in hospitals is extremely complex, partially because of the complexity of nursing care and the fact that when patients need supplies and treatments, it is often through the nurse that these resources are consumed. In addition, patients' needs for nursing care change throughout hospitalization, so the calculation of nursing hours of care for even one patient is not a simple matter. Costs, whether based on an acuity-adjusted patient day approach or a DRG approach, can be either resource-based or based on direct care hours. If resource-based costing is done, resource consumption data must be collected for each patient or patient group. The problem with this approach is that nursing hours are very costly, and resource consumption may not adequately reflect nursing care hours. For example, a patient receiving an extremely expensive medication may not otherwise require more care than the average patient, but the resource consumption will be extremely high. On the other hand, a patient who requires many more hours of nursing care than average may not otherwise consume many resources. An example of this might be a patient who becomes extremely agitated or combative due to an untoward drug reaction. Such a patient may need three or four nurses to restrain him or her until either the reaction passes or another medication counteracts the side effects of the first drug. But otherwise, that patient may use very few resources.

An hourly approach entails applying a standard charge per hour of nursing care consumed to each patient or patient group. The hourly charge includes all nursing costs. In this case, only hours of care are collected or, more typically, the hours are calculated based on the patient's acuity score. Data related to resources consumed are not used for costing nursing services. The hourly approach is used by most lawyers and accountants in their practices.

If nurse managers want to budget the appropriate number of staff and other resources for the patients they expect to encounter, they must know the cost of providing nursing care to various types of patients. The characteristics of patients that make a difference in the cost of providing nursing is crucial. In order to cost by nursing hours of care, the following questions must be answered: What are the key determinants of how much nursing care a patient needs? Can patients be grouped by nursing resource requirements? What costing approaches exist and how technically and financially feasible are they? These issues are the subject of this chapter.

■ WHY STUDY THE COST OF NURSING SERVICES?

The original impetus for developing advanced methods of costing nursing services was a desire to "take nursing out of the room-and-board side of the ledger and put it on the revenue-producing side."[1] Historically, nursing has not been treated as a

---

[1] Shaffer, Franklin A. (1985). *Costing out Nursing: Pricing Our Product.* New York, NY: National League for Nursing, p. 5.

revenue center in health care. Instead, it has been included in the per diem charge in hospitals, along with hotel-type costs for room and meals or in the overall fee for most other types of health care organizations. This has created many misconceptions. Some administrators view nursing costs as a burden—a substantial outlay that does not generate revenue.

Such a perspective is clearly incorrect. The presence of the nursing staff and the quality of nursing care offered are critical factors in attracting patients to an institution. In fact, medical services traditionally provided in hospitals that can be provided without the benefit of the intensive nursing services have all been moved to the outpatient setting—and most outpatient settings are extremely dependent upon expert nursing services to operate. Without quality nursing care there would be no revenue. Nevertheless, without some costing mechanism superior to the one historically used, nursing cannot be treated as a revenue center. This causes the "burden" view to persist.[2] To address this problem, many researchers started trying to develop costing methods that would allow nursing to become a revenue center.

The more nurse managers understand the nature of the nursing services that are provided to patients and what it costs to provide those services, the better the position they are in to control those costs. Many health care organizations are in critical financial positions because the profit margins are very low, even for most successful hospitals. Although profit margins of 10% to 15% are not out of the ordinary for manufacturing and retail businesses, average hospital profit margins range from a low of –33% to a high of 5.8%, and the highest profit margins in the industry were just over 10% (Bazzoli, 2006; Griffith et al., 2006; Solucient, 2006). To survive, health care facilities must know which patients generate profits and which generate losses. Even if they feel morally bound not to turn away patients who generate losses, added knowledge can allow them to focus marketing attention on patients who are profitable. The profits made from those patients can then support the care of the remaining patients. Therefore, efficient management requires that nurse managers understand costs by type of patient.

■ CURRENT COSTING APPROACHES

The essence of the costing problem is that in most hospitals, nursing costs are charged to patients as part of the daily room rate rather than being charged separately on the patient's bill. As a result, all patients receive the same charge for nursing care services. In terms of providing management with an understanding of the cost implications of various patients, this provides extremely poor information. It implicitly assumes that all patients consume exactly the same amount of nursing care, even though different patients have different nursing care requirements.

Why has costing for nursing care taken this direction to begin with? In order to charge different amounts to different patients, it must be possible to determine varying amounts of resource consumption for the various patients. In some areas it would be virtually impossible to measure differential consumption. For example, how much of the chief financial officer's time is consumed by each patient? One would be hard-pressed to show that patients receive differing amounts of benefit from the chief financial officer. Even if they did, it would be impossible to measure.

---

[2] There are political and power issues related to this "burden" view. However, they are beyond the scope of this book.

In the case of nursing, however, patients do consume different amounts of nursing resources. This is particularly true for inpatient settings because nursing requirements vary considerably with individual patients. Nevertheless, until the decade of the 1980s, measuring differential consumption was if not impossible, at least too costly to consider. Hospitals are faced with two extreme alternatives. One choice is to take the total annual cost of nursing care and divide that by the number of patients treated for the year to come out with an average cost per patient. At the other extreme, the hospital could hire a data collector to follow each nurse and determine exactly how much of that nurse's time was used by each patient. Figure 18-1 reflects this extreme choice. Alternative A is a simple and inexpensive approach at one extreme. Alternative Z is an extremely detailed and expensive approach at the other extreme.

What hospital could afford to assign a data collector to each nurse to observe how much of the nurse's time was being devoted to each patient? The value of information should always justify its cost. Alternative Z in Figure 18-1 is too costly to undertake. Figure 18-2 adds a compromise. In most cases, a patient with a 3-day length of stay would consume less nursing care than a patient with a 15-day length of stay. If total nursing care costs are divided by total patient days, patients who are in the hospital for more days can be assigned more nursing cost than patients who are in the hospital for fewer days. This is Alternative B. It is still not nearly as precise and accurate an approach as Alternative Z. However, it is not much more expensive than Alternative A, and it provides a much better approximation of the nursing care costs of a variety of patients.

However, under Alternative B, the approach most hospitals use, the nursing cost is assumed to be the same for all patient days. More days imply more cost, but for the same number of patient days, all patients are assumed to use the same amount of nursing care. Although this is much better than Alternative A, it is still a poor measure of nursing cost. The varying acuity levels of patients mean that there are varying amounts of nursing care per patient day.

■ SOLUTIONS FOR THE COSTING PROBLEM

Computerization of the Costing Process

How can the cost of each individual patient be better measured without having an accountant follow every nurse? One solution that many hospitals are beginning to examine is computerization. The addition of computers, not only at nursing stations but also next to each bedside, is seen by many nurses to be the future for all hospitals. Many hospitals have already installed bedside computer terminals.

There are a variety of uses for such computers. Although full computerization of all paperwork, such as nursing and physician records of care, laboratory and radiology results, dietary and other clinical services, is proceeding in many hospitals throughout the country, systems have not yet been used to track nursing activity and to cost out nursing care. Much of the work nurses do to improve the quality and safety of patient care is cognitive and not easily captured by a computer. For example, when a nurse goes into a patient's room to start an IV or to hang a new IV bag, a strict evaluation of the time required will not take account of the fact that the nurse also looks at the patient's skin, feels the temperature of the skin and the elasticity of the skin as an assessment of hydration and nutrition, looks at the patient's face for

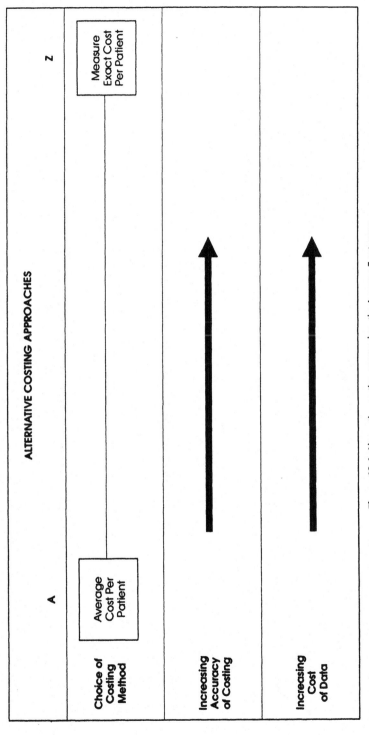

Figure 18-1 Alternative costing approaches: the A versus Z extremes.

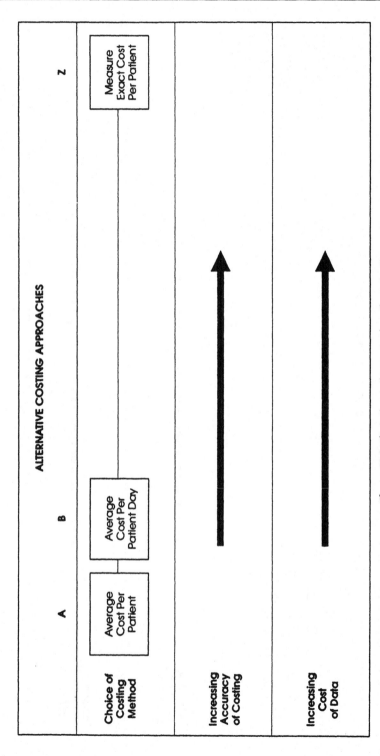

Figure 18-2 Alternative costing approaches: Alternative B.

signs of distress, talks to the patient, and performs other activities that are not recorded in a note about starting or hanging an IV.

The major reason so many management engineers' attempts to determine the amount of nursing time per patient have failed is that engineers are not trained in patient assessment, so they have no idea of the importance of that type of work. When they design staffing algorithms that exclude time for those activities, there are two bad results. First, patient mortality rates increase because nurses are assigned to so many patients that they no longer have time for those cognitive and assessment activities (Aiken et al., 2002; Aiken, Smith, & Lake, 1994). Second, costs increase because nurses are so dissatisfied with the quality of their work and the lack of time to provide the quality patient care they learned in school that they leave the hospital and sometimes the profession. Therefore, computers will be much better able to assist in measuring the nursing resources expended on each patient when algorithms are developed that account for the cognitive and assessment work of nurses. At that point, the computer should be able to track sophisticated data on nursing resource usage by patient.

In Figure 18-3, computers have been added to the continuum from low-accuracy, low-cost information to high-accuracy, high-cost information. This alternative has been labeled Y. With computers, nurses record not only when they are with each patient but also what they are doing for each patient. The specific cost of the nurse giving care can be associated with the patient by having the computer multiply the time spent by the salary of the particular nurse providing the care. When nurses are doing some indirect activities, such as documenting a patient's care, the computer can also assign that cost to the appropriate patient because the documentation is being done on the computer.

The system will need a fast way to record the data so that it does not greatly increase the documentation work of the nurse. Radio frequency identification (RFID) chips may eventually assist with that task. An RFID chip embedded in the nurse's name tag can be detected by a sensor in the door frame. The sensor is a data receiver that transmits information to the computer. Specifically, it records the times of the nurse's entry into and exit from the patient's room and links that information with the patient's hospital ID number. (This technology is not yet sufficiently advanced to determine whether it can be used for patients in double rooms or in other situations in which the patient is not in a private room.) Links between the Nurse Activity Program and the electronic patient record allow the nurse to record the patient care activities via voice data entry or screen formats that provide a menu of nursing care activities. The nurse can then very quickly record the care provided during that visit using voice data entry, a touch screen, or a mouse click. RFID technology for such uses is still under development. However, the Wal-Mart company is investing in developing the programming and technology to advance RFID technology to the individual product level. When those advances are completed, RFID chips will allow much finer tracking than is possible at present. This means that RFID technology cannot yet be used to track nurse-patient time measurements, but this technology deficit will be rectified by the year 2010 or sooner.

Substantial progress is currently being made in a variety of areas to ease the input of data into the computer. Uniform price codes (bar coding) have become more widely used for a variety of supplies consumed by health care organizations. Many employee identification cards now carry a magnetic strip containing the employee number in computer-readable form. This allows nurses to slide their cards into the

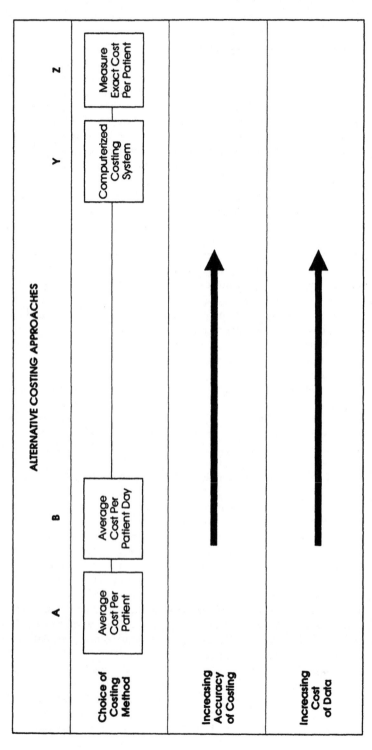

Figure 18-3 Alternative costing approaches: Alternative Y.

computer to identify themselves. However, the magnetic strips will probably be replaced with RFID chips in the near future. Light pens have been replaced by touch-sensitive screens. Such screens allow the user to simply touch a particular item on the screen to select menu choices and enter data. The result of progress in computer software design is that bedside terminals or other computers could be programmed to capture accurately most of the costs (both the direct costs and many of the indirect costs) of providing nursing care to specific patients.

Note that Alternative Y is close to Alternative Z in several respects. The data to be gained are potentially accurate and clearly can be patient-specific. When a patient requires the presence of a nurse at the bedside for substantial amounts of time, that cost will be captured passively, that is, without the nurse's having to document nursing care time along with activities in the patient's records. Future systems may well be programmed to assign different patients costs (and ultimately charges) based on their differing consumption of nursing resources. Even if payment methodologies change such that charges are no longer relevant (e.g., if national health insurance is implemented in the United States), there will still be a need to calculate the costs of nursing care because any payment methodology, regardless of the payer, ultimately requires an accounting of the costs of care.

Current Solutions

Another approach to estimating the cost of nursing care is a *patient classification system*. Patient classification systems require rating patients based on their likely nursing resource requirements according to their acuity. Sicker patients requiring more nursing care are assigned higher acuity or higher classification levels. Many hospitals have developed their own systems, and several commercial systems are widely used in hospitals throughout the United States. Patients are rated on scales, such as 1 to 5. Patient classification systems were discussed in Chapter 8.

Nonhospital health care organizations also have a variety of approaches for classifying patients by resource consumption. However, they often focus on physician time or total resources. Work is needed to improve the ability to assess nursing resource consumption by various types of patients in various types of health care organizations.

Patient classifications are not perfectly accurate measures of the resources needed for each patient. Some patients classified as level 2 patients will require more care than level 2 calls for, and some level 2 patients will require less care than would be expected based on that classification. However, if the system is functioning reasonably well, average patient resource consumption will match that which is expected on the basis of the classification system. And certainly it would generally be expected that a level 2 patient will consume resources closer to the level 2 average than to the level 1 average or the level 3 average.

If a mechanism to cost out patients based on their patient classification can be established, it will not provide the precise accuracy of Alternative Z. It will not even provide the Alternative Y accuracy that a computer system can generate. However, it can create a new alternative, called X (see Figure 18-4). Alternative X is inaccurate in that all patients are assigned the same nursing cost for a day at the same classification level. If two patients are both level 2 on a given day, their costs are assumed to be the same, even though it is known that they will probably not consume exactly the same nursing resources. However, Alternative X is much more accurate than Alternatives A and B. Alternative B assumes that the cost is the same per patient day for all patients, regardless of acuity.

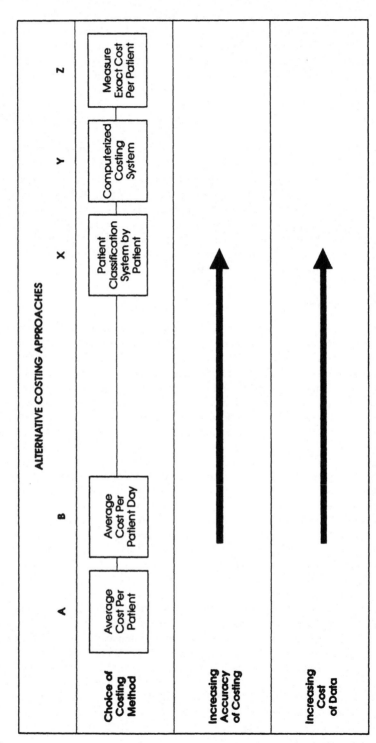

Figure 18-4 Alternative costing approaches: Alternative X.

Alternative X is an improvement because the cost is considered to be the same per patient day only for patients on the same acuity level. Different costs are assigned to patient days at different acuity levels. Users of Alternative X must recognize that the information has some degree of inaccuracy. However, the system may be accurate enough, given the current high costs of using either Alternative Y or Z. Therefore, patient classification systems can be the basis for a system that allows for more accurate estimates of the costs a hospital incurs for nursing care for different types of patients.

Somewhere between X and Y on the scale from A to Z, one could place workload measurement tools. These are variants of patient classification. Workload measurement tools attempt to determine the nursing care time required for each individual patient each day. The approach of these tools is to identify the time required for each of the types of nursing interventions that take up most of the nurses' time. Each patient is evaluated each day to determine which interventions are needed. Thus, such tools can track required care hours specific to each patient. This is contrasted with patient classification systems that use an average hour figure for all patients within a broad category or level of care.

Such an approach is not as sophisticated as Alternative Y, in which the actual care hours are entered into the computer as the patient receives the care. It is likely that some interventions will take longer than typical for some patients and less time for others. Therefore, the cost ultimately assigned to the patient will be based on average times, not actual times. However, the approach to workload measurement is more sophisticated than that of Alternative X, which uses average nursing care hours for all patients in a given patient classification category.

It would appear that some hospital administrators understand less about the importance of nursing care than does the public at large. As a result of public concerns about patient safety and quality of nursing care, 11 states have enacted laws or regulations that govern nurse-patient ratios, and another 18 states have introduced similar legislation (ANA, 2005)

The traditional model of paying for nursing services makes the implicit assumption that there is a strong association between medical care (e.g., DRGs) and the intensity of nursing care. Recent research has demonstrated the fallacy of that assumption. A study by John Welton (2006) found highly variable consumption of nursing resources among patients in the same specialty units. Therefore, the reality is that nurses do discriminate among patient care requirements and provide different levels of nursing care to patients. Given the growing body of evidence that nursing care levels and patient mortality rates are negatively correlated (Aiken et al., 2002; Aiken, Smith & Lake, 1994; Altman, Clancy, & Blendon, 2004; IOM, 2003; Needleman & Buerhaus, 2003; Stanton & Rutherford, 2004), the public and governmental demand that adequate levels of nursing care be provided in hospitals will undoubtedly continue to grow. The demand to provide better measures of nursing care and to provide the optimal level of nursing care so as to obtain desired patient outcomes will tend to encourage the use of technology to document both the need and the amount of nursing care delivered.

■ WHY CHANGE THE COSTING APPROACH?

The mere fact that the ability to improve costing now exists does not in itself explain why a nurse manager would want to improve costing. What is to be gained from having a more accurate measure of the varying costs of nursing care for different types of patients?

One argument sometimes offered is that separate costing for different types of patients will allow for *variable billing*. Variable billing refers to the fact that the amount billed to each patient per patient day or per treatment varies. Instead of simply charging all patients the same amount per day for their nursing care, different patients will be charged different amounts based on their differing resource consumption. Once the variable costs of caring for patients are known, they can be charged accordingly.

To the extent that patients are treated on a *prospective payment* basis, such as capitation or DRGs, variable billing holds little appeal. On the other hand, in most states, at least some patients are charged for the services they receive on a fee-for-service basis. In these cases, variable billing may be a way to better justify bills and, in some cases, increase overall revenues. Variable billing may be beneficial to nursing because it shows in a dramatic way the specific contribution that nursing makes to the overall revenue structure of the organization.

Variable billing is not the only advantage of better costing. A critical benefit of improved costing of nursing services is that the organization can generate information for better management decisions. Is a particular service too costly? What price can be bid for a Health Maintenance Organization (HMO) or a Preferred Provider Organization (PPO) contract? Health care costing has long been based on averages and cross-subsidizations. In the current environment, errors in the calculation of costs become more serious as negotiations for discounted prices become more intense. Thus, if the organization's managers are mistaken about the resources that a particular class of patient consumes, the ramifications can be serious. Less averaging of costs is more acceptable today than it was in the past. This means that managers are being pushed to increase the accuracy of the costing line in Figure 18-4, even though this also moves in the direction of increased cost of data acquisition.

In addition, as costing becomes more specific and more accurate, not only is it possible to deal better with pricing problems, but managers can be more efficient in managing costs as well. Another important advantage of specific costing is that it facilitates product line management. Specific product lines such as obstetrics, burn care, heart surgery, and solid organ transplant programs can be emphasized and expanded, or deemphasized and reduced or eliminated, depending on the profitability of that product line. Control of budgets improves as other measures of expected cost become available. Flexible budget systems can provide better analysis and control of costs, and productivity can be monitored better if more is known about costs. It is possible to assess how costs should change based on the changing numbers of patient days. It is also possible for information about the cost per patient for a given DRG to be used to assess the change in total costs as the number of patients in each DRG changes.

■ SHOULD COSTING BE LINKED TO DIAGNOSIS RELATED GROUPS?

If health care organizations are going to move in the direction of more accurate costing of nursing services, one of the critical questions is to determine how to categorize the cost. Should there be one nursing cost for medical patients and another for surgical patients? Should the cost be determined for men as opposed to women, or for young people as opposed to old people? Should there be one nursing cost for each type of patient based on the ICD or CPT[3] code? Should the cost be found by DRG or based on Medicare outpatient ambulatory groupings?

The problem managers are faced with is the definition of the product of nursing care. What is it that nursing produces? If a nurse changes a dressing or gives a patient a medication, are those the products of nursing care? Probably most people would consider those activities to represent only intermediate products. The ultimate product is the care of the patient, not any one part of that care.

However, health care organizations treat many different kinds of patients. They do not have only one final product: care of a patient. They have many final products represented by the various patients nurses give care to. Yet currently, all patients are costed for nursing care as if they were the same. This should be changed so that better control of costs can be achieved. Final products must be defined so that nurse managers can assess the cost of each one. Patients could be divided into categories called Nursing Resource Groupings (NRGs). Ideally, the patients would be divided into homogeneous NRGs based on the amount of nursing care consumed. Any patient in one NRG would consume a set of nursing resources similar to that of any other patient in that grouping.

What should be the basis for costing nursing services in the interim, until a NRG-type system is in use? One approach is to fall back on Alternative X. A patient classification system can be used to determine how many days of nursing a given patient is likely to need at each classification level. If the cost of each day at each classification level (discussed later in this chapter) can be determined, the manager can add up the costs to determine the patient's total nursing care costs. This requires determining the patient classification for every patient for every day. However, many hospitals already perform that task for the purposes of daily nurse staffing. Some hospitals will feel that the advantages of being at Alternative X on the costing accuracy scale are sufficient to warrant this investment in data collection. And if the hospital is already collecting daily patient acuity data, the approach carries the advantage of obtaining two measures from one -collection effort. Doing this improves not only costing but also improves the benefit realized from that data collection effort (see Chapter 14).

However, many health care providers do not want to spend the resources needed to classify every patient every day or to classify every treatment or visit. The alternative is to take a sample of patients from each DRG or other categorization and determine the average nursing cost for patients in each DRG or category, based on a sampling approach. All patients within a specific DRG will not consume the exact same nursing resources for each day at a specific patient classification level. Nor will all patients in one DRG have the same number of patient days at each classification level or even have the same total number of patient days. The same is true regardless of the patient categorization system used. This approach is based on an **average** length of stay and an **average** number of days at each patient classification level, as well as **average** nurse resource consumption within each patient classification level. As a result, the **average** amount of nursing resources for each type of DRG can be found. This must be considered a gross measure, and the variability about the mean

---

[3] ICD or International Classification of Disease codes and CPT or Current Procedural Terminology codes are the official codes that describe diseases treated and procedures performed. These codes are used for medical patient classification and for billing.

will be large. Several studies have found DRGs to be a weak predictor of nursing resource consumption as compared with other patient classification systems.

For example, if a hospital uses a nursing classification system that has a scale from 1 to 5, a group of patients from each DRG can be sampled to find out, on average, how many days of the patients' stays were at level 1, how many at level 2, and so on. The averaging of all patients in a given DRG at a given hospital does not provide a measurement alternative that is accurate enough to be labeled W on the scale of A to Z. Such an estimate of cost would probably be considered to be R on such a scale. It would not be nearly as accurate as X, but it would be substantially more accurate than Alternatives A and B. This new alternative R (see Figure 18-5) would be substantially less expensive than Alternatives X, Y, or Z.

Thus, it seems that DRGs or similar groupings or categorizations, although perhaps not ideal for the purpose of costing nursing care, are adequate categorizations for the assignment of average differential nursing costs. Many hospital decisions are based on particular DRGs or clusters of DRGs, so the DRG-based cost information generated is of considerable management value. Organizations caring for ambulatory patients similarly will have to find a workable system of grouping patients that improves the accuracy of costing while being relevant for decision making.

■ A SPECIFIC APPROACH TO COSTING NURSING SERVICES

Nursing care costs consist of the staff costs for direct patient care, the staff costs for indirect patient care (preparing for and cleaning up after nursing interventions, communications with the physicians and other hospital departments about patient care, watching monitors, etc.), patient care related costs (e.g., patient and unit supplies), supervisory and clerical costs of the unit (supervisors, secretaries, monitor technicians, etc.), and overhead (allocated from other departments). Note that the cost of nursing care is more than just the hourly salary and benefits of the nurse giving care at the bedside. Nursing management, assessment, planning, evaluating, teaching, and discharge planning are also critical elements of nursing care. Additionally, supplies, support staff, and overhead are elements of overall nursing care costs. A manager could try to determine the costs of each of these elements separately for each category of patient or could do the costing in a more aggregate fashion.

Start with the assumption that all nursing department costs are aggregated.

The key element that allows for improved costing of nursing services for hospitals is that patient classification systems for nursing care requirements are currently in place in almost every hospital. Without such systems, patients consume varying amounts of resources, but the manager has no way to measure the differential consumption. With a classification system, once a patient has been classified, the manager has some idea about the nursing resources that patient will consume.

For example, suppose that a nursing unit has the following hypothetical patient classification resource guidelines:

Acuity Level	Hours of Care
1	3.0
2	4.0
3	4.8
4	6.6
5	9.0

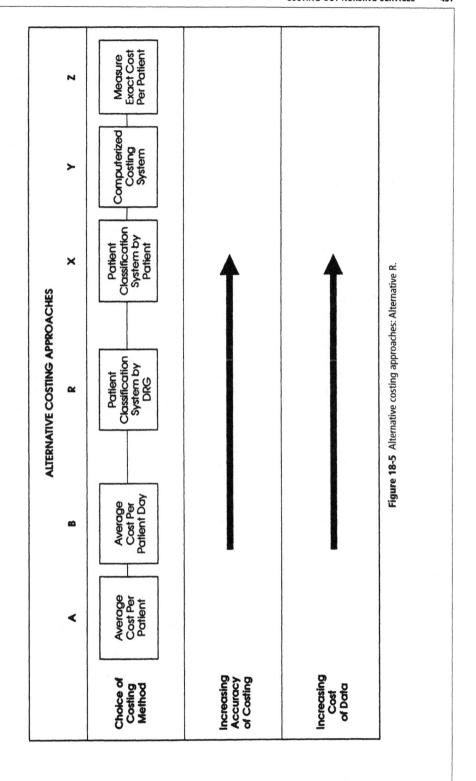

Figure 18-5 Alternative costing approaches: Alternative R.

In developing the patient classification system, various clinical indicators are used to determine whether a patient should be classified as a 1, 2, 3, 4, or 5. Once a patient has been classified, the classification system tells how many hours of nursing care should be required to treat that patient. In this example, a patient classified as a 4 would typically require on average 6.6 hours of care.

Note that the scale is not proportional. A patient classified as a 2 does not require exactly twice as many hours as a 1. A level 1 patient needs 3 hours of care, whereas a level 2 patient needs 4 hours. Rather than double, this is only 33% more care. A level 3 patient needs 4.8 hours. This is 20% more than a level 2. A level 4 patient requires 38% more care than a level 3. As one moves from level to level, the amount of additional care does not change in proportion. It changes based on the specific classification system and the clinical needs of a patient at each level in that system. In large part, this is because all patients require a minimum amount of care. In that minimum are included such items as admitting and discharging the patient; obtaining vital signs every 4 to 12 hours, depending upon the unit guidelines; managing medical orders; obtaining tests; administering basic medications; supervising the administration of IV medications; and other such tasks that are required for virtually every hospitalized patient (excluding patients in mental health units). As a patient's acuity rises, those same care activities are required, but additional care is required too, such as more frequent assessment of vital signs, more complex medications, multiple IVs, more laboratory and radiology tests, and so forth. But the basic care package is provided to every patient. Therefore, the changes in acuity levels cannot produce linear or exponential linear changes in hours of nursing care.

This complicates the cost calculation. If the scale were strictly linear, one could add up all the patient days at each level and divide into the total nursing cost to get a cost per unit of patient classification. For example, suppose the unit had one patient day that was a level 1, one patient day that was a 3, and one patient day that was a 4. The total of 1 + 3 + 4 is 8. If total nursing costs were $2,000, then the cost per patient classification unit would be $250 (i.e., $2,000/8). The cost for a patient day classified as a 4 would be $1,000 (4 × $250).

However, because the scale is not linear, it is necessary to create a relative value unit (RVU) scale. This scale allows determination of how much care each level requires relative to the care needed for a typical level 1 patient. A patient classified as a 1 will be given a value of 1 on the relative value scale. Each other classification level would then be calculated in relative proportion. This can be accomplished by dividing the required hours of care for each level by the number of hours required for level 1. For example:

$$\frac{\text{Level 2}}{\text{Level 1}} \quad \frac{4.0 \text{ hours}}{3.0 \text{ hours}} = 1.33$$

Therefore, the relative value assigned to classification level 2 is 1.33. This value of 1.33 represents the fact that a level 2 patient consumes 33 more nursing care hours than a level 1 patient. Continuing for all classification (acuity) levels:

Acuity Level	Hours of Care	RVU
1	3.0	1.00
2	4.0	1.33
3	4.8	1.60
4	6.6	2.20
5	9.0	3.00

Assuming the following information, the reader will be able to see how the RVU system can be used to develop cost information:

Total nursing costs:		$250,000	
Number of patient days			
at each acuity level:	Level	1: 100 days	
		2: 220 days	
		3: 350 days	
		4: 110 days	
		5: 40 days	

The first step is to determine the total amount of work performed by the nursing department. This is done by multiplying the RVUs for each acuity classification level by the number of days at that level. Using the number of patient days given above and the RVUs calculated above, the total RVUs would be:

Acuity Level	Patient Days	×	RVU	=	Total RVUs
1	100	×	1.00	=	100.00
2	220	×	1.33	=	292.60
3	350	×	1.60	=	560.00
4	110	×	2.20	=	242.00
5	40	×	3.00	=	120.00
	820				1,314.60

There were 1,314.6 units of nursing work performed. One can divide this into the total nursing cost to find the cost for each RVU of nursing work.

$$\frac{\text{Total Nursing Costs}}{\text{Total RVUs}} = \text{Cost per RVU}$$

$$\frac{\$250,000.00}{1,314.60} = \$190.17 \text{ per RVU}$$

Here one can see that the nursing cost for a patient for 1 day with classification 1 would be $190.17. The cost for a patient with classification 4 would be $190.17 multiplied by 2.20 (the RVU for classification level 4).

How would a manager calculate the nursing cost for a patient from admission to discharge? Suppose that the average DRG 128 patient had a length of stay of 7 days, with 2 days classed as a 1, 4 days classed as a 2, and 1 day classed as a 4. The nursing cost for DRG 128 would then be:

Acuity Level	Patient Days	×	RVU	×	Cost per RVU	=	Total Cost
1	2	×	1.00	×	$190.17	=	$380.34
2	4	×	1.33	×	190.17	=	1,011.70
3	0	×	1.60	×	190.17	=	0.00
4	1	×	2.20	×	190.17	=	418.37
5	0	×	3.00	×	190.17	=	0.00
	7						$1,810.41

Would all patients in a given DRG be expected to consume the same resources? Not really, but the manager can still be confident that an approach such as this, on average for any given DRG, will provide a much more accurate assignment of cost than simply assigning to every patient in a nursing unit the same daily cost for nursing care.

■ LIMITATIONS OF THE RELATIVE VALUE UNIT APPROACH

Patient Classification Versus Other Workload Measurement

The purpose of the RVU approach to patient classification is to provide a workable costing approach accessible to the majority of health care organizations in the country. However, it does not generate perfectly accurate measures of cost and is subject to a variety of limitations.

For example, the idea of an alternative to patient classification was discussed earlier. If a workload measurement tool is in place in a hospital and is being used on an ongoing basis to categorize the resource needs of each patient each day, it can be used to provide cost information that is potentially more accurate. Rather than being limited to perhaps 5 patient classification levels for a given med/surg unit, such an approach collects indicators of hours of resource consumption for each patient. It is more patient-specific than the RVU approach. Putting such an approach in place and following through with it on a continuous basis may be a considerable undertaking. However, if it is used, costing is made potentially easier.

Under such an approach, the required interventions for each patient are translated into required hours of care. Total nursing care costs for direct and indirect expenses must be calculated as with the RVU system. Dividing total nursing costs by total hours of care generates a cost per hour of care. This cost per hour can be multiplied by the required hours of care for each patient for each day as determined by the system. This will give the cost per patient for each day in the hospital. If aggregate information is desired by DRG, it can be obtained by averaging the costs of each patient in that DRG. However, the majority of hospitals do not have patient-specific work measurement systems in place. Many ambulatory settings do not have an adequate classification system to use to improve costing accuracy. They may have to leapfrog directly to a computerized system to achieve accurate costing.

Indirect Nursing Costs

A problem with both the RVU and more detailed work measurement systems, as described so far, is that in this chapter it has been assumed implicitly that all nursing costs vary in proportion to the hours of nursing care. Does that make sense for indirect costs? For example, will a sicker patient who requires more direct nursing care also require more indirect nursing care? More charting time? More supplies? More administrative and clerical support? More overhead? The answers to these questions depend on the specific situation of your institution.

For example, is it true that secretarial costs will be greater for patients that are more acutely ill? It may well be that a simple per diem allocation is a more appropriate way to allocate such costs. Costing could therefore be improved by dividing total nursing costs between those costs that vary with nursing care hours (such as RN staff and LPN staff and perhaps clinical supplies) and those costs that do not vary with nursing care hours (such as office supplies, nurse manager time, and secretarial time). The costs that vary with nursing care hours would be allocated by the RVU or work measurement approaches described earlier. The other costs could be divided by total patient days and assigned to patients based on their number of patient days.

Staffing Mix

A significant problem is the fact that most nursing classification systems provide required hours of care but do not specify the mix of care. If 30% of all nursing care hours are provided by LPNs, it is assumed that 30% of the care for each patient is provided by LPNs.

It is possible that one patient at level 2 might require 4 hours of RN care while another might require 3 hours of LPN care and only 1 hour of RN care. Obviously, both patients do not consume the same amount of nursing care resources, even if they consume the same number of hours of care. Therefore, there will be some distortion of costs unless the hospital uses a system that indicates not only how many hours of care are needed but also how many hours of care by staff type.

This problem is not unique to costing, however. It represents a weakness of patient classification systems. If the organization does not know the required mix of care providers, the classification system is not going to be useful for staffing decisions. Part of this problem stems from the fact that different organizations have varying views about which functions can be done by various types of staff. However, over time, one can expect that classification systems will improve. As they do, this mix problem should become less serious.

In the meantime, managers could attempt to separate the cost of RNs from the costs of LPNs and aides and assign those costs to patients separately. Special studies could be undertaken for each DRG to determine whether care was biased toward more than an average amount of RN care or toward more than an average amount of LPN care. Then the cost of nursing care for that DRG could be adjusted accordingly.

How complex are managers willing to make the costing system? Health care organizations must decide how much refinement they are willing to make to their costing systems, realizing that generally the more accurate the costing system is, the more expensive it is. Some managers believe that the historical average nursing cost per patient day is so inaccurate that an RVU-based system is a tremendous improvement, even with the problems cited here.

We have used a hospital as an example. The same principles apply whether the cost determination is for nursing care delivered in a hospital, nursing home, outpatient setting, or patient's home. However, in home care the costing is simplified by the fact that patient records explicitly indicate the level of staff that provided the care.

■ PRODUCT-LINE COSTING AND BUDGETING

One result of the work done on costing nursing services is that it is possible to group all patients of one type and find an average cost for that type of patient. In other words, *product-line* costing is feasible with this method. A product line is a group of patients with some commonality that allows them to be grouped together, such as a common diagnosis. In a similar approach, it is now common for organizations to focus on one disease, so-called disease management. Often an organization cannot eliminate one product in a product line without eliminating the entire product line. For example, if a hospital sells its bypass pump because it is losing money on bypass surgery, it will no longer be able to do heart valve surgery. They are both part of the open-heart surgery product line.

Many people believe that managers should be given hospital-wide responsibility for both the revenues and the expenses related to specific patient product lines.

For example, a manager might be responsible for the revenues related to the obstetrics product line. The manager is accountable for both the variance in the number of discharges and the revenue per discharge. Of course the manager would be responsible for the budgeted and actual costs of the product line as well.

Before one takes the step of costing by product line or budgeting by product line, it is necessary to question what the information will be used for. In terms of running a nursing unit, will knowledge of the cost for all patients in a given DRG be useful? The answer to that question depends a great deal on the types of decisions that a manager or organization faces.

Suppose that a hospital is trying to decide whether to accept a group of cardiac patients from an HMO at a discounted price. Knowing the costs for that type of patient would certainly be advantageous in the negotiating process. Often, product-line calculations include nursing costs simply as part of the overall per diem cost. The organization can have much better information about various types of patients if it relies on the costing procedures discussed earlier in doing product-line calculations.

Direct Care Hours

The direct care hours approach to product-line budgeting consists of dividing the patients in a given nursing unit into product lines, determining the number of hours of care required for each product line, and aggregating that information to find the total hours of care needed so as to include them in the budget. This is a straightforward approach to using product-line information to improve budgeting capability. It represents an alternative to using acuity-adjusted patient days for determining nurse staff requirements.

Consider calculation of direct care costs for a hospital product line. In this approach, the first step is to separate all patients in a unit into specific groups. These groups, or product lines, might or might not conform to DRGs. The next step is to determine how many patients are expected in the coming period in each group. This information can be generated using the forecasting techniques discussed in Chapter 6. Using historical information, forecasting can also be used to predict the average length of stay of the patients in each group.

Once the manager has predictions of the number of patient days in each group and the average length of stay, those two numbers can be multiplied to determine the total number of patient days expected in each product line. The number of patient days can be multiplied by the expected average direct care hours per patient day (HPPD) for patients in the product line so as to generate the total hours of direct care needed for each specific product line. The total direct care hours for each product line can then be aggregated to determine the total direct care hours needed for the unit for the coming year. Based on this information, the unit's budget for staff can be prepared. Table 18-1 presents a simplified example of this process. In this example, sufficient staff must be budgeted to provide 24,300 direct care hours. The benefit of this process is that it has the potential to provide accurate information about the resources needed by the unit.

The major difficulty with this process is determining an accurate measure of average direct care hours per patient day by product line. If this information is inaccurate, the resulting total direct care hours needed will be inaccurate as well. Gaining information about the actual average direct care hours per patient day can be accomplished using any of a number of the costing methods discussed in this chapter.

TABLE 18-1 Product-Line Budgeting for Direct Care Hours

	Forecast Volume of Patients	Forecast Average Length of Stay	Expected Patient Days	Expected Hours per Patient Day	Total Hours of Direct Care
Product Line 1	200	3	600	5	3,000
Product Line 2	50	5	250	6	1,500
Product Line 3	100	4	400	3	1,200
Product Line 4	300	7	2,100	6	12,600
Product Line 5	500	3	1,500	4	6,000
					24,300

If an accurate forecast of patient days by patient classification level cannot be generated, planning the budget based on a forecast of the number of patients in each product line may be extremely helpful.

Total Nursing Cost by Product Line

The discussion of direct care hours focuses on product-line budgeting primarily to help in preparing a budget for the amount of nursing staff needed for a unit. It is possible to think of product-line budgeting as a more complete approach to budgeting all the costs for a nursing unit or department. Such an approach is also more helpful for providing the organization with information on the total costs for nursing care for patients in each product line.

This approach to product-line costing has already been discussed earlier in this chapter, when the hypothetical costs for a DRG 128 patient were calculated. Using the RVU approach to patient costing, it was demonstrated in the example that the average costs for a patient in this product line would be $1,810.41. In the example, it was assumed that the actual total costs of the unit were known. Based on these total costs, the cost of having provided care to a DRG 128 patient was calculated.

If one were to use budgeted costs instead of actual costs, one could project the budgeted or anticipated costs for treating a patient in each given DRG or product line. Such information would be useful for a wide variety of managerial decisions, such as whether to expand capacity for treating patients in a particular product line.

Standard Treatment Protocols

A central article on product-line costing established an even more far-reaching approach to the topic.[4] This approach centers on the idea that hospitals treat patients by providing them with a large number of intermediate products. By carefully examining each department, one can make a list of the various intermediate products produced by that department. For example, a laboratory department produces different types of lab tests. Based on this approach, the set of intermediate products consumed

---

[4] Cleverley, William O. (1987). Product-costing for health care firms. *Health Care Management Review.* 12(4), 39-48.

by the average patient in a specific product line can be used to determine the costs of that product line. The set of intermediate products consumed by a patient in each product line is referred to as the standard treatment protocol (STP) for that product line.

In this system, each intermediate product is called a service unit (SU). A chest radiograph would be one type of service unit produced by the radiology department. A patient who has three chest radiographs receives three of this service unit. A standard cost profile (SCP) must be established for each SU. This profile indicates the cost of producing that service unit.

Conceptually, this seems straightforward. The patient care provided by each department is broken down into SUs. The cost of each SU is determined. The average number of each SU from each department is found for each product line. Then the SUs consumed for a product line are multiplied by their cost to determine the total costs for patients in that product line.

A difficulty with the approach is determining SUs for nursing units. One could try to break down nursing care into the various specific activities and then relate those to SUs. Administering a medication could be an SU. Taking a patient's vital signs could be an SU. Charting information about a patient could be an SU. At some point, when hospital computer information systems are adequately sophisticated, it would be possible to disaggregate nursing care and assign it to patients in this manner, or to directly measure at least some nursing activity through the use of RFID chips and room-based readers. It would then be possible to determine the average number of vital signs taken for a patient in a specific product line. For most hospitals, it is not currently cost-effective to collect such detailed levels of information. However, nursing SUs could be based on patient classification. Thus, a patient day at level 3 could be an SU. A day at level 4 would be a different SU. When the STP is established, it would consider which nursing SUs are typically consumed and how many of each. The costs for those SUs could be determined using the RVU method discussed earlier.

This method is an ambitious approach to product-costing and budgeting. It is used in more health care organizations each year. It creates the ability to have detailed information from all parts of the organization, including nursing, about each product line. The management implications of such information are significant. By examining all the SUs consumed in each department, a team of clinicians might be able to find ways to provide care more efficiently. SUs with lower SCPs might be substituted for more expensive ones. Ways might be found to reduce the number of SUs in various departments. If one considers product-line costing broadly, as a tool to use in managing the organization's product lines, it can be seen that the potential benefits of product-line costing and budgeting are significant.

Another approach that is starting to be discussed in the health insurance industry involves the idea of cost per patient outcome for a specific diagnosis. As the emphasis on quality and patient care outcomes intensifies, it is conceivable that insurance companies may penalize hospitals, nursing homes, and other health care facilities for some kinds of poor care outcomes. For example, they might refuse to pay for the extra days and treatments required as a result of a nosocomial infection. Or they might pay less than the full costs for such treatment. As the rate of hospital-acquired infections (such as Staphylococcus and Clostridium difficile) increases, the amount of treatment and the average length of stay due to those problems increases.

If the focus on quality is used as the basis for payments to hospitals, the definition of what third-party payers will pay for may well change from a DRG to something reflective of good quality of care for that DRG. With recent research that demonstrates lower mortality and complication rates when there is one nurse to every four patients on a medical unit rather than for one nurse to every eight patients, not only the insurance companies but also legislators, nurses, and the public in general have become more demanding about the amount of nursing care provided to hospitalized patients (Aiken et al., 1994; Aiken et al., 2002; Dorr, Horn, & Smout, 2005; Needleman & Buerhaus, 2003).

Summary and Implications for Nurse Managers

Improving the costing of nursing services has become important to nurse managers for several reasons. One reason is that improved cost information can be used to obtain an improved understanding of the contribution that nursing makes to the organization as a whole. A second reason is that the information generated by improved costing can be used to help managers make effective decisions and better control the costs of providing nursing services. Third, periodic nursing shortages make it more important to understand the nursing resources needed by patients. Costing information is also useful for examining changes in the way nursing care is provided. For example, the cost impacts of primary versus team nursing or of using different levels of staff can be examined.

The most accurate costing system requires continuous observation of all nurses by data collectors. The cost of such highly accurate costing is prohibitive. However, one can think of a continuum of costing methods. Less expensive methods provide less accurate data; more expensive methods provide more accurate data.

Over time, bedside computerization may become inexpensive enough to be introduced to most hospitals. Also over time, software programs will be developed and perfected to make using the computers easy and efficient. At the time of the writing of this book, however, the majority of hospitals did not have such systems in place. On the other hand, many hospitals are experimenting with such systems. If demonstration projects can show the bedside computer to be a cost-effective tool for nursing, it will not be long before costing can be done routinely at the bedside and nurses' stations.

In the meantime, patient classification systems can be used to improve substantially the assignment of nursing costs to patients in an economical way. Combining classification with an RVU system is relatively simple. Once this has been done, all nursing costs can be allocated based on the RVU system or some costs can be allocated using RVUs while other costs are assigned to patients based on patient days or some other approach. Each hospital must decide how much refinement to the RVU approach is worthwhile. Other health care organizations are likely to follow hospital advancements. However, some may decide to leapfrog directly to sophisticated computerized costing systems.

It is important to stress that the RVU approach suggested here is not perfect. It has a number of limitations and weaknesses. However, the nurse manager must decide whether these weaknesses are so significant that the method should not be used, in light of the fact that the costs generated, although not perfectly accurate, are likely to be a substantial improvement over costing methods that have been used historically.

Costing out nursing services provides a tool that is extremely useful for product-line costing and budgeting. Information about product-line costs can show management where profits are being made and where losses are accruing. Product-line information can aide managers substantially in understanding which patients place the greatest burden on the unit and in helping the organization to make appropriate decisions regarding changes in the organization's mix of patients.

References and Suggested Readings

Aiken, L., Clarke, S., Sloane, D., Sochalski, J., Silber, J. (2002). Hospital nurse staffing and patient mortality, nurse burnout, and job dissatisfaction. *Journal of the American Medical Association.* 288(16), 1987-1993.

Aiken, L., Smith, H., Lake, E. (1994). Lower Medicare mortality among a set of hospitals known for good nursing care. *Medical Care.* 32(5), 771-787.

Altman, D., Clancy, C., Blendon, R. (2004). Improving patient safety—Five years after the IOM Report. *New England Journal of Medicine.* 351(20), 2041-2043.

Barfield, J., et al. (1997). *Cost Accounting: Tradition and Innovations.* Minneapolis: West Publishing.

Bazzoli, F. (2006). Survey: Hospital margins drop. *Healthcare IT News.* Downloaded on January 10, 2007; http://www.healthcareitnews.com/story.cms?id=4440.

Dorr, D., Horn, S., Smout, R. (2005). Cost analysis of nursing home registered nurse staffing times. *Journal of the American Geriatrics Society,* 53(5), 840-845.

Finkler, S.A., Ward, D.R., Baker, J. (2007). *Essentials of Cost Accounting for Health Care Organizations,* ed 3. Sudbury, MA: Bartlett & Jones.

Griffith, J., Patullo, A., Alexander, J., Jelinek, R., Foster, D. (2006). Is anybody managing the store? Trends in healthcare performance. *Journal of Healthcare Management.* 51(6), 392-405.

Hansen, D., Mowen, M. (1997). *Cost Management,* ed 2. Cincinnati: South-Western Publishing.

Heshmat, S. (1997). Managed care and the relevant costs for pricing. *Health Care Management Review.* 22(1), 82-85.

Institute of Medicine. (2003). *Keeping Patients Safe: Transforming the Work Environment of Nurses.* Washington, D.C.: National Academies Press.

Needleman, J., Buerhaus, P. (2003). Nurse staffing and patient safety: Current knowledge and implications for action. *International Journal for Quality in Health Care.* 15(4), 275-277.

Needleman, J., Buerhaus, P., Stewart, M.,Zelevinski, K., Soeren, M. (2006). Nurse staffing in hospitals: Is there a business case for quality? *Health Affairs.* 25(1), 204-211.

Pappas, S. (2007). Describing costs related to nursing. *Journal of Nursing Administration.* 37(1), 32-40.

Rohloff, R. (2006). Full-time equivalents: What needs to be assessed to meet patient care and create realistic budgets. *Nurse Leader.* 4(1), 49-54.

Rothberg, M., Abraham, I., Lindenauer, P., Rose, D. (2005). Improving nurse-to-patient staffing ratios as a cost-effective safety intervention. *Medical Care.* 43(8), 785-791.

Solucient Industries. (May 1, 2006). Majority of U.S. hospitals showed no appreciable change in hospital-wide performance since 2000. *News Release, Solucient Industries.*

Spetz, J. (2005). The cost and cost-effectiveness of nursing services in health care. *Nursing Outlook.* 53(6), 305-309.

Stanton, M., Rutherford, M. (2004). *Hospital Nurse Staffing and Quality of Care.* Rockville, MD: Agency for Healthcare Research and Quality.

Welton, J. (2006). Paying for nursing care in hospitals. *American Journal of Nursing.* 106(11), 67-69.

Welton, J., Fischer, M., Degrace, S., Zone-Smith, L. (2006). Nursing intensity billing. *Journal of Nursing Administration.* 36(4), 181-188.

Welton, J., Unruh, L., Halloran, E. (2006). Nurse staffing, nursing intensity, staff mix, and direct nursing care costs across Massachusetts hospitals. *Journal of Nursing Administration.* 36(9), 416-425.

West, D.A., Hicks, L.L., Balas, E.A., West, T.D. (1996). Profitable capitation requires accurate costing. *Nursing Economic$.* 14(3), 150, 162-170.

Sample Budget Forms and Instructions

APPENDIX CONTENTS

Guide to Abbreviations Used Above in Form Numbers

BD	Budget Detail
C	Capital
F	FTE
NS	Nonsalary
P	Personnel
PCU	Patient Care Unit
RE	Revenue and Expense
S	Salary
V	Volume
W	Workload

■ GENERAL INSTRUCTIONS

All budget worksheets are to be completed and returned to the Budget Office. Use N/A to indicate any worksheets or areas of worksheets that do not apply to your area of responsibility. Each individual sheet must be:

- Identified by responsibility center number and name
- Identified with the fiscal year for which the budget is projected and
- Signed and dated by the manager completing the worksheet

■ VOLUME, REVENUE, AND WORKLOAD

A. Patient Day Volume/Revenue (BD/V1)

This worksheet is used for calculating patient day revenue by type of accommodation. Total budgeted patient days for individual patient care units are determined jointly by the Budget Office, the Admitting Department, and the Nursing Department. FOR YOUR INFORMATION ONLY, the following data appear on this worksheet:

- 7-Month YTD Budget—budgeted volume for this type for the period July 1 through January 31
- 7-Month YTD Actual—actual volume for this type for the period July 1 through January 31
- Annual Budget—total budgeted volume for this type for this fiscal year
- Projected Actual—straight-line volume projection for this year based on this year's actual through April, calculated as follows:

$$\frac{\text{7-month YTD Actual}}{7} \times 12$$

Note that these projections are simply the result of arithmetic calculations and are intended only to assist you in making your own projections. Your judgment and knowledge of your department must determine the appropriate budget projections for your area of responsibility.

1. Label and fill in the column FY _____ Budget with your projection for the coming year.
2. Fill in the column Charge per Day using the most current hospital rate book to identify the correct charge.
3. Calculate the Total Revenue by multiplying the FY _____ Budget by the Charge per Day.
4. Add the totals to calculate the Total Revenue for the cost center.

B. Other Volume/Revenue (BD/V2)

This worksheet is used for calculating revenue generated by supplies or services that are charged in addition to room revenue. FOR YOUR INFORMATION ONLY, the following data appear on this worksheet:

- 7-Month YTD Budget—budgeted volume for this type for the period July 1 through January 31
- 7-Month YTD Actual—actual volume for this type for the period July 1 through January 31

- Annual Budget—total budgeted volume for this type for this fiscal year
- Projected Actual—straight-line volume projection for this year based on this year's actual through April, calculated as follows:

$$\frac{\text{7-month YTD Actual}}{7} \times 12$$

Note that these projections are simply the result of arithmetic calculations and are intended only to assist you in making your own projections. Your judgment and knowledge of your department must determine the appropriate budget projections for your area of responsibility.

1. Label and fill in the column FY _____ Budget with your projection for the coming year.
2. Fill in the column Charge per Unit using the most current hospital rate book to identify the correct charge.
3. Calculate the Total Revenue by multiplying the FY _____ Budget by the Charge per Day.
4. Add any line items to your cost center that you anticipate will occur in the coming year but that are not on this report.
5. Delete any line items that currently show actual or budget volume but that you do not expect to occur in the coming year.
6. Add the totals to calculate the Total Revenue for the cost center.
7. Explain briefly at the bottom of the page or on the reverse side your rationale for adding or deleting any line items.

C. Workload (PCU/W1)

This worksheet is used to calculate nursing workload on the inpatient units using the existing patient classification system.

1. Complete Current ADC using the most recent year-to-date patient classification data for this cost center.
2. Complete the Projected Change column based on your analysis of trend data and identification of anticipated changes in your patient population.
3. Calculate Revised ADC as Current ADC ± Projected Change.
4. Calculate Projected Workload as Revised ADC times Relative Value.
5. Total all columns as indicated and calculate Average Acuity using formula on worksheet.
6. Include a brief discussion of the factors that led to the determination of the Projected Change.

BD/V1

PATIENT DAY VOLUME / REVENUE BUDGET WORKSHEET

FY _____

RESPONSIBILITY CENTER: 611 GENERAL SURGERY

BUDGETED DAYS _____

TYPE	7-MONTH YTD BUDGET	7-MONTH YTD ACTUAL	ANNUAL BUDGET	PROJECTED ACTUAL	FY BUDGET	CHARGE PER DAY	TOTAL REVENUE
Semiprivate	4,473	4,918	7,702	8,431			
Private	1,378	2,371	1,635	954			
Isolation	170	292	146	85			
TOTAL	6,021	5,957	10,365	10,212			

BD/V2

OTHER VOLUME / REVENUE BUDGET WORKSHEET

RESPONSIBILITY CENTER: 611 GENERAL SURGERY

FY _____

TYPE	7-MONTH YTD BUDGET	7-MONTH YTD ACTUAL	ANNUAL BUDGET	PROJECTED ACTUAL	FY BUDGET	CHARGE PER DAY	TOTAL REVENUE
Discharge Visit	438	497	750	852			
ECG Portable	262	222	450	381			
Standby Equip	204	197	350	338			
TOTAL							

PCU/W1

WORKLOAD BUDGET WORKSHEET

FY _____

RESPONSIBILITY CENTER: _____

PATIENT TYPE	CURRENT ADC	PROJECTED CHANGE	REVISED ADC	RELATIVE VALUE	PROJECTED WORKLOAD
1	_____	_____	_____	0.4	_____
2	_____	_____	_____	1.0	_____
3	_____	_____	_____	2.0	_____
4	_____	_____	_____	4.4	_____
Total	_____	_____	_____		_____

Workload_____ ÷ ADC_____ = Average Acuity_____

Discussion:

■ FTEs AND SALARY EXPENSE

NOTE: Description of the method for determining FTEs requested must accompany the budget worksheets for FTEs and salary expense. Format for this description may vary by department and division. For the inpatient nursing units using the existing patient classification system, the Personnel Budget Worksheets (PCU/P1 and PCU/P2) will be completed for each responsibility center. In all calculations, an FTE is equal to 2,080 hours.

A. Position/Hours/FTE (BD/F1)

This worksheet is used to identify by specific position title the number of positions and the related hours and FTEs, both straight time (S/T) and overtime (O/T) to be budgeted for each cost center. The worksheet represents the current authorized budget for this cost center (including any adjustments that were approved during the current fiscal year):

- **Curr Auth Positions**—number of positions currently authorized in this position category
- **Position Title**—description of position as it appears in the personnel position files
- **ST Hours**—straight-time hours authorized for this position
- **ST FTE**—straight-time FTEs authorized for this position, calculated by dividing ST hours by 2,080
- **OT Hours**—overtime hours authorized for this position
- **OT FTE**—overtime FTEs authorized for this position, calculated by dividing OT hours by 2,080
- **Total Hours**—straight time plus overtime hours
- **Total FTEs**—straight time plus overtime FTEs

All columns are totaled, and the calculations for converting authorized hours to FTEs are shown at the bottom of the form.

1. Identify positions, hours, and FTEs to be requested for the cost center for the coming fiscal year (descriptions to accompany this worksheet).
2. Compare requests by position with current authorized and change authorized positions, hours, and FTEs to reflect requests.
3. If a position is requested that does not appear on the worksheet, it can be added on any available blank line. Positions that are no longer required should be crossed out.
4. Total all columns and complete calculations labeled Projected at bottom of form.

B. Base Salary (BD/S1)

This worksheet is used to calculate the base salaries generated by the FTEs described in the previous worksheet. There is a separate worksheet for each position title, and additional blank worksheets are available if a position that is new to the cost center is to be added. The worksheet lists by name all staff currently employed in that position category and in that cost center, and also includes:

- FTE—the portion of a full-time equivalent that the employee fills
- Shift—the usual shift that the employee is scheduled to work

- Base Hourly Rate—the rate at which the employee is currently being paid; does not include any increases that are scheduled for this fiscal year but that have not yet been added to the employee's salary
- Base Annual Salary—base hourly rate times 2,080 hours times FTE

Totals for the position category appear at the bottom of the worksheet.

1. Correct the data for current employees to reflect what will actually be in effect at the end of this fiscal year:
   - Correct FTE and shift designations if necessary
   - Change Base Hourly Rate and Base Annual Salary for any employee who will receive a salary increase
   - Delete any employees who will terminate or transfer out
   - Add any employees who will be hired or transferred in
2. Add as Vacant (Current) any positions that are currently vacant and include the FTE, Shift, Base Hourly Rate, and Base Annual Rate anticipated for those positions.
3. Add as Vacant (New) any additional positions that are being requested and include the FTE, Shift, Base Hourly Rate, and Base Annual Rate anticipated for those positions.
4. Correct the totals for the position category. *Totals in each position category must correspond with the S/T totals for the position listed on the Position/Hours/FTE Budget Worksheet (BD/F).*

C. Differential Budget Worksheet (BD/S2)

This worksheet is used to identify the expenses for those differentials paid to employees for working particular shifts, such as evenings, nights, weekends, or holidays, or under special conditions, such as on call. Refer to the Personnel Manual for the policy on payment of differentials and to the current Wage and Salary Guidelines for the differential rates.

1. Calculate differentials for each position category individually (exception: differentials may be combined for full-time and part-time staff with the same position title—e.g., Unit Aide FT and Unit Aide PT).
2. For evenings, nights, weekends, and on call, calculate from staffing patterns the required number of Hours/Week. Multiply by 52 to determine the Annual Hours.
3. Enter the Rate for each differential type, and multiply by Annual Hours to determine the Total $$$.
4. For Holiday, calculate the number of staffed hours required for each of the recognized organizational holidays, and enter under Annual Hours.
5. Since the holiday differential rate is 50% of base rate, it is necessary to determine the average base rate for the position category. This is calculated using the totals for the position category determined on the Base Salary Budget Worksheet, using the following formula:

$$\frac{\text{Total base salary}}{(\text{FTEs} \times 2{,}080)} = \text{Average hourly salary}$$

Average hourly salary $\times$ 0.5 = Holiday differential rate

6. Enter the Rate for Holiday and multiply by Annual Hours to determine the Total $$$.
7. Sum all Total $$$ amounts to determine Total This Position.

D. Overtime (BD/S3)

This worksheet is used to determine the overtime expenses corresponding to the hours and FTEs identified on the Position/Hours/FTE Budget Worksheet (BD/F1). Overtime expense is calculated separately for each position title. Overtime is paid at 50% above combined (base + differential) hourly rate. Budget calculations must therefore include both of these types of dollars. The formulas for calculating overtime are detailed on the worksheet and use the following data for the individual position category:

- Overtime Hours—from Position/Hours/FTE Budget Worksheet (BD/F1)
- Total S/T FTE—from Position/ Hours/FTE Budget Worksheet (BD/F1)
- Total Base Salary—from Base Salary Budget Worksheet (BD/S1)
- Total Differential—from Differential Budget Worksheet (BD/S2)

E. Salary Expense (BD/S4)

This worksheet is used to total the salary expenses by position category for the cost center. Each position title represented on the Position/Hours/FTE Budget Worksheet (BD/F1) must be represented. For each position category, enter the following:

- Base Salary—from Base Salary Budget Worksheet (BD/S1)
- Differential—from Differential Budget Worksheet (BD/S2)
- Overtime—from Overtime Budget Worksheet (BD/S3)

Sum the amounts across each line for the Total for the individual position category. Sum the columns for the Total for each expense type and for the cost center. Leave all salaries at this year's rates. The Budget Office will adjust for raises once the percentages have been determined.

PCU/P1

PERSONNEL BUDGET WORKSHEET   Page 1

FY _____

RESPONSIBILITY CENTER: _____

Bed Complement _____ Total Patient Days _____ % Occupancy _____

ADC _____ × Average Acuity _____ = Average Workload _____

Average Workload _____ × Target HPW _____ = Hours/24 Hours_____

Hours/24 Hours_____ ÷ 8 = Shifts/24 Hours _____

DAILY STAFFING PATTERN
Variable Staff (Preliminary):

SHIFT DISTRIBUTION		_____%	_____%	_____%	
Mix	Position	7–3	3–11	11–7	Total
%	Staff Nurse				
%	LPN/LVN				
%	Patient Care Technician				
%	Nursing Asst				
	Total				

Variable Staff (Adjusted):

SHIFT DISTRIBUTION		_____%	_____%	_____%	
Mix	Position	7–3	3–11	11–7	Total
%	Staff Nurse				
%	LPN/LVN				
%	Patient Care Technician				
%	Nursing Asst				
	Total				

Support Staff:

Position	7–3	3–11	11–7	Total
Secretary				
Unit Aide (M–F)				
Total				

Fixed Staff: Nurse Manager _____ Clinical Specialist_____

PCU/P2

PERSONNEL BUDGET WORKSHEET   Page 2

FY _____

CALCULATION OF NONPRODUCTIVE TIME

Factor for days off and nonproductive time:

YTD as of _____

(a) Total paid hours _____

(b) Total paid nonproductive hours _____ (sick + vacation + holiday + other paid nonworked)

(c) Total paid productive hours (a) − (b) _____

(d) % paid nonproductive (b) ÷ (c) _____(convert % to decimal)

(e) Factor $1 \times 1.4 \times 1(d) = 1 \times 1.4 \times$ _____

CALCULATION OF TOTAL REQUIRED FTEs

CATEGORY	SHIFT/24 HOUR	FACTOR (e)	TOTAL FTEs REQUIRED	BUDGET FTE	
				ST	OT
Nurse Manager					
Clinical Specialist					
Staff Nurse					
LPN/LVN					
Patient Care Technician					
Nursing Assistant					
Secretary					
Unit Aide (M–F)					
Total					

BD/F1

POSITION/HOURS/FTE BUDGET

FY _____

RESPONSIBILITY CENTER: 611 GENERAL SURGERY

CURR AUTH POSITIONS	POSITION TITLE	ST HOURS	ST FTE	OT HOURS	OT FTE	TOTAL HOURS	TOTAL FTE
1	Nurse Manager	2,080	1.0	—	—	2,080	1.0
1	Clin Specialist	2,080	1.0	—	—	2,080	1.0
13	Staff Nurse FT	27,040	13.0	1,040	0.5	28,080	13.5
8	Staff Nurse PT	8,320	4.0	—	—	8,320	4.0
3	LPN/LVN FT	6,240	3.0	208	0.1	6,448	3.1
1	LPN/LVN PT	832	0.4	—	—	832	0.4
3	Nsg Asst FT	6,240	3.0	624	0.3	6,864	3.3
3	Nsg Asst PT	1,248	0.6	—	—	1,248	0.6
4	Secretary FT	8,320	4.0	208	0.1	8,528	4.1
2	Secretary PT	1,664	0.8	—	—	1,664	0.8
2	Unit Aide FT	4,160	2.0	—	—	4,160	2.0
1	Unit Aide PT	832	0.4	—	—	832	0.4
42	Total	69,056	33.2	2,080	1.0	71,136	34.2

CURRENTLY AUTHORIZED

$$\text{ST FTE} = \frac{69{,}056}{2{,}080} = 33.2$$

$$\text{OT FTE} = \frac{2{,}080}{2{,}080} = 1.0$$

$$\text{TOTAL FTE} = \frac{71{,}136}{2{,}080} = 34.2$$

PROJECTED

$$\text{ST FTE} = \frac{}{2{,}080} =$$

$$\text{OT FTE} = \frac{}{2{,}080} =$$

$$\text{TOTAL FTE} = \frac{}{2{,}080} =$$

BD/S1

BASE SALARY BUDGET WORKSHEET

FY _____   Page ___ of ___

RESPONSIBILITY CENTER: 611 GENERAL SURGERY
POSITION CATEGORY: STAFF NURSE PART TIME

NAME	FTE	SHIFT	BASE HOURLY RATE	BASE ANNUAL SALARY
Briggs, Martha	0.2	3–11	$17.99	$ 7,484
Coram, Amy	0.5	11–7	17.73	18,439
Douglas, Ida	0.5	7–3	21.44	22,298
Francis, Jamie	0.5	7–3	15.21	15,818
Howells, Robert	0.5	3–11	19.37	20,145
Martins, Mary	0.8	3–11	22.85	38,022
Ridley, George	0.5	7–3	18.22	18,949
Westbury, Vickie	0.5	11–7	16.24	16,890

Total This Position Category:

Positions   8

FTEs   4.0   Base Salary $158,045

BD/S2

DIFFERENTIAL BUDGET WORKSHEET

FY _____

RESPONSIBILITY CENTER: _____

Page ___ of ___

Position Title: _____

DIFFERENTIAL TYPE	HOURS/WEEK	ANNUAL HOURS	RATE	TOTAL $$$
Evening				
Night				
Weekend				
Holiday				
On Call				
			Total This Position: $	

Position Title: _____

DIFFERENTIAL TYPE	HOURS/WEEK	ANNUAL HOURS	RATE	TOTAL $$$
Evening				
Night				
Weekend				
Holiday				
On Call				
			Total This Position: $	

BD/S3

OVERTIME BUDGET WORKSHEET

FY _____

RESPONSIBILITY CENTER: _____   Page ____ of ____

Position Title _____ Overtime Hours _____

Total S/T FTE _____ × 2,080 hours = _____Total Hours

Total Base Salary _____ + Total Differential _____

= _____ Combined Total

Combined Total _____ ÷ Total Hours _____

= _____ Combined Hourly Rate

Combined Hourly Rate _____ × 1.5 × Overtime Hours _____

= _____ Overtime Total

Position Title _____ Overtime Hours _____

Total S/T FTE _____ × 2,080 hours = _____Total Hours

Total Base Salary _____ + Total Differential _____

= _____ Combined Total

Combined Total _____ ÷ Total Hours _____

= _____ Combined Hourly Rate

Combined Hourly Rate _____ × 1.5 × Overtime Hours _____

= _____ Overtime Total

BD/S4

SALARY EXPENSE BUDGET WORKSHEET

FY _____

RESPONSIBILITY CENTER: _____

POSITION TITLE	BASE SALARY	DIFFERENTIAL	OVERTIME	TOTAL
TOTAL				

■ NONSALARY EXPENSE

This portion of your budget packet is used to describe the anticipated nonsalary expenses for the coming year. These include all of the 611 (Supply) and 911 (Interdepartmental) expense accounts that appear on your monthly responsibility center revenue and expense statements. The Revenue and Expense Budget Worksheet (BD/RE1) can be used to identify the accounts in which you have incurred expenses for the current year and in which you may wish to budget expenses for the coming year. FOR YOUR INFORMATION ONLY, the following data appear on this worksheet:

- 7-Month YTD Actual—actual expense for this account for the year-to-date (YTD) period July 1 through January 31
- Annual Budget—total budgeted expense for this account for this fiscal year
- 12-Month Projection—straight-line expense projection for this year based on this year's actual through April, calculated as follows:

$$\frac{\text{7-month YTD Actual}}{7} \times 12$$

Note that these projections are simply the result of arithmetic calculations and are intended only to assist you in making your own projections. Your judgment and knowledge of your department must determine the appropriate budget projections for your area of responsibility.

A. Revenue and Expense (BD/RE1)

This worksheet summarizes the projected revenue and expense in all categories for the next fiscal year.

1. Revenue
   - Enter total from Patient Day Volume/Revenue Budget Worksheet (BD/V1) on account line 010 Routine
   - Enter total from Other Volume/Revenue Budget Worksheet (BD/V2) on account line 020 Other
2. Salary Expense—from Salary Expense Budget Worksheet (BD/S4), enter:
   - Base Salary Total on account line 010 Salaries—Regular
   - Overtime Total on account line 020 Salaries—Overtime
   - Differential Total on account line 030 Salaries—Differentials
   - Leave other expense lines blank; the Budget Office will calculate other fringe benefit amounts
3. Supply Expense—enter appropriate amount for each account line; this must be consistent with the total expense calculated on the corresponding Nonsalary Expense Budget Worksheet (BD/NS1).
4. Interdepartmental Expense—enter appropriate amount for each account line; this must be consistent with the total expense calculated on the corresponding Nonsalary Expense Budget Worksheet (BD/NS1).
5. The Budget Office will calculate totals and contributions when all expenses have been identified.

B. Nonsalary Expense (BD/NS1)

This worksheet is used to describe the elements included in the budget projections for each type of expense. A separate sheet is used for each nonsalary (supply or interdepartmental) account that is budgeted for more than $2,000.

For some nonsalary accounts, the amount to be budgeted may be determined by volume and related to volume changes from this year. For this type of expense, budget may be calculated using the formula:

$$\frac{\text{This Year YTD \$\$\$ Expense}}{\text{This Year's Volume}} \times \text{Next Year's Volume} = \text{Next Year's Expense}$$

If so, the formula with the appropriate numbers is entered on the worksheet. Any adjustments that must be made to this result should be clearly explained. For other accounts, it may be more appropriate to list out on the specific items or activities that will generate the expense (e.g., in the Equipment or Seminar/Meetings accounts). A brief narrative is also acceptable for those accounts that are not clearly described by either of the above methods.

Budget all nonsalary accounts in this year's dollars. The Budget Office will adjust for inflation as needed when these rates are determined.

BD/RE1

REVENUE AND EXPENSE BUDGET WORKSHEET

FY _____

RESPONSIBILITY CENTER: 611 GENERAL SURGERY

ACCOUNT NUMBER/ DESCRIPTION	FY 08 7-MONTH YTD ACTUAL	FY 08 ANNUAL BUDGET	FY 08 PROJECTED ACTUAL	FY 09 BUDGET PROJECTION
311. Revenue				
010 Routine	($3,244,410)	($5,556,030)	($5,561,846)	
020 Other	(27,590)	(47,893)	(47,297)	
Total Operating Revenue	($3,272,000)	($5,603,923)	($5,609,143)	
411. Salary Expense				
010 Salaries - Regular	$ 730,881	$1,292,966	$1,252,939	
020 Salaries - Per Diem	2,758	0	4,728	
030 Salaries - Overtime	40,128	62,288	68,791	
040 Salaries - Differentials	97,995	170,419	167,991	
050 FICA	61,285	107,316	105,060	
060 Health Insurance	62,125	111,842	106,500	
070 Pension	19,855	35,816	34,037	
090 Other	17,228	29,092	29,534	
Total Salary Expense	$1,032,255	$1,809,738	$1,769,580	
611. Supply Expense				
010 Patient Care Supplies	$ 41,692	$ 62,023	$ 71,472	
020 Office Supplies	1,907	3,070	3,269	
030 Forms	3,111	5,560	5,333	
040 Supplies Purchased	1,210	1,935	2,074	
050 Equipment	1,553	2,903	2,662	
060 Seminars/Meetings	1,163	2,258	1,994	
070 Books	145	258	249	
080 Equipment Rental	385	1,703	660	
090 Miscellaneous	388	968	665	
Total Supply Expense	$ 51,554	$ 80,677	$ 88,378	
911. Interdepartmental Expense				
010 Central Supply	$ 7,828	$ 13,995	$ 13,419	
020 Pharmacy	9,527	17,019	16,332	
030 Linen/Laundry	16,046	28,678	27,507	
040 Maintenance	977	4,515	1,675	
060 Telephone	1,962	3,225	3,363	
070 Photocopy	124	323	213	
090 Miscellaneous	165	194	283	
Total Interdepartmental Expense	$ 36,629	$ 67,948	$ 62,793	
Total Operating Expense	$1,120,438	$1,958,363	$1,920,751	

BD/NS1

NONSALARY EXPENSE BUDGET WORKSHEET

FY _____

RESPONSIBILITY CENTER _____   Page ___ of ___

Account Number _____ Description _____

Current Year Budget $_____ Projected Actual $_____

Calculation/itemization for budget request:

Total budget request $_____

■ CAPITAL EQUIPMENT AND CONSTRUCTION

The capital budget identifies those requested items that are capitalized and charged to depreciation rather than to regular operational accounts. Items that must be capitalized include:

- Individual items (equipment, furniture, etc.) with a unit cost of $2,000 or more (including installation costs) and a life expectancy of 2 years or more
- Items purchased in bulk with a total cost of $2,000 or more and a life expectancy of 2 years or more (even if the cost of the individual item is less than $2,000)
- Construction, maintenance, and renovations in excess of $7,500 and
- Computer software products with a cost of $20,000 or more (including installation costs)

All capital budget requests are to be listed on the Capital Budget Worksheet (BD/C1). In addition, any capital requests with a total cost of $5,000 or greater will require a separate Capital Justification Worksheet (BD/C2).

A. Capital Budget (BD/C1)

List each item on this form, completing the information required in each column:

1. Priority—assign a priority number to each request, using 1 for the highest priority number. Items do not need to be listed in priority order as long as the priorities are clearly identified
2. Type—enter one of the following codes:
   - CR—construction or remodeling
   - RE—item that replaces an existing item in the department
   - RU—item that replaces and upgrades an existing item in the department
   - AS—item that is in addition to similar items already available within the department and
   - AN—item that is an addition and not currently available in the department
3. Equipment Quantity—identify how many of this item are requested.
4. Description—provide a simple description of the item or project, including relevant model numbers, etc.
5. Unit Cost—enter the price of a single one of this item, or the total cost of the project.
6. Extended Cost—calculate unit cost × equipment quantity.
7. Comments—include any additional information that will be useful in evaluating the request.

B. Capital Justification (BD/C2)

This form must be completed for each priority on the Capital Budget Worksheet (BD/C1) whose extended cost is $7,500 or greater. Attach additional pages if necessary, and identify them clearly with the responsibility center and priority number.

1. Description—include a brief but complete description of the item or project, including the proposed location.
2. Justification—provide a thorough justification for the item or project, including implications if funding is not made available.

3. Construction Costs—these should be reviewed with the Planning and Engineering Departments, as well as with any other affected services; enter date of cost estimates and name and title of individual providing this estimate.
4. Equipment Costs—include both purchase price and installation costs; attach vendor's proposal if available.
5. Impact on Operational Costs—describe and quantify as much as possible the incremental costs associated with this item or project, including salaries, fringes, maintenance contracts, utilities, supplies, or interdepartmental expenses.
6. Impact on Revenue—describe and quantify as much as possible the incremental revenue that could be generated as a result of this item or project.

BD/C1

CAPITAL BUDGET WORKSHEET

FY ____

Page ____ of ____

RESPONSIBILITY CENTER ____

PRIOR. #	TYPE CR/RE/RU AS/AN	EQUIP. QTY	DESCRIPTION	UNIT COST	EXTENDED COST	COMMENTS

BD/C2

CAPITAL JUSTIFICATION FORM

FY _____

RESPONSIBILITY CENTER _____   PRIORITY ITEM # _____

Description of Item or Project:

Justification:

Construction Costs: **Equipment Costs:**

Fees   _____   Purchase Price   _____

Construction   _____   Installation   _____

Contingency   _____

Total   _____

Date of Estimate _____   By _____

Impact on Operational Expenses:

Impact on Revenues:

Index

Page numbers in *italics* refer to illustrations; page numbers followed by a b refer to boxes; page numbers followed by a t refer to tables.

CPSIA information can be obtained at www.ICGtesting.com
Printed in the USA
LVOW04s2113020815

448518LV00016B/174/P